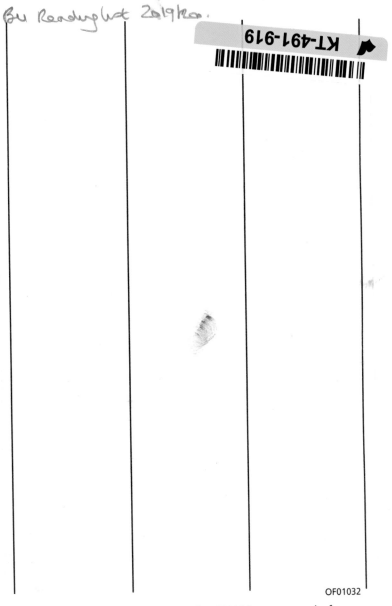

Legal Aspects of Physiotherapy

To Carmel

Legal Aspects of Physiotherapy

Second Edition

Bridgit Dimond

MA, LLB, DSA, AHSM, Barrister-at-law
Emeritus Professor of the University of Glamorgan

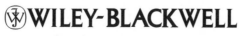

A John Wiley & Sons, Ltd., Publication

This edition first published 2009
© 1999, 2009 Bridgit C. Dimond

Blackwell Publishing was acquired by John Wiley & Sons in February 2007.
Blackwell's publishing programme has been merged with Wiley's global Scientific, Technical,
and Medical business to form Wiley-Blackwell.

First published 1999
Second edition 2009

Registered office
John Wiley & Sons Ltd, The Atrium, Southern Gate, Chichester, West Sussex, PO19 8SQ, United Kingdom

Editorial offices
9600 Garsington Road, Oxford, OX4 2DQ, United Kingdom
2121 State Avenue, Ames, Iowa 50014-8300, USA

For details of our global editorial offices, for customer services and for information about how
to apply for permission to reuse the copyright material in this book please see our website at
www.wiley.com/wiley-blackwell.

The right of the author to be identified as the author of this work has been asserted in accordance
with the Copyright, Designs and Patents Act 1988.

Library of Congress Cataloging-in-Publication Data
Dimond, Bridgit.
  Legal aspects of physiotherapy / Bridgit Dimond. – 2nd ed.
      p. cm
  Includes bibliographical references and index.
  ISBN 978-1-4051-7615-6 (pbk. : alk. paper)   1. Physical therapy—Law and legislation—Great Britain.
  2. Physical therapists—Legal status, laws, etc.—Great Britain.   I. Title.

KD2968.T47D565   2009
344.4104'1—dc22
2008052869

A catalogue record for this book is available from the British Library.

Set in 10/12 pt Palatino by Graphicraft Limited, Hong Kong
Printed in Singapore by Ho Printing Singapore Pte Ltd

1   2009

Contents

Foreword

I warmly welcome the brand new edition of Bridgit Dimond's very comprehensive guide to the legal issues affecting physiotherapy clinical practitioners, managers, teachers and students.

Gone are the days when practitioners could think that legal issues were nothing to do with the way they treated patients, kept records, behaved towards other staff, managed services or trained as students. Ignorance is no defence before the law, nor is it if you are faced with being struck off the UK professional register by the Health Professions Council because of your lack of knowledge.

Bridgit Dimond's new book is by far the best legal source book for physiotherapists ever published. It is very readable and well laid out with clear conclusions, questions and exercises to reinforce the practical legal information which is up to date with current developments (it even includes a guide to the recent NHS Constitution).

I can highly recommend this new guide to the law for physiotherapists which is very well researched. It should be on the bookshelf of every physiotherapy department, NHS manager, private practice or student reading list.

Phil Gray
Chief Executive
Chartered Society of Physiotherapy

February 2009

Preface

Much has changed in the 9 years since the first edition was published. New Acts of Parliament, new cases, new organisations within the Department of Health, a new registration body in the Health Professions Council have led to an almost complete rewriting of the original work. However, the aims still remain the same: to bring to the physiotherapist an understanding of the legal principles which relate to her practice across a wide spectrum of specialties, illustrated through actual cases and fictional, yet realistic situations to which she can relate. It is hoped that the result will be of practical assistance to her understanding of the constraints and opportunities of the legal context within which she works.

Bridgit Dimond

Acknowledgements

This book could not have been written without the unstinted help of so many physiotherapists and officers of the CSP. It is perhaps unfair to mention some by name, but I must acknowledge the invaluable help of the following (in alphabetical order): Nikki Adams, Leonie Dawson, Paul Donnelly, Frances Fitch, James Greenwood, Laura Henderson, Jill Higgins, Annie Karim, Linda Knott, Robert Ledger, Carmen Rowland, Margaret Revie, Marion Rutter, Sue Smith, Jane Thomas, Pippa White, Sandra Wickham, Siobhan Williams. Others who have assisted include Austin Dorrity. My special thanks are due to Samantha Molloy, the CSP librarian who could not have been more helpful in assisting me in making use of the CSP resources.

Once again I acknowledge with thanks the encouragement and forbearance of my family, particularly Bette who read the typescript and prepared the index.

My special thanks are due to Carmel Richards for her support and encouragement and to whom this book is dedicated.

Abbreviations

ABI	Association of British Insurers	CAM	complementary and alternative medicines
ABPI	Association of the British Pharmaceutical Industry	CCAM	Council for Complementary and Alternative Therapies
A&E	accident and emergency		
ACAS	Advisory, Conciliation and Arbitration Service	CCP	collaborative clinical care profiles
ACPC	Area Child Protection Committee	CDI	community dependency index
		CE	Conformité Européenne (marking following EC Directive 93/68/EEC)
ADL	activities of daily living		
ADR	alternative dispute resolution		
ADR	adverse drug reaction	CHAI	Commission for Health Audit and Inspection (known as the Healthcare Commission)
AIDS	aquired immune deficiency syndrome		
AMHP	approved mental health professional	CHC	Community Health Council
		CHP	Council for Health Professions
ASW	approved social worker	CHRE	Council for Healthcare Regulatory Excellence (formerly CRHCP)
BAOT	British Association of Occupational Therapists		
BCMA	British Complementary Medicine Association	CIGLC	Clinical Interest Group Liaison Committee
BERR	Department for Business Enterprise and Regulatory Reform (replacing the DTI)	CI/OG	Clinical Interest and Occupational Group
		CNST	Clinical Negligence Scheme for Trusts
BMA	British Medical Association		
BNF	British National Formulary	COSHH	Control of Substances Hazardous to Health [Regulations]
BP	blood pressure		
CA	Court of Appeal		
CAB	Citizen's Advice Bureau	CPA	care programme approach

CPA	Consumer Protection Act 1987	EC	European Community
CPAUIA	Commissioner for Protection Against Unlawful Industrial Action	ECHR	European Court of Human Rights
		ECP	extended care practitioner
CPD	continuing professional development	ECT	electroconvulsive therapy
		EEA	European Economic Area
CPN	community psychiatric nurse	EHR	electronic patient record
CPPIH	Commission for Patient and Public Involvement in Health	EL	executive letter
		ELS	existing liabilities scheme
CPR	cardiopulmonary resuscitation	EOC	Equal Opportunities Commission
CPS	Crown Prosecution Service		
CPSM	Council for Professions Supplementary to Medicine	EPP	expert patient programme
		EPR	electronic patient record
CQC	Care Quality Commission	ERG	external reference group
CRE	Commission on Racial Equality	ESP	extended scope practitioners
CRHCP	Council for the Regulation of Health Care Professionals (now see CHRE)	FACS	fair access to care services
		FHSA	Family Health Services Authority
CRTUM	Commissioner for the Rights of Trade Union Members	FT	NHS Foundation Trust
		GMC	General Medical Council
CSAG	clinical standards advisory group	GMS	general medical services
		GP	general practitioner
CSCI	Commission for Social Care Inspection	GPFH	GP fundholder
		GPwSI	general practitioner with special interests
CSIP	Care Services Improvement Partnership	GSCC	General Social Care Council
CSP	Chartered Society of Physiotherapy	GSL	general sales list
		HAI	hospital acquired infection
DBERR	Department for Business, Enterprise and Regulatory Reform	HASAW	Health and Safety at Work etc. Act 1974
		HASC(CHS)A	Health and Social Care (Community Health and Standards) Act 2003
DCSF	Department for Children, Schools and Families		
DfES	Department for Education and Skills	HC	health circular (from Department of Health)
DFG	disabled facilities grants	HCHS	Hospital and Community Health Services
DGH	district general hospital		
DH	Department of Health	HFEA	Human Fertilisation and Embryology Authority
DISC	disability information and study centre	HIV	human immunodeficiency virus
DN(A)R	do not (attempt) resuscitate(ation)	HL	House of Lords
DPA	Data Protection Act 1998	HMSO	Her Majesty's Stationery Office (now the Stationery Office)
DSS	Department of Social Security		
DWP	Department for Work and Pensions	HPA	Health Protection Agency
		HPC	Health Professions Council

HRSW	Health Related Social Worker	MHRA	Medicines and Healthcare Products Regulatory Agency (since 1 April 2003)
HSC	Health Services Commissioner (Ombudsman)		
HSE	Health and Safety Executive	MHRT	Mental Health Review Tribunal
HSG	Health Service Guidance	MND	motor neurone disease
HTA	Human Tissue Authority	MREC	Multi-Center Research Ethics Committee
ICAS	Independent Complaints Advocacy Service		
		MRSA	methicillin-resistant *Staphylococcus aureus*
ICM	Institute of Complementary Medicine		
		NAA	National Assistance Act
ICP	integrated care pathway	NAESC	National Association for the Education of Sick Children
ICRS	Integrated Care Records Service		
		NAHAT	National Association of Health Authorities and Trusts (now Confederation of HAs and Trusts)
ICS	integrated children's system		
ICT	information communication technology		
IM&T	information management and technology	NAI	non-accidental injury
		NAO	National Audit Office
IMCA	independent mental capacity advocate	NCAA	National Clinical Assessment Authority
IMHA	independent mental health advocate	NCSC	National Care Standards Commission
ISA	Independent Safeguarding Authority	NDC	National Disability Council
		NHSME	National Health Service Management Executive
ISIP	Integrated Service Improvement Programme		
		NFR	not for resuscitation
IV	intravenous	NFR	neurophysiological facilitation of respiration
JCC	Joint Consultative Committee		
JP	Justice of the Peace	NHS	National Health Service
LA	local authority	NHS FT	NHS Foundation Trust
LAC	local authority circular	NHS LA	NHS Litigation Authority
LEA	Local Education Authority	NHSU	NHS University
LHB	Local Health Board (Welsh equivalent of PCT)	NICE	National Institute for Health and Clinical Excellence
LINKS	Local Involvement Networks	NIHR	National Institute for Health Research
LOLER	Lifting Operations and Lifting Equipment Regulations		
		NMC	Nursing and Midwifery Council
LPA	lasting power of attorney		
LPC	Low Pay Commission	NMW	national minimum wage
LREC	Local Research Ethics Committee	NPFIT	National Programme for Information Technology
LSP	Local Strategic Partnership or Local Service Provider	NPRN	National Physiotherapy Research Network
MDA	Medical Devices Agency (see MHRA)	NPSA	National Patient Safety Agency
		NRES	National Research Ethics Service (Replaced COREC in 2007)
MHAC	Mental Health Act Commission		

NSF	National Service Framework	PPE	personal protective equipment
NSPCC	National Society for the Prevention of Cruelty to Children	PPiF	Patient and Public involvement Forums
NVQ	national vocational qualification	PRN	as required (of medicines)
		PSM	profession supplementary to medicine
OECD	Organisation for Economic Co-operation and Development	PUWER	Provision and Use of Work Equipment Regulations
Ofsted	Office for Standards in Education	PVS	persistent vegetative state
		PwSI	practitioner with special interests
OFV	opportunities for volunteering scheme	QA	quality assurance
		QBD	Queens Bench Division (of the High Court)
OGC	Office for Government Commerce	QC	Queen's Counsel
OOS	Occupational Overuse Syndrome	QOF	Quality and Outcomes Framework
OPD	out-patient department	RCN	Royal College of Nursing
OSC	Overview and Scrutiny Committee	REC	Research Ethics Committee
OT	occupational therapist	RIDDOR	Reporting of Injuries Diseases and Dangerous Occurrences Regulations
OTC	over the counter		
PACE	Physiotherapy Access to Continuing Education	RMO	Responsible Medical Officer
PALS	Patient Advice and Liaison Service	RPSGB	Royal Pharmaceutical Society of Great Britain
PBC	practice-based commissioning or prudential borrowing code	RSC	Rules of the Supreme Court
		RSI	repetitive strain injury
PC	Privy Council	SAP	single assessment process
PCC	Professional Conduct Committee	SCIE	Social Care Institute for Excellence
PCMH	Plea and Case Management Hearing	SCPHN	Specialist Community Public Health Nurse
PCT	primary care trust	SENDIST	Special Educational Needs and Disability Tribunal
PGD	patient group directions	SEU	social exclusion unit
PIAG	Patient Information Advisory Group	SHA	Strategic Health Authority
		SHAPE	Strategic Health Asset Planning and Evaluation
PMS	primary medical services contract	SOAD	second opinion appointed doctor
POM	prescription only medicine		
POVA	protection of vulnerable adults	SRSC	safety representative and safety committee
PPA	Prescription Pricing Authority		
PPC	Preliminary Proceedings Committee	SRV	social role valorisation
		SSD	social services department
PPC	Professional Practice Committee	SSI	Social Services Inspectorate
		SWD	short wave diathermy

TCEWS	Transforming Community Equipment and Wheelchair Services
TENS	transcutaneous electrical nerve stimulation
TU	Trade Union
UKCC	United Kingdom Central Council for Nursing, Midwifery and Health Visiting (replaced by the NMC)
UKCP	United Kingdom Council for Psychotherapy
WDC	Workforce Development Confederation
WHC	Welsh Health Circular

Clinical interest and occupational groups of the Chartered Society of Physiotherapy (CI/OGs)

Acupuncture Association of Chartered Physiotherapists (AACP)

Association of Chartered Physiotherapists in Animal Therapy (ACPAT)

Association of Chartered Physiotherapists in the Community (ACPC)

Association of Chartered Physiotherapists in Cystic Fibrosis (ACPCF)

Association of Chartered Physiotherapists in Energy Medicine (ACPEM)

Association of Chartered Physiotherapists in Cardiac Rehabilitation (ACPICR)

Association of Chartered Physiotherapists interested in Electrotherapy (ACPIE)

Association of Chartered Physiotherapists in Independent Healthcare (ACPIHC)

Association of Chartered Physiotherapists interested in Neurology (ACPIN)

Association of Chartered Physiotherapists in Reflex Therapy (ACPIRT)

Association of Chartered Physiotherapists in Management (ACPM)

Association of Chartered Physiotherapists in Occupational Health and Ergonomics (ACPOHE)

Association of Chartered Physiotherapists in Orthopaedic Medicine (ACPOM)

Association of Chartered Physiotherapists in Oncology & Palliative Care (ACPOPC)

Association of Chartered Physiotherapists for People with Learning Disabilities (ACPPLD)

Association of Chartered Physiotherapists in Respiratory Care (ACPRC)

Association of Chartered Physiotherapists in Sports Medicine (ACPSM)

Association of Chartered Physiotherapists in Therapeutic Riding (ACPTR)

Association of Chartered Physiotherapists in Women's Health (ACPWH)

Chartered Physiotherapists working with Older People (AGILE, formerly ACPSIEP)

Association of Orthopaedic Chartered Physiotherapists (AOCP)

Association of Paediatric Chartered Physiotherapists (APCP)

British Association of Bobath Trained Therapists (BABTT)

British Association of Chartered Physiotherapists in Amputee Rehabilitation (BACPAR)

British Association of Hand Therapists (BAHT)

Association of Chartered Physiotherapists interested in Massage and Soft Tissue Therapies (CPMaSST)

Chartered Physiotherapists in Mental Healthcare (CPMH)

Chartered Physiotherapists Promoting Continence (CPPC)

Craniosacral Therapy Association of Chartered Physiotherapists (CTACP)

Chartered Physiotherapists working as Extended Scope Practitioners (ESP)

Hydrotherapy Association of Chartered Physiotherapists (HACP)

International Support Group for Chartered Physiotherapists (ISG4CP)

Manipulation Association of Chartered Physiotherapists (MACP)

McKenzie Institute of Mechanical Diagnosis and Therapeutic Practitioners (MIMDT)

Medico-Legal Association of Chartered Physiotherapists (MLACP)

Organisation of Chartered Physiotherapists in Private Practice (Physio First)

Physiotherapy Pain Association (PPA)
Physiotherapy Research Association (PRS)

Unrecognised groups include:
HIV clinical interest group (CPIHIV)
Military Medicine (ACPIMM)
Bobath Tutors (BBTA)

Burn Care (BURNS)
Paediatric management (PPIMS)
Spinal Injury Lead Clinicians (SIUPLC)
Vestibular rehabilitation (ACPVR)
Visual Impairment (AVICP)
Yoga (YOGA)

1 Introduction

Why does a physiotherapist need to know the law?

Typical situation

A 20-year-old girl, Sandra, was injured in a road accident when a lorry went out of control and crashed into her as she was walking along the pavement. She survived with severe brain damage and was transferred to a neurosurgical unit. The consultant neurologist warned the parents that she might never recover fully and in fact might stay in a persistent vegetative state. The nurses however encouraged the parents to be more optimistic and gave them contact addresses for voluntary organisations. Her father thought it might be best if she was taken off the ventilator, but her mother wanted all possible treatment and care to continue. Sandra remained in a coma for several months, during which time she had intensive physiotherapy. She developed a severe pressure sore as a result of a splint which had been badly applied at the time of the accident. She slowly recovered consciousness and had suffered a severe left sided hemiplegia. She moved to a specialist rehabilitation unit, returning home for the weekends. Her parents paid for her to have private physiotherapy at the weekends. The occupational therapist recommended that she should have a bed downstairs and should use a hoist for bathing. Sandra refused since she was determined to be independent. She was however concerned that her compensation following the road accident might be reduced the more she persevered in her exercises. She was also hoping to be able to drive a specially adapted car but, since she suffered epileptic fits following the brain injury, was advised to wait till these were clearly under control. Later she ended in-patient treatment, returning to the centre for check-ups and relying upon local physiotherapists for her care. They liaised with the centre.

Legal issues which arise

The facts describe a situation well known to many physiotherapists and repeated in various guises across the country every day. On examination however it gives rise to numerous legal issues. Some of them are shown in Figure 1.1 together with the chapters where that particular legal issue is discussed.

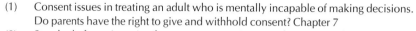

> (1)   Consent issues in treating an adult who is mentally incapable of making decisions. Do parents have the right to give and withhold consent? Chapter 7
> (2)   Standard of care in caring for a comatose patient. At what point and on the basis of what circumstances can active treatment be withdrawn? What rights do the relatives have? Chapters 10 and 25
> (3)   Giving information to relatives about prognosis and about voluntary groups. Chapter 7
> (4)   Liability for causing pressure sores and for treating them. Chapter 10
> (5)   Manual handling implications when a client refuses to use a hoist. Chapter 11
> (6)   Duty of carers when a patient with uncontrolled epilepsy wishes to drive a car. Chapter 16
> (7)   Duty of staff if patients are incapable of driving because of conditions such as epilepsy but refuse to accept their advice. Chapters 7, 10 and 16
> (8)   Entitlements to NHS and Social Services care. Chapters 20–24
> (9)   Financial support for disabled. Chapter 20
> (10) Rights to have specially adapted wheelchairs and cars. Chapter 15
> (11) Compensation following a road traffic accident. How it is calculated and the extent to which it will be reduced if a patient puts more effort into recovery? Chapter 10
> (12) Who would have administered the finances if she had remained in a comatose state but had been awarded substantial compensation? Chapter 22

Figure 1.1   Legal issues arising from Sandra's situation

Physiotherapists and the law

Figure 1.1 shows only a few of the legal issues that can confront the physiotherapist in one particular case. It provides the justification for this book that aims to explain within the context of physiotherapy the law which applies to physiotherapists' practice. Physiotherapists need to have sufficient familiarity with the basic principles of law, so that when they are in a difficult situation they know immediately the laws that apply and the point at which they need to seek expert advice. Information from the Professional Advice Service within the Professional and Development Unit of the Chartered Society of Physiotherapy (CSP) shows that over 1000 queries are received each year on issues which have legal implications covering consent, employer/employee relations, the duty of care, confidentiality, social services, documentation, patients' rights, the NHS organisation and many other topics which show the need for physiotherapists to have some understanding of the law. All these issues are covered in this book.

Research was undertaken by Herman Triezenberg[1] to identify present and future ethical issues arising in physical therapy practice. Sixteen issues were raised: six involving patients' rights and welfare, five professional issues and five business and economic factors. Of these, 13 had never been discussed in previous physical therapy literature. The list is shown in Figure 1.2. It will be noted that each ethical issue also raises legal questions. The fact that the respondents to his questionnaires were US citizens is reflected in the number of topics relating to the financial relationship between therapist and patient and the dangers of exploitation and fraud. Legal issues arising from private practice are considered in Chapter 19. In a commentary on the research Ruth Purtilo,[2] Director of the Center for Health Policy and Ethics, Creighton University, Omaha states:

> The more physical therapists can do to create a broad base of understanding about the ethical issues facing the profession, the more likely we are to enter the new millennium prepared to make a meaningful contribution.

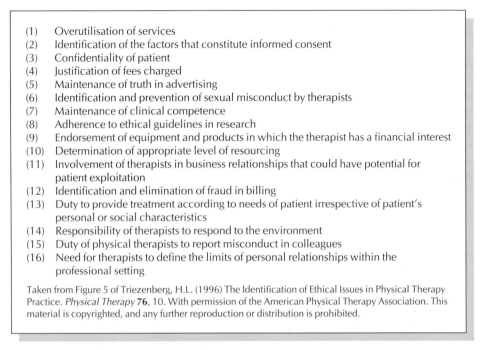

(1)   Overutilisation of services
(2)   Identification of the factors that constitute informed consent
(3)   Confidentiality of patient
(4)   Justification of fees charged
(5)   Maintenance of truth in advertising
(6)   Identification and prevention of sexual misconduct by therapists
(7)   Maintenance of clinical competence
(8)   Adherence to ethical guidelines in research
(9)   Endorsement of equipment and products in which the therapist has a financial interest
(10)   Determination of appropriate level of resourcing
(11)   Involvement of therapists in business relationships that could have potential for patient exploitation
(12)   Identification and elimination of fraud in billing
(13)   Duty to provide treatment according to needs of patient irrespective of patient's personal or social characteristics
(14)   Responsibility of therapists to respond to the environment
(15)   Duty of physical therapists to report misconduct in colleagues
(16)   Need for therapists to define the limits of personal relationships within the professional setting

Taken from Figure 5 of Triezenberg, H.L. (1996) The Identification of Ethical Issues in Physical Therapy Practice. *Physical Therapy* **76**, 10. With permission of the American Physical Therapy Association. This material is copyrighted, and any further reproduction or distribution is prohibited.

Figure 1.2   Ethical issues in physical therapy practice

Exactly the same point could be made about a legal understanding.

Definition of physiotherapy

A Royal Charter was granted in 1920 to the body which later became the Chartered Society of Physiotherapy and established as the only recognised examining and professional body for physiotherapists in the UK. It was authorised to:

promote a curriculum and standard of qualification for persons engaged in the practice of massage, medical gymnastics, electrotherapeutics and kindred methods for treatment [and] to make and maintain lists of persons considered to be qualified to practise in such methods of treatment.

The new Curriculum Framework drafted by the CSP in 1996 and updated in 2002[3] defines physiotherapy as:

A health care profession concerned with human function and movement and maximising potential. It uses physical approaches to promote, maintain and restore physical, psychological and social well-being, taking account of variations in health status. It is science-based, committed to extending, applying, evaluating and reviewing the evidence that underpins and informs its practice and delivery. The exercise of clinical judgment and informed interpretation is at its core.

Anne Parry points out the dangers of researchers defining physiotherapy in a minimalist way, i.e. by limiting it to exercise therapy, massage and physical applications, and then concluding that it is ineffective.[4] She urges 'Complain vociferously when "physiotherapy" is misused. If you don't care, no one else will.'

Once need for a physiotherapist has been determined, the physiotherapist will:

• agree long- and short-term goals with the patient, carer and team;

- determine the cost-effective type, frequency, duration, progression and mix of skills needed;
- give a degree of priority to the case;
- take the case on to the case load when a full care regime can be undertaken;
- continue to re-assess and review the treatment plan;
- discharge the patient when goals are met or progress is optimal;
- take full legal responsibility for his/her care.[5]

All these stages have legal implications which will be covered in this book.

The definition used in the CSP website is as follows:

> Physiotherapy is a heath care profession concerned with human function and movement and maximising potential. Physiotherapists work in a wide variety of health settings such as intensive care, mental illness, stroke recovery, occupational health and care of the elderly. Physiotherapy is certainly far more than fixing musculoskeletal sports injuries although that is perhaps the most common perception of the profession.

In the revised paper on the Scope of Professional Practice 2008, the definition of the scope of practice of physiotherapy is based on the four pillars (massage, exercise, electrotherapy and kindred forms of treatment) and is:

> any activity undertaken by an individual physiotherapist that may be situated within the four pillars (see above) of physiotherapy practice where the individual is educated, trained and competent to perform that activity. Such activities should be linked to existing or emerging occupational and/or practice frameworks acknowledged by the profession, and be supported by a body of evidence.

The Paper states that:

> Physiotherapy applies broad boundaries to its professional practice via the four pillars of practice contained within the Royal Charter.

Whilst the first three pillars are narrowly related to specific treatment interventions, the fourth pillar (i.e. kindred forms of treatment) is suitably broad to allow physiotherapists to expand their expertise according to patient need.

In considering the scope of practice of the individual physiotherapist the Information Paper states that:

> Members may choose to work as either a generalist or a specialist practitioner, and may choose to practice within the first three pillars or practice, or they may wish to extend their practice into the fourth pillar of practice and develop further clinical skills aimed at enhancing patient care.

The CSP is the final arbiter about the nature of the practice of individual members and whether what they perform is identifiable as physiotherapy. Should there be a challenge to an individual's activity/competence, the CSP would be required to confirm that the individual was working within their personal scope of practice. Providing there is the evidence of an individual's competence to undertake the role/activity in question, and that the activity sits within the four pillars of practice, the individual would be covered by their PLI (Public Liability Insurance) as working within the scope of the profession.

This paper and the legal implications following from extending the scope of physiotherapy practice are considered in Chapter 4.

History of physiotherapy

Physiotherapy has ancient origins. In a review of the use of physiotherapy in health and lung conditions Diana Innocenti[6] discusses how massage and gymnastics were practised in the ancient world and were documented in China by Kong-Fu at around 3000 BC. There is also evidence of the use of massage and gymnastics for the improvement of health in Greece at around 700 BC. John Hutchinson presented his research on lung volumes and spirometry to the Royal Medical and Chirurgical Society on 28 April 1846. Allen Mason's many articles on the history of individual aspects of physiotherapy practice provide an amusing insight into its ancient past and into the different forms of treatment.

The modern development of the profession that led to state registration of physiotherapy practice probably begins with the establishment of the Society of Masseurs in 1894. Jane Wicksteed has researched the history of the Chartered Society of Physiotherapy from 1894–1945[7] and describes how the original founders, nurses or midwives by training but all practising as masseuses, were anxious to establish their credibility as masseuses in the eyes of the public. They therefore set up a Council and Society, establishing examinations and membership rules and sought support from doctors as patrons and external examiners.

The development of the Society in the twentieth century illustrates the way in which new groups and new practices were assimilated within the main structure. In 1900 the Society became incorporated and linked in with Swedish physical exercises or gymnastics. New training schools were established and popularity increased. In 1916 Queen Mary became patron of the Society. In 1920 a Royal Charter was awarded and the Chartered Society of Massage and Medical Gymnastics (CSMMG) was formed with the amalgamation of the Incorporated Society of Trained Masseurs and the Institute of Massage and Remedial Gymnasts, the chairman being a member of the medical profession. Light and electrotherapy and hydrotherapy were added to the syllabus and examinations. In 1942 the name of the Chartered Society of Physiotherapy was adopted when the CSMMG and the Incorporation of Physiotherapists amalgamated. In 1986 the Chartered Society merged with the Society of Remedial Gymnastics and Recreational Therapy and 726 remedial gymnasts became members of the CSP.[8] In 1960 physiotherapists obtained state registration under the Professions Supplementary to Medicine Act 1960. In 2002 the Health Professions Council became the registration body for those professions

which came under the Council for Professions Supplementary to Medicine and its role in registration, professional conduct and education is considered in Chapters 3, 4 and 5 respectively. In 1977 the autonomy of the profession was recognised in a Health Circular[9] and this has ultimately led to physiotherapists providing a direct access service to patients within specific specialties.

CSP strategy for 2005–10[10]

The CSP Vision and Mission for 2005–10 set three strategic priorities: building core services, putting members at the heart of the CSP and raising the profile and influence of the profession and the CSP with each strategic priority having the following strategic objectives:

- Building core services:
  - Strategic objective 1: robust foundations and infrastructure
  - Strategic objective 2: define and promote the membership package
  - Strategic objective 3: robust foundation for clinical practice and service delivery
  - Strategic objective 4: continue to improve the quality of our core services
  - Strategic objective 5: ensure diversity principles are integral to CSP service delivery
  - Strategic objective 6: understanding the issues facing the different countries
  - Strategic objective 7: partnerships with other organisations
- Putting members at the heart of the CSP:
  - Strategic objective 8: develop our representative structures
  - Strategic objective 9: support to members in influencing local health decision-making
  - Strategic objective 10: develop interactive CSP
- Raising the profile and influence of the profession and the CSP:
  - Strategic objective 11: raise the understanding of the general public

■ Strategic objective 12: ensure that physiotherapy is 'at the table' when decisions are made.

The future

In May 2008 the CSP published a consultation paper on the future of physiotherapy.[11] The CSP wished to take advantage of the sixtieth anniversary of the NHS to make explicit its vision for the contribution of physiotherapy to the health and wellbeing of the UK population over the coming years and also its role in working with stakeholders to deliver this vision. The paper identifies the main changes and drivers affecting health and wellbeing services including designing and delivering services around service user need; improving access to services with 7-day cover and self-referral to a wider range of practitioners; more diverse settings for the delivery of health and social care including the voluntary and leisure sectors; greater integration of health, social care and education; new modes of planning and commissioning services; personal responsibility for health and wellbeing; self-care and self-management of long-term conditions; government drive to address health inequalities; skills no longer unique to one professional group; more effective use of support workers; greater focus on performance and quality management; practice to be founded on robust evidence, evaluation and continuing professional development; development of competencies; differences across the separate countries within the UK; technological advances and developments; demographic changes; changing systems of regulation and increasing significance of global issues in health and social care need and service delivery. The paper expands on the ways in which the physiotherapy workforce (defined as physiotherapists and support workers in diverse roles including clinicians, managers, educators and researchers) must develop to achieve this vision. It also sets out the role of the CSP in preparing new curriculum guidance in conjunction with education providers and employers and in setting out a new physiotherapy framework.

A new Code of Practice and Conduct is to be prepared which will move away from a rules-based approach towards an ethical standards-oriented framework. The new Code will define professionalism, define evidence-based scope of practice, provide a resource to support members in their professional activity, define what people should be able to expect from physiotherapy and its workforce; provide bench marks against which members can self-assess their standards of practice, conduct and service delivery and reflect the full range of practice and settings. The emphasis in the new Code will be on individual responsibility for decision making and professional development; working with clients as equals and coping with uncertainty. The finalised paper is to be published in the summer of 2008 and will be followed by stage 2 and the development of new resources and tools overseen by an expert Steering Group.

The Darzi Review published its final recommendations in July 2008 in time for the sixtieth anniversary of the NHS. The reports are considered in Chapter 28.

Clinical interest and occupational groups of the CSP

The breadth of physiotherapy practice is supported by clinical interest groups and occupational groups within the CSP. They have been described by Ruth Dubbey[12] as serving

> as a forum for physiotherapists to encourage, promote and facilitate interchange of thoughts and ideas as well as providing expertise with education, practice and research in their specialty.

There are over 50 recognised clinical interest and occupational groups (CI/OGs) and many more non-recognised groups representing the diverse interests and specialties of physiotherapists. Criteria for a CI/OG to be recognised by the CSP were developed by the Professional Practice Committee in 1992 and were re-examined as part of the review of the CI/OGs during 2000. The criteria agreed by the Professional Practice

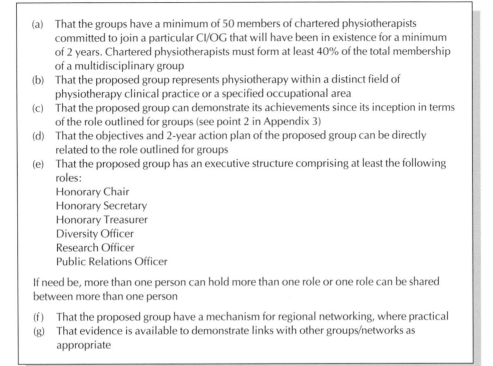

(a)   That the groups have a minimum of 50 members of chartered physiotherapists committed to join a particular CI/OG that will have been in existence for a minimum of 2 years. Chartered physiotherapists must form at least 40% of the total membership of a multidisciplinary group

(b)   That the proposed group represents physiotherapy within a distinct field of physiotherapy clinical practice or a specified occupational area

(c)   That the proposed group can demonstrate its achievements since its inception in terms of the role outlined for groups (see point 2 in Appendix 3)

(d)   That the objectives and 2-year action plan of the proposed group can be directly related to the role outlined for groups

(e)   That the proposed group has an executive structure comprising at least the following roles:
Honorary Chair
Honorary Secretary
Honorary Treasurer
Diversity Officer
Research Officer
Public Relations Officer

If need be, more than one person can hold more than one role or one role can be shared between more than one person

(f)   That the proposed group have a mechanism for regional networking, where practical

(g)   That evidence is available to demonstrate links with other groups/networks as appropriate

Figure 1.3   Criteria for recognition of a Clinical Interest and Occupational Group (CI/OG)[13]

Committee in March 2001 are shown in Figure 1.3. The procedure for recognition is shown in Figure 1.4. There exists a Clinical Interest and Occupational Group Liaison Committee, which meets four times a year at the CSP headquarters. At the time of writing no new groups are being recognised as a review is being undertaken of processes and resources. This work is expected to be finished by December 2008 and may result in a change of the recognition criteria.

Recent developments in terms of training etc. and continuing professional development (CPD) are considered in Chapter 5.

The diversity and range of treatments provided by the physiotherapist means that the laws covered in this book will be extensive and many specialist areas will be discussed. First however it is necessary to understand the basic structure, language and sources of law and it is this to which we turn in the next chapter.

Conclusions

The publication of the CSP Strategy for 2005–10, the Scope of Professional Practice in 2008 and Charting the Future should enable the practice of physiotherapy to develop extensively but safely in several new directions. In particular, the recognition that the former fixed boundaries between different professions will disappear will present both opportunities and significant challenges with many legal implications. The role of the registered physiotherapist as a supplementary prescriber of medicines is considered in Chapter 15. Eventually physiotherapists may be recognised as independent prescribers. Such developments, once perhaps seen as an extremely unlikely part of physiotherapy practice, are a natural extension within the fourth pillar of 'kindred activities'.

(1) Groups seeking recognition will be invited to complete a pro-forma (Appendix 3) to submit evidence to the Professional Practice Committee (PPC)

(2) Recognition is granted for 5 years

(4) Re-recognition process

    (4.1) Every 5 years the form that was filled in for recognition will need to be completed again

    (4.2) The form will be sent out at least 6 months in advance, to make sure that the group has adequate time to meet and discuss what they have achieved in the past 5 years

    (4.3) Once the form has been returned to the administrative assistant, the form will be put forward to the Professional Practice Committee (via the CIGLC) for consideration

    (4.4) In the case of the form not being returned within 3 months of the re-recognition date (9 months after the form has been sent out), the group will no longer be recognised

Figure 1.4 Recognition process and re-recognition process for clinical interest and occupational groups

Questions and exercises

1 How would you define the core work of the physiotherapist?

2 To what extent do you consider it is appropriate to describe a physiotherapist as 'supplementary to medicine'? Consider this in relation to the extended scope practitioner that is considered in Chapter 4.

3 Do you consider the personal beliefs and philosophies of the physiotherapist are relevant to her work? To what extent, if any, should they be taken into account by a prospective employer or client?

4 What are the legal implications for the physiotherapist of the CSP paper Charting the Future of Physiotherapy and of the Darzi Review of the NHS (see Chapter 28)?

References

1 Triezenberg, H.L. (1996) The Identification of Ethical Issues in Physical Therapy Practice. *Physical Therapy* **76**, 10, 1097–1098.

2 Purtilo, R. (1996) Invited Commentary. *Physical Therapy* **76**, 10, 1107–1108.

3 The Chartered Society of Physiotherapy (2002) *Curriculum Framework for Qualifying Programmes in Physiotherapy*. The Chartered Society of Physiotherapy, London.

4 Parry, A. (1997) Choice Treatment for Physiotherapy, *Physiotherapy* **83**, 6, 277.

5 Squires, A., Hastings, M. (1997) Physiotherapy with Older People: Calculating Staffing Need. *Physiotherapy* **83**, 2, 58–64.

6 Innocenti, D. (1996) An Overview of the Development of Breathing Exercises into the Specialty of Physiotherapy for Heart and Lung Conditions. *Physiotherapy* **82**, 12, 681–693.

7 Wicksteed, J.H. (1948) (reprinted by the CSP in 1994 to celebrate the centenary) *The Growth of a Profession*. Edward Arnold, London.

8 Barclay, J. (1994) *In Good Hands: the History of the Chartered Society of Physiotherapists 1894–1994*. Butterworth Heinemann, Oxford.

9 Department of Health and Social Services (1977) *Relationship Between the Medical and Remedial Professions*. HC (77)33. DHSS, London.

10 Chartered Society of Physiotherapy (2005) *Strategy for 2005–10*. CSP, London.

11 Chartered Society of Physiotherapy (2008) *Charting the Future of Physiotherapy*. Position Paper Draft. CSP, London.

12 Dubbey, R. (1996) Clinical Interest Groups. *Physiotherapy* **82**, 5, 283–284.

13 Chartered Society of Physiotherapy (2004) *Clinical Interest and Occupational Handbook*. CSP London.

2 The Legal System

Law can be perplexing to those who have never studied it. The jargon, the complexity of a lawyer's answer to the simplest question, can place a significant barrier between the ordinary health professional and the law practitioner. However, any health professional or health service manager has to work within the context of the law, and therefore has to know the basic legal principles which constrain or empower him/her. He/she also needs to have a clear understanding of the point at which it is essential to bring in legal advice and support. This chapter is aimed at providing an introduction to the basic terms which are used and a description of the framework within which the law is implemented. The Glossary provides an explanation of some of the technical terms that are used. Each member of the Chartered Society of Physiotherapy receives a legal package setting out their basic entitlements and insurance cover. A similar package is provided for those members of the profession who are self-employed and are members of Physio First (see Chapter 19) The following topics will be covered:

- Sources of law
- Civil and criminal law
- Civil and criminal courts
- Types of civil action
- Public and private law
- Legal personnel
- Procedure in civil courts
- Procedure in criminal courts
- Accusatorial system
- Law and ethics
- Guidance on conduct and procedures

Sources of law

Law derives from two main sources: statute law and the common law. These are illustrated in Figure 2.1.

Statute law

Statute law is based on legislation passed through the agreed constitutional process. Legislation of the European Community now takes precedence over the Acts of Parliament of the United Kingdom Government. This country must observe the Treaties of the European Community, and is

Statute Law	Common Law
EC Regulations	**EC Court rulings**
Acts of Parliament/Statutes	**House of Lords** – cases on important
made by House of Commons	points of law
House of Lords	**Court of Appeal**
Royal Assent	**High Court/Crown Court**
Statutory Instruments	Decisions binding on basis of rules of
made by relevant Ministry	precedent and hierarchy
laid before Parliament	
Statutes and statutory instruments as well as previous cases are interpreted by judges and the decisions become part of the common law	

Figure 2.1   Derivation and sources of law

bound by Regulations made by the European Council and the European Commission. These have direct application to Member States. This is in contrast to the European Directives, which must be incorporated into UK law to be effective (although they do apply directly to state authorities).

Draft legislation in the form of a bill is introduced into either the House of Lords or House of Commons, sometimes by the Government and sometimes by a private member, and follows a recognised procedure by way of hearings, committee stages and the report stage. Eventually, following agreement by both Houses and the signature of the Queen, it becomes an Act of Parliament. The actual date it comes into force will either be set out in the Act itself or will be determined at a later date by Statutory Instrument. The Act of Parliament may provide for powers to be delegated to ministers and others to enact detailed supplementary rules. These are known as Statutory Instruments. They must be formally placed before Parliament before coming into effect.

Common law

Decisions by judges in courts create what is known as the common law. A recognised hierarchy of the courts determines which previous decisions are binding on courts hearing similar cases. The European Court of Justice based in Luxembourg can hear cases between member states on European law, such as quota disputes or applications by domestic courts for a ruling on a particular point of law.

Figure 2.2 shows the civil court system and Figure 2.3 shows the criminal court system.

A recognised system of reporting of judges' decisions ensures certainty over what was stated and the facts of the cases. The main principles which are set out in a case are known as the *ratio decidendi* (reasons for the decision). Other parts of a judge's speech which are not considered to be part of the *ratio decidendi* are known as *obiter dicta* (things said by the way). Only the *ratio decidendi* is directly binding on lower courts, but the *obiter dicta* may influence the decision of judges in later court cases. It may be possible for judges to 'distinguish' previous cases and not follow them on the grounds that the facts are significantly different. For example before the Occupier's Liability Act 1984 was passed, which defined the liability of an occupier of premises towards trespassers, liability was based on decisions made by judges on particular facts. Cases which involved harm to children (where the occupier had been held liable) were held not to be binding on judges hearing cases involving adults, so that occupiers were not liable to an adult trespasser. The earlier cases relating to children were 'distinguished'.

Judges are however bound by statute and if case law results in an unsatisfactory situation, then this may be remedied by amending the existing legislation through the parliamentary

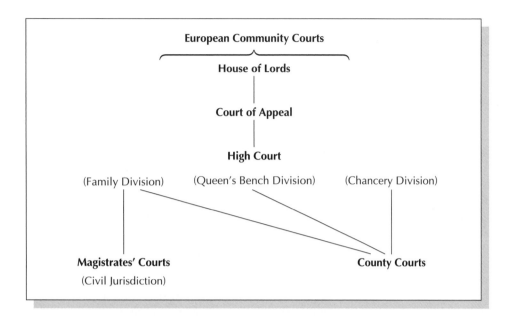

Figure 2.2   Simplified diagram showing the hierarchy of the civil courts

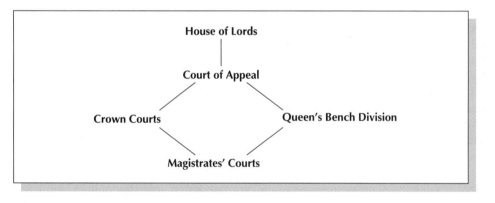

Figure 2.3   The hierarchy of the criminal courts

process. Statutes nevertheless have to be interpreted by judges in court cases if disputes arise in relation to what the statute means. Thus law develops through a mix of statutory promulgation and common law decision making.

Procedure for judicial review

The decisions of judicial and administrative bodies can be challenged by an application to the Queen's Bench Division for the decision or adjudication to be reviewed. Thus if a person detained under the Mental Health Act 1983 were to appeal unsuccessfully to a Mental Health Review Tribunal (MHRT) and considered that the decision not to discharge him/her was based upon a failure to apply the correct law or because the principles of natural justice were infringed (e.g. the chairman was prejudiced against him personally), he/she could apply to the Queen's Bench Division of the High Court, for the decision of the MHRT to be reviewed.[1] However, this procedure is not recommended where an

Act of Parliament lays down a specific procedure for challenging the decision of a statutory body. For example in the case of *Gossington* v. *Ealing Borough Council*,[2] Mr Gossington applied for judicial review of the decision of London Borough of Ealing to provide him with only 5 hours of home help per week instead of the original 10 hours. The judge held that, since the Act provided for an application to the Secretary of State if a local authority fails to carry out its statutory functions, the applicant had not exhausted the other available routes open to him to remedy the wrong he felt that he had suffered, and therefore the application for judicial review was refused.

The Human Rights Act 1998

The European Convention on Human Rights (1950) provides protection for the fundamental rights and freedoms of all people. The UK is a signatory as are many European countries which are not members of the European Community. Thus Norway is a signatory to the European Convention on Human Rights but not a member of the European Community. It is enforced through the European Court of Human Rights, which meets in Strasbourg. However, following the passing of the Human Rights Act 1998 most of the Articles will be directly enforceable in the UK courts in relation to alleged infringement by a public authority or an organisation that performs a public function. The Articles included in the Human Rights Act 1998 are shown in Appendix 1. An introduction to the Human Rights Act together with guidance on its provisions and the cases which have been heard in relation to the articles is available from the Ministry of Justice (replacing the Department of Constitutional Affairs) website.[3] For further discussion on the Human Rights Act see Chapter 6.

Other international charters relating to health

This country is also a signatory to, or has recognised, many other International Charters which recognise rights in a variety of fields. These include the UN Convention on the Rights of the Child, the UN Convention on the Elimination of All Forms of Discrimination against Women, the Universal Declaration of Human Rights, the Declaration of Helsinki developed by the World Health Organization in 1964 (relating to research practice). These Charters are not directly enforced in this country, though their principles may be contained in statutory or common law, and reflected in guidance provided by the Department of Health and professional bodies and organisations.

Civil and criminal law

The civil law covers the law which governs disputes between citizens (including corporate bodies) or between citizens and the state. Thus contract law and the law of torts (civil wrongs excluding breach of contract), rights over property, marital disputes and the wrongful exercise of power by a statutory authority all come under the civil law.

Criminal law relates to actions that can be followed by criminal proceedings in which an accused is prosecuted. The sources of criminal law are both statutory and the common law: thus the definition of murder derives from a decision of the courts in the seventeenth century, whereas theft is defined by a 1968 Act of Parliament as amended by subsequent legislation.

Examples of some of the principal differences between a civil case and a criminal case are shown in Figure 2.4.

There is an overlap between civil and criminal wrongs: thus touching a person without his/her consent may be a civil wrong, known as trespass to the person. It may also be a crime, i.e. a criminal assault or battery. Similarly, driving a car carelessly may lead to criminal proceedings for driving without due care and attention but if someone was injured as a result would also lead to civil proceedings for negligence, as it is almost certain that the driver would have been in breach of a duty of care owed to that person. In one

	Criminal hearings	**Civil hearings**
Basis of action	A charge of a criminal offence	An alleged wrong by one person against another
Action brought by	Crown Prosecution Service (CPS) – occasionally a private prosecution	The person wronged [the claimant (formerly known as plaintiff)] or if a child, a person on his/her behalf
Standard of proof	Beyond reasonable doubt	Balance of probabilities
Facts decided by	Magistrates Courts the magistrate(s) Crown Court the jury	The judge
Law applied by	Magistrates Courts the magistrate(s) Stipendiary magistrate or lay magistrates advised by legally qualified clerk Crown Court the judge	The judge(s)

Figure 2.4 Differences between civil and criminal hearings

case where a patient alleged that an unregistered physiotherapist had raped and indecently assaulted her, the police decided not to prosecute. However, the patient brought a civil action for assault and obtained compensation of over £25 000, including an amount representing aggravated damages because the defendant put her through the harrowing ordeal of having to appear in court.[4]

In another case, Dr Adomako, an anaesthetist, failed to realise that during an operation a tube had become disconnected, as a result of which the patient died. He was prosecuted in the criminal courts and convicted of manslaughter.[5] There would also be liability on him and his employers in the civil courts for his negligence in causing the death of the patient (see Chapter 10). Both criminal proceedings and civil proceedings could thus arise from the same set of facts or incidents.

The Law Commission[6] recommended that the law should be changed to enable it to be made easier for corporations and statutory bodies to be prosecuted for manslaughter. Notable disasters such as the capsizing of the *Herald of Free Enterprise*, which led to 187 deaths, and the King's Cross underground fire in 1987 (31 deaths), the Piper Alpha oil platform disaster (167 deaths) and the Paddington Rail crash in 1999 (31 deaths) were not followed by successful prosecutions of the organisations involved. The Corporate Manslaughter and Corporate Homicide Act 2007 was intended to ensure that organisations responsible for such deaths were held criminally responsible.

Corporate Manslaughter and Corporate Homicide Act 2007

The Act abolishes the common law offence of corporate manslaughter by gross negligence and replaces it with statutory offences which can be committed by specified organisations if its activities are managed or organised in a way which (a) causes a person's death, and (b) amounts to a gross breach of a relevant duty of care owed by the organisation to the deceased. An organisation is guilty of an offence under this section only if the way in which its activities are managed or organised by its senior management is a substantial element in the breach of the duty of care. The organisations specified include

- Negligence
- Nuisance
- Defamation
- Breach of statutory duty
- Trespass (to the person, goods or land)
- Breach of contract

Figure 2.5   Civil actions

'corporations' and also the Department of Health. The duty of care is defined widely and includes duties to a detained patient, but excludes any duty of care owed by a public authority in respect of a decision as to matters of public policy (including in particular the allocation of public resources or the weighing of competing public interests). Duty of care also excludes emergency responses carried out by an NHS body or ambulance service. The jury determines if there has been a gross breach of the duty of care beyond reasonable doubt. On conviction, the organisation can be fined, subjected to remedial order and required to publish details of the offence, the fine and the remedial action ordered. A prosecution under health and safety laws can proceed at the same time as a prosecution for corporate manslaughter. Individuals cannot be prosecuted under the Act, but they are liable to a common law prosecution for manslaughter and if gross negligence that caused the death is established can be convicted of manslaughter. (See the case of the anaesthetist above.[5]) Following conviction, a company could be given an unlimited fine.

Types of civil action

Figure 2.5 illustrates some of the kinds of civil action that may be brought. In this book we are principally concerned with the law relating to negligence, breach of statutory duty and trespass to the person, but the physiotherapist should also be aware of the civil law relating to defamation and nuisance.

Public and private law

Another distinction in the classification of laws is that of public and private law. Figure 2.6 illustrates the difference between the two.

Public law deals with those areas of law where society intervenes in the actions of individuals. In contrast, private law is concerned with the behaviour of individuals or corporate bodies to each other. The Children Act 1989 covers both private law and public law relating to children: care proceedings, protection orders, child assessment orders are part of public law; orders in relation to children made following divorce or

Public Law
Matter of public concern e.g.

- Protection of children
- Public nuisance
- How statutory duties are carried out

Private Law
Matter arising between individuals (people or organisations) e.g.

- Purchasing a house
- Suing for personal injury
- Suing for breach of contract

Figure 2.6   Differences between public and private law

nullity, such as with whom the child is to live, are part of private law. Thus the report by Lord Laming into the death of Victoria Climbié[7] was concerned with public law: the duty of social services departments to take action to protect children. In contrast, a dispute over whether consent has been given for a child to have treatment would be part of private law.

Scotland and Northern Ireland

This book describes the law that applies to England and Wales. This for the most part also applies to Scotland and Northern Ireland, but there are some differences since there are specific statutory provisions for these countries and Scots common law has different roots. Devolution of power from Westminster is increasing the differences in law across the countries of the UK.

Legal personnel

If patients believe that they have a claim for compensation because of the actions or omissions of health professionals, after possibly seeking advice from their local patient advocacy and liaison service (PALS) (in Wales Community Health Councils have been retained) (see Chapter 14), they could ask a solicitor to take the case. A solicitor is a professionally qualified person (usually a degree in law or a degree followed by the Common Professional Examination, followed by completion of the Law Society's professional examinations and completion of a set time in supervised practice) who tends to have direct contact with the client. The solicitor may seek the opinion of a barrister (known as counsel) on liability and the amount of compensation. A barrister will usually have a degree in law or a degree followed by the Common Professional Examination and must complete the examinations set by the Council for Legal Education. The barrister must be a member of an Inn of Court and complete a term of apprenticeship known as pupillage. Traditionally the barrister has had the role of conducting the case in court and preparing the documents that are exchanged between the parties in the run up to the court hearing (known as the pleadings). However, increasingly the right of solicitors to represent the client in court has been extended until it is now possible for solicitors with special training and recognition to undertake the work of advocacy formerly undertaken by barristers alone. Many see the final result of this development to be a single legal profession.

Procedure in civil courts

Figure 2.7 sets out a summary of the stages that take place in civil litigation in the High Courts. In 1996 Lord Woolf[8,9] conducted an inquiry to determine how access to justice could be simplified and speeded up, and the main changes are discussed in Chapter 10. Major reforms in civil proceedings consequent upon the Woolf recommendations came into force in April 1999. The Rules of Civil Procedure can be accessed via the Ministry of Justice website or via the Open Government website.[10]

For personal injury claims under £1000 and other civil claims under £3000 the claim would normally be heard in the small claims court through a process of arbitration. Above these amounts and for claims up to £50 000 the claim could be heard in the County Court. Above £50 000 the claim would usually be heard in the High Court.

Procedure in criminal courts

Figure 2.8 sets out the stages that would be followed in a criminal prosecution of an offence triable only on indictment. The magistrates, who are either lay people known as justices of the peace (JPs) sitting in threes (the bench) or legally qualified persons known as stipendiary magistrates (who sit alone), can only hear charges which relate to offences known as summary offences or offences such as theft which can be

Pre-action protocol must be followed. Pre-hearing procedure depends upon whether the case is assigned to the small claims tract; the fast track or the multi-track. (see the rules on civil procedure)[16].

Writ/claim form is issued: *this commences a civil action in the High Court*

Statement of claim

to set out the basic issues

Defence

Further and Better Particulars

to clarify the issues

Interrogatories (formal questions)

Discovery (disclosure) of Documents

so each party knows the other's case

Exchange of experts' reports

Payment into court (if appropriate)   *a formal offer of settlement*

Summons for directions

Hearing: Opening speeches

Examination in chief

presentation of facts by witnesses of fact and opinion by experts on behalf of the claimant

Cross-examination

Re-examination

Closing summary

Decision by judge

Appeal

Enforcement of judgment (if appropriate)

Figure 2.7   Procedure in the civil courts

Committal: in Magistrates Court
Crown Court trial:
Plea and Case Management Hearing
Arraignment of jury
Plea is taken
Prosecution opening address

Prosecution witnesses	examination in chief
	cross-examination
	re-examination
Defence witnesses	examination in chief
	cross-examination
	re-examination

Final speeches – prosecution and defence summarise the case
Judge address to the jury – explaining the law
Jury retire and consider verdict – to decide on the facts
Finding of guilt or innocence – by jury
Sentencing if guilty verdict – by judge

Figure 2.8   Procedure in a criminal case

heard either as summary offences or on indict-ment (i.e. which are triable either way). Only the crown court (with judge and jury) can hear charges of offences which can only be made on indictment (indictable only offences). Such offences are the most serious, e.g. murder, rape, grievous bodily harm, and other offences against the person. The magistrates however have a limited gate-keeping role in relation to these offences. Once the magistrates decide that an 'either way' offence should be tried in the Crown Court, it will be sent there directly and a date for the plea and case management hearing agreed. Indictable only cases are transferred to the Crown Court immediately (i.e. at first appearance before the magistrates), and sometimes before witness statements are taken. At this preliminary hearing a timetable will be set for the service of the pro-secution evidence, service of defence statements and a date for the Plea and Case Management hearing (PCMH). In criminal cases the Crown Prosecution Service (CPS) has the responsibility for preparing the case, including statements, wit-nesses, etc., for the prosecution in criminal cases.

Accusatorial system

A feature of the legal system in this country is that it consists of one side tasked with the responsibility of proving that the other side is guilty, liable or at fault of the wrong or crime alleged. This is known as an 'accusatorial' sys-tem (or sometimes 'adversarial') and applies to both civil and criminal proceedings, as can be seen from the stages illustrated in Figures 2.7 and 2.8. In criminal cases the prosecution attempts to show beyond reasonable doubt that the accused is guilty of the offence with which he/she is charged. The magistrates, or the jury in the crown court, determine whether the pro-secution has succeeded in establishing the guilt of the accused, who is presumed innocent until proved guilty. In civil proceedings, the claimant (formerly known as the plaintiff), i.e. the person bringing the action, has to establish on a balance of probability that there has been negligence, trespass, nuisance or whatever civil wrong is

alleged. In civil cases (apart from defamation), there is no jury and the judge has the respons-ibility of making a decision on disputed facts and determining whether the claimant has succeeded in establishing the civil wrong. (The Health and Social Care Act 2008 contains pro-vision for the civil standard of proof, instead of the criminal standard, to be used in fitness to practise proceedings held by the regulatory bodies and therefore the Health Professions Council (HPC) (see Chapter 3).

In this accusatorial system of law, one party to a case confronts the other party and the role of the judge is to chair the proceedings, intervening where necessary in the interests of justice and clarifying points of law and procedure. It con-trasts with the system of law that is known as 'inquisitorial', where the judge plays a far more active role in determining the outcome. An example of an inquisitorial system in the UK is the coroner's court. Here the coroner is respon-sible for deciding which witnesses would be relevant to the answers to the questions which are placed before him by statute (i.e. the identity of the deceased and how, when and where he came to die). The coroner asks the witnesses questions in court and decides who else can ask questions and what they can ask. As a result of this 'inquisition', he/she, or a jury if one is used, determines the cause of death. (See Chapter 25 on the role of the coroner.)

Some may feel that an inquisitorial system of justice is fairer since the outcome of the accusatorial system may depend heavily upon the ability of the barristers representing the party in court. However, the strengths of the accusat-orial system probably outweigh the weaknesses; there are after all many challenges to the decisions of the coroners. The effect of the Woolf reforms in civil cases is the adoption of a case management approach to civil claims in order to speed their progress and reduce the costs. The adversarial system has been kept, but in certain cases expert witnesses are agreed between the parties or are appointed by the court. These reforms are considered in Chapters 10 (Negligence) and 13 (Giving Evidence in Court). They were implemented in April 1999.

Law and ethics

Law is both wider and narrower than the field of ethics. On the one hand the law covers areas of practice which may not be considered to give rise to any ethical issue, other than the one whether the law should be obeyed; for example, to park in a no parking area would not appear to raise many ethical issues other than the decision to obey or to ignore the law. On the other hand there are major areas of health care which raise significant ethical questions where there appears to be little law. For example, a chaplain visiting a patient in hospital might appear to raise solely ethical issues, but the Information Commissioner has ruled that a chaplain is not a health professional and therefore has no right to be notified of patients belonging to that religion without the consent of the patient. The elective ventilation of a corpse in order to keep the organs alive for transplant purposes raised considerable ethical issues for health professionals and relatives, but provided the requirements of the Human Tissue Act and the Transplant Acts were satisfied there was formerly no legal issue but considerable ethical ones. The legal situation has now been changed however by section 47 of the Human Tissue Act 2004, which enables a person to take steps for the purpose of preserving the part for use for transplantation. At any time a practice which is considered to be contrary to ethical principles can be challenged in court and, on the basis of any existing statute law or decided cases, the judge will determine the legal position.

Situations may arise where a health professional considers the law to be wrong and contrary to his/her own ethical principles. In such a case he/she has to decide personally what action to take, in full awareness that he/she could face the effects of the criminal law, a civil action, disciplinary procedure by his/her employer and professional proceedings by his/her registration body. In certain cases the law itself provides for conscientious objection. Thus no one can be compelled to participate in an abortion unless it is an emergency situation to save the life of the mother (Abortion Act 1967). Similar provisions apply to activities in relation to human fertilisation and embryology, where the Human Fertilisation and Embryology Act 1990 provides a statutory protection clause.

The Law Commission in its report on Mental Incapacity[11] drafted legislation to cover advance refusals of treatment but considered it would be inappropriate to have a conscientious objection clause for a health professional to ignore the existence of the previously declared wishes of the patient. A health professional may have strong ethical views about the need to save the life of an adult who lacks the mental capacity to make his or her decisions at the present time, but who made an advance directive refusing treatment in the specified circumstances that now exist (e.g. nasogastric feeding). However, the health professional has no right to overrule the patient's valid and relevant advance refusal. The Mental Capacity Act 2005 has made provision for the recognition of advance decisions and there is no provision for any conscientious objection (see Chapter 25).

It is inevitable that any discussion of the function of physiotherapy should be concerned with the ethical or philosophical beliefs of the therapist who is providing the treatment and it is essential that the physiotherapist understands the extent to which the law is in harmony with his/her ethical beliefs and values.

Guidance on conduct and procedures

Rules of professional conduct

Both the Health Professions Council[12] and the Chartered Society of Physiotherapy[13] have issued a Code of Conduct and Rules governing professional practice. These are not in themselves directly enforceable in a court of law, but could be used as evidence in civil or criminal proceedings that their reasonable professional standards of practice have not been followed. An allegation of a breach of the Rules could also be used as a basis for professional conduct proceedings, for which the ultimate sanction is removal from the Health Professions Council's Register. This is discussed in Chapter 4.

Charters and their enforcement

Recent years have seen an increase in the publication of charters across both the public and private sector. In July 1992 the Citizen's Charter was published and it was followed by a Patient's Charter, with different editions being published by the different parts of the UK. Since then health authorities and NHS Trusts have prepared their own charters for their patients.

These charters are not legally enforceable in themselves, except insofar as they recognise existing legal rights. Thus every patient is entitled to have a reasonable standard of care and this is enforceable whether or not it is included in a charter (see Chapter 10). Charters do however provide to the public a measure of the quality of service which it can expect, and a failure could always lead to a complaint being made (see Chapter 14). The implementation of the standards set out in charters is monitored by the individual NHS Trusts and primary care trusts (PCTs) and health authorities and by the government. They have to a certain extent been replaced by the setting of standards in the National Service Frameworks, which are considered in Chapter 17. The Government at the present time is recommending a constitution for the NHS and this is discussed in Chapter 28.

Other guidance

Many other organisations and public bodies issue guidance for professional conduct and procedures for the provision of health care. The National Health Service Executive and Department of Health issue circulars and executive letters providing advice for health and social services organisations and staff. These do not have the direct force of law but it is expected that they are to be followed. Thus in 1997 the High Court ruled against the North Derbyshire Health Authority, which had refused to fund the purchase of beta-interferon for the treatment of multiple sclerosis.[14] The judge found that the health authority had knowingly failed to apply national guidance in an NHS circular. It cannot be assumed however that the guidance is always correct in law, and in R v. *Wandsworth Borough Council*[15] the court held that ministerial guidance was contrary to the law as stated in statute.

Directions issued by the Secretary of State under statutory powers, e.g. under the National Health Service and Community Care Act 1990 (as re-enacted in the NHS Act 2006), are directly enforceable against health organisations through the default mechanisms provided for in the legislation.

Conclusions

The variety of the sources of law and perplexity as to what a law is can be very confusing, but it is helpful for professionals when confronted with a statement that 'the law says . . .', to seek an explanation whether the basis for the assertion is a statute or decision of a court or whether it is derived from a charter or professional code of practice or, as often may be the case, a pronouncement which has no proper foundation in law at all.

Questions and exercises

1 A client has consulted you about the possibility of bringing a claim for compensation. What advice would you give him/her on the procedure which would be followed and the steps which he/she should take?

2 Draw up a diagram that illustrates the difference between civil and criminal procedure.

3 Turn to the glossary and study the definitions of legal terms included there.

4 In what ways do you consider that conflict between ethical beliefs and the law should be resolved?

References

1   *R* v. *Hallstrom, ex parte W; R* v. *Gardener, ex parte L* [1986] 2 All ER 306.

2   *Gossington* v. *Ealing Borough Council* (CA) 18 November 1985, Lexis transcript.

3   www.justice.gov.uk

4   *Miles* v. *Cain* 25 November 1988, Lexis transcript.

5   *R* v. *Adomako* [1995] 1 AC 171; [1994] 3 All ER 79.

6   Law Commission (1996) *Report on Criminal Prosecutions*. The Stationery Office, London.

7   http://www.victoria-climbie-inquiry.org.uk

8   Lord Woolf (January 1996) *Access to Civil Justice Inquiry Consultation Paper*. HMSO, London.

9   Lord Woolf (July 1996) *Access to Justice Final Report*. HMSO, London.

10 www.open.gov.uk/lcd/civil/procrules_fin/crules.htm

11 Law Commission Report (1995) *Mental Incapacity*. No. 231. HMSO, London.

12 Health Professions Council (2003 revised 2008) *Standards of Conduct, Performance and Ethics*. HPC, London.

13 Chartered Society of Physiotherapy (2002) *Rules of Professional Conduct* CSP, London.

14 *R* v. *North Derbyshire Health Authority* [1997] 8 Med LR 327.

15 *R* v. *Wandsworth Borough Council, ex parte Beckwith* [1996] 1 All ER 129 (discussed in Dimond, B. (1997) *Legal Aspects of Care in the Community*, pp. 465–466. Macmillan, Basingstoke).

16 www.justice.gov.uk/civil/procrules

Section A

Professional Issues

3 Registration and the Role of the Statutory Bodies

In this chapter we consider the statutory basis of physiotherapy in the UK and the provisions for registration. We also discuss the role of the Health Professions Council (HPC), which replaced the Council for Professions Supplementary to Medicine (CPSM) and the Physiotherapy Board in 2002. The following topics will be covered:

- Statutory basis of the HPC
- Registration machinery
- Private practitioners
- Non-registered professionals
- The future

The CPSM was established under the Professions Supplementary to Medicine Act 1960. It was an independent, self-regulating, statutory body, and a board for each of the professions that it regulated reported to it. A review of the Professions Supplementary to Medicine Act 1960 was undertaken by JM Consulting Ltd under a steering group chaired by Professor Sheila McLean. Following a consultation document issued in October 1995, a report[1] was published in July 1996. Two broad areas were identified as requiring reform:

- the weaknesses in the powers provided by the 1960 Act;
- the weaknesses in the statutory bodies and working arrangements.

It made significant recommendations for reform, including the establishment of a Council for Health Professions, the establishment of statutory committees (with the power for Council to set up other non-statutory committees) and the protection of title. Its main recommendations are shown in Figure 3.1.

A consultation paper was published in August 2000,[2] which invited comments within 3 months on the legislative proposals. It stated that modernising professional self-regulation should be seen as a component part of a wider strategy to modernise the whole of the NHS to help deliver better health and faster, fairer care. A draft order was published in April 2001[3] and was issued as a statutory instrument in 2002.[4]

Statutory basis of the HPC

The CPSM was replaced in 2002 by the HPC, which at present covers the professions shown in Figure 3.2. Practitioner psychologists are to

(1)   A new statutory body should be established with new powers
(2)   Legislation should allow for the growth in the number of professions
(3)   The purpose of the new legislation should be the protection of the public
(4)   Professions to be covered should be based on the potential for harm arising from either invasive procedures or the application of unsupervised judgment by the professional which can substantially impact on patient/client health or welfare
(5)   All the professions under the CPSM should be included
(6)   Other professional groups may be eligible
(7)   Protection of common title for all of the regulated professions should be established
(8)   The new statutory body should have more effective and flexible powers
(9)   The government, through the Secretary of State or Privy Council, should continue to provide oversight and the ultimate court of appeal, but with reduced involvement in policy and administrative matters
(10)   The normal costs of the regulatory body should be funded from registration fees

Figure 3.1   Basic recommendations of the review body on the 1960 Act

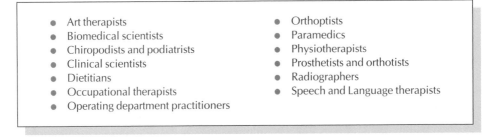

- Art therapists
- Biomedical scientists
- Chiropodists and podiatrists
- Clinical scientists
- Dietitians
- Occupational therapists
- Operating department practitioners
- Orthoptists
- Paramedics
- Physiotherapists
- Prosthetists and orthotists
- Radiographers
- Speech and Language therapists

Figure 3.2   Professions covered by the Health Professions Council

become a registered profession under the HPC in proposals contained in a draft order for consultation published in 2008[5] and more professions may be added to the aegis of the HPC in the future.

The HPC reports to the Privy Council (PC). The HPC appoints a Registrar, who runs a secretariat for the HPC, administering the registration scheme and providing support services. The President of the HPC is appointed by the members for a term of 4 years. The Council agreed at its meeting in December 2004 on the role of the President. This would include providing strong non-executive leadership, and encouraging open and proactive accountability to the public and professions, to chair meetings of the Council, set the chief executive's objectives and monitor his/her performance against these objectives.

Activities of the HPC

Under the Health Professions Order 2001,[4] which was enacted under the powers set out in section 60 of the Health Act 1999, the HPC has the principal functions of establishing from time to time standards of education, training, conduct and performance for members of the relevant professions and to ensure the maintenance of those standards. In addition other functions may be provided by order of the Privy Council. The functions of the HPC are set out in Schedule 3 to the 1999 Health Act and are not transferable by Order to another body.[6] They are shown in Figure 3.3 Other functions are set out in the Health Professions Order 2001, which can be downloaded from the Office of Public Sector Information website.[7]

- Keeping the Register of members admitted to practise
- Determining standards of education and training for admission to practise
- Giving advice about standards of conduct and performance
- Administering procedures (including making rules) relating to misconduct, unfitness to practise and similar matters

Figure 3.3 Functions of the HPC as set out in Schedule 3 to the Health Act 1999

The Health Professions Order states (Article 3(4)) that the main objective of the Council in exercising its functions

shall be to safeguard the health and wellbeing of persons using or needing the services of registrants.

Article 3(5) of the Health Professions Order states that

(5) In exercising its functions, the Council shall:
  (a) have proper regard to the interests of all registrants and prospective registrants and persons referred to in paragraph (4) in each of the countries of the United Kingdom and to any differing considerations applying to the professions to which this Order applies and to groups within them; and
  (b) co-operate wherever reasonably practicable with:
    (i) employers and prospective employers of registrants,
    (ii) persons who provide, assess or fund education or training for registrants or prospective registrants, or who propose to do so,
    (iii) persons who are responsible for regulating or coordinating the regulation of other health or social care professions, or of those who carry out activities in connection with the services provided by those professions or the professions regulated under this Order,
    (iv) persons responsible for regulating services in the provision of which registrants are engaged.

Composition of the Health Professions Council

The Council is constituted in accordance with Part I of the First Schedule to the Health Professions Order. The Council consists of:

(a) 13 members who are appointed by the Council on being elected under the election scheme made under paragraph 2 (referred to in this Order as 'registrant members');

(b) 13 members who are appointed by the Privy Council (referred to in this Order as 'lay members');

and

(c) 13 members appointed by the Council on being elected under the election scheme made under paragraph 2 (referred to in this Order as 'alternate members').

(2) The Council shall appoint an alternate member for each registrant member.

(3) An alternate member has the same functions as a registrant member but he may attend a Council meeting in his capacity as an alternate member and vote, only if his corresponding registrant member is unable to do so.

Each profession registered with the HPC has both a registrant member and an alternate member.

Committees of the Health Profession Council

The HPC is required to have four committees known as:

(a)   the Education and Training Committee
(b)   the Investigating Committee
(c)   the Conduct and Competence Committee
(d)   the Health Committee.

These four committees are referred to in the Order as 'the statutory committees' (and the last three are also known as Practice Committees) and each of the statutory committees shall have the functions specified in the Order. The Education and Training Committee is considered in Chapter 5, and the role of the other three statutory committees – the Practice Committees – in Chapter 4.

The Council has the power to establish such other committees as it considers appropriate in connection with the discharge of its functions, and may, in particular, establish professional advisory committees whose function is to advise the Council and its statutory committees (whether on the request of the Council or otherwise) on matters affecting any relevant profession, and may delegate any of its functions to them, other than any power to make rules.

The HPC committee structure is shown on its website[8] and in addition to the statutory committees consists of audit, communications, finance and resources, approvals and registration (the last two being subcommittees of the Education and Training statutory committee).

All statutory committees are to be chaired by a member of Council and each Committee will have at least one lay member. They will make recommendations and decisions in consultation with the Council.

Registration machinery

The HPC has the responsibility of setting up registration machinery and has a statutory duty to appoint a Registrar. In accordance with the provisions of this Order the Council shall establish and maintain a register of members of the relevant professions.

(2)   The Council shall from time to time:
   (a)   establish the standards of proficiency necessary to be admitted to the different parts of the register being the standards it considers necessary for safe and effective practice under that part of the register; and
   (b)   prescribe the requirements to be met as to the evidence of good health and good character in order to satisfy the Education and Training Committee that an applicant is capable of safe and effective practice under that part of the register.

Article 6(1) states that the register shall be divided into such parts as the Privy Council may by order determine, on a proposal by the Council or otherwise, and in this Order, references to parts of the register are to the parts so determined.

(2)   There shall be one or more designated titles for each part of the register indicative of different qualifications and different kinds of education or training and a registrant is entitled to use whichever of those titles, corresponding to the part of the register in which he is registered, is appropriate in his case.

The Register will show, in relation to each registrant, such address and other details as the Council may prescribe. The required details prescribed by Council were set out in the Rules that came into force on 9 July 2003.[9] These include:

- The full name of the registrant
- His registration number
- His last known home address (but this shall not be included in any published version of the register without her consent) and
- Any qualification of the registrant which has led to his registration

The Registrar may also enter on the Register any other information that is material to a registrant's registration. The Registrar is required to keep the register in a form and manner which guards against falsification and shall take all reasonable steps to ensure that only he and such persons as have been authorised by him in writing for the purpose shall be able to amend the register or have access to the version of the register which contains entries which are not included in the published version of the register.

Protected titles

Each of the professions registered with the HPC has a protected title. Article 39 states that an offence is committed if a person with intent to deceive (whether expressly or by implication):

(a) falsely represents himself to be registered in the register, or a particular part of it or to be the subject of any entry in the register;
(b) uses a title referred to in Article 6(2) to which he is not entitled;
(c) falsely represents himself to possess qualifications in a relevant profession.

The protected title for the professions covered in this book are: physiotherapist and physical therapist. Protection means that an offence is committed if a person uses such a title if he or she is not registered with the HPC. It is also an offence to imply that a person is one of the professions that the HPC regulates. For example if someone states that they provide physiotherapy services when they are not on the HPC register, an offence is committed. An individual can use the title if their application is being processed under the HPC grandparenting scheme or are in the HPC appeal process.

Under Article 7(1) after consultation with the Education and Training Committee, the HPC is required to make rules in connection with registration and the register, and as to the payment of fees. The rules shall, in particular, make provision as to:

(a) the form and keeping of the register;
(b) the procedure for the making, alteration and deletion of entries in the register;
(c) the form and manner in which applications are to be made and the fee to be charged –
     (i)   for registration, renewal of registration and readmission to the register,

(ii)   for the making of any additional entry in the register, and
(iii) for registration to lapse;
(d) the documentary and other evidence which is to accompany applications of the kind mentioned in sub-paragraph (c).

Rules relating to parts of entries in the Register came into force on 9 July 2003.[10] Schedule 1 sets out the different parts.

The standards of proficiency required for the registration of a physiotherapist can be seen on the HPC website[11] (see Chapter 5).

Access to register

The Council is required to make the register available for inspection by members of the public at all reasonable times and to publish the register maintained by it in such manner, and at such times, as it considers appropriate (Article 8(1) and (2)).

(3) Any copy of, or extract from, the published register shall be evidence (and in Scotland sufficient evidence) of the matters mentioned in it.
(4) A certificate purporting to be signed by the Registrar, certifying that a person:
     (a) is registered in a specified category;
     (b) is not registered;
     (c) was registered in a specified category at a specified date or during a specified period;
     (d) was not registered in a specified category, or in any category, at a specified date or during a specified period; or
     (e) has never been registered,

shall be evidence (and in Scotland sufficient evidence) of the matters certified.

The articles make provision relating to the requirements for registration, together with the appropriate professional qualifications, the payment of fees, renewal of registration and readmission and lapse of registration.

Application to be registered

A person seeking admission to a part of the register shall be registered if the application is made in the prescribed form and manner and he/she:

- satisfies the Education and Training Committee that he/she holds an approved qualification awarded:
  - less than 5 years ago;
  - more than 5 years, but he/she has met specified requirements as to additional education, training, and experience;
- satisfies the Education and Training Committee that she meets the Council's prscribed requirements as to safe and effective practice;
- has paid the prescribed fee.

Good character and good health

The Rules[9] which came into force on 9 July 2003 require the applicant to provide a reference as to the good character of the applicant by a person who is not a relative of the applicant and is a person of standing in the community, such as a registered professional, doctor, solicitor, accountant, bank manager, JP head of the educational college or religious official. (A Character Reference Form is provided under Schedule 3 to the Rules.) The person who signs the character reference must confirm that they have known the applicant for at least 3 years and they do not know of any reason why they should not practise their profession 'with honesty and integrity'.

The applicant must also provide a reference to the physical and mental health of the applicant from a person who is not a relative but is the applicant's doctor. (A Health Reference Form is provided under Schedule 4 to the Rules.) Alternative arrangements are laid down where these requirements are not possible. Only a doctor registered with the General Medical Council or the appropriate regulatory body if outside the UK can complete a health reference. A detailed document about information on the health reference has been published by the HPC and is available on its website.[12] It covers the situation where a prospective registrant has had health problems or has a disability. The HPC has consulted on two sets of guidance in relation to its health, disability and registration policy and managing fitness to practice.

Procedural rules

Provisions for renewal of registration and re-admission require the applicant to meet any set requirements for continuing professional development within the specified time.

The Rules[9] cover the procedure to be followed in applications for registration and provisions for amendments to the register and for renewal of registration. Rules also cover the circumstances in which a registered professional's name may be removed from the register on his/her own application or after the expiry of a prescribed period.

Provision is made for the definition of approved qualifications and European Economic Area qualifications.

Appeals

Appeals can be made under Article 37 against the decisions of the Education and Training Committee where an application for registration, re-admission or renewal or the inclusion of an additional entry has been refused or where specific conditions have been imposed on an applicant. There is also a right of appeal if the name of a registered professional has been removed on the grounds that he/she is in breach of a condition in respect of continuing education. The appeal lies to the Council.

Under Article 38 an appeal can be made from any decision of a Practice Committee or any decision of the Council under Article 37 to the appropriate court. Proposals for a Health Professions Independent Appeals Tribunal were not included in the final statutory instrument

(Health Professions Order 2001 S.I. 2002/254). Rules relating to appeals on registration matters came into force on 9 July 2003.[13] These cover the service of documents, the period during which an appeal can be made, the notice appeal, acknowledgement by the Council of the appeal notice, notice of hearing and the duties of parties and representatives to inform Council if they intend to attend. The Council can hear the Appeal itself (with a quorum of seven, with registrants and lay members but the registrants cannot exceed the number of lay members by more than one) or appoint an Appeal Panel (with at least three persons, one of which must be registered in the same part of the Register as the appellant, one of which must not be a registrant under the HPC or General Medical Council (GMC), and (where the health of the professional is in issue) a registered medical practitioner. A preliminary meeting can be held in private with the parties. The Appeal panel can determine an appeal without an oral hearing and may take into account written representations. A hearing can take place without the presence of the appellant, provided that the Appeal Panel is satisfied that all reasonable steps have been taken to give notice of the hearing to the appellant. The hearing should be held in pubic unless the Appeal panel is satisfied in the interests of justice or for the protection of the private life or the health professional, the complainant any person giving evidence or of any patient or client, the public should be excluded from all or part of the hearing. The Rules cover the order of the proceedings and the procedure to be followed.

Grandparenting

Interim arrangements were set up in preparation for a time when the title physiotherapist would become a legally protected title which enabled those who had not followed an approved course to take advantage of the HPC grandparenting arrangements under which advice was provided for their becoming recognised as registered professionals. A helpline was set up by the HPC

(Grandparenting information line 0845 300 4720). A review by the HPC of the grandparenting process between July 2003 and July 2005 concluded that although it was a challenging process it was successful in protecting the public. The experience gained from the process would guide the HPC in running grandparenting periods for any future professions to come under its regulation.

Re-registration

Published in February 2007, the government's White Paper 'Trust, Assurance and Safety: the Regulation of Health Professionals in the 21st Century'[14] recommended that all health professionals should be subject to some kind of check on their continued fitness to practise. This is often known as 'revalidation'. Some of the recommendations of the White Paper are shown in Figure 3.4. The HPC has set up a professional liaison group (PLG) to explore the issue of continuing fitness to practise, including the White Paper recommendations. The Health and Social Care Act 2008 includes provisions for enactment of some of these recommendations (see below). The HPC's requirements for continuing professional development are considered in Chapter 5.

Registration of additional professional groups

The HPC, which replaced the Council for the Professions Supplementary to Medicine (see earlier), has the power to recognise new registered professions and has published guidelines setting criteria on opening new parts of the Register.[15] Each applicant organisation must:

- cover a discrete area of activity displaying some homogeneity;
- apply a defined body of knowledge; practise based on evidence of efficacy;
- have at least one established professional body that accounts for a significant proportion of that occupational group;
- operate a voluntary register;

(1) **Securing independence of the regulators**
    Parity of membership between lay and professional members
    Professional concerns not to dominate their work
    All councils to become more accountable to Parliament, presenting annual reports to the UK Parliament or to the Devolved Assembly legislatures
    Council members to be independently appointed
    Councils to become smaller and more-board like, with greater consistency of size and role across the professional regulatory bodies
    The Council for Healthcare Regulatory Excellence (CHRE), to take on a stronger and more independent role in providing expert advice on professional regulation;
    No mergers, for the time being, of the professional regulatory bodies
    The Government will review these arrangements in 2011
    The Government will work with the pharmacy profession to establish a General Pharmaceutical Council
(2) **Revalidation reforms**
    All the statutorily regulated health professions to have in place arrangements for the revalidation of their professional registration through which they can periodically demonstrate their continued fitness to practise
(3) **Proposals to deal with local concerns including the use of separate lists of professionals held by each primary care trust**
(4) **Fitness to practise hearings**
    All Fitness to practice panels to use the civil standard of proof, with its sliding scale, rather than the criminal standard
    CHRE to have enhanced powers to scrutinise the regulators' handling of fitness to practise cases
    CHRE to develop common protocols for local investigations across all the regulators, with guidance to employers on when such cases should be referred to the national regulator
    The extension of the National Clinical Assessment Service (NCAS) to other health professionals to be investigated
    A national advisory group to develop a national strategy and to advise on measures to ensure appropriate prevention and early intervention for health professionals
    New independent body to establish a central list of people, vetted and approved for all adjudication panels, chosen by the Appointments Commission for their expertise and specifically trained to undertake these duties in a fair and impartial manner
(5) **Non-medical professional regulatory bodies should continue to be responsible for the educational standards of the professionals they regulate**
(6) **proposals relating to the professional registers and the extension of the information held on them for patients, the public, employers and the professions**
    CHRE to be asked to recommend a single standard definition of good character, working with the regulatory bodies, and encompassing wider work within Europe to promote information sharing on the good character of professionals who cross national borders
    Closer cooperation and coordination to be established between regulators and employers when a health professional enters employment for the first time
(7) **Statutory regulation proposals**
    For applied psychologists, several groups of healthcare scientists, psychotherapists and counsellors and other psychological therapists statutory regulation to be introduced
    Criteria to be developed by a UK working party to determine which roles of emerging professions should eventually be statutorily regulated
    No new statutory regulators to be established except for pharmacists
    Harmonisation across the regulators of regulatory practice and legislative provisions so that they all have the most up-to-date and comprehensive duties and powers

Figure 3.4 Recommendations of the White Paper Trust, Assurance and Safety

- have defined routes of entry to the profession;
- have independently assessed entry qualifications;
- have standards in relation to conduct, performance and ethics;
- have fitness to practice procedures to enforce those standards;
- be committed to continuous professional development.

Over 53 organisations have sought statutory registration from the HPC, including the Acupuncture Regulatory working group, the British Society of Clinical Hypnosis and the Craniosacral Therapy Association of the UK. Once the Council has approved an application, an HPC recommendation and an accompanying report to regulate the profession is submitted to the Secretary of State. If the Secretary of State agrees with the application, an order will be drawn up under Section 60 of the Health Act 1999, submitted for consultation, if necessary, amended and then placed before Parliament. In practice however the registration of professions which come under the complementary and alternative medicine umbrella is likely to become the remit of the new Complementary and Natural Healthcare Council (see Chapter 27).

Council for Health Care Regulatory Excellence

As a result of the NHS Reform and Health Care Professions Act 2002 (sections 25–29) a Council for the Regulation of Health Care Professionals (CHRE) (the Council) has been set up (now known as the Council for Healthcare Regulatory Excellence (CHRE)) which oversees the work of nine regulatory bodies including the HPC, GMC and NMC (Nursing and Midwifery Council). The CHRE is a corporate body with the following functions:

- to promote the interests of patients and other members of the public in relation to the performance of their functions by the GMC, GDC, NMC, HPC and other health professional registration bodies;
- to promote best practice in the performance of those functions;
- to formulate principles relating to good professional self-regulation, and to encourage regulatory bodies to conform to them; and
- to promote cooperation between regulatory bodies; and between them, or any of them, and other bodies performing corresponding functions.

The five functions on which it assesses performance of the regulatory bodies are:

- Standards and Guidance
- Registration
- Fitness to Practise
- Education
- Governance and External Relations.

In fulfilling these functions the CHRE published a critical review of the Nursing and Midwifery Council in 2008.[16] The report identified serious weaknesses in the NMCs governance and culture, in the conduct of its Council, its ability to protect the interests of the public through the operation of fitness to practise processes and its ability to retain the confidence of key stakeholders. It makes recommendations to the NMC and to the Department of Health. Each regulatory body has a statutory duty to cooperate with the CHRE in carrying out its investigations.

Powers of the Council

The Council has the powers to do anything which appears to it to be necessary or expedient for the purpose of, or in connection with, the performance of its functions. Examples are given in the Act as to what this could include:

- investigate and report on the performance by each regulatory body of its functions;
- recommend changes to the way in which the regulatory body performs any of its functions.

The Council will not however be able to do anything in relation to a case of any individual who is the subject of proceedings before a regulatory body or about whom an allegation has been made to the regulatory body.

Schedule 7 of the NHS Reform and Health Care Professions Act 2002 makes provision for the finer detail of the Council, such as its membership, appointment and procedure.

Directions to a regulatory body

Each regulatory body must cooperate with the Council. If the Council considers that it would be desirable to do so for the protection of members of the public, it may direct a regulatory body to make rules. Rules made under these directions must be approved by the Privy Council or by the Department of Health before coming into force. The regulatory body must comply with the directions of the Council.

Investigation of complaints about a regulatory body

Regulations may also be made by the Secretary of State on how the Council can investigate complaints made to it about the way in which a regulatory body has exercised any of its functions. These regulations may cover: who is entitled to complain, the nature of complaints which the Council must or need not investigate, matters which are excluded from the investigation, requirements to be complied with by the complainant, making of recommendations and reports by the Council, confidentiality of information supplied to or obtained by the Council, the use which the Council may make of such information, payments to persons in connection with investigations and privilege in relation to any matter published by the Council in the exercise of its functions under the regulations. The regulations can also cover powers to be given to the Council requiring persons to attend

before it, give evidence or produce documents and the admissibility of evidence in accordance with the rules of civil proceedings in the High Court.

Referral of a professional conduct decision to the High Court

Where the Council is of the view that a decision by the regulatory body in professional misconduct proceedings as specified in the Act is unduly lenient or a relevant decision should not have been made and that it would be desirable for the protection of members of the public for the Council to take action, the Council may refer the case to the High Court (or Court of Session in Scotland) (S.29 NHS Reform and Health Care Professions Act 2002). The High Court has the power to dismiss the case, allow the appeal and quash the relevant decision, substitute any other decision for the decision of the Committee or person concerned or remit the case to the committee or other person concerned to dispose of the case in accordance with directions from the Court. Some of the cases taken up by the CHRE in relation to physiotherapy registrants are considered in Chapter 4. The CHRE has published a digest of feedback points from the CHRE's consideration of cases under S.29.[17] The CHRE has also published guidance on sexual boundary violations by health professionals,[18] which can be downloaded from the CHRE website.[19]

The existence of the overarching Council is leading to greater uniformity in standards, professional practice, discipline and other procedures across all registered health professions. The Health and Social Care Act 2008 will change the make-up of CHRE's governing Council, which will become smaller and there will no longer be respresentation from the regulators on the Council. The Act also gives the CHRE new responsibilities such as auditing the early stages of regulators' fitness to practise procedures.

Future regulation of the health professions

A review of non-medical regulations was published in 2004 (Foster review)[20] to which the CSP responded.[21] The CSP had two fundamental concerns about the proposals: 1. the employer-led approach to regulation and the focus on those working in the NHS and 2. the use of the Knowledge and Skills Framework as the regulatory tool. The CSP supported the proposal not to merge the regulatory bodies and also to extend the scope of regulation to include healthcare support workers and new roles in healthcare. The White Paper Trust, Assurance and Safety – the Regulation of Health Professionals in the 21st century[22] set out provisions for reforms to the regulation of health professions. Many of its regulations have been included in the Health and Social Care Act 2008. The Act contains the following provisions:

- the establishment of a new regulator for hospitals, care homes and social services to be known as the Care Quality Commission (this is considered in Chapter 17);
- reforms of the system of professional regulation to ensure it earns and sustains the confidence of patients, professionals and Parliament;
- all healthcare professional regulatory bodies to use the civil, rather than criminal, standard of proof (see below);
- creates an independent adjudicator to undertake independent and objective formal adjudication for the professional regulatory bodies;
- ensures that all healthcare organisations employing or contracting with doctors appoint a 'responsible officer' to work with the GMC to identify and handle cases of poor; professional performance by doctors
- updates the Public Health (Control of Disease) Act 1984 with the aim of providing a more effective and proportionate response to infectious disease (see Chapter 11);

- extends financial support to mothers-to-be from the twenty-ninth week of pregnancy (see Chapter 17).

Civil standard of proof

One of the more significant changes contained in the Health and Social Care Act is the proposal to introduce the civil standard of proof of a balance of probabilities into the procedures of health care regulatory bodies instead of the criminal standard of beyond reasonable doubt. The effect of this should be to make it easier to achieve a finding of unfitness to practice of a registrant and thus provide greater protection for the public.

Private practitioners

The only difference between private practitioners and others is that the former are not employees. They may in fact be employers in their own right. No difference is made in the registration procedure between those who are employed and those who are in private practice. Chapter 19 is concerned with the legal aspects of private practice.

Non-registered physiotherapists

Since the implementation of the protected title provisions and the creation of an offence a non-registered physiotherapist is a contradiction in terms. The earlier legislation under which NHS and Local Authorities could only employ registered physiotherapists is now redundant. Unless a physiotherapist is registered with the HPC she would be unable to use the title of physiotherapist and would be committing an offence if she claimed to be providing physiotherapist services without the appropriate registration. This is an important protection for the public since there has in the past been a lack of understanding by the general public about the significance of the term 'registered status'.

Confirmation of this lack of understanding is shown by the words of a judge in a case where an unregistered physiotherapist was charged with assault on a patient.[23] The judge said:

> Although the Defendant is not a physiotherapist of the Chartered Institute [sic.] and he does not hold himself out as such, he has considerable experience and has had some training in physiotherapy principally through the Football Association. Soccer has been his great love and remains so. He is not a trickster in physiotherapy. Eamonn Martin, the international athlete and Olympic competitor, was one of his regular patients.

The judge did not refer to the lack of the professional code of practice and assessed level of training and competence which all registered practitioners and Chartered Society members must have.

The protection of title provided by the Health Professions order is an important development in safeguarding the public. The following account of an incident involving the offence of wrongly using the protected title is taken from the Health Professions Council Newsletter.[24]

Fake 'physio' cautioned by Essex Police for misuse of protected title

A man claiming to be a 'registered physio' was arrested last month and cautioned by Essex Police. He was not registered with the HPC as a physiotherapist and was using business cards that stated 'registered physio'. He was working in the Essex area when arrested, and accepted a police caution for fraud. The HPC provided a statement to the police to confirm that he wasn't registered. Kelly Johnson, Director of Fitness to Practise, commented, 'We are delighted with the outcome of this case and to have worked so closely and effectively with Essex Police to

ensure the public are adequately protected.' Health professionals who wish to practise in the UK using a protected title such as 'physiotherapist' or 'dietician' must, by law, be registered with us and meet our standards for their professional skills, training, behaviour and health. For a full list of protected titles and more information, please see our website.[25]

Support workers

The registered practitioner is increasingly expected to work with support from non-registered practitioners known variously as health support workers, care assistants, physiotherapy assistants and other titles. There have been discussions taking place over recent years on the possibility of bringing these support workers under the umbrella of one of the registration bodies such as the Nursing and Midwifery Council or the Health Professions Council. In its White Paper[22] the Department of Health looked at research in Scotland on the regulation of support workers and made the following comments:

> The Scottish model is that induction standards focus on generic public protection concepts such as confidentiality, dignity, advocacy, and similar core concepts and values apply to all HCSWs employed in the NHS, regardless of their role. The Government in England will evaluate the results of the Scottish pilot study and consider the way forward with stakeholders. The Government will consider whether there is sufficient demand for the introduction of statutory regulation for any assistant practitioner roles at levels 3 and 4 on the Skills for Health Career Framework. This will be subject to the same mechanisms for determining need, suitability and readiness as for the other emerging professions.

The legal aspects relating to the supervision of the activities of non-registered practitioners and delegation to them are considered in Chapter 10 on negligence.

Conclusions

The Shipman Inquiry and in particular recommendations contained in the fifth Shipman Report[26] has led to a political determination to provide greater public protection from health professional abuse and incompetence. Recommendations from the White Paper[22] have led to significant changes to the regulation of health professionals which are contained in the Health and Social Care Act 2008. It remains to be seen how effective these changes are in ensuring effectively and efficiently regulated healthcare professions.

✎ Questions and exercises

1 Do you consider that the abolition of the CPSM and the establishment of the HPC provides sufficient protection for the public and the health professional?

2 You are invited to become a member of the HPC. What duties would you expect to perform and what training would you wish to receive?

3 Do you consider that the functions of the registered physiotherapist should be protected rather than just the title?

References

1 JM Consulting Ltd (1996) *The Regulation of Health Professions: Report of a Review of the Professions Supplementary to Medicine Act 1960 with Recommendations for New Legislation*. JM Consulting Ltd, Bristol.

2 NHS Executive (2000) *Modernising Regulation The New Health Professions Council: A Consultation Document*. Department of Health, London.

3 Department of Health (2001) *Establishing the new Health Professions Council*. DH, London.

4 The Health Professions Order 2001 SI 2002 No 254.

5 Health Care and Associated Professions (Miscellaneous Amendments) No 2 Order 2008.

6 Health Act 1999 Schedule 3 paragraph 8(2).

7 www.opsi.gov.uk

8 www.hpc-uk.org/aboutus

9 The Health Professions Council (Registration and Fees) Rules Order of Council 2003 SI 2003 No 1572.

10 The Health Professions (Parts of and Entries in the Register) Order of Council 2003 SI 2003 No 1571.

11 http://www.hpc-uk.org/education/docs/HPC_physiotherapists

12 www.hpc-uk.org/publications

13 The Health Professions Council (Registration Appeals) Rules Order of Council 2003 SI 2003 No 1579.

14 Department of Health (2007) White Paper. *Trust, Assurance and Safety: the Regulation of Health Professionals in the 21st Century*. Cmnd 7013. DH, London.

15 http://www.hpc-uk.org/aboutregistration/new/criteria

16 Council for Healthcare Regulatory Excellence (2008) *Performance Review on the NMC*. CHRE, London.

17 Council for Healthcare Regulatory Excellence (2008) *Protecting the Public: Learning from Fitness to Practise*. CHRE, London.

18 Halter, M., Brown, H., Stone, J. (2007) *Sexual Boundary Violations by Health Professionals – An Overview of the Published Empirical Literature*. CHRE, London.

19 www.chre.org.uk

20 Department of Health (2006) *Healthcare Professional Regulation: Public Consultation on Proposals for Change*. DH, Leeds.

21 Chartered Society of Physiotherapy (2006) *Response to the Review of Regulation of Non-medical Healthcare Professions*. CSP, London.

22 White Paper. (2007) *Trust, Assurance and Safety – the Regulation of Health Professionals in the 21st Century*. Cmnd 7013.

23 *Miles* v. *Cain* 25 November 1988, Lexis transcript.

24 Health Professions Council News letter Issue 1 – December 2007.

25 http://www.hpc-uk.org/aboutregistration/protectedtitles

26 The Shipman Inquiry (2004) Fifth report. *Safeguarding Patients: Lessons from the Past – Proposals for the Future*. Command Paper CM 6394 December Stationery Office. Available from: www.the-shipman-inquiry.org.uk/reports.asp

4 Professional Conduct Proceedings

In the last chapter we considered the law relating to the statutory bodies set up to control entry on to the register and the functions and constitutions of the machinery for professional regulation set up under the Health Professions Council (HPC). In this chapter we consider the regulation of professional discipline. The Chartered Society of Physiotherapy (CSP) has prepared a guide for members on HPC investigations.[1] (An appendix includes guidelines on providing a written statement to the HPC Investigating panel.) The following areas will be discussed:

- Health Professions Council
- Role of the Chartered Society of Physiotherapy (CSP)
- Code of ethics and professional practice
- Scope of professional practice
- Post-registration control and supervision
- Insurance and indemnity
- The future

Health Professions Council

Duties in respect of conduct and fitness to practise

Part V of the Order establishing the HPC,[2] sets out the provisions for Fitness to Practice procedures for health professionals registered under the HPC. The HPC is required to establish three Practice Committees: an Investigating Committee, the Conduct and Competence Committee and the Health Committee. In relation to Fitness to Practice, the Order requires the HPC to:

- establish and keep under review the standards of conduct, performance and ethics expected of registrants and prospective registrants and give them such guidance on these matters as it sees fit;
- establish and keep under review effective arrangements to protect the public from persons whose fitness to practise is impaired.

Rules relating to the constitution of Practice Committees came into force on 23 May 2003.[3] These relate to the appointment of the members and chairman, tenure of the members, vacancies, standards for members and meetings.

Allegations

A procedure is laid down for dealing with allegations made against a registered person to the effect that his/her fitness to practice is impaired by reason of:

- misconduct;
- lack of competence;
- a conviction or caution in the UK for a criminal offence (or a conviction elsewhere for what would also be a crime in England or Wales);
- his/her physical or mental health;
- a determination by a UK statutory body responsible for a health or social care profession that he/she is unfit to practise that profession (or a determination by a licensing body elsewhere to the same effect.

Screeners

Allegations can be referred to a panel of screeners and at least two of them (with one lay person and one registrant from the professional field of the person under scrutiny) shall consider whether the allegation is well founded. The Council has made rules relating to the appointment and functions of the screeners that came into force on 9 July 2003.[4] Under these rules where a panel comprises two screeners a case may only be closed if made by a unanimous decision but where a panel comprises more than two screeners it may be made by a majority verdict. A Practice Committee may request screeners to mediate in a case, and in this case, a panel shall undertake mediation with the aim of dealing with an allegation without it being necessary for the case to reach the stage at which the Health Committee or Conduct and Competence Committee would arrange a hearing. There is no set procedure for the mediation.

Investigating Committee

The Investigating Committee (Article 26) investigates any allegation referred to it following a set procedure. If the committee considers that there is a case to answer it must notify in writing with reasons the registered professional concerned and the person making the allegation. It has powers, where it concludes that there is a case to answer, to undertake mediation, refer the case to screeners for them to undertake mediation, to the Health Committee or the Conduct and Competence Committee.

Rules of procedure for the Investigating Committee came into force on 9 July 2003.[5] Where an allegation is referred to the Committee it shall, at the same time that it sends the notice to the health professional send him/her a copy of the standards of conduct, performance and ethics. The Investigating Committee can seek such advice or assistance as it thinks fit, but cannot interview the health professional unless he/she consents, or take account of any document or other material which the health professional has not had the opportunity to comment upon.

Conduct and Competence Committee

The Conduct and Competence Committee, after consultation with the other Practice Committees, shall consider:

- any allegation referred to it by the Council, screeners, the Investigating Committee of the Health Committee;
- any application for restoration referred to it by the Registrar.

Procedure rules for the Conduct and Competence Committee came into force on 9 July 2003.[6] The Conduct and Competence Committee can refer any allegation to the Health Committee (see below) when it appears to the Committee that an allegation which it is considering would be better dealt with by the Health Committee. The Rules cover the possibility of a preliminary meeting in private with their parties, further investigations carried out by the Committee including:

- asking the health professional to provide a written description of his/her practice;
- inspecting a sample of the health professional's patient or client records (this can only be carried out with the consent of the patient or client, unless the records are provided in a form from which the patient or client cannot be identified);
- inviting the health professional to take a test of competence;
- interviewing the complainant, the health professional and any person nominated by the health professional.

Where the Committee has found that the health professional has failed to comply with the standards of conduct, performance and ethics established by the Council,[7] the Committee may take that failure into account, but such failure shall not be taken of itself to establish that the fitness to practise of the health professional is impaired.

The rules include the following provisions:

- The proceedings of the Conduct and Competence Committee shall be held in public unless the Committee is satisfied that, in the interests of justice or for the protection of the private life of the health professional, the complainant, any person giving evidence or of any patient or client, the public should be excluded from all or part of the hearing.
- The rules of admissibility of evidence in civil proceedings apply unless the Committee is satisfied that the admission of evidence is necessary in order to protect members of the public.
- Where the health professional has been convicted of a criminal offence, a certified copy of the certificate of conviction is admissible as proof of that conviction.
- The Committee may require evidence to be given on oath or affirmation.

- The Committee may adjourn the proceedings from time to time as it thinks fit.
- The Committee may require any person (other that the health professional) to attend a hearing and give evidence or produce documents.
- The Chairperson shall explain the order of proceedings to the parties, and unless it is decided to the contrary, the following is the usual procedure:
  - The chairman invites the solicitor to present the case against the health professional and to give the evidence in support of that case.
  - Any witnesses are called by the solicitor, examined by him, cross-examined by the health professional or his/her representative, and may be re-examined by the solicitor and may be questioned by the Committee.
  - The health professional may address the Committee and give evidence on his/her fitness to practise.
  - Witnesses may be called by the health professional, examined in chief by the health professional or his/her representative, cross examined by the solicitor, and re-examined by the health professional or his/her representative and may be questioned by the Committee.
  - The solicitor may address the Committee again.
  - The health professional or his/her representative may address the Committee.
- Where the health professional is neither present nor represented at a hearing, the Committee may nevertheless proceed with the hearing if it is satisfied that all reasonable steps have been taken to service the notice of hearing.
- The Committee is required to notify the health professional and complainant of its decision and the reasons for reaching that decision and shall inform the health professional of his/her right to appeal.
- Proceedings for hearing applications for restoration to the Register are also established.

The Health Committee

The Health Committee shall consider any allegation referred to it by the Council, screeners, the Investigating Committee or the Conduct and Competence Committee and also any application for restoration referred to it by the Registrar. Article 29 sets out the procedure to be followed. Procedural rules for the Health Committee have been established by Order in Council and came into force on 9 July 2003.[8] These rules cover the service of documents, the power of the Health Committee to refer a case to the Conduct and Competence Committee, the action to be taken by the Health Committee if an allegation is referred to it. Its powers are similar to that of the Conduct and Competence Committee (see above) but in addition it can invite the health professional to undergo a medical examination by a registered medical practitioner nominated by the Health Committee. The usual order of proceedings of the Health Committee is similar to that of the Conduct and Competence Committee. The Health Professional can also hear the case in the absence of the health professional if it is satisfied that all reasonable steps have to been taken to serve notice on the health professional. A similar procedure is established for the Health Committee to hear applications for restoration to the Register.

Assessors

Articles 30 to 35 cover further procedural details, including the appointment of legal assessors who have the general function of giving advice to screeners, the statutory committees or the Registrar on questions of law. Rules relating to legal assessors came into force on 9 July 2003.[9] These require any advice given by the legal assessor to be given in the presence of every party, or person representing a party, in attendance at the hearing, unless the Council or Committee has begun to deliberate on its decisions and considers that it would be prejudicial to the discharge of its functions for the advice to be tendered in the presence of the parties or their representatives. In this latter case as soon as possible after completion of the deliberations, the legal assessor is required to inform the parties of the advice he gave and subsequently record that advice in writing. Where the Council fails to accept the advice of the legal assessor, a record shall be made of the advice and a copy of that given to the parties.

Medical assessors can also be appointed to give relevant advice. Additional rules relating to the functions of assessors came into force on 9 July 2003[10] and these enable legal and medical assessors to be present at any Part V hearing by a Practice Committee, to be present at any appeal hearing held by the Council and the legal assessor, if present, can inform the Practice Committee or Council of any irregularity in its consideration of the matter or in the conduct of the proceedings; the medical assessor, if present, can inform the Practice Committee or Council and the parties to the proceedings, if it appears to him/her that, without his/her advice, a mistake may be made in judging the medical significance of information or the absence of information.

Appeals

An appeal from any decision of a Practice Committee lies to an appropriate court. Earlier proposals for the establishment of a Health Professions Independent Appeals Tribunal were not contained in the final order.

Fitness to practise

This is defined by the HPC as involving more than just competence in a registrant's chosen profession. It also includes health and character as well as the necessary skills and knowledge to do their job safely and effectively. Registrants must also be trusted to do their job legally.[11] Impairment of fitness to practise may include misconduct, lack of competence, a conviction or caution for a criminal offence, the physical or mental health of the registrant and a decision reached by another regulatory responsible for health care. Anonymous complaints may be considered if they relate to serious and credible concerns about a registrant's fitness to practise and the HPC considers that it is appropriate to take further action. In the Annual Fitness Report of the HPC for 2006/7 there were 52 complaints to the HPC about physiotherapists, which constituted 16.1% of total complaints (79 complaints in 2005–6). There were 40 670 registrants, which formed 22.9% of total number on the HPC register. The HPC report noted that in cases concerning physiotherapists, most complaints have been about clinical competence. It had also seen more complaints of a sexual nature in this profession. Complaints may come from a variety of sources, including members of the public, other registrants, patients and their families, employers, managers and the police.

The complaints about physiotherapists whose hearings have been held include:

Pornography	Outcome of hearing	Caution
Inaccurate patient records	Outcome of hearing	Caution
Record keeping and other issues	Outcome of hearing	Caution
Inappropriate comments to colleagues	Outcome of hearing	Suspension
Relationship with a patient	Outcome of hearing	Conditions of practice
Theft from employer	Outcome of hearing	Strike off
Health	Outcome of hearing	Suspension

In 2006–7 three physiotherapists were struck off, three suspended, three cautioned, one given a conditions of practice order, two no further action taken and in three cases the allegations were not well founded. Four physiotherapists were unrepresented and 11 represented. The HPC is obliged to inform the Council for Healthcare Regulatory Excellence (CHRE) (see Chapter 3) about cases that have been considered by the panels of the CCC not to be well founded. In the case involving one of the physiotherapists,

the CHRE considered that the decision of the panel was unduly lenient and the case was referred to the High Court and a hearing is awaited. In another case involving a physiotherapist where the allegations were not well founded, the panel found that the registrant admitted that she displayed a lack of competence in her employment, but she had insight into her problems and had taken measures to ensure that her practice was up to standard. She had completed a course by the time of the hearing and the panel was satisfied that her fitness to practise was not impaired. The Director of Fitness to Practise of the HPC concluded her report by reminding readers that the fitness to practise proceedings involve only a tiny proportion of the health professionals on the HPC register.

The following is a case heard in December 2007 and published on the HPC website.[12]

A physiotherapist was appointed as a senior 2 post in November 2005, but never practised in that capacity because his managers and peers did not deem him competent to do so. The HPC Conduct and Competence Committee found that on several occasions he had demonstrated a lack of basic care and that his professional judgments and clinical decision making skills were inadequate. He failed to adapt techniques for individual patient needs and did not keep adequate records. He also showed a lack of insight into his shortcomings.

The panel imposed a suspension order for 1 year.

In another case a physiotherapist was suspended from practice for 1 year for failing to meet the required level of English language proficiency required by the HPC.[13]

A physiotherapist was struck off for lack of competency and misconduct. He had cancelled a patient's appointment so that he could go home early and then led his colleagues to believe that it was the patient who had cancelled the appointment. It was reported that the registrant had left work early on a number of occasions. He failed to follow the Trust's rehabilitation protocol. His employers carried out an audit of five of his patients and concluded that there was a low average assessment, very poor subjective/objective analysis and record keeping. In his records he had missed a number of red flag conditions, which ought to have merited immediate referral to specialists.

Interim orders

If the investigating panel feels that the allegation is serious enough that the public might need some type of immediate protection, the panel might make an application for an interim order. A hearing will then take place often at short notice. The panel will consist of a chairperson, a person in the same profession as the registrant under investigation, and a lay person and a legal assessor. In hearings of the Health Committee, a registered doctor will also be on the panel. The solicitor for the HPC will present the case, calling witnesses to support the allegation. The registrant or their representative may cross-examine the witnesses. The panel may ask questions. The registrant will then present his or her case calling witnesses and/or making statements to the panel. If the allegation is considered to be proven the panel will declare it to be well founded.

Sanctions available

- no further action to be taken;
- mediation (a consensual process appropriate where issues between the health professional and the screeners are unresolved. Only available if the alternative would be no further action);
- caution order (can last for between 1 to 5 years);
- conditions of practice order (for a specific period not exceeding 3 years. It could require supervised practice and/or further training);
- suspend registration (for up to a year);
- striking off order (only imposed in very serious circumstances in order to protect the public. It may not be made in respect of an allegation relating to competence or health

unless the registrant has been continuously suspended, or subject to a conditions of practice order, for a period of 2 years at the date of the decision to strike off. Striking off is a sanction of last resort for serious, deliberate or reckless acts involving abuse of trust such as sexual abuse, dishonesty or persistent clinical failure. Striking off should be used where there is no other way to protect the public, for example, where there is a lack of insight, continuing problems or denial.

Guidance for panel members on the sanctions to be imposed was given by the HPC in September 2007.[14] The HPC emphasises the sanctions are not intended to be punitive. Panels must give appropriate weight to the wider pubic interest considerations, which include:

- the deterrent effect to other health professionals;
- the reputation of the profession concerned;
- public confidence in the regulatory process.

Review of conditions of practice or suspension order

These orders will be reviewed shortly before they are due to end. In the case of a conditions or practice order, the review panel will look for evidence that the registrant has met the conditions such as a report from a supervisor or evidence that the registrant has received further training. In the case of a suspension order, the review panel will look for evidence that the problems that led to the suspension have now been dealt with. The panel must be satisfied that the public is adequately protected. If they are not satisfied, they could continue the conditions of practice or suspension order or they could replace the suspension order with a conditions of practice order. If they feel that a registrant has not met the terms of a conditions of practice order, they could replace it by a suspension order of by a striking-off order. The following list summarises the action that the review panel can take:

- confirm the order;
- extend the period for which the order has effect (but a conditions of practice order may not be extended by more than 3 years at a time or a suspension order by more than 1 year at a time);
- replace the order with one it could have made at the time it made the order being reviewed;
- make a conditions of practice order which takes effect when a suspension order expires;
- reduce the duration of an order (but a caution order may not be reduced to a duration of less than one year);
- revoke or vary any condition imposed by the order;
- revoke the order.

Review of striking-off order

Article 33(2) of the Health Professions Order 2001 specifies that, unless new evidence comes to light, an application for restoration to the register may not be made within 5 years of the date of the order.

The Health Professions Council and employers

The HPC would expect cooperation from employers in relation to the fitness to practice of registered professionals. Employers would be expected to inform the HPC if disciplinary proceedings are being taken against a registrant and there is evidence to suggest that a person's ability to practice their profession may be impaired. Other registrants have a duty under the HPC Standards of Conduct, Performance and Ethics to bring concerns about a fellow registrant to the attention of the HPC. The HPC would seek to work with employers on a collaborative, case by case basis. The HPC has statutory powers to compel those involved (other than the registrant) to provide information and it is a criminal offence to refuse to do so. It is therefore able to pursue lines of inquiry that may not be open to an employer.[11]

Role of the Chartered Society of Physiotherapy

Most registered physiotherapists join the CSP, although there are a few who do not become chartered even though they are registered. The CSP has its own regulations for membership and any member struck off by the HPC would lose the right to remain a member of the CSP.

The CSP plays an important part in working with the HPC in the setting and maintenance of educational standards, which are discussed in Chapter 5. It also has a significant role in the preparation of standards on professional conduct. The Rules are considered below. It has also issued other guidance and free information sheets on a variety of topics, many of which are referred to in the relevant chapters of this book. In addition, the many Clinical Interest and Occupational Groups (considered in Chapter 1) have issued guidance for their members.

Code of ethics and professional practice

Health Professions Council standards of conduct, performance and ethics

The HPC published standards of conduct, performance and ethics for its registered practitioners in 2003. In 2006 it decided to review the standards to ensure they continued to be fit for purpose and that they conformed to the expectations of the public, registrants and other stakeholders. A consultation document was published on the revised standards which had been drawn up on the basis of the following broad principles that the standards should:

- focus where possible on providing guidance to registrants based on our expectations of their behaviour;

- be based on overarching principles with some further detail on key points (with more detailed guidance available elsewhere, if necessary);
- be applicable to all registrants (as far as possible) including those engaged in research, clinical practice, education and roles in industry;
- be written in broad terms to accommodate changes in best practice, technology, legislation and in wider society.

Following the consultation a revised standards of conduct, performance and ethics came into force in July 2008.[7] The new standards expand on 14 duties of the registrant, which are:

Your duties as a registrant. The standards of conduct, performance and ethics you must keep to:

(1) You must act in the best interests of service users.
(2) You must respect the confidentiality of service users.
(3) You must keep high standards of personal conduct.
(4) You must provide (to us and to any other relevant statutory regulator) any important information about conduct and competence.
(5) You must keep your professional knowledge and skills up to date.
(6) You must act within the limits of your knowledge, skills and experience and, if necessary, refer the matter to another practitioner.
(7) You must communicate properly and effectively with service users and other practitioners.

(8) You must effectively supervise tasks that you have asked others to carry out.
(9) You must get informed consent to give treatment (except in an emergency).
(10) You must keep accurate records.
(11) You must deal fairly and safely with the risks of infection.
(12) You must limit your work or stop practising if your performance or judgment is affected by your health.
(13) You must behave with honesty and integrity, and make sure that your behaviour does not damage the public's confidence in you and your profession.
(14) You must make sure that any advertising is accurate.

These standards of conduct, performance and ethics are accompanied by standards of proficiency published by the HPC.

The Rules of Professional Conduct[15]

In addition to the HPC standards, conduct, performance and ethics, the CSP had published its own Rules for its members. The Rules are not law in the sense that a breach of their provisions would lead directly to criminal or civil proceedings, but such a breach could be used in evidence in professional conduct or other proceedings where the activities of a physiotherapist were in question. The Rules cover the topics shown in Figure 4.1.

The principles on which the Rules are based are reflected in the Society's *Service Standards*

(1) Scope of practice
(2) Relationships with patients
(3) Confidentiality
(4) Relationships with professional staff and carers
(5) Duty to report
(6) Advertising
(7) Sale of services and goods
(8) Personal and professional standards

Figure 4.1 Rules of professional conduct[15]

of *Physiotherapy Practice*[16] and *Core Standards of Physiotherapy Practice*,[17] both of which also include criteria to provide measures of how these principles and standards are being adhered to.

A Code of Conduct has also been prepared for physiotherapist assistants,[18] which is discussed in Chapter 10.

The CSP has also issued guidance on standards of business conduct.[19] This applies to physiotherapists wherever they practice (see Chapter 19 for the physiotherapist in private practice) and covers the topics of:

- conflict of interests
- conflict of stance/position
- changes in employment status
- restrictive clauses
- incentives
- favouritism
- gifts and hospitality.

Receipts of gifts from clients

This is one area of professional practice which frequently concerns health professionals. Clients/patients are often grateful for the help they have received and wish to make a small gesture in recognition of this. Most Trusts have policies prohibiting the receipt of gifts except under strict procedures. These might include accepting a gift to a department or unit rather than to an individual and ensuring that any gift is notified to a senior manager and a record is made. It is, of course, axiomatic that the gift should not have any influence on the standard of care provided or lead to any priority for that patient which is not justified on clinical grounds. Any large gift should be dealt with through the unit manager's office since it may become part of the charitable funds held in trust by the Health Authority or Trust. Similarly, if a patient indicates that they wish to make a bequest in a will, the solicitors of the trust should be involved to ensure that there is no question of undue influence and that the patient receives independent advice. The HPC Code requires the registered practitioner or the

prospective registrant under principle 3 to keep high standards of personal conduct; under principle 14 to behave with integrity and honesty; and under principle 17 to make sure that his/her behaviour does not damage his/her profession's reputation – all of which could relate to the unauthorised receipt of gifts.

Scope of professional practice

The basic principle which underlies professional practice is stated in the sixth principle of the HPC Standards of conduct, performance and ethics:

> You must act within the limits of your knowledge, skills and experience and, if necessary, refer the matter to another professional.

Similarly Rule 1 of the *Rules of Professional Conduct* (2002) of the CSP states:

> Chartered physiotherapists shall only practice to the extent that they have established, maintained and developed their ability to work safely and competently and shall ensure that they have appropriate professional liability cover for that practice.

The principle will apply not only to their basic practice but also to any extension in the scope of that practice.

There is increasing pressure on physiotherapists to expand their field of activities. On the one hand, many are attracted by the uses of complementary therapies as an adjunct to their practice. They are therefore acquiring training in such therapies as acupuncture, reflexology, aromatherapy and similar fields. The legal implications of this are considered in Chapter 27. On the other hand, some physiotherapists are being asked by their employers and managers to undertake activities not usually associated with the core physiotherapy role. The guidance issued by the CSP in 1994[20] cited such tasks as injections, phlebotomy, electrocardiography, suturing and acting as a clinical assistant in filtering patients for orthopaedic, rheumatology and neurological clinics. This guidance must now be reviewed in the light of the paper *Scope of Professional Practice* published by the CSP in 2008 (see below).

Specific guidance was given by the CSP for chartered physiotherapists working as extended scope practitioners[21] (known as ESPs). ESPs are clinical physiotherapy specialists with an extended scope of practice. They see patients referred for assessment, clinical diagnosis and management of neuromusculoskeletal disorders. Some of the extended role activities they can undertake include:

- requesting investigations (X-rays, scans, blood tests, etc.);
- using the results of investigations to assist clinical diagnosis and appropriate management of patients;
- listing for surgery and referring to other medical and health care professionals.

The CSP in conjunction with other healthcare professional bodies (RCN, Society and College of Radiographers, General Chiropractic Council, General Osteopathic Council and NHS alliance and the Royal College of Radiologists have published an information sheet on clinical imaging requests from non-medically qualified professionals (November 2006 published by the Royal College of Nursing). It sets out the policy position that radiographers can accept requests from non-medically qualified referrers, provided that the referrer is adequately trained and remains competent to refer and that there are written local agreements and protocols. The eligibility criteria for physiotherapists to act as ESPs are that physiotherapists are able to demonstrate that they:

- are currently registered with the HPC and CSP;
- have completed IR(ME)R (Ionising Radiation (Medical Exposure) Regulations 2000) training and any additional local clinical imaging training in accordance with the training section of this guidance;
- have evidence of education/training to achieve competence in:
  - history taking

- physical examination
- formulating a diagnosis and being aware of varied differential diagnoses
- advanced communication
- advanced clinical reasoning and decision making

- understand their professional accountability arising from the current CSP *Rules of Professional Conduct* 2002, *Core Standards of Physiotherapy Practice* and medico-legal issues arising from their extended role;
- are aware of boundaries to their knowledge and competence;
- undertake continuing professional development activities to maintain their competence, including updating training within the latest IR(ME)R guidelines;
- have knowledge to request the appropriate investigations for their patients, understand findings of radiological investigations and reports, and have the ability to act on them;
- are fully familiar with current, local clinical imaging protocols;
- undertake evaluation of their clinical imaging referrals regularly.

Requesting clinical images is within the scope of Chartered Physiotherapists working to the CSP rules of professional conduct and as such covered by the professional liability insurance of the CSP membership.

Does the expansion in the role of the physiotherapist raise the standard even for those who are not trained in these areas? This is an issue which is considered in Chapter 15 in relation to prescribing medicines. Here it is considered in relation to requesting X-rays.

Situation: should the physiotherapist have realised?

A patient was referred by her GP for an X-ray of her lumbar spine, which was given a NAD (nothing abnormal discovered) report by the radiologist. The physiotherapist who was treating was concerned at her lack of progress and decided that further investigations should be carried out. It was subsequently discovered that she had multiple metastatic deposits within her lumbar spine and pelvis. Subsequently it was found that the original X-ray report was wrongly reported. In this situation the physiotherapist had been trained in the requesting of X-rays and knew when further diagnostic examinations should be carried out. What however if the physiotherapist had not requested further investigations? Would she be liable for the delay in diagnosis?

The answer can be found by determining the reasonable standard of practice of a physiotherapist in that situation, i.e. the Bolam test (see Chapter 10). It is probable that all physiotherapists should have a basic understanding of the need for fresh avenues of investigation if their treatment does not appear to be succeeding, whether or not they have received the additional training in the requesting and reporting on X-rays. However, liability for the further delay in diagnosis because the physiotherapist had not requested the further investigations earlier is unlikely to be upheld. In this scenario there would appear to be a breach of the duty of care by the original reporting radiologist. As in all situations, it is essential that the physiotherapist understands the limits of his/her competence and knows when to refer the patient on to a consultant or for further diagnostic tests.

The CSP guidance lists the considerations that should be taken into account when setting up an ESP post. It also stresses the importance of clear protocols for the role of the ESP and the importance of evaluation and audit of the ESP post. The use of expanding the scope of practice in orthopaedics is considered below and in Chapter 20. This guidance on ESPs must now be reconsidered in the light of the paper on the Scope of Professional Practice published by the CSP in 2008 (see below).

An article by Sally Roberts[22] reviews the professional implications of the scope of the practice of physiotherapy and identifies action physiotherapists can take to ensure that they are practising within the scope of physiotherapy.

One of the greatest difficulties for practitioners in entering into a new area of expertise is knowing when they are competent to practise in this field. Unless there is a system of accreditation for individual training courses the practitioner does not know the strengths and limitations of any training course they follow. Since the individual is personally accountable, it is suggested that developments in the scope of professional practice should be through a mix of education/training and supervised practice. In addition, in areas of uncertainty over both the recommended practice and also whether a particular activity is within the scope of expanded practice, it is useful to check with colleagues over their knowledge and experience. For example, physiotherapists working in the field of orthopaedics might be asked by a consultant to 'work up' patients prior to surgery – specifically the anterior cruciate ligament reconstructions and also shoulder stabilisation and rotator cuff repairs. The following questions have arisen:

- Does anyone routinely see this category of patients immediately pre-op in order to strengthen, work on proprioception, stability, etc.? Are there any procedures, protocols, existing evidence of research-based practice?

Responses from colleagues and evidence of research could lead to a recognised standard of professional practice in this area.

It is important to ensure that any extended practice is research based. Research by Paula Kersten et al.[23] concluded that the widespread introduction of ESP roles in physiotherapy had been largely concerned with service demands as opposed to quality of care, patient-related outcomes or cost implications. The authors state:

It is paramount that the expansion of ESP roles, driven by policy, goes hand in hand with robust research in order to strengthen the evidence base for ESP in physiotherapy. Investment in training for therapists entering into and developing these roles is urgently required to ensure that they are equipped to practice safely and have the skills to evaluate their effectiveness.

In an article examining the role of the physiotherapist in emergency departments, the authors question whether their activities are more correctly seen, not as extended scope, but as 'advanced' scope of practice, where the physiotherapist uses advanced clinical skills in a new work setting, such as the emergency department.[24]

Self-referral and the scope of professional practice

The ability of patients to secure direct access to physiotherapy advice and treatment enables a more efficient use of physiotherapy services but at the same time presents challenges to the physiotherapist in determining the boundaries to his/her competence. Research in Scotland found that self-referral was cost effective and clinically effective and popular with physiotherapists.[25] The authors have also studied the effects of direct access to physiotherapy services in primary care and concluded that the limited evidence so far available does not support the concern that direct access would result in a demand with which the profession would be unable to cope. The results suggest that direct access could improve patient access, which is in keeping with the aspirations of current primary care development.[26] A guide has been written for therapists on self-referral by two of the authors of the research.[27] At the time of writing the DH has six pilot schemes across England designed to evaluate self-referral to physiotherapists. An information pack is available on the DH website.

Orthopaedics (an example of extended role practice)

An interesting example of the extended role of the physiotherapist in specialist clinics was given by Durrell.[28] She showed how an appropriately trained physiotherapist can act in selecting referrals from a general case mix and request and interpret investigations (such as blood tests, X-rays and scans), forming a working diagnosis and planning patient management. The issues that arise from this extended activity include:

- consent from the patient that the referral is to a physiotherapist and not a doctor;
- responsibility for the patient being with the physiotherapist once an appointment is booked;
- the importance of good communication with the consultant and GP;
- open access to medical advice, including an immediate opinion if necessary, and cross-referral;
- adequate training for the physiotherapist to undertake these activities;
- agreement on the scope of professional practice between doctors and physiotherapists;
- appropriate professional liability cover;
- the employer's agreement over the expansion to ensure their vicarious liability (see Chapter 10) for these activities;
- guidelines and protocols need to be developed to cover the increasing number of extended role activities.

The experience of physiotherapy extended scope practitioners in orthopaedic outpatient clinics was evaluated in an article by Lesley Jane Dawson and Fery Ghazi.[29] They stated that the most crucial point to emerge was the importance of the relationship between the medical team and extended-scope practitioners. They recommended further study of the experiences of the extended-scope practitioner in primary care, a rapidly developing area, where the post holder does not have the benefit of consultant support.

Sue Thomas[30] describes how the use of skilled chartered physiotherapists as the first line assessment of orthopaedic patients has speeded up the referral process in orthopaedics. The Medicines Act has been amended to enable physiotherapists to become non-medical prescribers under the Act. This is considered in Chapter 15

The scope of physiotherapist practice 2008

In January 2008 the CSP published its seminal work on the scope of professional practice for the physiotherapist. The Royal Charter outlined the four aspects, known as pillars, of practice that a physiotherapist might use as massage, exercise, electrotherapy and kindred forms of treatment. The CSP paper *Scope of Professional Practice*[31] stated that:

> Whilst the first three pillars are narrowly related to specific treatment interventions, the fourth pillar is suitably broad to allow physiotherapists to expand their expertise according to patient need.

In modern healthcare, skills are no longer unique to one professional grouping and there is a growing blurring of professional boundaries so it is now therefore inappropriate to publish a list of activities that are deemed 'in' or 'out' of scope of practice; instead activities should be linked to the four pillars of physiotherapy practice.

The CSP puts forward the following definition:

> Therefore, the scope of practice of physiotherapy is defined as any activity undertaken by an individual physiotherapist that may be situated within the four pillars of physiotherapy practice where the individual is educated, trained and competent to perform that activity. Such activities should be linked to existing or emerging occupational and / or practice frameworks acknowledged by the profession, and be supported by a body of evidence.

It sees itself as the arbiter over whether an activity comes within the scope of practice:

> Should there be a challenge to an individual's activity/competence, the CSP would be required to confirm that the individual was working within their personal scope of practice. Providing there is the evidence of an individual's competence to undertake the role/activity in question, and that the activity sits within the four pillars of practice, the

individual would be covered by their PLI as working within the scope of the profession.

It further states that:

> Consequently a physiotherapist may practice any activity that falls within the remit of the four pillars of practice, provided that they are appropriately educated, trained and competent to practice in the way that they do. Their practice must be both lawful and reasonable and the physiotherapist should be insured to practice. The way a physiotherapist practices should have the overall aim of being of benefit to identified patient/population needs, their practice should be recognised as fitting within an existing or emerging occupational or practice framework recognised by the profession and there should be a body of evidence to support the activity.

On Extended Scope Practice the CSP states that:

> Extended scope practice falls under the fourth pillar of practice and requires additional training and development beyond that acquired during undergraduate or immediate postgraduate training. Mentoring, training and supervision of such activities tends to be given to the member by another registered professional e.g. a doctor, in reflection of the fact that many of the activities in question were previously performed by medical practitioners e.g. requesting and interpreting medical imaging, pathology tests etc. Provided the member is competent in the activity, can demonstrate that the activity is linked to the Charter's four pillars of practice, and the Curriculum Framework/World Congress of Physical Therapy definitions of physiotherapy, such activity will now be covered by the CSP's PLI cover, subject to the terms of the policy.

'Kindred forms of treatment'

This phrase is the key to the acceptability of any expansion in the scope of practice of the physiotherapist. But kindred in relation to massage, exercise and electrotherapy is extremely wide. Some touching of the patient perhaps is the only limitation, but even this may not be a useful boundary since all professional/patient contact involves communication and therapy.

- What have physiotherapists taken on as expanded role activities?
  - requesting investigations (X-rays, scans, blood tests, etc.);
  - using the results of investigations to assist clinical diagnosis and appropriate management of patients;
  - listing for surgery and referring to other medical and health care professionals;
  - taking direct referrals in orthopaedic clinics;
  - non-medical prescribing.
- What activities could they not undertake?
  - any activity where the law requires another health professional to undertake that activity, e.g. roles specified by the law such as by the Mental Health Act; certification of death; Abortion Act;
  - any activity where they have not had the appropriate training and therefore lack the required competence;
  - any activity which contravenes the Rules and Standards of the HPC or the CSP;
  - any activity where their employer refuses to agree to that coming within the scope of their practice or in the course of employment;
  - any activity which the CSP does not consider to be part of the practice of a physiotherapist;
  - any activity which is not covered by personal liability insurance.

A cystic fibrosis clinic

This will be taken as an example of the potential scope of the physiotherapist on the assumption that he/she has received all the necessary training, supervision and is competent. The physiotherapist could administer the nebuliser, make up the necessary medicines, give an injection, refer to the doctor, request X-rays, consider medication for the future and prescribe it (providing the rules of supplementary prescribing or patient group directions were followed – see Chapter 15), put in place a cannula, listen to the chest, carry out percussion and drainage, prescribe oxygen, advise on diet, advise on exercise and lifestyle. What else is needed?

- Could they admit as an in-patient?
- Could they refer for surgery?

The answer to these questions depends upon the collaborative arrangements within the hospital, which may permit a physiotherapist to admit a patient, but not enable the patient to be referred for surgery without prior approval from a surgeon.

Complementary therapies and the physiotherapist

Acupuncture, aromatherapy, reflexology, and many complementary and alternative therapies can clearly be seen as coming within the definition of 'kindred activities'. However, is the physiotherapist who practises acupuncture still a physiotherapist, or has he/she become an acupuncturist and is there any difference? Should the physiotherapist be qualified as a registered acupuncturist in order to use acupuncture? Is it possible to be qualified in just a few acupuncture activities but not be an acupuncturist?

Standards and the HPC

The HPC explicitly recognises the fact that a registrant's scope of practice will change over time and the practice of experienced registrants often becomes more focused and specialised than that of newly registered colleagues. It states in its standards of proficiency (which can be found on the HPC website):[32]

Your particular scope of practice may mean that you are unable to continue to demonstrate

that you meet all of the standards that apply for the whole of your profession. (Bold in HPC document.)

As long as you make sure that you are practising safely and effectively within your given scope of practice and do not practise in the areas where you are not proficient to do so, this will not be a problem.

It is thus important, especially for senior physiotherapists, to recognise those areas where they are no longer competent and accept that more junior staff may have a wider scope of practice.

The employer's responsibility

The concept of vicarious liability is discussed in Chapter 10, where it is pointed out that the activities of the negligent employee must be in the course of employment in order for the employer to be held vicariously liable. If there is written evidence of the employer's agreement to these expanded roles, then the argument that the employee was not acting in the course of employment while undertaking these activities is unlikely to succeed. However, even where there is no written evidence of the employer's agreement, the employer could still be held vicariously liable for any harm that results on the basis of the wider definition of 'course of employment' used by the House of Lords in the case of *Lister* v. *Hesley Hall*[33] (see Chapter 10).

Collaborative practice

Physiotherapists, unlike many other professions supplementary to medicine, have since 1977,[34] seen themselves as able to take direct referrals (i.e. other than through a doctor) and the CSP has been concerned to protect this power. Thus in a collaboration[35] with occupational therapists and speech and language therapists there was a reassurance from the then Secretary of State for Health, Virginia Bottomley (Appendix D to the article), that the NHS reforms of 1990 were not intended to restrict referral to physiotherapists, so that physiotherapists could continue to accept referrals from sources other than consultants and GPs.

It should be borne in mind when the expansion of the scope of professional practice of the physiotherapist is being considered that there may well be many overlaps with the professional ambitions of other health professions including nurses and occupational therapists. Collaboration with these groups therefore becomes extremely important. The document referred to covers collaborative practice in the following areas:

- professional organisations
- education
- undergraduate education
- research, clinical research and evaluation
- manpower planning and support workers
- staff retention and job satisfaction.

Close collaborative practice between professions was also envisaged by the Department of Health in its White Paper *The New NHS: Modern Dependable*.[36]

Legal consequences of negligence in undertaking extended scope activities

Negligence in undertaking extended scope activities could lead to fitness to practise proceedings before the HPC; disciplinary proceedings before an employer; civil proceedings brought by any person who has as a consequence been harmed with the employer being sued because of its vicarious liability or where the physiotherapist is self-employed by civil action against him/her personally. In addition, where death or serious injury has occurred there could be a criminal prosecution of the employee or of the NHS organisation. Under the Corporate Manslaughter and Corporate Homicide Act 2007 the NHS organisation could be prosecuted following a death (see Chapter 2).

Post-registration control and supervision

Once physiotherapists are qualified and registered they are professionally accountable for their actions and are not subject to any system of professional supervision comparable with the statutory supervision of the midwife. They are expected to provide the reasonable standard of care the patient is entitled to have (see Chapter 10) and it would be no defence for them to argue that they were only recently qualified and that was why negligence occurred. In practice, however, senior colleagues provide support for junior staff and would ensure that some form of supervision and training was in place. It is, of course, more difficult in those work areas where a physiotherapist would be working on his/her own. Schemes for continuing education and training are considered in Chapter 5.

Commissioning work

The CSP has published guidance for its members on making a business case so that they can attract existing and new work.[37] The CSP points out that as NHS commissioning becomes a reality, physiotherapists will no longer be able to measure the effectiveness of their work purely on the quality of clinical outcomes; they will also need to demonstrate that the services they provide are value for money and help to achieve wider health targets and outcomes.

Insurance and indemnity

It is essential that any physiotherapist should ensure that he/she is covered in relation to the possibility of claims for compensation. If he/she is employed, he/she will be covered by the vicarious liability of the employer, provided that the situation giving rise to the claim occurs while he/she is working in the course of his/her employment. However, if he/she does work outside the course of his/her employment or as a self-employed physiotherapist he/she would be personally responsible for the payment of any compensation (see further Chapter 10 on negligence and Chapter 19 on private practice).

In its 2002 *Rules of Professional Conduct* in guidance on Rule 1 (see earlier) the CSP suggests that:

Physiotherapists should ascertain from their employer the level and extent of that vicarious responsibility at the start of their employment. It is important that members do not extend their practice in such a way that is unknown or unacceptable to the employer. This could mean that, if an incident occurs in respect of that modality and litigation follows, the employer may not accept liability. Some independent hospitals and other employers do not cover their employees.

It should perhaps be pointed out that vicarious liability is not determined by the employer but by the law. If an activity is defined according to common law as coming within the course of employment, then an employer can be held liable for any harm caused by the negligent act of an employee, even though the employer were to protest that the employee was not working in the course of employment according to his definition. 'In course of employment' has been given a very wide definition by the House of Lords when it held that an employer was liable for sex assaults committed on pupils by a warden since they were undertaken in the course of employment[38] (see Chapter 10).

The CSP has contracted with MPS Risk Solutions for insurance cover for its members. Its policy document which can be downloaded from the CPS website covers the following topics:

- about MPS Risk Solutions Limited
- complaints procedure
- claims procedure
- the insurance contract
- the cover
  - Section A – malpractice
  - Section B – good Samaritan acts
  - Section C – professional indemnity

- ■ Section D – libel and slander
- ■ Section E – public liability
- ■ Section F – products liability
- limit of indemnity
- indemnity to employees
- indemnity to principal
- general exclusions
- claims conditions
- cancellation
- governing law
- words with special meanings.

Members can also download the policy and the certificate of insurance giving the schedule of cover. Members should be aware of the exclusions from cover since these include any claim or investigation arising from any services rendered by any person while under the influence of intoxicants or narcotics and also any claim or investigation arising from allegations of actual or attempted sexual relations, sexual contact or intimacy, sexual harassment or sexual exploitation whether under the guise of treatment or not, or in the course of treatment or not. (This latter exclusion does not apply to the successful defence of such a claim.)

For details on education, reference should be made to Chapter 5, and for the law relating to teaching and research, Chapter 25.

Conclusions

Standards of professional practice are constantly increasing and the onus is on the professional personally to ensure that his/her competence is maintained and that he/she upholds the reasonable standards of professional practice. He/she therefore has the responsibility of ensuring that he/she obtains the necessary training and instruction to remain competent and to develop safely in new areas of practice. The CSP publication the *Scope of Physiotherapy Practice* should ensure that the physiotherapist can develop and enhance his/her skills competently and safely. It is hoped that this publication could be followed by procedures and protocols covering those new

areas where physiotherapists are extending their scope of practice to ensure that appropriate governance arrangements are in place within the organisation. The HPC has laid down rules relating to continuing professional development that registrants must satisfy in order to be eligible for re-registration. It has established a programme for the audit of continuing professional development (CPD) of registrants. Physiotherapists will be audited just prior to renewing their registration in April 2010 but are expected to comply with the standards from their introduction in July 2006.[39]

The CSP has published guidance on the HPC's CPD standards.[40] The HPC has established itself as a significant force in the protection of the public and in establishing clear standards of practice of its registrants. However, as a consequence of the Government's White Paper *Trust, Assurance and Safety* and the Health and Social Care Act 2008 significant changes are planned in the regulation of health care professionals (see Chapter 3).

Questions and exercises

1   A colleague tells you that she has been reported to the Health Professions Council for unfitness to practice. Advise her on the procedure that will be followed and how she could defend herself.

2   Do you consider that the following conduct by a registered physiotherapist should be the subject of professional conduct proceedings:
    (a)   a parking fine
    (b)   an offence of shoplifting
    (c)   being cited in a divorce as an adulterer
    (d)   being found guilty of a breach of the peace following a New Year's Eve party?

3   Explain the legal situation in relation to insurance cover for an employed and a self-employed physiotherapist.

References

1   Chartered Society of Physiotherapy (2006) *Member Guide of HPC Investigations*. CSP, London.

2   Health Professions Order 2001 Statutory Instrument 2002/254.

3   The Health Professions Council (Practice Committees) (Constitution) Rules Order of Council 2003 SI 2003 No 1209.

4   The Health Professions Council (Screeners) Rules Order of Council 2003 SI 2003 No 1573.

5   The Health Professions Council (Investigating Committee) (Procedure) Rules Order of Council 2003 SI 2003 No 1574.

6   The Health Professions Council (Conduct and Competence Committee) (Procedure) Rules Order of Council 2003 SI 2003 No 1575.

7   Health Professions Council (2003 revised 2008) *Standards of Conduct, Performance and Ethics*. HPC, London.

8   The Health Professions Council (Health Committee) (Procedure) Rules Order of Council 2003 SI 2003 No 1576.

9   The Health Professions Council (Legal Assessors) Order of Council 2003 SI 2003 No 1578.

10 The Health Professions Council (Functions of Assessors) Rules Order of Council 2003 SI 2003 No 1577.

11 www.hpc-uk.org/complaints

12 www.hpc-uk.org/mediaandevents/pressrelease/index.asp?id=227 3 December 2007.

13 www.hpc-uk.org/mediaandevents/pressrelease/index.asp?id=224 7 November 2007.

14 Health Professions Council (2007) *Indicative Sanctions Policy*. HPC, London.

15 Chartered Society of Physiotherapy (2002) *Rules of Professional Conduct*. CSP, London.

16 CSP Professional Affairs Department (2005) *Service Standards of Physiotherapy Practice*. CSP, London.

17 Chartered Society of Physiotherapy (2005) *Core Standards of Physiotherapy Practice*. CSP, London.

18 Chartered Society of Physiotherapy (2002) *Physiotherapy Assistants Code of Conduct*. CSP, London.

19 CSP Professional Affairs Department (1995) *Standards of Business Conduct*. No. PA 26. CSP, London.

20 CSP Professional Affairs Department (1994) *Physiotherapists Working Outside the Scope of Physiotherapy Practice*. No. PA 21. CSP, London.

21 CSP Professional Affairs Department No. PA 29. *Chartered Physiotherapists Working as Extended Scope Practitioners*. CSP, London.

22 Roberts, S. (2005) The Scope of Practice of Physiotherapy. *In Touch* **113**, 27–30.

23 Kersten, P. *et al.* (2007) Physiotherapy Extended Scope of Practice – Who is Doing What and Why? *Physiotherapy* **93**, 235–242.

24 Anaf, S., Sheppard, L.A. (2007) Physiotherapy as a Clinical Service in Emergency Departments: a Narrative Review. *Physiotherapy* **93**, 243–252.

25 Holdsworth, L.K., Webster, V., McFayden, S. (2007) What are the Costs to NHS Scotland of Self-referral to Physiotherapy. *Physiotherapy* **93**, 3–11.

26 Holdsworth L., Webster V. (2004) Direct Access to Physiotherapy in Primary Care: Now? – and Into the Future? *Physiotherapy* **90**, 64–72.

27 Holdsworth L., Webster V. (2006) *Patient Self Referral: A Guide for Therapists*. Radcliffe Publishing, Oxford.

28 Durrell, S. (1996) Expanding the scope of physiotherapy: clinical physiotherapy specialists in consultants clinics. *Manual Therapy* **4**, 210–213.

29 Dawson, L.J., Ghazi, F. (2004) The Experience of Physiotherapy Extended Scope Practitioners in Orthopaedic Outpatient Clinics. *Physiotherapy* **90**, 210–216.

30 Thomas, S. (1994) Speeding up the referral process in orthopaedics. NHS Executive VFM Update No. 11, June.

31 Chartered Society of Physiotherapy (2008) *Scope of Professional Practice*. CSP, London.

32 www.hpc-uk.org

33 *Lister & Others* v. *Hesley Hall Ltd* [2001] UKHL 22 [2002] 1 AC 215; The Times Law Report, 10 May 2001; [2001] 2 WLR 1311.

34 Department of Health and Social Services (1977) *Relationship Between the Medical and Remedial Professions*. HC (77)33. DHSS, London.

35 Chartered Society of Physiotherapy, the College of Occupational Therapists and the College of Speech and Language Therapists (no date) *Promoting Collaborative Practice*. CSP, COT, CSLT, London.

36 DoH (1997) *The New NHS: Modern Dependable*. HMSO, London.

37 Chartered Society of Physiotherapy (2007) *Making the Business Case*. CPS, London.

38   *Lister & Others* v. *Hesley Hall Ltd* [2001] UKHL 22 [2002] 1 AC 215; The Times Law Report, 10 May 2001; [2001] 2 WLR 1311.

39   Health Professions Council (2004) *Standards for Continuing Professional Development.* HPC, London.

40   Chartered Society of Physiotherapy (2006) *Health Professions Council (HPC) Standards for Continuing Professional Development CPD 39.* CSP, London.

5 Education and the Physiotherapist

This chapter is concerned with the statutory provisions for controlling the education of the physiotherapist both pre- and post-registration. (Reference should be made to Chapter 26 on the legal aspects of teaching and research.) The following issues will be considered:

- Health Professions Council
- Role of Chartered Society of Physiotherapists
- Approval of education providers and programmes
- External placement for clinical training
- Post-registration education
- Supervision and mentoring
- The future

Health Professions Council

The HPC was launched in April 2002 replacing the Council for Professions Supplementary to Medicine and its Professional Boards (see Chapter 3). Under the Health Act 1999 one of the statutory duties of the HPC, which is not transferable by Order to another body, is determining the standards of education and training for admission to practice.

Education and Training Committee of the Health Professions Council

One of the statutory committees that must be set up by the HPC is an Education and Training Committee. This advises the Council on the performance of the Council's functions in relation to:

- establishing standards proficiency;
- establishing standards and requirements in respect of education and training for both registration and continuing professional development (CPD);
- giving guidance on education and training standards to registrants, employers and others.

The Council is required to establish from time to time:

- the standards of education and training necessary to achieve the standards of proficiency it has established;
- the requirements to be satisfied for admission to such education and training which may

include requirements as to good health and good character.

The Education and Training Committee shall ensure that universities and other institutions are notified of the standards and requirements and shall take appropriate steps to satisfy itself that those standards and requirements are met. The Education and Training Committee can approve courses of education or training, qualifications, institutions, such tests of professional competence, education, training and experience which would lead to the award of additional qualifications, which would be recorded in the register. The Council is required to publish a statement of the criteria that will be taken into account in deciding whether to give approval. The Council is also required to maintain and publish a list of the courses of education or training, qualifications and institutions that are or were approved under the Order.

The HPC has set out the standards of proficiency it considers necessary for safe and effective practice under each part of the HPC Register. The standards of proficiency required for the registration of a physiotherapist can be seen in full on the HPC website.[1] The introduction to the standards of proficiency states that:

> These are the standards we have produced for the safe and effective practice of the professions we regulate. They are the minimum standards we consider necessary to protect members of the public.

The standards include generic standards for all professions regulated by the HPC and profession-specific standards for each regulated profession. They are set out under the following headings: expectations of a health professional, the skills required for the application of practice and knowledge, understanding and skills.

Approval of education providers and programmes

The Education Department of the HPC has since September 2004 been carrying out approval visits to education providers and programmes throughout the UK. A panel from the HPC consisting of one education executive and two visitors – at least one of whom is from the same part of the Register as the professional with which the programme is concerned. Following the visit the panel may recommend a programme to the Education and Training Committee for one of the following:

- to approve the programme;
- to set conditions on the programme, all of which must be met before the programme can be approved;
- to not approve the programme;
- to withdraw approval of the programme.

In the event of either of the last two recommendations being made, the graduates of the programme will not be entitled to register with the HPC and as such will not be able to practise in the UK using one of the titles protected by the HPC.

A new approval process has been introduced to allow an independent review of programmes for regulatory purposes and ensure rigour surrounding the outcomes of the approvals event. The HPC Visitors need to be satisfied that the education provider and its programmes meet the HPC Standards of Education and Training to ensure that graduates meet the HPC Standards of Proficiency to allow eligibility for registration with the HPC. The main areas where the new Approvals process differs from the previous systems are:

- that, as far as possible, the new procedures will align with and build upon existing approval and quality assurance processes already used by education providers;
- programmes will be approved on an open-ended basis subject to satisfactory annual monitoring returns. (The HPC reserves the right to visit a programme when problems are apparent.)
- the introduction of a unified approach to allow multiple-professional approvals to be incorporated into a single approvals event;

- where required, formal approval of new education providers will now be achieved at the same time as programme approval;
- annual monitoring will adopt a lighter touch by reporting by exception and according to an education provider's own annual monitoring timetable, using their own documentation where available;
- following feedback from the HPC consultation process, the Annual Monitoring Review will be extended to include a Cyclical Review, which will take place according to the education provider's own internal programme review timetable. No Annual Monitoring Report will be required in a year where Cyclical Review occurs;
- the HPC will no longer visit clinical/practice placements. Quality assurance (QA) of such placements will be the responsibility of the education provider, to be evidenced by the inclusion into an education provider's own quality assurance mechanisms for QA systems which ensure that the HPC Standards of Education and Training and Standards of Proficiency are being met within clinical/practice placements. The HPC reserves the right to visit clinical/practice placements;
- the HPC will no longer approve the appointment of external examiners. Instead, its Visitors will look for evidence that at least one external examiner is from the relevant part of the Register.

Higher Education Funding Council and Quality Assurance Agency

The Higher Education Funding Council, which has the responsibility of providing public funds for teaching provision in colleges, is also legally responsible for ensuring that the quality of education is assessed in the universities and colleges it funds. It therefore contracts with the Quality Assurance Agency (QAA) on an annual basis to devise and implement quality assurance methods. The QAA reviews the quality of all publicly funded higher education teaching provision in England. The QAA carries out two methods of quality assurance: institutional audit in higher education institutions and an integrated Quality and Enhancement review of higher education delivered in further education colleges.

Role of the Chartered Society of Physiotherapy

The CSP supports the work of the HPC in developing the criteria for the recognition of courses for registration. The CSP published Competencies and Competence Frameworks: Skills for Health and the Competence agenda in 2006. The paper Using Competences and Competence Frameworks was intended to accompany the former document. The latter looks at practical issues involved in using competences with case studies.

External placement for clinical training

While the theoretical content of the training and education will take place largely within universities or colleges of higher education, it is necessary for the colleges to agree placements for clinical training and instruction with NHS Trusts and social services departments (SSDs).

A memorandum of agreement is drawn up between college and Trust or SSD, to set down the basic principles behind the placement. It should cover:

- the number of students to be taken by the Trust/SSD
- the liability for any harm caused *by* the student
- the liability for any harm caused *to* the student.

It should also clarify the duties of the clinical instructor. Some agreements may now include payment for the clinical placements from the college to the Trust/SSD or even from the Trust to the college – third year students may be valuable members of the multidisciplinary team.

The NHS Knowledge and Skills Framework and the Development Review Process

The NHS Knowledge and Skills Framework and the Development Review Process (NHS KSF)[2] was published in 2004. It defines and describes the knowledge and skills which NHS staff need to apply in their work in order to deliver quality services. It provides a single, consistent, comprehensive and explicit framework on which to base the review and development for all staff. It is at the heart of the career and pay progression strand of the Agenda for Change (see Chapter 17). It is made up of six core dimensions: communication; personal and people development; health, safety and security; service improvement; quality and equality and diversity. The other 24 dimensions are specific and are grouped under health and well-being; estates and facilities; information and technology, and general. The purposes of the NHS KSF is to facilitate the development of services so that they better meet the needs of users and the public; support effective learning and development of individuals and teams; and promote equality for and diversity of all staff.

Post-registration education/continuing professional development

As in pre-registration training and education, the colleges, the HPC and the CSP are concerned to maintain standards of competence in the profession. The HPC defines CPD as

> a range of learning activities through which health professionals maintain and develop throughout their career to ensure that they retain their capacity to practice safely, effectively and legally within their evolving scope of practice.[3]

The HPC has published standards for CPD that are available from its website and monitors compliance with these standards through audit. From 1 July 2006 all registrants are required to engage in CPD and must record their activities in their portfolio, and if selected for audit must complete the CPD profile, which will then be assessed by CPD assessors.

Chartered Physiotherapists are directed that they should only

> practise to the extent that they have established, maintained and developed their ability to work safely and competently and shall ensure that they have appropriate professional liability cover for that practice.
>
> (first rule of the CSP Professional
> Conduct Rules revised in 2002)

CPD is therefore a professional obligation.

The CSP is therefore concerned with post-registration professional development and in 1996 undertook a review of its existing post-qualifying education, known as physiotherapy access to continuing education (PACE). The principal recommendations were that CPD should replace PACE as the umbrella term for the Society's initiatives on post-qualifying learning. In addition it recommended that physiotherapists providing post-qualifying education should make links with higher education institutions to develop, deliver and gain recognition for their programmes and the CSP should explore the feasibility of accrediting its members' professional development.[4]

In April 2007 the CSP joined with 10 other health professional associations to publish a joint statement on CPD for health and social care practitioners.[5] The aim of the joint statement was to influence health and social care policymakers, commissioners and employers to provide enhanced CPD support for health and social care practitioners. The document expected that a minimum 6 days (45 hours) per year for protected CPD time should be granted above existing statutory and mandatory training and formal study leave arrangements. The time for CPD includes time for the documentation of learning outcomes, alongside direct involvement in CPD activities.

A policy statement was issued by the CSP on CPD in September 2007, which stated that CPD should be seen as a systematic, ongoing structured process of maintaining, developing and enhancing skills, knowledge and competence both professionally and personally in order to improve performance at work. It states that the CSP policy on CPD:

1. adopts an outcomes-based approach with a focus on achievement
2. links learning with enhancement of quality of patient care, service delivery and professional excellence while ensuring public safety
3. is obligatory through the Rules of Professional Conduct and Code of Conduct
4. is based on individual responsibility, trust and self-evaluation
5. recognises a range of learning activities
6. expects the establishment and maintenance of a portfolio of learning
7. requires access to information and appropriate resources based on equity
8. encourages professional support, networking and collaboration
9. CPD is the work-oriented aspect of lifelong learning.

It is the responsibility of the individual practitioner to maintain his or her post-registration competence, experience and knowledge.

Situation: leave refused

A physiotherapist asks if she can have paid time off to develop her skills in manipulation. She is told that the department is too busy to allow her to have the paid time off, and she should use her holiday entitlement to attend the course. What is the law?

In the absence of a contractual right to have paid time off for CPD, it would be difficult for the physiotherapist to insist upon receiving paid time off. However, in serious cases (for example where it is essential for the employee's work to be trained in a specific area) it may be possible for the employee to argue that the employer is in fundamental breach of contract in failing to give her the opportunity to be trained and competent to do the job for which she is employed. This

would amount to a situation of constructive dismissal and is discussed in Chapter 17. Care must be taken since the employer would try and argue that the employee voluntarily resigned and it was not in fundamental breach of the contract of employment.

If the Trust or SSD is unwilling to fund post-registration courses or study leave, individual practitioners may have to be prepared to meet the cost themselves. The joint statement on CPD for health and social care practitioners[5] envisaged that 6 days of CPD should be permitted per year, but this is not yet a statutory or contractual right. It is up to the discretion of the employer what CPD can be funded, but it is hoped that the joint statement will achieve its aim of influencing commissioners and employers in recognising the importance of CPD.

Supervision and mentoring

It cannot be assumed that only full-time clinical teachers have responsibilities in education and training. Increasingly, the colleges are looking for practitioners to provide not only clinical supervision for pre-registration students, but also a mentoring role for students and newly qualified registered staff. The responsibilities of the senior practitioner in relation to supervision and delegation cannot be underestimated and reference should be made to Chapter 10 on this topic. The CSP revised its overview of mentoring in 2005.[6] This publication looks at the roles and responsibilities involved in mentoring, the qualities of a mentor, the benefits of mentoring and mentoring in practice. It states that:

Mentoring can be a valuable support mechanism, focussing on growth and development in the broadest context and can form part of CPD. The relationship aims to empower the mentee to enable them to become independent learners, with both partners learning during and from the process. The mentor develops a range of transferable skills which can be used for other CPD activities.

The mentoring relationship is based on open-ness, trust, confidentiality and shared beliefs and values.

Conclusions

The HPC has established clear standards for pre-registration and CPD for its registrants and in the case of physiotherapists is receiving strong support from the CSP. One of the challenges for the future, when many registrants will be trained to undertake activities normally associated with other registered health professions, will be to ensure that individual competence is defined, evaluated and monitored.

✏️ **Questions and exercises**

1 Define a development plan to ensure your continued professional competence.
2 What improvements do you consider could be made in ensuring the integration of theoretical and clinical training for the pre-registration student?
3 Design a protocol that could be used for those physiotherapists who act as mentors for junior colleagues.

References

1 http://www.hpc-uk.org/education/docs/HPC_physiotherapists.
2 Department of Health (2004) *The NHS Knowledge and Skills Framework and the Development Review Process*. DH, London.
3 www.hpc-uk.org
4 Gosling, S. (1996) From PACE to CPD. *Physiotherapy* **82**, 499–501.
5 Chartered Society of Physiotherapy and others (2007) *Joint Statement on Continuing Professional Development for Health and Social Care Practitioners*. CSP, London.
6 Chartered Society of Physiotherapy (2005) *Mentoring – An Overview*. CPD 35. CSP, London.

Section B

Client-Centred Care

6 Rights of Clients

In this Section we consider the rights of the client. First we take an overview of the basic statutory and common law rights. The next chapter looks at consent to treatment and information to be given to the client, and the remaining chapters consider confidentiality and the right of access to health records and freedom of information.

In this chapter the following topics are considered:

- Statutory basis of the client's rights
- The right to care and treatment
- Charters and target setting
- Questionable claims

Statutory basis of the client's rights

The Human Rights Act 1998 introduced a statutory duty on public authorities and organisations exercising functions of a public nature to recognise the Articles of the European Convention on Human Rights. These are shown in Appendix 1. It will be noted that there is no specific right to access health care that is free at the point of delivery, but questions of rights to treatment have arisen in relation to the right to life (article 2) and the right not to be subjected to inhuman or degrading treatment (article 3). Further information on human rights can be found on the Ministry of Justice website and, in addition, since 2003 the National Health Service Litigation Authority (NHSLA) has provided a 'Human Rights Act Information Service' to the NHS. One of the central aims of this service is to minimise the cost to the NHS of obtaining legal advice in relation to the Human Rights Act 1998 by providing NHS bodies with access to a centrally coordinated information service and also to encourage the sharing of good practice in this area.[1] The service provides a quarterly newsletter and a series of case sheets.

Public authorities and organisations exercising functions of a public nature must recognise and implement the human rights set out in the European Convention on Human Rights (see Appendix 1). In June 2007 the House of Lords[2] decided, in a majority decision, that private care homes under contract with local authorities for the provision of places were not exercising functions of a public nature for the purposes of the Human Rights Act. This has led to an understandable reaction from many charities concerned with the care of vulnerable adults that overriding legislation be passed. Provision is made in the Health and Social Care Act 2008 for care homes to be brought within the definition of public authority for the purposes of Human Rights. The High Court held that a housing trust, which was a registered social landlord could be a public body for the purposes of the Human Rights Act 1998.[3] The Court held that the nature of its activities and the context within which it operated was a very different situation from an ordinary commercial business. It was heavily subsidised by the government and played a role in the implementation of government policy.

Rights to health care and social care derive from the legislation shown in Figure 6.1 and

from the common law (see Chapter 2 and the glossary for an explanation of these terms).

Some of these Acts are considered in more detail in the chapters covering specific client groups.

Absolute or discretionary rights

It should be noted that very few statutes bestow absolute rights on clients or patients. The National Health Service Act 1977 (as re-enacted in Section 1 of the National Health Service Act 2006) re-enacted the duty of the Secretary of State to continue to promote in England and Wales a comprehensive health service designed to secure improvement:

- National Health Service Act 1977 (based on the National Health Service Act 1946)
- National Assistance Act 1948
- Health Service and Public Health Act 1968
- Chronically Sick and Disabled Persons Act 1970
- National Health Service Act 1977
- Disabled Persons (Service, Consultation and Representation Act 1986)
- Health and Social Services and Social Security Adjudications Act 1983
- Mental Health Act 1983 (as amended by the Mental Health Act 2007)
- Children Acts 1989 and 2004
- National Health Service and Community Care Act 1990
- Disability Discrimination Act 1995
- Carers (Recognition and Services) Act 1995
- Data Protection Act 1998
- Community Care (Residential Accommodation) Act 1998
- Health Act 1999
- Care Standards Act 2000
- Carers and Disabled Children Act 2000
- NHS Reform and Health Care Professions Act 2002,
- Community Discharge (Delayed Discharges) Act 2003
- Health and Social Care (Community Health and Standards) Act 2003
- Human Tissue Act 2004
- Mental Capacity Act 2005
- National Health Service Act 2006
- Safeguarding Vulnerable Groups Act 2006
- Mental Health Act 2007
- Health and Social Care Act 2008

Figure 6.1 Statutes giving rights to health care and social care

- in the physical and mental health of the people of those countries
- in the prevention, diagnosis and treatment of illness.

Under Section 2 of the 2006 NHS Act the Secretary of State has the following powers.
The Secretary of State may:

a. provide such services as he considers appropriate for the purpose of discharging any duty imposed on him by this Act;
b. do anything else which is calculated to facilitate, or is conducive or incidental to the discharge of such a duty.

The duty under Section 1 left much to his/her discretion as can be seen from Figure 6.2.

The rights recognised by the statutes and common law are summarised in Figure 6.3. These are covered in the chapters that follow.

Enforcement of rights

These rights can be enforced by the individual patient in many ways through administrative and judicial machinery.

Administrative machinery includes the following:

- complaint through the set procedure (see Chapter 14)
- inquiry by Secretary of State
- independent inquiry.

Judicial remedies include the following:

- an action for negligence – when harm has occurred (see Chapter 10);
- an action for trespass to the person – where treatment has been given without consent (see Chapter 7);

3(1)   The Secretary of State must provide throughout England, to such extent as he considers necessary to meet all reasonable requirements:

(a)   hospital accommodation;
(b)   other accommodation for the purpose of any service provided under this Act;
(c)   medical, dental, nursing ophthalmic and ambulance services;
(d)   such other facilities for the care of pregnant women, women who are breast feeding and young children as he considers are appropriate as part of the health service;
(e)   such other services or facilities for the prevention of illness, the care of persons suffering from illness and the after-care of persons who have suffered from illness as he considers are appropriate as part of the health service;
(f)   such other services as are required for the diagnosis and treatment of illness.

3(2)   For the purposes of the duty in subsection (1) services provided under

(a)   Section 83(2) (primary medical services), Section 99(2) (primary dental services) or Section 115(4) (primary ophthalmic services) or
(b)   a general medical services contract, a general dental services contract or a general ophthalmic services contract

must be regarded as provided by the Secretary of State.

3(3)   This section does not affect Chapter 1 of Part 7 (pharmaceutical services)
Other services which the Secretary of State has a duty to provide are set out in Schedule 1 of the NHS Act 2006 and include the medical inspection of pupils, contraceptive services provision of vehicles for disabled persons, microbiological services and research activities.
Part 4 of the 2006 NHS Act covers primary medical services; Part 5 the provision of dental services; Part 6 ophthalmic services and Part 7 pharmaceutical services.

Figure 6.2   Discretionary duties of the Secretary of State: Section 3(1) of NHS Act 2006.

- To receive care and treatment (not absolute)
- To receive a reasonable standard of care and treatment
- To give or withhold consent to treatment and/or care
- To confidentiality
- To access health and personal social services records
- To complain
- To receive rights recognised in the Human Rights Act 1998
- To receive information about the public authorities in accordance with the Freedom of Information Act 2000

Figure 6.3   Summary of client rights in the NHS and under social services

- an action for breach of statutory duty – where it is alleged that a statutory authority has not fulfilled its duties;
- an action for judicial review of the decisions of a statutory authority or other administrative body.

In addition, there are many organisations with powers of inspection over health and social services to which complaints may be made which could lead to inspections and investigations. These include:

- *the Healthcare Commission
- *the Mental Health Act Commission
- *the Commission for Social Care Inspection
- the Health and Safety Inspectorate
- Environment, Trading and Food Standards Inspectorates .

*These organisations have been amalgamated in the Care Quality Commission under the Health and Social Care Act 2008

The right to care and treatment

Unenforceable rights

As can be seen from Figure 6.2 there is not an absolute right to obtain treatment under the NHS. In the inevitable situation where resources are finite and demand outmatches supply, providers and purchasers have to weigh up the priorities. Where individual patients have sought

to enforce the statutory duty to provide services, the courts have refused to intervene unless there is evidence that there has been a failure to make a reasonable decision about the allocation of resources. Thus, patients who brought an action for breach of statutory duty against the Secretary of State for Health and the Regional and Area Health Authorities on the grounds that they had waited too long for hip operations failed in their claim.[4]

Jamie Bowen, a child suffering from leukaemia, was refused a course of chemotherapy and a second bone marrow transplant on the grounds that there was only a very small chance of the treatment succeeding and therefore it would not be in her best interests for the treatment to proceed. The Court of Appeal upheld the decision of the health authority[5] as they were unable to fault its process of reasoning and allowed the appeal.

The Master of the Rolls (Sir Thomas Bingham) stated:

> While I have every sympathy with B, I feel bound to regard this as an attempt – wholly understandable, but nevertheless misguided – to involve the court in a field of activity where it is not fitted to make any decision favourable to the patient.

More recent cases however show that there are occasions where the court is prepared to intervene over a failure to provide resources. The following are some examples.

One case concerned three transsexuals who wished to undergo gender reassignment.[6] The health authority refused to fund such treatment on the grounds that it had been assigned a low priority in its lists of procedures considered to be clinically ineffective in terms of health gain. Under this policy, gender reassignment surgery was listed among others as a procedure for which no treatment, apart from that pro-vided by the authority's general psychiatric and psychology services, would be commissioned, save in the event of overriding clinical need or exceptional circumstances. The transsexuals sought judicial review of the health authority's refusal and the judge granted an order quashing the authority's decision and the policy on which it was based. The health authority then took the case to the Court of Appeal, but lost its appeal. The Court of Appeal held that:

(1)   While the precise allocation and weighting of priorities is a matter for the judgment of the authority and not for the court, it is vital for an authority:
    (a)   to accurately assess the nature and seriousness of each type of illness;
    (b)   to determine the effectiveness of various forms of treatment for it;
    (c)   to give proper effect to that assessment and that determination in the formulation and individual application of its policy.
(2)   The authority's policy was flawed in two respects:
    (a)   it did not treat transsexualism as an illness, but as an attitude of mind which did not warrant medical treatment;
    (b)   the ostensible provision that it made for exceptions in individual cases and its manner of considering them amounted to the operation of a 'blanket policy' against funding treatment for the condition because it did not believe in such treatment.
(3)   The authority was not genuinely applying the policy to the individual exceptions.

(4)   Article 3 and Article 8 of the European Convention on Human Rights (see Chapter 2) did not give a right to free health care and did not apply to this situation, where the challenge is to a health authority's allocation of finite funds. Neither were the patients victims of discrimination on the grounds of sex.

In one case[7] a woman was waiting for a hip replacement operation and went abroad for treatment after being told that she would have to wait a year for the operation on the NHS. She asked her local hospital in Bedford to pay for the trip under the E112 certificate scheme, but Bedford Primary Care Trust (PCT) refused on the grounds that the wait was within the government's waiting times guidelines. She brought an action for judicial review of the PCT's refusal, claiming that its decision was unlawful and infringed her rights under Articles 3 and 8 of the European Convention on Human Rights.

The judge held, based on Article 49 of the EC Treaty[8] (which prohibited restrictions on freedom to provide services within the Community) that prior authorisation for treatment by an NHS patient in another member state of the European Union at the expense of the NHS could be refused on the ground of lack of medical necessity only if the same or equally effective treatment could be obtained without undue delay at an NHS establishment. He also held that in assessing what amounted to undue delay, regard had to be had to all the circumstances of the specific case, including the patient's medical condition and, where appropriate, the degree of pain and the nature and extent of the patient's disability. Consideration of NHS waiting times and waiting lists were relevant, when having regard to all the circumstances. On the facts of the case, however, the claimant did not recover the money, since the local hospital had offered her an earlier operation. The Court of Appeal referred the case to the European Court of Justice for a preliminary ruling on the application of article 49 and article 22 of Regulation 1408/71.

The European Court of Justice held that:[9]

(1)   In order to be entitled to refuse to grant the authorisation referred to in Article 22(1)(c)(i) of that regulation on the ground that there is a waiting time for hospital treatment, the competent institution is required to establish that that time does not exceed the period which is acceptable on the basis of an objective medical assessment of the clinical needs of the person concerned in the light of all of the factors characterising his medical condition at the time when the request for the authorisation is made or renewed, as the case may be.

(2)   An NHS patient is entitled under Article 49 EC to receive hospital treatment in another Member state at the expense of that national service and refusal of prior authorisation cannot be based merely on the existence of waiting lists intended to enable the supply of hospital care to be planned and managed on the basis of predetermined general clinical priorities, without carrying out an objective medical assessment of the patient's medical condition, the history and probable cause of his illness, the degree of pain he/she is in and/or the nature of his/her disability at a time when the request for authorisation was made or renewed.

(3)   Where the delay arising from such waiting lists appears to exceed an acceptable time having regard to an objective medical assessment of the above mentioned circumstances, the competent institution may not refuse the authorisation sought on the grounds of the existence of those waiting lists, an alleged distortion of the normal order of priorities linked to the relative urgency of the cases to be treated, the fact that the hospital treatment provided under the national system in question is free of charge, the obligation to make available specific funds to reimburse the cost of treatment in another Member State and/or a comparison between the cost of that treatment and that of equivalent treatment in the competent Member State.

(4)   Article 49 EC must be interpreted as meaning that where the legislation of the competent Member State provides that hospital treatment provided under the national health service is to be free of charge, and where the legislation of the Member State in which a patient registered with that service was or should have been authorised to receive hospital treatment at the expense of that service does not provide for the reimbursement in full of the cost of that treatment, the competent institution must reimburse that patient, the difference (if any) between the cost, objectively quantified, of equivalent treatment in a hospital covered by the service in question up to the total amount invoiced for the treatment, provided in the host Member State and the amount which the institution of the latter Member State is required to reimburse under Article 22(1)(c)(i) of Regulation No 1408/71 (as updated) on behalf of the competent institution pursuant to the legislation of that Member State.

(5)   A patient who is authorised to receive treatment in another Member State or who is refused authorisation which is subsequently held to be unfounded, is entitled to receive both the costs of medical treatment and also the ancillary costs associated with cross-border movement for medical purposes provided that the legislation of the competent Member State imposes a corresponding obligation on the national system to reimburse in respect of treatment provided in a local hospital covered by that system.

In July 2008 the EU published a draft directive which would allow patients to seek cross-border heath care with their countries of residence paying the costs.[10] The draft directive is to be examined by the European Parliament and the Council of Ministers before being finalised. The stated aim of the EC was to lay down a framework on patients' rights to treatment abroad.

Refunding care provided outside the NHS

In a bizarre case a private medical services company, European Surgeries Ltd, arranged for a patient to have a contract operation performed by a German company. The patient paid European Surgeries Ltd, who paid the German Company. European Surgeries Ltd then sought judicial review of the Trust's refusal to reimburse the patient. The judge refused the application noting that the patient had never been in touch with the trust or requested payment, nor had the trust commissioned the service. The fact that the company wished to increase its business by telling customers that the trust would have to reimburse them was not a justifiable claim.[11]

Right to artificial insemination

The UK's policy on no artificial insemination was challenged by a prisoner who had been married while he and his partner were serving prison sentences. The husband had been convicted of murder and would not be released till 2009, when his wife would be 50. He therefore argued that the policy against artificial insemination was a breach of his article 8 rights to a private and family life, home and correspondence. The Grand Chamber of the European Court of Human Rights held that there was a breach of article 8 rights; prisoner's rights should not be automatically forfeited; the state's duty to protect children, did not extend to preventing potential parents conceiving in such circumstances; the policy did not allow for any real weighting of the public and private interests.[12]

Public and Private treatment

Recent concerns have centred around the extent to which NHS treatment and care which is free at the point of delivery could be supplemented by treatment which is privately funded. For example, breast cancer sufferers have been told that they will be denied NHS treatment if they pay privately for 'top-up' NHS drugs, and this is likely to lead to court action. It was reported that the NHS refused to pay for an operation to prevent migraines because the patient paid privately for earlier treatment.[13] Maureen Alder paid £13 000 for an operation to implant wires into her brain to prevent migraines. The batteries needed replacing and the NHS was not prepared to fund the cost. The South Gloucester Primary Care Trust is reported as saying that if someone elects to privately fund a treatment that is not funded by the PCT and no exceptional grounds have been agreed in advance, then the individual will remain responsible for funding any ongoing costs.

This issue is relevant to those physiotherapists who have a private practice. One of their patients admitted to hospital for a condition not treated by the private physiotherapist might ask if the private treatment can continue in the hospital. What is the situation if the hospital physiotherapist refuses to permit such continuing treatment, while not being prepared to provide it within the NHS? The issue has not yet been considered by the courts, but the NHS as occupier does have the right to control the terms on which persons are admitted on to the premises and could therefore refuse admission to private physiotherapists. Such a refusal should be on reasonable grounds and it is hoped that the private practitioner could develop an understanding with the NHS physiotherapist, particularly as NHS physiotherapy services become more limited (see Chapter 19).

The National Institute for Health and Clinical Excellence

The National Institute for Health and Clinical Excellence (NICE) was established to eradicate the postcode lottery in the provision of health services, so that following an analysis of research findings recommendations could be made about which medicines and services were clinically and cost effective and could therefore be made available on the NHS. In practice, however, the failure of NHS organisations to implement NICE recommendations has led to a diversity in the provision of services. For example, the British Heart Foundation following an audit reported that a postcode lottery for services existed, where 60% of those who need cardiac rehabilitation do not have access to it.[14] The CSP pointed out that the cost of a cardiac rehabilitation programme was £600 compared with £1400 per day in a cardiac unit and called for more funding for cardiac rehabilitation.

Guidance issued by NICE on restricting the use of specified drugs to treat Alzheimer's Disease to patients with moderate–severe levels of the disease was challenged in a court case in 2007.[15] Eisai Ltd sought judicial review of the processes followed by NICE in its assessment of the drugs. The judge found that NICE did appropriately take into account the benefits which the drugs brought to carers, it did reflect the costs of long-term care in its calculations, it did not breach principles of procedural fairness by providing a read-only version of the economic model, it was not irrational in concluding that there was no cumulative benefit to patients after 6 months' treatment with the drugs and its assessment and consideration of a 2000 Alzheimer's Disease study was not irrational. However, the judge did rule that NICE was in breach of its duties under the Disability Discrimination Act and the Race Relations Act by not offering specific advice regarding people with learning disabilities and people who lacked English as a first language in its technology appraisal guidance. As a consequence of the case, NICE was asked to revise its guidance within 28 days. The revised guidance can be seen on its website.[16] Subsequently the Court of Appeal ruled, in allowing Eisai's appeal, that procedural fairness required NICE to release a fully executable version of an economic model to those consulted in the course of an appraisal process and not simply a read-only version. To do otherwise would place drug companies at a significant disadvantage in challenging the reliability of those models.[17]

Concern was expressed at the publication of NICE draft guidelines in relation to the treatment of rheumatoid arthritis. It was proposing to reduce the options available by allowing patients to be given only one of a trio of highly effective drugs called anti-TNFs.[18] The protest included a letter to *The Times* from several signatories, including the CE of the CSP, who pointed out that the 40 000 patients who suffered from severe rheumatoid arthritis were facing incredible pain, which would reduce their working capability, and the NICE proposals were contrary to Darzi reviews (see Chapter 28).[19] NICE has stated that consultees had the opportunity to appeal against the draft and its final guidance would be published in February 2009.

The work of NICE is further considered in Chapter 10. The eradication of the postcode lottery for health care is recommended as part of the Darzi reforms, which are discussed in Chapter 28.

Another organisation for tackling inequalities in health care is the Equality and Human Rights Commission. It has written to strategic health authorities asking them to ensure that doctors and hospitals give equal priority to men. There is evidence of poorer male health: men are twice as likely to die from the 10 most common cancers that affect both sexes. Surgery opening hours are male-unfriendly. The Commission has the power to issue compliance orders to NHS trusts which persistently fail to provide equal care for men.[20]

Physiotherapists and resources

The inability to provide all the services the patient requires is a major concern of physiotherapists. This mismatching between needs and supply of services may never reach court, but physiotherapists are aware when they do not have the resources to provide as intensive or extensive treatment as the patient would appear to require. For example, an audit of elderly care in-patient physiotherapy services revealed that patients received around half of the treatment that staff felt was necessary.[21] This issue is discussed further in Chapter 10 in the context of rationing and prioritising services.

Since the patient has no absolute right to receive treatment, the patient cannot insist that the care is provided by a specific member of staff (although the patient could probably require a member of staff of the same gender); nor could the patient insist on the provision of clinical treatment which was clinically contraindicated or not supported by professional opinion; nor, if the physiotherapist was of the view that continued treatment in a chronic condition was no longer effective, could the patient insist on receiving it. The patient could however refuse to accept treatment from a student (but probably not from a physiotherapy assistant if the activity is within his/her sphere of competence) and normally the patient's consent would be requested in advance to the presence of and care by students.

The right of the health professional to use his/her professional discretion in refusing to provide treatment which he/she considers to be inappropriate for the patient has been reinforced by a decision of the Court of Appeal in a case where Leslie Burke challenged the GMC's guidelines on withholding treatment.

The Burke case

Leslie Burke, a patient suffering from a degenerative brain condition brought an action against the GMC arguing that their guidance[22] to doctors on 'Withholding and Withdrawing Life-Prolonging Treatment: Good Practice in Decision Making' was illegal. Counsel for the GMC argued that there is no obligation to provide treatment that would enable a patient to survive a life-threatening condition regardless of the suffering involved in the treatment and regardless of the quality of life the patient would experience thereafter. She also stated that no evidence existed that Mr Burke would ever be denied life-prolonging treatment. Withdrawing artificial feeding and hydration in his case would be entirely inappropriate.[23]

Mr Burke won his case before the High Court. The judge granted judicial review holding that once a patient had been admitted to an NHS hospital there was a duty of care to provide and go on providing treatment, whether the patient was competent or incompetent or unconscious. This duty of care, which could not be transferred to anyone else, was to provide that treatment which was in the best interests of the patient. It was for the patient if competent to determine what was in his/her best interests. If the patient was incompetent and had left no binding and effective advance directive, then it was for the court to decide what was in his/her best interests. To withdraw artificial feeding and hydration at any stage before the claimant finally lapsed into a coma would involve clear breaches of both Articles 8 and 3 because he would thereby be exposed to acute mental and physical suffering. The GMC guidelines were therefore in error in emphasising the right of the claimant to refuse treatment, but not his right to require treatment.

The GMC appealed against this ruling and the Court of Appeal's reserved judgment was given on 29 July 2005.[24] The Court of Appeal held that doctors are not obliged to provide patients with treatment that they consider to be futile or harmful, even if the patient demands it. Autonomy and the right of self-determination do not entitle the patient to insist on receiving a particular medical treatment regardless of the nature of the treatment. However, where a competent patient says that he or she wants to be kept alive by the provision of food and water, doctors must agree to that. Not to do so would result in the doctor not merely being in breach of duty in the law of negligence but guilty of the criminal offence of murder.

The right to refuse a specific patient for treatment on conscientious grounds

Rule 2.4 of the Rules of Professional Conduct 2002 recognises the situation when a physiotherapist is reluctant to treat a particular patient because of conscientious or moral objections. It emphasises that these objections must be recognised and discussed with an experienced colleague. This would also be the situation where the patient's behaviour towards the physiotherapist is unacceptable (e.g. salacious behaviour which makes the physiotherapist feel uncomfortable when treating the patient). Guidance also suggests that if, in the therapist's opinion, a patient may be dangerous or unstable, treatment can be withheld. In the employed setting, referral to, or the seeking of advice from, an experienced colleague is important.

However, the Rules state that if the reason for not wishing to treat a patient is because of his/her sex, religion, race, sexual orientation or medical condition it is unlikely that any change of physiotherapist would be appropriate or should be tolerated.

It should be pointed out that any such discrimination by a physiotherapist would be illegal under recent regulations, which are considered in Chapter 17.

Enforceable rights

Some rights to care are however enforceable. These arise in circumstances of:

- a failure to provide a general practitioner;
- a failure to provide appropriate emergency services in an accident and emergency department.

Here the claim would be based upon the duty to ensure that a reasonable standard of care was provided (see Chapter 10 on negligence). In the case of primary care medical services, a person can apply to the PCT (in Wales the local health board) to be placed on the list of a general practitioner.

Duty to follow DH guidelines

In July 1997 the High Court ruled against North Derbyshire Health Authority, which had refused to fund the purchase of beta-interferon in the treatment of multiple sclerosis.[25] In its press announcement following the decision, a spokeswoman for the authority stated that the drug had not yet been supported by clear research findings on its effectiveness. It lost the case because the health authority had failed to follow DH guidelines in the supply of the drug to patients with multiple sclerosis. On the other hand, even following ministerial guidelines to the letter would not render an authority immune from a successful claim being made against it. In *R* v. *Wandsworth Borough Counci*[26] the Court found that the guidance itself was incorrect.

Charters and target setting

Effect of the charters and targets

In the past there have been national charters for patients in both secondary and primary care; and many hospitals, community health services and GP practices and patient associations have prepared their own charters. In recent times the Department of Health has set targets, including times for admission or out-patient appointments. These give certain assurances to clients and patients that services will be provided within set times and to a specific quality. However, these charters or targets do not bestow legal rights and the client or patient cannot enforce them unless the services they offer are already part of the law. For example, the client might be advised that full information will be given to him or her about the range of services available and about any contra-indications or side effects. Should a health professional fail to give the appropriate information and the client suffers harm of which he/she had not been warned, then the client would have a legal right of action. However, this would not be on the basis of the charter or target, but because of an existing common law right to be given appropriate information as part of the duty of care owed by the health professional to the client (see Chapter 7). The Government is proposing an NHS Constitution, which may give legal rights to patients to enforce healthcare provisions. It is discussed in Chapter 28.

The effect of the European Court of Justice in the Bedford case[9] (see above), may lead to those who are waiting in excess of the national waiting times targets or whose clinical condition indicates that they should be treated earlier than the target maximum waiting times may be able to obtain treatment in another EC state and being reimbursed the costs of treatment.

A patient could also complain to the NHS Trust and this could reach the Healthcare Commission and eventually the Health Service Commissioner (See Chapter 14). The patient could also complain to the strategic health authority or PCT because of the Trust's failure to comply with the targets or standards set by the Department of Health and therefore with the NHS agreement it has with the strategic health authority or PCT.

Where the client is receiving private health care under a contract agreed with a physiotherapist in private practice, then a charter might be seen as part of the agreement and the client may then be able to sue for breach of contract (see Chapter 19).

Questionable claims

Physiotherapists may be confronted by clients who, in contrast to those who are ignorant of their rights, are anxious to exploit the system for any benefits that are obtainable. This can be seen from a letter to the *British Journal of Occupational Therapy* by Rosemary Barnitt.[27] Her point is that in undertaking research into ethical dilemmas experienced by several hundred occupational therapists and physiotherapists, she is 'surprised by the number who have found themselves being referred "patients" with apparently substantial physical disabilities, but who turn out to have insignificant or no health problems'. She gave an example of a referral to a social services occupational therapist of a man in a wheelchair who had requested home adaptations. On assessment, the therapist felt that the man could walk and function normally but had chosen to take on a disabled role. She asked for information

about this phenomenon and followed up with a letter 5 months later in the same journal[28] saying that she had over 40 letters and telephone calls on this subject.

The requirement for the physiotherapist to follow the professional standards of assessment (and not be biased in favour of the claimant or defendant) in making reports to be used in court action is considered in Chapter 13.

Situation: unjustified claims

A physiotherapist has been providing home treatment to a patient following a stroke. She is anxious that the treatment should be continued in the outpatient department, but the patient says that he is not able to attend because of his disability which prevents him leaving the house. She subsequently hears from a colleague that the patient was seen in a supermarket. Can the physiotherapist refuse to provide physiotherapy services at home?

There are of course limited resources for health care which must be used justly and wisely. Abuse or unjustified expenditure in one area limits resources for use elsewhere and may mean that justifiable claims are not met. In this situation, the patient should be advised that he must attend the clinic in order to receive his treatment and that transport will be made available. If the patient is mentally competent and decides that he is not prepared to attend then that is his decision (see Chapter 18 on care in the community).

Conclusions

This is a complex area of law, partly because there has been no attempt, as yet, to codify the rights to which a patient/client is entitled nor has there been any attempt to ensure that such a code is enforceable through the legal system. The establishment of a constitution for the NHS is currently on the political agenda and is considered in Chapter 28. At present any potential litigant therefore has first to ascertain if the wrong which he/she claims to have suffered is one recognised by the common law or statute law and then to take advice on the means of enforcement. The following chapters cover patient/client separate rights which are currently recognised in law and enforceable in the courts. Chapter 14 covers the procedures relating to complaints and to the enforcement mechanism for standards within NHS.

✍️ Questions and exercises

1 What client rights in health and social care do you consider that the law should recognise?
2 There will never be the resources to meet all demands upon health and social services. What criteria would you draw up to determine priorities for patients to receive physiotherapy services?
3 What do you consider are the advantages of the Human Rights Act 1998? (see Appendix 1)
4 What would the advantages be in establishing a constitution for the NHS?

References

1 www.nhsla.com/HumanRights
2 *YL* v. *Birmingham City Council* [2007] UKHL 22. *The Times*, 21 June 2007.
3 *R (Weaver)* v. *London and Quadrant Housing Trust*. The Times Law Report, 8 July 2008 QBD.
4 *R* v. *Secretary of State for Social Services, ex parte Hincks and others*. (1979) *Solicitors Journal*, 29 June, 436.
5 *R* v. *Cambridge and Huntingdon Health Authority, ex parte B* [1995] 2 All ER 129.
6 *North West Lancashire Health Authority* v. *A, D and G* [1999] Lloyd's Rep Med (1999) 2 CCL Rep 419; [2000] 1 WLR 977.
7 *R (Watts)* v. *Bedford Primary Care Trust and Another* [2003] The Times Law Report, 3 October 2003; EWHC 2228; [2004] EWCA Civ 166.
8 (Previously Article 59) EC Treaty (OJ 1992 C224/6).
9 *Watts* v. *Bedford Primary Care Trust and the Secretary of State for Health* Case C-372/04 May 2006.
10 Charter, D. (2008) Patients to Travel for treatment in Europe and the NHS will pay. *The Times*, 3 July, p. 16.
11 *European Surgeries Ltd* v. *Cambridgeshire Primary Care Trust* [2007] EWHC 2758; [2008] P.I.Q.R.P8 QBD.
12 *Dickson* v. *United Kingdom* (44362/04) [2007] 3 F.C.R. 877.
13 Templeton, S.-K. (2008) Pensioner Who Went Private is Refused NHS Op. *The Sunday Times*, 18 May.
14 British Heart Foundation (2007), *National Audit of Cardiac Rehabilitation; Annual Report 2007*. BHF, London.
15 *Eisai Ltd* v. *National Institute for Health and Clinical Excellence (Alzheimer's Society and Shire Pharmaceuticals Ltd Interested parties)* [2007] EWHC 1941.
16 http://guidance.nice.org.uk/TA111
17 *R (on the application of Eisai)* v. *National Institute for Health and Clinical Excellence and Shire Pharmaceuticals Ltd and the Association of the British Pharmaceutical Industry* [2008] EWCA Civ 438; The Times Law Report, 7 May 2008.
18 Hawkes, N. (2008) Restricting Arthritis Drugs a 'Prescription for Pain'. *The Times*, 21 July, 5.
19 Ros Meer Director of Arthritis and Musculoskeletal Alliance and others. Letter to the Editor Arthritis Drugs Get People Back to Work. (2008) *The Times*, 26 July.
20 Templeton, S.-K. (2008) NHS ordered to end care bias against men. *The Sunday Times*, 25 May.
21 David, C., Noon, J., Abdulla, A. (1998) An Audit of Elderly Care In-patient Physiotherapy Services. *Agility*, January, 13–16.
22 General Medical Council (2002) Withholding and Withdrawing Life Prolonging Treatment: Good Practice in Decision Making. GMC, London.
23 Horsnell, M. (2004) Feeding a Terminal Patient 'Is Treatment'. *The Times*, 28 February.
24 *R. (on the application of Burke)* v. *General Medical Council and Disability Rights Commission and Official Solicitor to the Supreme Court* [2004] EWHC 1879; [2004] Lloyd's Rep. Med 451; [2005] EWCA Civ 1003, 28 July 2005.

25 R. v. *North Derbyshire Health Authority, ex parte Fisher* [1997] 8 Med LR 327.

26 R. v. *Wandsworth Borough Council, ex parte Beckwith* [1996] 1 All ER 129 (discussed in Dimond, B. (1997). *Legal Aspects of Care in the Community*, pp. 465–6, Macmillan, Basingstoke).

27 Barnitt, R. (1995) Letter to the Editor on 'Ethical Dilemmas'. *British Journal of Occupational Therapy*, **58**, 2, 78.

28 Barnitt, R. (1995) Letter to the Editor. *British Journal of Occupational Therapy*, **58**, 7, 308.

7 Consent and Information Giving

This chapter covers the legal issues relating to consent to treatment. It will be concerned with those issues which arise in relation to the mentally competent adult and the provisions of the Mental Capacity Act 2005, which provides a framework for decision making in relation to those over 16 years of age who lack the requisite capacity to make specific decisions. The laws relating to consent in the case of children, the mentally ill, older people and those with learning disabilities are covered in the chapters in Section E dealing with those specialist client groups. The topic of disclosure is considered in Chapter 8 on confidentiality. The following topics are considered in this chapter:

- Basic principles
- Trespass to the person
- Mental Capacity Act 2005
- Duty to inform

Basic principles

There are two distinct aspects of the law relating to consent to treatment. One is the actual giving of consent and the possibility that a trespass to the person has occurred because the patient did not give consent to the treatment. The other is the duty to give information to the patient prior to the giving of consent. The absence of consent could result in the patient suing for trespass to the person. The failure to provide sufficient relevant information could result in an action for negligence. These two different legal actions will be considered separately. Rule 9 of the Standards of conduct, performance and ethics of the Health Professions Council (HPC)[1] states:

> You must get informed consent to give treatment (except in an emergency)

The HPC guidance on the rule states that:

> You must explain to the patient, client or user the treatment you are planning on carrying out, the risks involved and any other treatments possible. You must make sure that you get their informed consent to any treatment you do carry out. You must make a record of the person's treatment decisions and pass this on to all members of the health or social-care team involved in their care. In emergencies, you may not be able to explain treatment, get consent or pass on information to other members of the health or social-care team.

However, you should still try to do all of these things as far as you can.

If someone refuses treatment and you believe that it is necessary for their well-being, you must make reasonable efforts to persuade them, particularly if you think that there is a significant immediate risk to life. You must keep your employers' procedures on consent and be aware of any guidance issued by the Department of Health or other appropriate authority in the country in which you practise.

Trespass to the person

A trespass to the person occurs when an individual either apprehends a touching of his/her person (an assault) or the individual is actually touched (a battery) and has not given consent. The person who has suffered the trespass can sue for compensation in the civil courts (and a prosecution could also be brought in criminal cases).

In civil cases, the victim has to prove:

- the touching or the apprehension of the touching;
- that it was a (potentially) direct interference with his/her person.

The victim does not have to show that harm has occurred. This is in contrast to an action for negligence in which the victim must show that harm has resulted from the breach of duty of care (see Chapter 10).

Defences to an action for trespass to the person

The main defence to an action for trespass to the person is that consent was given by a mentally competent person. In addition there are two other defences in law which are:

- statutory authorisation under the Mental Health Act 1983 (as amended by the Mental Health Act 2007) (discussed in Chapter 21);

- statutory authorisation under the Mental Capacity Act 2005 (see below).

Consent

For consent to treatment to be valid, the person giving it must be mentally competent. A child of 16 and 17 has a statutory right to give consent. A child below 16 may give consent if 'Gillick competent' (see Chapter 23). The consent must be given without any duress or force or deceit.

Competence and capacity

It will be seen below that in the case of *Re T*[2] the Court of Appeal emphasised the duty of the health professional to ensure that a person who was refusing a necessary treatment had the capacity to do so. Where there is any doubt about the competence of an individual to give a valid consent there are considerable advantages if the capacity to give a valid consent could be checked by a person who is not involved in the treatment which is being recommended. This person should record his/her actions and observations.

The Mental Capacity Act (MCA) 2005 provides a statutory definition of capacity to give consent, which is specific to the decision that has to be made (i.e. a person may have the mental capacity to give consent to one decision (e.g. what clothes he/she should wear), but not to another decision (e.g. whether to have an appendectomy).

Section 1(2) of the MCA recognises as a basic principle that:

> A person must be assumed to have capacity unless it is established that he lacks capacity.

This presumption can be rebutted on a balance of probabilities (i.e. the civil standard of proof) if there exists an impairment or disturbance in the functioning of the mind or brain and this impairment or disturbance results in an inability to make or communicate decisions. The MCA defines a lack of mental capacity as follows:

A person lacks capacity for the purposes of the MCA in relation to a matter:

if at the material time he is unable to make a decision for himself in relation to the matter because of an impairment of, or a disturbance in the functioning of, the mind or brain.

The impairment or disturbance can be permanent or temporary.

The MCA thus requires a two-stage test of the lack of mental capacity: the existence of an impairment or functioning in the mind or brain and secondly an inability to make or communicate decisions as a result of this defect.

The MCA Section 2(3) states that a lack of capacity cannot be established merely by reference to:

(a)   a person's age or appearance, or
(b)   a condition of his, or an aspect of his behaviour, which might lead others to make unjustified assumptions about his capacity.

Superficial assumptions cannot therefore be the basis of a decision on whether a person has the requisite mental capacity.

Under Section 3(1) of the MCA a person is unable to make a decision for himself if he is unable:

(a)   to understand the information relevant to the decision,
(b)   to retain that information,
(c)   to use or weigh that information as part of the process of making the decision, or
(d)   to communicate his decision (whether by talking, using sign language or any other means).

This follows closely the definition of mental incapacity used in a case where a patient detained in Broadmoor Hospital under the Mental Health Act 1983 refused to consent to a life-saving operation to amputate his leg. The judge in applying the definition concluded that the patient did have the requisite mental capacity to make a decision and his refusal must therefore be accepted.[3]

Section 3(2) of the MCA stated that a person is not to be regarded as unable to understand the information relevant to a decision if he/she is able to understand an explanation of it given to him in a way that is appropriate to his circumstances (using simple language, visual aids or any other means). This requirement could be resource intensive since high technology equipment may be necessary to assist persons with certain types of brain damage to communicate.

Under Section 3(3) the fact that a person is able to retain the information relevant to a decision for a short period only does not prevent him/her from being regarded as able to make the decision.

This would enable persons who have intermittent competence to make decisions during those short breaks of competence.

What information must the person making the decision be able to understand? This information is defined by the MCA in Section 3(4) as including information about the reasonably foreseeable consequences of:

(a)   deciding one way or another, or
(b)   failing to make the decision.

Once an assessment has concluded that a person has the mental capacity to make a specific decision then that person can make a decision for a good reason, a bad reason or no reason at all. The fact that the decision is unwise is not grounds for overruling the person's right to make the decision. However, too many unwise decisions may be grounds for reviewing the assessment of capacity in order to confirm that the person has the requisite mental capacity.

On the other hand, if the assessment is that the person lacks the requisite mental capacity, then decisions must be made in that person's best interests and the MCA provides guidance on how these decisions should be made including the appointment of an independent mental capacity advocate. The other provisions of the MCA are considered in later chapters of this book. (Lasting Powers of Attorney Chapter 24; advance decisions Chapter 25; the Court of Protection and its deputies and new criminal offence of wilful neglect and ill treatment Chapter 22.)

A *Code of Practice*,[4] which was prepared by the Department of Constitutional Affairs is available from its successor, the Ministry of Justice, which provides guidance on the implementation of the MCA.

Different ways of giving consent

Consent can be given by word of mouth, in writing or can be implied, i.e. the non-verbal conduct of the person may indicate that he/she is giving consent. All these forms of giving consent are valid, but where procedures entail risk and/or where there is likely to be a dispute over whether consent was given it is advisable to obtain consent in writing. It is then easier to establish in a court of law that consent was given.

Although consent can be given by word of mouth or by non-verbal communication, there are a few situations where consent must be recorded in writing by law, and Chapter 21 covers the provision of the Mental Health Act 1983 and consent by detained patients. It must be emphasised that where consent is recorded in writing, that document is evidence that consent has given. The actual consent is the state of mind of the person agreeing to have the treatment. The Report of the Inquiry into children's heart surgery at the Bristol Royal Infirmary emphasised the importance of openness and trust between health professionals and patients.[5] It also made significant recommendations on obtaining consent which included the following:

- In a patient-centred healthcare service patients must be involved, wherever possible, in decisions about their treatment and care.
- Information should be tailored to the needs, circumstances and wishes of the individual.
- We note and endorse the recent statement on consent produced by the DH reference guide to consent for examination and treatment (DH 2001). It should inform the practice of all healthcare professionals in the NHS and be introduced into practice in all trusts.

- The process of informing the patient, and obtaining consent to a course of treatment, should be regarded as a process and not a one-off event consisting of obtaining a patient's signature on a form.
- The process of consent should apply not only to surgical procedures but also to all clinical procedures and examinations that involve any form of touching. This must not mean more forms: it means more communication.
- As part of the process of obtaining consent, except when they have indicated otherwise, patients should be given sufficient information about what is to take place, the risks, uncertainties, and possible negative consequences of the proposed treatment, about any alternatives and about the likely outcome, to enable them to make a choice about how to proceed.

Application to physiotherapy

In practice there are many physiotherapy activities and treatments that cannot proceed without the cooperation of the patient and consent to the involvement is often implied from the patient's non-verbal communication. In such cases, therefore, trespass to the person actions are unlikely. The focus is more likely to be on the nature of the information that is made available before the consent is given and the possibility of an action for breach of the duty of care to inform (see below).

Care should however always be taken if it is necessary to examine patients or have physical contact with them to ensure that the patient consents to this contact and continues to consent. When a physiotherapist is seeing a patient over a course of treatment, he/she might record VCG in his/her records, i.e. verbal consent given. What is the legal value of such a record? Imagine if subsequently the patient denied that consent had been given and claimed that a trespass to his or her person had taken place, would VCG have any weight in court? Clearly, in the absence of witnesses, it is one person's word against another. The claimant would have the burden of proving on a balance of probabilities that there was a trespass to his/her person. The treatment should have begun with written evidence that consent was given. In each subsequent visit the physiotherapist should have reassured him/herself that the patient was still giving consent to the treatment and documented that confirmation.

Consent for intimate examinations

Physiotherapists are particularly concerned when they are required to carry out intimate examinations on their patients. Often in even basic care the physiotherapist might have to ask a patient to undress completely. In such circumstances it is advisable for the patient to be warned about this possibility before they attend, so that they can be prepared and bring with them a friend or chaperon. If such examination is necessary and it is a male physiotherapist who is working in the department, a female patient should be given a choice over whether she is to be attended by a male physiotherapist or not. If she agrees, the male physiotherapist should ensure that he is chaperoned and watch carefully for any signs that would suggest that a female colleague should take over. It must be remembered that this is also to protect the male physiotherapist from any allegations in such circumstances. Guidance on the use of chaperones is given in Rule 2.5 of the *Rules of Professional Conduct* 2002, which refers to the document issued by the Industrial Relations Department of the Chartered Society of Physiotherapy (CSP) Chaperoning and Related Issues, which covers the identification of groups of members who may be particularly vulnerable to allegations of indecent or inappropriate behaviour; specific measures that can be taken to minimise the risk of such allegations being made; consent and documentation; and treatment techniques which may lead to an increased risk of such allegations. The HPC has also published guidance on sexual boundary violations by Health Professionals.[6]

In some conditions it may be necessary for the physiotherapist to carry out a pelvic floor examination, which would require vaginal examination and occasionally rectal examination. (See guidance by CSP for post-graduate physiotherapists on pelvic floor and vaginal or ano-rectal assessment 2005.[7]) The patient should be clearly informed about what this examination would entail and specific consent to this should be obtained, preferably in writing. Although consent by word of mouth would be valid in law, it would be more difficult to establish in court where it may be one person's word against another's. Rule 2 of the CSP *Rules of Professional Conduct*[8] states that the use of tick boxes is no longer acceptable and whereas a signature on a consent form does not itself prove that consent is valid, the point of the form is to record the patient's decision, and also increasingly the discussions that have taken place. It suggests that there are some specific physiotherapy procedures where it may help to have written consent:

> movements of force to the cervical spine, vaginal and rectal examinations, nasopharyngeal and tracheal catheter suction with competent patients and exercise tolerance tests for patients with cardiac conditions. When written consent is required and forms are used, some indication of the information given, the options offered and how consent was received should be included to ensure that the form has legal credibility.

Clinical and Occupational Groups may provide guidance on this issue, and employers may already have policies which must be followed for particular interventions.

CSP guidance on consent PA 60 updated August 2005 sets out why consent is important, what is a valid consent, why consent must be voluntary, why there must be sufficient information, if patient lacks capacity, children and young people, obtaining and documenting consent.

There are clear advantages for the physiotherapist in obtaining consent in writing from the patient at the beginning of any treatment plan.

At this time the physiotherapist can explain to the patient the nature and extent of the treatment, its likely effects and any side effects or inherent risks. If it is the intention to use electrotherapy or manipulation, the physiotherapist could explain any risks of the treatment and also obtain the consent of the patient in writing. If at any time, the treatment plan is significantly changed, this may be reflected in a new written consent by the patient.

Consent forms

It will be noted that many physiotherapy treatments will be given without any written evidence of consent. Where, however, it is feared that there may be significant risks of substantial harm or there is likely to be any dispute whether consent was given, it is advisable for consent to be obtained in writing. The NHS Management Executive has issued guidance updated by the Department of Health in 2001 and to be revised following the MCA on consent to treatment[9-11] it gives a form in the appendix that can be used for the consent for treatments given any health professions. This should act as a reminder that the relevant information should be given to patients for them to give valid consent and ensure that all the requisite details are recorded. The Department of Health forms can be used by any health professional and adapted for use for specific treatments.

The NHS Management Executive also recommends that a form could be completed when an adult who lacks mental capacity to give consent to treatment is provided with care in the absence of consent (see below). This form could be adapted for completion by the physiotherapist.

Withdrawal of consent

- What if someone wishes to leave hospital?

It is a principle of consent that a person who has given consent (and has the requisite mental capacity) can withdraw it at any time, unless there is a contractual reason why this is not so. This means that if people wish to leave hospital contrary to their best interests then, unless they lack the capacity to make a valid decision, they are free to go. Clearly there are advantages in obtaining the signature of such patients that the self-discharge or refusal to accept treatment is contrary to clinical advice, but if they refuse to sign a form that they are taking discharge contrary to clinical advice, that refusal must be accepted. It would in such a case be advisable to ensure that there is another professional as a witness to this and that a careful record is made by both professionals.

Refusal to consent

The Court of Appeal set out the basic principles of self-determination of the mentally competent adult in the case of *Re T*.[2] However, it also emphasised the importance of the health professional ensuring that any refusal to give consent to life-saving treatment and care was valid.

Case: *Re T*

A woman suffering from complications after childbirth had made it clear that she would not wish to have a blood transfusion. She was very much under the influence of her mother, a Jehovah's Witness. When it became evident that she would need blood to stay alive, the Court allowed the application of the cohabitee and father for blood to be given. This was on the grounds that her refusal was not valid. This decision was confirmed by the Court of Appeal.

The Court of Appeal laid down the following propositions.

(1) *Prima facie* every adult has the right and capacity to decide whether or not he/she will accept medical treatment, even if a refusal may risk permanent injury to his/her health or even lead to premature death. It matters not whether the reasons for the

refusal are rational or irrational, unknown or even non-existent. However, this presumption of capacity is rebuttable.

(2) An adult may be deprived of his/her capacity to decide either by long-term mental incapacity or retarded development, or by temporary factors such as unconsciousness or confusion or the effects of fatigue, shock, pain or drugs.

(3) If an adult patient did not have the capacity to decide at the time of purported refusal and still does not have that capacity, it is the duty of the doctors to treat him/her in whatever way they consider (in the exercise of their clinical judgment) to be in his/her best interests. (This common law principle is now incorporated in the Mental Capacity Act 2005 – see below).

(4) Doctors faced with a refusal of consent have to give very careful and detailed consideration to what was the patient's capacity to decide at the time when the decision was made.

(5) Doctors must also consider if the refusal has been vitiated because of the will of others who have sought to persuade the patient to refuse. If his/her will has been overborne, the refusal will not represent the true decision.

(6) In all cases doctors will need to consider what is the true scope and basis of the refusal.

(7) Forms of refusal should be redesigned to bring the consequences of a refusal forcibly to the attention of patients.

(8) In cases of doubt as to the effect of a purported refusal of treatment, where failure to treat threatens the patient's life, doctors and health authorities should not hesitate to apply to the courts for assistance. (Since October 2007 and the implementation of the Mental Capacity Act 2005, this court will now be the Court of Protection.)

The right of the adult mentally competent person to refuse food was upheld in the case of a prisoner who had gone on hunger strike.

Although the prisoner was diagnosed as suffering from a personality disorder he was held to be of sound mind so that the law required the Home Office, prison officers and doctors to accept his refusal to take food or drink.[12] This case overruled a case where suffragettes who went on hunger strike were force fed[13] and the defence of acting out of necessity was applied. It is now clear that this defence is only available when the adult lacks the requisite mental capacity (see below).

The principle of the right of self-determination if the adult is mentally competent has subsequently been considered and extended by the Court of Appeal in two cases where a compulsory caesarean had been carried out. In the first case,[14] where the pregnant woman suffered from needle phobia and would not agree to an injection preceding the caesarean, the court held the needle phobia to be so acute as to render her mentally incapable and therefore it was declared that doctors performing a caesarean, acting in her best interests, would not be acting illegally.

The Court of Appeal laid down principles to assist clinicians in treating a pregnant woman:

- In cases where the competence of the mother to make a decision is in doubt, the doctors are advised to seek a ruling from the High Court on the issue of competence. (Since October 2007, application would be made to the Court of Protection under the MCA.)
- Those involved with the pregnancy should identify a potential problem as early as possible so that both hospital and patient can seek legal advice.
- The need for an emergency application to court should be avoided as far as is possible.
- Both parties should be represented, unless the mother refuses. An unconscious mother should be represented by the guardian *ad litem*.
- The Official Solicitor should be notified of all applications.
- There should be some evidence of the lack of competence of the patient (not necessarily from a psychiatrist).

The facts of the second case[15] are shown below.

Case: *St George's Healthcare National Health Service Trust* v. *S*

S was diagnosed with pre-eclampsia and advised that she needed urgent attention, bedrest and admission to hospital for an induced delivery. Without that treatment the health and life of both herself and the unborn child were in real danger. She fully understood the potential risks but rejected the advice. She wanted her baby to be born naturally.

She was then seen by an approved social worker and two doctors in relation to compulsory admission to hospital under Section 2 of the Mental Health Act 1983 for assessment. They repeated the advice that she had been given and she refused to accept it. On the basis of the written medical recommendations of the two doctors the approved social worker applied for her admission to hospital for assessment under Section 2 of the Mental Health Act 1983. Later that day, again against her will, she was transferred to St George's Hospital. In view of her continuing adamant refusal to consent to treatment an application was made *ex parte* on behalf of the hospital authority to Mrs Justice Hogg, who made a declaration that the caesarean section could proceed, dispensing with S's consent to treatment. The operation was carried out and a baby girl delivered. S was then returned to Springfield Hospital and 2 days later her detention under Section 2 of the Mental Health Act was ended.

She then sought judicial review of her detention, the High Court judgment and the caesarean operation.

The Court of Appeal held that the Mental Health Act 1983 could not be deployed to achieve the detention of an individual against his/her will merely because her thinking process was unusual, or even apparently bizarre and irrational, and contrary to the view of the overwhelming majority of the community at large. A woman detained under the Act for mental disorder could not be forced into medical procedures unconnected with her mental condition unless her capacity to consent to such treatment was diminished. The Court of Appeal was not satisfied that S was lawfully detained under Section 2 of the Mental Health Act 1983 because she was not suffering from mental disorder of a nature or degree which warranted her detention in hospital for assessment. Although on the face of the documents her admission would appear to have been legal, her transfer to St George's Hospital was unlawful and at any time she would have been justified in applying for a writ of *habeas corpus*, which would have led to her immediate release. The declaration made by the High Court judge should not have been made on an *ex parte* basis (i.e. without representation of the woman) and was unlawful.

The difference between the two cases is that in the first case the woman was held, as a result of the extreme needle phobia, to be mentally incompetent, and therefore the caesarean could be carried out in her best interests without her consent, whereas in the second case S was not to be held mentally incompetent, and therefore the compulsory caesarean was a trespass to her person. In neither case did the Court consider the rights of the fetus to influence the decision making. The fetus is not regarded in law as a legal personality until birth. Until then the wishes of a mentally competent pregnant woman will prevail whatever the effect on the unborn child.

The existence of a mental illness will not automatically mean that people are incapable of giving a valid refusal of consent to treatment in their best interests, as in the case of *Re C*,[16] where a patient in Broadmoor was considered to have the capacity to refuse a leg amputation that doctors had advised him was indicated as a life-saving measure. An injunction (see glossary) was ordered against any doctors carrying out an amputation on him without his consent.

The principles established by the Court for consent to be seen as competent were:

- comprehending and retaining treatment information;
- believing it; and
- weighing it in the balance to arrive at a choice.

In applying this test to C the judge was completely satisfied that the presumption that C had the right of self-determination had not been replaced. Although his general capacity had been impaired by schizophrenia, he had understood and retained the treatment information, and believed it and had arrived at a clear choice. (See Chapter 21 for further details of the law of consent and the mentally ill.)

Refusal of ventilation

The principles laid down in the case of St George's Healthcare National Health Service Trust were applied by the President of the Family Division in a case where a woman was on life support and was protesting about this ventilation.[17]

Miss B suffered a ruptured blood vessel in her neck that damaged her spinal cord. As a consequence she was paralysed from the neck down and was on a ventilator. She was of sound mind and knew that there was no cure for her condition. She asked for the ventilator to be switched off. Her doctors wished her to try out some special rehabilitation to improve the standard of her care and felt that an intensive care ward was not a suitable location for such a decision to be made. They were reluctant to perform such an action as switching off the ventilator without the court's approval. Miss B applied to court for a declaration to be made that the ventilator could be switched off.

The only issue before Dame Elizabeth Butler-Sloss, President of the Family Division, was did Ms B have the requisite mental capacity to refuse this life-saving treatment? Two psychiatrists gave their expert opinion that she did have the capacity to refuse treatment and in the light of that the judge found in her favour and held that placing her on ventilation against her wishes was a trespass to her person. The following principles were laid down:

- There was a presumption that a patient had the mental capacity to make decisions whether to consent to or refuse medical or surgical treatment offered.

- If mental capacity was not an issue and the patient, having been given the relevant information and offered the available option, chose to refuse that treatment, that decision had to be respected by the doctors, considerations of what the best interests of the patient would involve were irrelevant.

- Concern or doubts about the patient's mental capacity should be resolved as soon as possible by the doctors within the hospital or other normal medical procedures.

- Meanwhile, the patient must be cared for in accordance with the judgment of the doctors as to the patient's best interests.

- It was most important that those considering the issue should not confuse the question of mental capacity with the nature of the decision made by the patient, however grave the consequences. Since the view of the patient might reflect a difference in values rather than an absence of competence the assessment of capacity should be approached with that in mind and doctors should not allow an emotional reaction to or strong disagreement with the patient's decision to cloud their judgment in answering the primary question of capacity.

- Where disagreement still existed about competence, it was of the utmost importance that the patient be fully informed, involved and engaged in the process, which could involve obtaining independent outside help, of resolving the disagreement since the patient's involvement could be crucial to a good outcome.

- If the hospital were faced with a dilemma that doctors did not know how to resolve, this must be recognised and further steps taken as a matter of priority. Those in charge must not allow a situation of deadlock or drift to occur.

- If there was no disagreement about competence, but the doctors were for any reason unable to carry out the patient's wishes, it was their duty to find other doctors who would do so.

- If all appropriate steps to seek independent assistance from medical experts outside the hospital had failed, the hospital should not hesitate to make an application to the High Court or seek the advice of the Official Solicitor.
- The treating clinicians and the hospital should always have in mind that a seriously physically disabled patient who was mentally competent had the same right to personal autonomy and to make decisions as any other person with mental capacity.

It was reported on 29 April 2002 that Ms B had died peacefully in her sleep after the ventilator had been switched off. The principles set out in the Ms B case must now be seen in the light of the Mental Capacity Act 2005.

Mental Capacity Act 2005

The Mental Capacity Act 2005 resulted from over 10 years of discussions and consultations designed to fill the vacuum in statute law on decision making on behalf of a mentally incapacitated adult (i.e. a person over 16 years). The Law Commission had published draft legislation in 1995 in a Mental Incapacity Bill.[18] This was followed by a further consultation document: *Who decides?*[19] And then by a report setting out proposals for change.[20] A draft Bill was prepared[21] and subjected to scrutiny by a Joint Committee of Parliament.[22] The Mental Capacity Bill received royal assent in April 2005 but was not brought fully into force until October 2007. The Act covers the following subjects:

- Basic principles (see below)
- Definition of capacity (see above)
- Acting in the best interests of an adult lacking mental capacity (see below)
- Bournewood safeguards (see Chapter 21)
- Independent Mental Capacity Advocates (see Chapter 22)
- Lasting powers of attorney (see Chapter 25)
- Advance decisions (see Chapter 25)

- Court of Protection, deputies, visitors, Office of Public Guardian (see Chapter 22)
- Criminal offence of wilful neglect and ill treatment (Chapter 22)
- Code of Practice (see below).

Basic principles

Section 1 of the MCA sets out the basic principles that apply for the purposes of the Act. They are shown in Box 7.1.

Box 7.1   Basic principles of the Mental Capacity Act 2005.

- A person must be assumed to have capacity unless it is established that he/she lacks capacity.
- A person is not to be treated as unable to make a decision unless all practicable steps to help him/her to do so have been taken without success.
- A person is not to be treated as unable to make a decision merely because he/she makes an unwise decision.
- An act done, or decision made, under this Act for or on behalf of a person who lacks capacity must be done, or made, in his/her best interests.
- Before the act is done, or the decision is made, regard must be had to whether the purpose for which it is needed can be as effectively achieved in a way that is less restrictive of the person's rights and freedom of action.

These principles would apply to all persons who are likely to be caring for or making decisions on behalf of those who may lack the requisite mental capacity.

Mental capacity

The MCA sets out a definition of mental capacity, which is considered earlier. This replaces previous case law but will in time become itself the subject of judicial decision making as disputes arise as to how this decision is to be applied or interpreted.

Best interests

Where, but only where, the patient lacks the capacity to give consent to treatment, treatment can proceed on the basis that it is in the best interests of that individual. This is laid down by the Mental Capacity Act 2005, which replaces the right at common law (i.e. judge-made law) to act out of necessity in the best interests of the

mentally incompetent person. Where the health professional acts in the best interests of a person lacking the requisite mental capacity, he or she would not be committing a trespass to the person. The common law ruling was made by the House of Lords in the case of *Re F*.[23] In that case the House of Lords declared that it was lawful for doctors to sterilise a mentally handicapped person who lacked the capacity to give a valid consent provided that they acted in her best interests. The court did, however, require a reference to the court to be made in future cases, and a Practice Direction[24] was issued.

Section 4 of the MCA outlines the steps that must be taken into account in determining the best interests of a person incapable of making a specific decision and is shown in Box 7.2.

Box 7.2   Section 4 of the Mental Capacity Act 2005: acting in the best interests.

4. (1)   In determining for the purposes of this Act what is in a person's best interests, the person making the determination must not make it merely on the basis of
(a)   the person's age or appearance, or
(b)   a condition of his, or an aspect of his behaviour, which might lead others to make unjustified assumptions about what might be in his best interests.

4. (2)   The person making the determination must consider all the relevant circumstances and, in particular, take the following steps.

4. (3)   He must consider
(a)   whether it is likely that the person will at some time have capacity in relation to the matter in question, and
(b)   if it appears likely that he will, when that is likely to be.

4. (4)   He must, so far as reasonably practicable, permit and encourage the person to participate, or to improve his ability to participate, as fully as possible in any act done for him and any decision affecting him.

4. (5)   Where the determination relates to life-sustaining treatment he must not, in considering whether the treatment is in the best interests of the person concerned, be motivated by a desire to bring about his death.

4. (6)   He must consider, so far as is reasonably ascertainable
(a)   the person's past and present wishes and feelings (and, in particular, any relevant written statement made by him when he had capacity),
(b)   the beliefs and values that would be likely to influence his decision if he had capacity, and
(c)   the other factors that he would be likely to consider if he were able to do so.

4. (7)   He must take into account, if it is practicable and appropriate to consult them, the views of
    (a)   anyone named by the person as someone to be consulted on the matter in question or on matters of that kind,
    (b)   anyone engaged in caring for the person or interested in his welfare,
    (c)   any donee of a lasting power of attorney granted by the person, and
    (d)   any deputy appointed for the person by the court, as to what would be in the person's best interests and, in particular, as to the matters mentioned in subsection (6).

4. (8)   The duties imposed by subsections (1) to (7) also apply in relation to the exercise of any powers which
    (a)   are exercisable under a lasting power of attorney, or
    (b)   are exercisable by a person under this Act where he reasonably believes that another person lacks capacity.

4. (9)   In the case of an act done, or a decision made, by a person other than the court, there is sufficient compliance with this section if (having complied with the requirements of subsections (1) to (7)) he reasonably believes that what he does or decides is in the best interests of the person concerned.

4. (10)   'Life-sustaining treatment' means treatment which in the view of a person providing health care for the person concerned is necessary to sustain life.

4. (11)   'Relevant circumstances' are those
    (a)   of which the person making the determination is aware, and
    (b)   which it would be reasonable to regard as relevant.

Determining the best interests of a person lacking the requisite mental capacity could be a slow and lengthy process and it is helpful if each department has a pro forma to ensure that the correct steps have been taken and full consultation has taken place with those able to give information on the matters listed in Section 4(6). As in the assessment of mental capacity, no superficial assumptions should be made on the basis of a person's appearance, so in determining what are a person's best interests, reliance cannot be based solely on a person's age, appearance or behaviour or condition.

Restraint

The MCA (apart from the Bournewood safeguards – see below and Chapter 21) permits limited restraint to be used but only in specified circumstances. These circumstances are shown in Box 7.3.

Box 7.3   Use of restraint and the Mental Capacity Act 2005 Section 6: conditions.

The first condition is that D reasonably believes that it is necessary to do the act in order to prevent harm to P.

The second is that the act is a proportionate response to

    (a)   the likelihood of P's suffering harm, and
    (b)   the seriousness of that harm.

(4)   For the purposes of this section D restrains P if he
    (a)   uses, or threatens to use, force to secure the doing of an act which P resists, or
    (b)   restricts P's liberty of movement, whether or not P resists.

If the conditions set out in Box 7.3 are satisfied then limited restraint could be used if it is in a person's best interests.

The Bournewood safeguards

The House of Lords, in the case of *R* v. *Bournewood Community and Mental Health NHS Trust*,[25] held that the common law power to act out of necessity in the best interests of the patient also included the right to admit adult mentally incapacitated patients to psychiatric hospital. It overruled a decision of the Court of Appeal that such patients had to be detained under the Mental Health Act 1983 where this applied. However, the European Court of Justice[26] overruled the House of Lords holding that the detention of a person incapable of consenting to admission other than under the Mental Health Act was contrary to their human rights as set out in article 5. The Government was therefore compelled to fill the gap revealed by this decision and did so by amending the Mental Capacity Act 2005 to provide measures which are known as the Bournewood safeguards. These are considered in Chapter 21.

Code of Practice

The MCA (S 42 (1)) places a duty upon the Lord Chancellor to provide a Code or Codes of Practice for the guidance of the following persons or covering certain topics:

(a)   persons assessing whether a person has capacity in relation to any matter
(b)   persons acting in connection with the care or treatment of another person
(c)   donees of lasting powers of attorney
(d)   deputies appointed by the court
(e)   persons carrying out research in reliance on any provision made by or under the Act (and otherwise with respect to Sections 30–34)
(f)   independent mental capacity advocates
   (f)a   persons exercising functions under Schedule A1 (i.e. the Bournewood safeguards)
   (f)b   representatives appointed under Part 10 of Schedule A1
(g)   with respect of the provisions of Sections 24–26 (advance decisions and apparent advance decisions), and
(h)   with respect to such other matters concerned with this Act as he thinks fit.

The Code of Practice came into force in April 2007 and is to be updated to incorporate guidance on the Bournewood safeguards. It can be accessed on line at the Ministry of Justice's website.[27]

Situation: who decides?

> An elderly man had a stroke and decisions had to be made about his ongoing treatment. The Consultant asked his daughter if she would give consent for him to have an operation.

In this situation, the Mental Capacity Act 2005 now applies. If the father is incapable of making his own decisions and has not drawn up an advance decision applicable to the current situation (see Chapter 25) or appointed a donee under a lasting power of attorney to make decisions on his behalf (see Chapter 25) then action must be taken in his best interests. The daughter does not herself have the legal right to give or withhold consent on behalf of her father but the person making the decision (and this would be the clinician responsible for the treatment) must ascertain what are in the best interests of the patient and find out from relatives and others close to the patient what the views and opinions of the patient would have been had he been able to make his own decisions. In Chapter 25 the case of Tony Bland[28] the Hillesborough victim in a persistent vegetative state and the decision to discontinue artificial feeding is considered.

Duty to inform

As part of the duty of care owed in the law of negligence the professional has a duty to inform the patient about the significant risks of substantial harm which could occur if treatment were to proceed.

If the harm has not been explained to the patient and the harm then occurs, the patient can claim that, had he/she known of this possibility, he/she would not have agreed to undergo the treatment. The patient could then bring an action in negligence. To succeed the patient would have to show:

- that there was a duty of care to give specific information;
- the defendant failed to give this information and in so doing was therefore in breach of the reasonable standard of care which should have been provided;
- as a result of this failure to inform, the patient agreed to the treatment; and
- subsequently suffered the harm.

The leading case is that of Sidaway,[29] where the House of Lords stated that the professional was required in law to provide information to the patient according to the Bolam test, i.e. the standard of the reasonable practitioner following the accepted approved standard of care (see Chapter 10).

Causal link between the failure to notify of reasonably foreseeable risks and the injury sustained

In 2002 the House of Lords had to decide if the claimant was required to prove that had she been told of the risks she would not have agreed to the proposed treatment which resulted in the harm of which she should have been warned.

Case: *Chester* v. *Afshar* (2002)[30]

The patient suffered from severe back pain and gave consent to an operation for the removal of three intravertebral discs. The neurosurgeon failed to give a warning to her about the slight risk of post-operative paralysis that the patient suffered following the operation. The trial judge held that the doctor was not negligent in his conduct of the operation, but was negligent in failing to warn her of the slight risk of paralysis which she suffered. He also held that, had she been aware of the risk, she would have sought advice on alternatives to surgery and the operation would not have taken place when it did, if at all. He therefore held that there was a sufficient causal link between the defendant's failure to warn and the damage sustained by the claimant and that link was not broken by the possibility that the claimant might have consented to surgery in the future. He gave judgment for damages to be assessed. The defendant appealed to the Court of Appeal which dismissed the appeal. The defendant then appealed to the House of Lords which by a majority verdict dismissed his appeal.

The House of Lords held that the claimant had shown that she had been notified of the risk of paralysis, which in fact occurred, she would have had to think further about undergoing the surgery and therefore she had established a causal link between the breach and the injury she had sustained and the defendant was liable in damages.

To ensure that the patient understands the information which is given, there are considerable advantages in a written handout being provided (checking of course that the patient is literate). This would also assist if there were any dispute over the information having been given.

In Chapter 9 the duty of a doctor to give full information as a requirement by the General Medical Council (GMC) is considered.

Application to physiotherapy

The duty placed upon the physiotherapist is that he/she should ensure that the patient is given information about the significant risks of substantial harm which could arise from treatment. He/she would be judged by the standard of the reasonable practitioner in that situation with that specific patient. (This is further discussed in Chapter 10 on negligence.) This requires the physiotherapist to ensure that he/she maintains his/her competence and knowledge about current issues and research. It also requires the physiotherapist to make an assessment of the competence of clients to understand what they are being told, and to use language which conveys the necessary information accurately and effectively. In difficult situations it would be advisable for a physiotherapist to ask a colleague, possibly a psychologist, to provide an independent assessment of the mental competence of the patient.

Many of the clinical interest groups attached to the CSP have drawn up their own guidance and information on consent to treatment and risk assessment for their particular specialty. For example, the Manipulation Association of Chartered Physiotherapists in conjunction with the University of Nottingham[31] has drawn up an information document designed to assist clinicians in their clinical reasoning during their assessment of neck pain and headache in relation to potential neurovascular dysfunction. It includes a discussion on the real risk of arterial complications following manual therapy. This information would be vital to clinicians in fulfilling their duty of care to inform the patient about significant risks of substantial harm.

Lisa Roberts discusses an information leaflet provided for patients attending a musculoskeletal department.[32] She concludes that there are advantages in ensuring that any information leaflet is objectively scored for readability, peer reviewed for content, evaluated and tested by patients. She also emphasises the importance of periodic reinforcement of information given to patients. The leaflet discussed is available electronically from the author.

Research into written information given to patients after breast surgery led to a recommendation that the use of post-operative exercises should be commenced earlier.[33] The authors point to the lack of a date of publication for the information making it more difficult for the user to be sure that they are following up-to-date information.

Kim Jones discusses the problems involved in explaining rehabilitation theory to neurologically impaired patients and their families,[34] in particular explaining the concept of neural plasticity. She uses the analogy of a path between a house and a grain store through a cornfield to communicate to patients how rehabilitation can take place.

Debate arose over the information, including pictorial information, which should be given to patients about lymphoedema following publication of the book written by Michael Mason, *Living with Lymphoedema*. He argues that:

> most patients . . . request as much information as possible about their medical problems. Lymphoedema patients are no different. They want to know, among other things, the prognosis, the treatment and how bad their condition can become if left untreated. Once they have all of this information, patients are then in the position to make an informed decision about their treatment.[35]

This therefore justifies the use of before and after pictures. Most physiotherapists would probably accept that this is sound practice, providing the information is given sensitively.

Written information provided in a department should be reviewed critically to assess its readability by patients. Judith Chapman and John Langridge assessed the physiotherapy health education literature distributed by a physiotherapy service[36] and concluded that many leaflets were written at a level too high for the average comprehension of their patients. The authors recommend the use of an uncomplicated method for assessing reading levels of written materials.

Communication should of course be a two-way process and in a stimulating paper Barbara Martlew[37] describes a study in a day hospice to examine patients' perceptions of the problems caused by their terminal illness, the relevance and benefit of physiotherapy and the factors contributing to quality of life. Recommendations are made on the benefits of listening sensitively, of being aware of the underlying fear that symptoms indicate disease progression, and on utilising the quality of life indicators when setting goals for physiotherapy intervention.

Analysing the reasons why patients fail to attend for out-patient treatment can also provide an important way of improving communication with patients. Jane Armistead studied initial non-attendance rates for physiotherapy.[38] Rates of attendance were better if made by telephone than by post and referrals from GPs were more likely to lead to non-attendance than referrals from consultants. The author concludes that there is a need to 'provide a flexible, responsive service and stimulate the moral responsibility of the consumers.'

Questions and exercises

1   Analyse your practice in relation to obtaining consent from the patient and decide if it could be improved.

2   Draw up a form for consent to physiotherapy.

3   Prepare a hand out for the client/patient giving information about the nature of any specific treatment which you provide, setting out any inherent risks.

Conclusion

The physiotherapist must accept that the law now enshrined in the Mental Capacity Act 2005, recognises the autonomy of the mentally competent patient to decide whether or not to participate in treatment activities. The onus is on the health professional to inform the patient fully about the benefits and risks of the treatment. The implementation of the Mental Capacity Act 2005 means that there is now in place a statutory framework for decision making on behalf of those who lack the requisite mental capacity. Each department should have a copy of the Code of Practice to assist individual practitioners in the determination of capacity and the assessment of the individual's best interests. The GMC has updated its guidance on consent after collaborating with National Theatre actors who performed scenes which raised the issues of patients, carers and doctors. The guidance reflects the changing relationship between doctors and patients, with the decline in deference and demands for more information. The guidance, which is available on the GMC website, would be of value to physiotherapists.[39]

References

1   Health Professions Council (2004 reprinted 2007) *Standards of Conduct, Performance and Ethics*. HPC, London.

2   *Re T (Adult: Refusal of Medical Treatment* [1992] 4 All ER 649.

3   *C (re) (an adult) (refusal of medical treatment)* [1994] 1 All ER 819.

4   Department of Constitutional Affairs (2007) *Code of Practice*. Available from www.justice.gov.uk

5   Bristol Royal Infirmary Inquiry (Kennedy Report) (2001) *Learning from Bristol: the Report of the Public Inquiry into Children's Heart Surgery at the Bristol Royal Infirmary 1984–1995*. Command paper Cm 5207. The Stationery Office, London.

6   Halter, M., Brown, H., Stone, J. (2007) *Sexual Boundary Violations by Health Professionals – An Overview of the Published Empirical Literature*. CHRE, London.

7   Chartered Society of Physiotherapy for post graduate physiotherapists on pelvic floor and vaginal or ano-rectal assessment. PA 19A. Information paper October 2005.

8   Chartered Society of Physiotherapy (2002) *Rules of Professional Conduct*. CSP, London.

9   NHS Management Executive (1990) *A Guide to Consent for Examination and Treatment*. (HC(90)22 and HSG(92)32). Department of Health, London.

10   Department of Health (2001) *Reference Guide to Consent for Examination or Treatment*. DH, London. Available from www.dh.gov.uk/consent

11   Department of Health (2001) *Good Practice in Consent Implementation Guide*. DH, London.

12   *Secretary of State for the Home Department* v. *Robb* [1995] 1 All ER 677.

13 *Leigh* v. *Gladstone* (1909) 25 TLR 139.

14 *Re M B (Caesarian Section)* The Times Law Report, 18 April 1997; [1997] 2 FLR 426.

15 *St George's Healthcare National Health Service Trust* v. *S; R* v. *Collins and Others, ex parte S.* The Times Law Report, 8 May 1998. [1998] 3 All ER 673; *St George's NHS Trust* v. *S* (Guidelines) (No 2) [1999] Fam 26.

16 *Re C* (Adult: Refusal of Medical Treatment) [1994] 1 All ER 819.

17 *Re B (Consent to treatment: capacity),* The Times Law Report, 26 March 2002; [2002] 2 All ER 449.

18 Law Commission (1995) *Mental Incapacity.* HMSO, London.

19 Lord Chancellor (1997) *Who Decides?* Lord Chancellor's Office, Stationery Office, London

20 Lord Chancellor's Office (1999) *Making Decisions: The Government's Proposals for Decision Making on Behalf of Mentally Incapacitated Adults.* Stationery Office, London.

21 Department of Health Draft Mental Incapacity Bill. CM 5859 June 2003.

22 House of Lords and House of Commons Joint Committee on the Draft Mental Incapacity Bill Session 2002–3 HL paper 189-1; HC 1083-1.

23 *F* v. *West Berkshire Health Authority and another* [1989] 2 All ER 545.

24 Practice Note [1993] 3 All ER 222 (replaces previous Practice Note issued 1989).

25 *R* v. *Bournewood Community and Mental Health NHS Trust, ex parte L* (HL) [1998] 1 All ER 634.

26 *R* v. *Bournewood Community and Mental Health NHS Trust ex parte L* [1998] 3 All ER 289; [1999] AC 458; *L.* v. *United Kingdom* (Application No 45508/99) Times Law Report, 19 October 2004.

27 www.justice.gov.uk

28 *Airedale NHS Trust* v. *Bland* [1993] 1 All ER 821.

29 *Sidaway* v. *Bethlem Royal Hospital Governors* [1985] 1 All ER 643.

30 *Chester* v. *Afshar,* The Times Law Report, 13 June 2002; [2002] 3 All ER 552 CA; The Times Law Report, 19 October, 2004 HL; [2004] UKHL 41; [2004] 3 W.L.R. 927.

31 Manipulation Association of Chartered Physiotherapists and the University of Nottingham (2007) *Cervical Arterial Dysfunction and Manipulative Therapy.* Information Document. MACP, London.

32 Roberts, L. (2006) First Impressions: An Information Leaflet Provided for Patients Attending a Musculoskeletal Department. *Physiotherapy* **92**, 179–186.

33 Todd, J., Topping, A. (2005) A Survey of Written Information on the Use of Post-operative Exercises after Breast Cancer. *Physiotherapy* **91**, 87–93.

34 Jones, K. (1997) The Grain Store Analogy: Explaining Rehabilitation Theory to Neurologically Impaired Patients and their Families. *Physiotherapy,* **83**, 575–577.

35 Mason, M. (1996) Letter to the Editor: Facing the Frightful Facts. *Physiotherapy* **82**, 3, 216.

36 Chapman, J., Langridge, J. (1997) Physiotherapy Health Education Literature. *Physiotherapy,* **83**, 406–412.

37 Martlew, B. (1996) What Do You Let the Patient Tell You? *Physiotherapy,* **82**, 558–565.

38 Armistead, J. (1997) An Evaluation of Initial Non-attendance Rates for Physiotherapy. *Physiotherapy,* **83**, 591–596.

39 www.gmc-uk.org

8 Confidentiality

All physiotherapists, whether working in the public or private sector, have a duty to maintain the confidentiality of information obtained from or about the patient. This chapter explores the source of this obligation and the exceptions recognised in law to the duty. The following topics are considered:

- The nature of the duty
- The Data Protection Act 1998
- Exceptions to the duty of confidentiality
- Implications for the physiotherapist
- Link with ethical issues
- The future

The nature of the duty

The duty to respect patient confidentiality arises from a variety of sources that are set out in Figure 8.1.

The Rules of Professional Conduct:
HPC and CSP

Each registered professional has certain professional obligations that are enforceable through the fitness to practice machinery set up under the Health Professions Council.

Clause 2 of the HPC *Standards of Conduct, Performance and Ethics*[1] requires its registrants to:

> Respect the confidentiality of your patients, clients and users.

It amplifies this by requiring the registrant:

> to treat information about patients, clients or users as confidential and use it only for the purpose for which it was given. You must not knowingly release any personal or confidential information to anyone who is not entitled to it, and you should check that people who ask for information are entitled to it.
>
> You must only use information about a service user:
> To continue to care for that person; or
> For purposes where that person has given you specific permission to use the information.

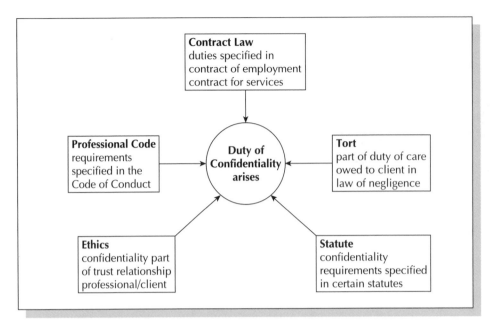

Figure 8.1   Sources of the obligation to respect the confidentiality of patient information

You must also keep to the conditions of any relevant data protection legislation and always follow best practice for handling confidential information. Best practice is likely to change over time, and you must stay up to date.

The HPC published a consultation document on confidentiality guidance for registrants in June 2007. The consultation has now ended and the final guidance awaited.[2]

Rule 3 of the Rules of Professional Conduct of the CSP[3] sets out the duty of the physiotherapist in relation to confidentiality:

Chartered physiotherapists shall ensure the confidentiality and security of information acquired in a professional capacity.

The commentary on Rule 3 points out that:

The Data Protection Act (1998) forms the legal framework for this Rule and a number of NHS circulars are also relevant. This Rule outlines the physiotherapist's responsibilities in relation to the confidentiality and security of information gained by him/her during the course of practice. All the information, which the patient gives to the physiotherapist, is treated in the strictest confidence. All personnel (e.g. clerical and reception staff) involved with patients in the delivery of a physiotherapy service should be made aware of and adhere to all aspects of this Rule.

It also points out that 'The Standards of Physiotherapy Practice, particularly Core Standards 3, 12, 13, 14 and 15 and Service Standards 19 and 20, provide explicit statements to assist physiotherapists in the practical application of all aspects of this Rule.'

Standard 3 relates to the confidentiality of information about the patient and sets eight criteria with guidance on each. These criteria include ensuring privacy for obtaining confidential information, obtaining the written consent of the patient before disclosing clinical information (including videos) for teaching purposes, ensuring the security in transmitting information.

The contract of employment/contract for services

The employed health professional also has an obligation to observe the confidentiality of patient information that derives from the contract of employment and is enforceable by the employer. This will usually be set out expressly in the contract of employment, but, even if the contract is silent on the topic, the courts may imply into it such a term. Should the health professional be in breach of this expressed or implied term, then the employer can take appropriate action through the disciplinary machinery. This may be simply counselling or an oral warning, or any of the stages in the disciplinary procedure may be invoked, depending on the circumstances. In serious cases, the employer may be considered justified in dismissing the employee. (In such a case if the employer has acted unreasonably and the employee has the necessary continuous service requirement (see Chapter 17) the employee could challenge the employer's action by an application to an employment tribunal for unfair dismissal.)

Those who work as self-employed professionals do not have an obligation to an employer but they do have a contract for services with their patients which may impose conditions relating to confidentiality. A confidentiality term may also be implied into the contract. Should the health professional be in breach of these contractual conditions, then the patient could bring an action in the civil courts and have the usual remedies for breach of contract (see Chapter 19 on the private practitioner).

The duty of care owed in the law of negligence

The health professional owes a duty to the patient to retain information given to her in confidence.

Case: *Furniss* v. *Fitchett* [4]

In this New Zealand case, the court upheld an action for damages in the tort of negligence for breach of confidence. A doctor treating the plaintiff had given to the patient's husband a letter about the patient's mental state, which was used by the husband's solicitor in matrimonial proceedings.

The doctor was held to be in breach of the duty of care which he owed to the patient.

Should the health professional be in breach of this duty, then the patient could bring an action against the employer of the health professional on the basis of its vicarious liability for the actions of an employee acting in course of employment.

One weakness of the patient's right of action in the law of negligence is that the patient has to prove harm. There may be potential, following unauthorised disclosure, for harm to arise, but until it does so arise the patient cannot obtain compensation. He/she might however obtain an injunction to prevent the disclosure.

Case: *X* v. *Y* [5]

The court ordered an injunction to be issued to prevent the disclosure by the press of the identity of doctors suffering from AIDS. Two GPs were diagnosed as having contracted AIDS. They received counselling in a local hospital while continuing with their medical practice. A journalist heard of the situation from an employee of the health authority and wrote an article for a national newspaper. The health authority sought an injunction to prevent any further disclosure of the information obtained from the patients' records. The judge granted the injunction on the grounds that the records of hospital patients, particularly those suffering from this appalling condition, should be as confidential as the courts could properly make them. He rejected the defendant's argument that it was in the public interest for the identity of these doctors to be known.

The judge did not however agree to the health authority's application for disclosure of the name of the employee who had given the information to

- Abortion Regulations 1991 (made under the Abortion Act 1967)
- NHS (Venereal Disease) Regulations 1974
- Human Fertilisation and Embryology Act 1990 [as amended by the Human Fertilisation and Embryology (Disclosure of Information) Act 1992]
- Data Protection Act 1998

Figure 8.2   Statutory prohibition against disclosure

the journalist. He held that the exceptions under section 10 of the Contempt of Court Act 1981 to the principle that the court cannot require disclosure from a journalist did not apply to the situation and the journalist was entitled to protect his source.

Another difficulty is that if a patient is wishing to preserve secrecy of information, then the danger of a court action is that the dispute will be brought into the open and the publicity will then defeat the patient's main objective. This perhaps explains why there are very few decided cases on confidentiality.

The duty set out in specific statutes

Figure 8.2 identifies the statutes that make it an offence to disclose specified information.

Where information is disclosed in breach of these statutory provisions, the holder of the records or the patient can initiate the appropriate enforcement machinery. The Data Protection Act 1998 is considered below. (See also Chapter 9 on the Data Protection Act provisions in relation to subject access.)

Human Rights Act 1998

Article 8 of the European Convention on Human Rights can be invoked where privacy has been invaded. The articles can be found in Appendix 1. Article 8 recognises the right to respect for private and family life:

1. Everyone has the right to respect for his private and family life, his home and his correspondence.

The right is however qualified by paragraph 2:

2. There shall be no interference by a public authority with the exercise of this right except such as is in accordance with the law and is necessary in a democratic society in the interests of national security, public safety or the economic wellbeing of the country, for the prevention of disorder or crime, for the protection of health or morals, or for the protection of the rights and freedoms of others.

The Court of Appeal held that there was a breach of Article 8 rights when a photographer took a photo covertly using a long-range lens in a public place of the baby son of the author J. K. Rowling without the consent of the parents and knowing that they would object on the child's behalf to the photo being taken.[6]

Article 8 can clash with Article 10, which recognises a qualified right of freedom of expression, and there have been several cases where celebrities have claimed Article 8 rights but the press have demanded freedom of expression under Article 10. For example in the case of Naomi Campbell, the House of Lords in a majority decision held that even though she had brought into the public domain the fact that she was being treated for drug addiction, certain information could still be kept confidential, including the time, form and place of the drug therapy and she was therefore entitled to damages against the Mirror Group Newspapers for that breach of confidence.[7] In this respect her right to privacy succeeded against the right to freedom of expression. Similarly, in a case brought by Max Mosley against the *News of the World*, which published accounts of his sado-masochistic sex sessions, the judge decided that there was no evidence of Nazi behaviour and his private rights under Article 8 should be upheld. There was no public interest which justified a breach of Article 8.[8]

The European Court of Human Rights held that secret interception by the Ministry of Defence of the external communications of Liberty were not dealt with adequately under the Interception of Communications Act 1985 with sufficient clarity to give individuals protection and there was therefore a breach of Article 8 rights.[9]

The trust obligation between health professional and patient

This duty was acknowledged by the House of Lords[10] in the case known as 'the Spycatcher case'. It was accepted that as a broad principle a duty of confidence arises:

- if information is confidential; and
- comes to the knowledge of a person where he or she has notice, or is held to have agreed, that the information is confidential, (with the effect that it would be just that he or she should be precluded from disclosing the information); and
- it is in the public interest that the confidentiality should be protected.

Clearly these principles would apply to information which the physiotherapist was given by or about a patient. The principles were applied in the case of *Stephens* v. *Avery*.[11]

Case: *Stephens* v. *Avery*

In this case concerning unconscionable disclosure the plaintiff and first defendant were close friends who freely discussed matters of a personal and private nature on the express basis that what the plaintiff told the first defendant was secret and disclosed in confidence. The first defendant passed on to the second and third defendants, who were the editor and publisher of a newspaper, details of the plaintiff's sexual conduct, including details of the plaintiff's lesbian relationship with a woman who had been killed by her husband. The plaintiff brought an action against the defendants claiming damages on the grounds that the information was confidential and was knowingly published by the newspaper in breach of the duty of confidence owed by the first defendant to the plaintiff.

In an action by the defendants to strike out the claim as disclosing no reasonable cause of action the defendants failed and appealed to the Chancery Division. They lost this appeal on the grounds that, although the courts would not enforce a duty of confidence relating to matters which had a grossly immoral tendency, information relating to sexual conduct could be the subject of a legally enforceable duty of confidence if it would be unconscionable for the person who had received information on the express basis that it was confidential subsequently to reveal that information to another.

Data Protection Act 1998

This Act, which replaces the 1984 Act, applies to manually held records as well as computerised records. The Information Commissioner is responsible for the enforcement of both the Data Protection and the Freedom of Information Acts.[12]

The European Directive on Data Protection[13] was implemented in this country by the Data Protection Act 1998 (DPA). Under the legislation, members had to establish a set of principles with which users of personal information must comply. The legislation also gives individuals the right to gain access to information held about them (see Chapter 9) and provides for a supervisory authority to oversee and enforce the law. NHS guidance on the Act was provided by a circular in March 2000.[14] The NHS Information Authority was abolished in April 2005 and its work undertaken by NHS Connecting for Health.[15] (*The Information Security Management: Code of Practice* prepared by the Department of Health (DH) is considered in Chapter 12.) An explanation of the Data Protection Act 1998 is also available from the Data Protection Commissioner now known as the Information Commissioner.[16] Good practice notes on the Data Protection Act are available from the Information Commissioner's website.[17]

The Data Protection Act 1998, unlike its 1984 predecessor, applies to manual records if they form part of a relevant filing system as well as to computerised records and provides tighter provisions on the processing of sensitive personal data. New rules for the transfer of personal data outside the European Community are set out.

The person responsible for the enforcement and overseeing of Data Protection legislation was known as the Data Protection Commissioner (the Registrar under the 1984 Act), but since that individual is now also responsible for the implementation of the Freedom of Information Act 2000 (see Chapter 9) he/she is now known as the Information Commissioner, with both Acts coming within his or her jurisdiction, together with the Environmental Information Regulations and the Privacy and Electronic Communications Regulations. Good practice notes, codes of practice and technical guidance notes on all this legislation are available on the Information Commissioner's website.[17] The Information Commissioner's Office has legal powers to ensure that organisations comply with the legal requirements and details of cases where these powers of enforcement have been used are available on the Information Commissioner's Office website.

An application for judicial review by the Secretary of State of an information tribunal decision that had quashed a ministerial certificate claiming exemption from providing subject access on grounds of national security failed. The High Court held that the Information Commissioner had the power to check whether an exemption was properly claimed.[18.]

The Data Protection Act 1998 lays down statutory principles, which are set out in Figure 9.1.

Terminology

'Data' means information which:

(a) is being processed by means of equipment operating automatically in response to instructions given for that purpose;

(b) is recorded with the intention that it should be processed by means of such equipment;

(c) is recorded as part of a relevant filing system or with the intention that it should form part of a relevant filing system;

(d) does not fall within paragraph (a), (b) or (c) but forms part of an accessible record as defined by Section 68.

'Personal data' (as defined in the DPA 1998) are data which relate to a living individual who can be identified (a) from those data, or (b) from those data and other information which is in the possession of, or likely to be in the possession of, the data controller – and includes any expression of opinion about the individual and any indications of the intentions of the data controller or any other person in respect of the individual. Guidance on the meaning of personal data was published by the Information Commissioner in August 2007,[17] and stated that information that is not personal data today may become personal data as technology advances. The Court of Appeal in 2003 in the case brought by Michael Durant against the Financial Services Authority defined personal data narrowly. Subsequently the Information Commissioner updated the guidance and says that information could count as personal data even if it does not include a person's name. For example:

> There will be circumstances where the data you hold enables you to identify an individual whose name you do not know and you may never intend to discover. Similarly, a combination of data about gender, age, and grade or salary may well enable you to identify a particular employee even without a name or job title.

'Sensitive personal data' are personal data consisting of information as specified in Section 2 of the 1998 Act. Section 2 includes racial or ethnic origins, political opinions and his/her physical or mental health or condition or sexual life.

'Data subject' is the individual who is the subject of the personal data.

'Data controller' means a person who, either alone or with others, determines the purposes for which and the manner in which any personal data are, or are to be, processed.

'Processing' includes obtaining, recording or holding information or carrying out any operation, including retrieval or consultation or use of the information, and disclosure (definition abbreviated by author).

The Data Protection Act 1998 imposes constraints on the processing of personal information in relation to living individuals. It identifies eight data protection principles that set out standards for information handling. (These can be seen in Figure 9.1.)

In the context of confidentiality, the most significant principles are:

- the first, which requires processing to be fair and lawful and imposes other restrictions;

- the second, which requires personal data to be processed for one or more specified and lawful purposes;
- the seventh, which requires personal data to be protected against unauthorised or unlawful processing and against accidental loss, destruction or damage.

The Data Protection Act prohibits processing unless conditions set out in two particular schedules are met. Schedule 2 conditions apply to all processing whereas Schedule 3 provides additional and more exacting conditions that only apply to the processing of sensitive personal data, such as health information. Schedule 2 is shown in Figure 8.3 and Schedule 3 is shown in Figure 8.4. The DH in its *NHS Code of Practice on Confidentiality* notes that

> The consent of the data subject is one of the conditions in each Schedule that might be satisfied. However only one condition in

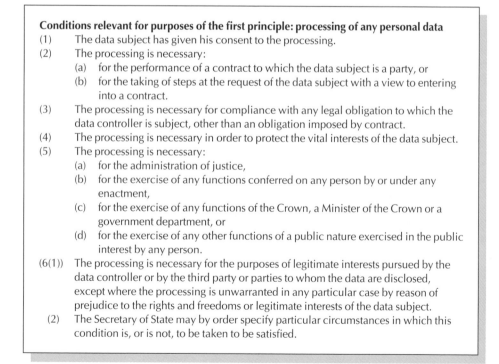

Conditions relevant for purposes of the first principle: processing of any personal data

(1)   The data subject has given his consent to the processing.

(2)   The processing is necessary:
    (a) for the performance of a contract to which the data subject is a party, or
    (b) for the taking of steps at the request of the data subject with a view to entering into a contract.

(3)   The processing is necessary for compliance with any legal obligation to which the data controller is subject, other than an obligation imposed by contract.

(4)   The processing is necessary in order to protect the vital interests of the data subject.

(5)   The processing is necessary:
    (a) for the administration of justice,
    (b) for the exercise of any functions conferred on any person by or under any enactment,
    (c) for the exercise of any functions of the Crown, a Minister of the Crown or a government department, or
    (d) for the exercise of any other functions of a public nature exercised in the public interest by any person.

(6(1)) The processing is necessary for the purposes of legitimate interests pursued by the data controller or by the third party or parties to whom the data are disclosed, except where the processing is unwarranted in any particular case by reason of prejudice to the rights and freedoms or legitimate interests of the data subject.

(2)   The Secretary of State may by order specify particular circumstances in which this condition is, or is not, to be taken to be satisfied.

Figure 8.3   Schedule 2 of the Data Protection Act 1998

Conditions relevant for purposes of the first principle: processing of sensitive personal data

(1) The data subject has given his explicit consent to the processing of the personal data.

(2(1)) The processing is necessary for the purposes of exercising or performing any right or obligation which is conferred or imposed by law on the data controller in connection with employment.

  (2) The Secretary of State may by order:

    (a) exclude the application of sub-paragraph (1) in such cases as may be specified, or

    (b) provide that, in such cases as may be specified, the condition in sub-paragraph (1) is not to be regarded as satisfied unless such further conditions as may be specified in the order are also satisfied.

(3) The processing is necessary:

    (a) in order to protect the vital interests of the data subject or another person, in a case where:

      (i) consent cannot be given by or on behalf of the data subject, or

      (ii) the data controller cannot reasonably be expected to obtain the consent of the data subject, or

    (b) in order to protect the vital interests of another person, in a case where consent by or on behalf of the data subject has been unreasonably withheld.

(4) The processing:

    (a) is carried out in the course of its legitimate activities by any body or association which:

      (i) is not established or conducted for profit, and

      (ii) exists for political, philosophical, religious or trade-union purposes,

    (b) is carried out with appropriate safeguards for the rights and freedoms of data subjects,

    (c) relates only to individuals who either are members of the body or association or have regular contact with it in connection with its purposes, and

    (d) does not involve disclosure of the personal data to a third party without the consent of the data subject.

(5) The information contained in the personal data has been made public as a result of steps deliberately taken by the data subject.

(6) The processing:

    (a) is necessary for the purpose of, or in connection with, any legal proceedings (including prospective legal proceedings),

    (b) is necessary for the purpose of obtaining legal advice, or

    (c) is otherwise necessary for the purposes of establishing, exercising or defending legal rights.

(7(1)) The processing is necessary:

    (a) for the administration of justice,

    (b) for the exercise of any functions conferred on any person by or under an enactment, or

    (c) for the exercise of any functions of the Crown, a Minister of the Crown or a government department.

  (2) The Secretary of State may by order:

    (a) exclude the application of sub-paragraph (1) in such cases as may be specified, or

    (b) provide that, in such cases as may be specified, the condition in sub-paragraph (1) is not to be regarded as satisfied unless such further conditions as may be specified in the order are also satisfied.

Figure 8.4   Schedule 3 of the Data Protection Act 1998

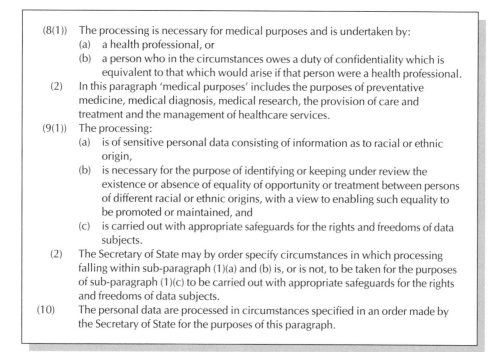

(8(1)) The processing is necessary for medical purposes and is undertaken by:
    (a) a health professional, or
    (b) a person who in the circumstances owes a duty of confidentiality which is equivalent to that which would arise if that person were a health professional.

(2) In this paragraph 'medical purposes' includes the purposes of preventative medicine, medical diagnosis, medical research, the provision of care and treatment and the management of healthcare services.

(9(1)) The processing:
    (a) is of sensitive personal data consisting of information as to racial or ethnic origin,
    (b) is necessary for the purpose of identifying or keeping under review the existence or absence of equality of opportunity or treatment between persons of different racial or ethnic origins, with a view to enabling such equality to be promoted or maintained, and
    (c) is carried out with appropriate safeguards for the rights and freedoms of data subjects.

(2) The Secretary of State may by order specify circumstances in which processing falling within sub-paragraph (1)(a) and (b) is, or is not, to be taken for the purposes of sub-paragraph (1)(c) to be carried out with appropriate safeguards for the rights and freedoms of data subjects.

(10) The personal data are processed in circumstances specified in an order made by the Secretary of State for the purposes of this paragraph.

Figure 8.4   *(cont'd)*

each Schedule needs to be satisfied and NHS bodies processing personal health information for legitimate medical purposes may satisfy a condition in each Schedule without needing to obtain patient consent. Medical Purposes is defined as including the purposes of preventative medicine, medical diagnosis, medical research, the provision of care and treatment and the management of healthcare services. Note however that, in addition to these schedules, there is a general requirement, within the Data Protection Act 1st principle, for all processing to be lawful. This includes meeting common law confidentiality obligations, which are likely themselves to require consent to be obtained.

The DH stated in November 2003 that it would ensure full compliance with the 8 Data Protection principles and would ensure that:

● There is someone with specific responsibility for Data Protection in the organisation.

Currently the nominated person is the Data Protection Manager.

● Everyone managing and handling personal information understands that they are contractually responsible for following good data protection practice, is appropriately trained to do so and is appropriately supervised.

● Anybody wanting to make enquiries about handling personal information knows what to do and these are promptly and courteously death with

● Methods of handling personal information are clearly described, a regular review and audit is made of the way personal information is managed and methods of handling personal information are regularly assessed and evaluated.

The Information Commissioner has published a booklet on the DPA and how to enforce the rights given by the Act.[19] It lists the following rights and in each case refers to a further publication from the ICO office where information on how to enforce that right is given:

(i)   The right to find out what information is held about you on computer and in some paper records. This is called the right of subject access.

(ii)   The right to find out what credit reference agencies report about you and how you correct mistakes on such reports.

(iii) The right to take steps to prevent your personal data being processed if the processing is likely to cause you or someone else to suffer substantial damage or substantial distress which is unjustified.

(iv)   The right to require the data controller not to use your personal data to market you with products, services or ideas.

(v)   The right (in some circumstances) to prevent decisions being taken about you which are based solely on automatic processing.

(vi)   The right to have inaccurate information amended or destroyed.

(viii) The right to claim compensation from the data controller, if damage or distress has been suffered as a result of a data controller failing to comply with the Act.

(ix)   The right to take legal proceedings against the data controller. These proceedings will usually commence in the County Court.

DNA databases

At the time of writing a case is before the European Court of Human Rights concerning the National DNA database. Two men from Sheffield, Michael Marper and S., have brought the case because they were arrested in 2001 and had their fingerprints and DNA samples taken. They were not convicted of any crime and argue that the samples should have been destroyed. Their case was rejected by the British courts and in February 2008 the European Court of Human Rights found in their favour.[20] There are concerns that the result of their success would

lead to more than $^{1}/_{2}$ million samples being removed from the database.[21]

In the meantime, the Information Tribunal held that police were breaking rules on the holding of personal details and that they should remove information about minor crimes from their records because storing it breached data protection laws.[22]

Caldicott Guardians

Dame Fiona Caldicott was appointed to chair a committee to make recommendations on confidentiality within the NHS. The Committee reported in December 1997 and included in its recommendations the need to raise awareness of confidentiality requirements, and specifically recommended the establishment of a network of Caldicott Guardians of patient information throughout the NHS. The Caldicott Guardian is a senior person responsible for protecting the confidentiality of patient and service-user information and enabling appropriate information sharing. He or she was seen to play a key role in ensuring NHS and Social Services organisations satisfied the higher practicable standards for handling patient identifiable information. Subsequently, a steering group was set up to oversee the implementation of the report's recommendations. A circular issued in 1999[23] gave advice on the appointment of the Guardians. Further details on the Caldicott Guardians, recommendations and a manual can be found on the DH website.[24] The principles set down in the Caldicott Report can be seen in Figure 8.5. The Caldicott principles also apply to social services.[25]

From 2003 it has been possible to download from the DH website a toolkit for guidance and assessment for all information governance areas.[26]

Patient Information Advisory Group

Section 60 of the Health and Social Care Act 2001 makes it lawful to disclose and use confidential patient information in specified circumstances

(i)   Justify the purpose.
(ii)   Don't use patient identifiable information unless it is absolutely necessary.
(iii) Use the minimum necessary patient identifiable information.
(iv)   Access to patient identifiable information should be on a strict need to know basis.
(v)   Everyone should be aware of their responsibilities.
(vi)   Understand and comply with the law.

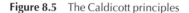

Figure 8.5   The Caldicott principles

where it is not currently practicable to satisfy the common law confidentiality obligations. This does not create new statutory gateways, so the processing must still be for a lawful function, but does mean that the confidentiality obligations do not have to be met, e.g. consent does not have to be obtained. Even where these powers apply however, the Data Protection Act 1998 also continues to apply. The Patient Information Advisory Group (PIAG) was established under the Health and Social Care Act 2001 to review any draft regulations issued under Section 60. The Health Service (Control of Patient Information) Regulations 2002 were the first regulations to be made under Section 60 of this Act, and support the operations of cancer registries and the Public Health Laboratory Services in respect of communicable diseases and other risks to public health. The PIAG has been replaced by the National Information Governance Board for Health and Social Care

National Information Governance Board for Health and Social Care

The Board was established under the Health and Social Care Act 2008 and replaces the Patient Information Advisory Group. Its duties are:

- to monitor the practice followed by relevant bodies in relation to the processing of relevant information;
- to keep the Secretary of State, and such bodies as the Secretary of State may designate by direction, informed about the practice being followed by relevant bodies in relation to the processing of relevant information;

- to publish guidance on the practice to be followed in relation to the processing of relevant information;
- to advise the Secretary of State on particular matters relating to the processing of relevant information by any person; and
- to advise persons who process relevant information on such matters relating to the processing of relevant information by them as the Secretary of State may from time to time designate by direction.

The Board must, in exercising its functions, seek to improve the practice followed by relevant bodies in relation to the processing of relevant information.

'Relevant information' is defined as:

- patient information;
- any other information obtained or generated in the course of the provision of the health service; and
- any information obtained or generated in the course of the exercise by a local social services authority in England of its adult social services functions.

'Patient information' means:

- information (however recorded) which relates to the physical or mental health or condition of an individual ('P'), to the diagnosis of P's condition or to P's care or treatment; and
- information (however recorded) that is to any extent derived, directly or indirectly, from that information whether or not the identity of the individual in question is ascertainable from the information.

Exceptions to the duty of confidentiality

All the sources of law which recognise that there is a duty of confidentiality also recognise that there will be exceptions where it is lawful to disclose confidential information. Thus Rule 3 of the CSP's Rules of Professional Conduct recognises exceptions to the duty of confidentiality where:

> the physiotherapist is required to do so under statutory authority or so directed by a competent legal authority such as a judge, solicitor representing the patient and acting with consent, or where it is necessary to protect the welfare of the patient or to prevent harm, or if it is (rarely) justified in the public interest. If there is any doubt, the Chartered physiotherapist should seek advice either from their line manager or the Chartered Society of Physiotherapy.

The main exceptions to the duty of confidentiality are shown in Figure 8.6.

Consent of the patient

The duty of confidentiality is in the interest of the patient and the patient therefore can give consent to disclosure which without that consent would be unlawful. The patient should be competent to give consent. In the case of a mentally incompetent adult, consent to disclosure could be given on the patient's behalf in the patient's best interests by a representative guardian or carer of the patient, following the principles set down in the Mental Capacity Act 2005. Where the patient is a child under 16 years, then the principles of the Gillick case would apply (see Chapter 23) and a mature competent child under 16 could give consent to disclosure of confidential information.

The consent of the patient or his/her representative would be a defence against any potential proceedings being brought against the health professional. It is essential that evidence is available that consent has been given. There are therefore considerable advantages in obtaining this consent in writing.

The patient has the right to withdraw consent unless the terms of the disclosure are contrary to this. For example, a patient may agree that a video could be made about his/her care and treatment. Considerable expense may then be incurred for the video to be produced. The patient may then decide that he/she does not wish the video to be shown. Whether or not this can then be prevented will depend upon the terms on which his/her agreement to the disclosure was obtained.

Where the patient specifically refuses to give his/her consent to the disclosure of his/her diagnosis to others, such as his/her relatives, this request should as far as possible be respected under the duty of confidentiality and only if a specific exception to the duty applies could the information be passed on.

- Consent of the patient
- Disclosure in the clinical care or in the interests of the patient
- Court order:

  - subpoena
  - under the Supreme Court Act 1981

- Statutory duty to disclose
- Disclosure in the public interest

Figure 8.6   Exceptions to the duty of confidentiality

For clinical care or in the interests of the patient

Health professionals working in a multidisciplinary setting need to share information about the patient in order to fulfil their duty of care to the patient. Indeed it could be said that if relevant information were not passed to other professionals caring for the patient and harm were to occur to the patient as a result of that failure, then the professional and her employer could be answerable to the patient in a negligence action.

Situation: unknown information

A physiotherapist is asked to undertake treatment for a patient but is refused access to the medical records of the patient. She sees the patient in the out-patient department and the patient fails to inform her that she is pregnant. As a consequence of her treatment, the patient miscarries. Had the physiotherapist had access to the medical records she would have been aware of the pregnancy. Is the physiotherapist liable for the miscarriage?

In this situation, the physiotherapist should, as part of her examination of the patient, have enquired about a possible pregnancy. If she failed to do so, she would have been negligent. If she asked, but the patient was not honest, then there should be no negligence on the physiotherapist's part. However, the fact that the physiotherapist does not have an automatic right of access to the patient's records is of concern.

Where information is disclosed to colleagues as part of the duty of care to the patient, care should be taken to ensure that it is relevant to and necessary for their responsibilities.

Situation: telling colleagues

A mother, who is hemiplegic following a stroke, is refusing care for herself when she needs it to look after her child appropriately. She forbids the physiotherapist to discuss her needs with colleagues.

In this situation, in the interests of the child, the mother must accept that the child's interests require information to be made available about the mother's needs but only insofar as it is relevant to her ability to care for the child. It could be pointed out to the mother sensitively that, if because of her own needs she is unable to give the necessary care to the child, then action may have to be taken under the Children Act 1989 to secure the wellbeing of the child.

Court order

Subpoena

The court has the right to ensure that information relevant to an issue being decided before it is made available in the interests of justice. Both criminal and civil courts therefore have the right to issue a subpoena (see glossary) for the necessary information to be produced before it. Other quasi-judicial proceedings such as inquiries may also have a right to subpoena information depending upon the statutory provisions under which they are established.

Where a court requires information, a health professional cannot refuse to comply on the grounds that the information was received in professional confidence. The courts do not recognise any privilege from disclosure attaching to the doctor or other health professional, or even a priest. The only exceptions recognised by the courts to their right to order disclosure are legal professional privilege and privilege on grounds of the public interest (e.g. national security).

Legal professional privilege This covers communications between clients and their legal advisers. The judge cannot order disclosure of such communications. The reason is that it is in the interests of justice for a client to be able to confide fully with legal advisers without fear that such communications could be ordered to be disclosed in court. Reports to legal advisers are also privileged from disclosure if the principal purpose for which they were written is in contemplation of litigation.

Sometimes there may be several purposes behind the preparation of a report, as in a report following a health and safety accident where the report can be used for both management purposes, in order to prevent a similar accident arising again, and legal purposes. This was the situation in the case of *Waugh* v. *British Railways Board*,[27] where the House of Lords held that if the predominant purpose behind the report was for advice and use in litigation, then it will be privileged from disclosure.

However, the court looks at the reality of the matter, not what is said.

In the case of *Lask* v. *Gloucester Health Authority*[28] the court considered the ruling in *Waugh* v. *British Railways Board* in the situation where the health authority claimed legal professional privilege in respect of confidential reports completed following an accident. However, on the facts of the matter the court held that, in spite of declarations by the health authority and solicitors to this effect, the documents were not covered by legal professional privilege.

Legal Professional privilege is recognised as an exception to the right of access under Section 42 of the Freedom of Information Act 2000 (see Chapter 9).

The court held in March 2008 that the mention of a document in a written statement did not constitute an automatic waiver of legal professional privilege so as to entitle the other party to inspect it.[29]

Public interest immunity is the other exception to the right of the judge to order disclosure of any document relevant to an issue before it. This covers such interests as national security. The privilege from disclosure is given under the sworn affidavit of a minister and can be overruled by the judge. Public interest immunity was considered by the Scott inquiry, which recommended that immunity certificates should not be issued in criminal proceedings if the liberty of the subject was at stake.

Disclosure ordered under the Supreme Court Act 1981

This Act enables disclosure to be made where the case involves a claim for personal injury or death in two distinct circumstances:

(a)   under Section 33, where disclosure can be ordered against a prospective *party* (the proposed plaintiff or defendant) *prior* to the writ/claim form being issued; and

(b)   under Section 34 against a third party (i.e. not directly involved in the case) after the writ/claim form has been issued.

Under Section 33 of the Supreme Court Act 1981, when disclosure is ordered against a person likely to be a party in a personal injury case before the writ/claim form is issued, it can be ordered to be made to the applicant's legal advisers and any medical or other professional advisers of the applicant or, if the applicant has no legal advisers, to any medical or other professional adviser of the applicant. The Wolf Reforms to the Civil Procedure Rules require greater openness between parties at an early stage of a case and there is less reliance upon the Supreme Court Act. The Civil Procedure Rules can be accessed on the internet.[30]

Situation: the physiotherapist as potential defendant

> If a client is suing in relation to an incident during the care by a physiotherapist his/her records could be ordered to be disclosed to the legal advisers or professional advisers of the client while they are deciding whether or not to bring a case to court.

After litigation has commenced by the issue of a writ/claim form, disclosure can be ordered under Section 34 of the Supreme Court Act 1981 against a person who is not likely to be a party to a case, if that person has information likely to be relevant.

Situation: disclosure ordered against a physiotherapist

The client of a physiotherapist is involved in a road traffic accident and sues the driver of the vehicle that caused the accident. This driver wished to have access to information about the client held by the physiotherapist relating to his care in order to determine the likely prognosis of the client. If, for example, there was concern that the patient was unlikely to make a full recovery as a result of the road accident, but that he suffered from severe disabilities anyway, these existing disabilities could affect both liability (i.e. whether the driver was 100% to blame or at all) and quantum (the amount of compensation).

An order can be made in the action for disclosure of the client's records even though it is in breach of the duty of confidentiality and against the client's interests. If it is the client who caused the accident and who is being sued an order could similarly be made against the physiotherapist to show, for example, that the client should not have been driving, but only after proceedings have been begun by the issue of a writ/claim form.

Statutory duty to disclose

Several statutes require disclosure to be made, whether or not the patient gives consent. They are shown in Figure 8.7.

Where these Acts are relevant to the work of the physiotherapist he/she should be fully conversant with the statutory requirements on disclosure and ensure that any disclosure which he/she makes can be justified in law.

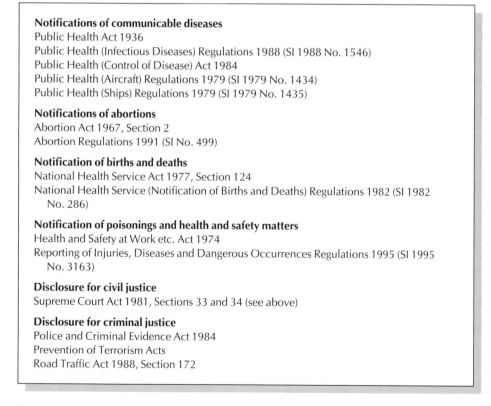

Notifications of communicable diseases
Public Health Act 1936
Public Health (Infectious Diseases) Regulations 1988 (SI 1988 No. 1546)
Public Health (Control of Disease) Act 1984
Public Health (Aircraft) Regulations 1979 (SI 1979 No. 1434)
Public Health (Ships) Regulations 1979 (SI 1979 No. 1435)

Notifications of abortions
Abortion Act 1967, Section 2
Abortion Regulations 1991 (SI No. 499)

Notification of births and deaths
National Health Service Act 1977, Section 124
National Health Service (Notification of Births and Deaths) Regulations 1982 (SI 1982 No. 286)

Notification of poisonings and health and safety matters
Health and Safety at Work etc. Act 1974
Reporting of Injuries, Diseases and Dangerous Occurrences Regulations 1995 (SI 1995 No. 3163)

Disclosure for civil justice
Supreme Court Act 1981, Sections 33 and 34 (see above)

Disclosure for criminal justice
Police and Criminal Evidence Act 1984
Prevention of Terrorism Acts
Road Traffic Act 1988, Section 172

Figure 8.7   Statutory provisions requiring disclosure to be made

Disclosure in the public interest

This is the most difficult exception to the duty of confidentiality. Professional registration bodies all recognise that in certain circumstances, disclosure without the patient's consent and contrary to his/her wishes may be justified.

In one decided case *W* v. *Egdell*[31] on the issue of disclosure in the public interest the Court of Appeal held that it was permissible for a psychiatrist who had been asked for a report by a patient who was seeking his discharge from detention under the Mental Health Act 1983 to send his report to the Mental Health Review Tribunal and the hospital without the consent of the patient.

Case: *W* v. *Egdell*

W was detained in a secure hospital under Sections 37 and 41 of the Mental Health Act 1983 following a conviction for manslaughter on the grounds of diminished responsibility. He had shot dead five people and two others required major surgery. He applied to a Mental Health Review Tribunal (MHRT) and obtained an independent medical report from Dr Egdell, who formed the view that W was suffering from a paranoid psychosis rather than paranoid schizophrenia. In the light of this report, W withdrew the application to the Tribunal. Dr Egdell had assumed that this report would be made available to the hospital and the Tribunal. He sought the permission of W to place his report before the hospital and he refused permission. Dr Egdell then sent the report to the managers asking them to forward a copy to the Home Secretary. He considered that his examination had cast new light on the dangerousness of W and it ought to be known to those responsible for his care and for the formulation of any recommendations for discharge.

Subsequently the Home Secretary referred W to an MHRT under the rules which require a hearing to be held at least every 3 years. The Home Secretary sent a copy of Dr Egdell's report to the Tribunal. W then issued writs against Dr Egdell, the hospital board, the Home Secretary, the Secretary of State for Health and the Tribunal, seeking injunctions preventing the defendants from using this material and claiming damages for breach of confidentiality.

The trial judge held that the court had to balance the interest to be served by non-disclosure against the interest served by disclosure. Since W was not an ordinary member of the public but a detained patient in a secure unit, the safety of the public should be the main criterion. Dr Egdell had a duty to the public to place the result of his examination before the proper authorities, if in his opinion, the public interest so required. The public interest in disclosure outweighed W's private interest.

The Court of Appeal supported this reasoning and stated:

A consultant psychiatrist who becomes aware, even in the course of a confidential relationship, of information which leads him, in the exercise of what the court considers a sound professional judgement, to fear that such decisions may be made on inadequate information and with a real risk of consequent danger to the public is entitled to take such steps as are reasonable in the circumstances to communicate the grounds of his concern to the responsible authorities.

Lord Justice Bingham

Other situations where disclosure in the public interest would be justified would include a situation where harm is occurring or likely to occur to a child or another person.

The multidisciplinary report

Certain professional groups including the CPSM participated with the British Medical Association and the Royal College of Nursing in drafting legislation to cover the use and disclosure of personal health information. In their report[32] public interest is defined as follows:

It shall be lawful for a qualified health professional to disclose personal health information where:

(a)   it relates to a patient for whom he [or she] has clinical responsibility, and

(b)   in the opinion of that professional disclosure is necessary in the public interest.

Disclosure in the public interest is necessary only where:

(a)   it relates to the prevention, detection or prosecution of a serious offence; or

(b)   it relates to the protection of public safety; or

(c)   failure to disclose would expose the patient or some other person to a real risk of death or serious harm.

The draft legislation also provided further safeguards against unauthorised disclosure by suggesting that a decision on whether or not disclosure should be made:

(i)   where the patient is being or has been treated in hospital as an in-patient or an out-patient under the care of a consultant, the disclosure decision must be taken by the consultant in charge of the patient's care; and

(ii)   where the patient is not or has not been treated by a doctor, by the qualified health professional employed by or in contract with the health service body concerned who is responsible at the time of the decision for the particular aspect of the patient's care.

This latter clause could clearly involve the physiotherapist. It would therefore be advisable for physiotherapists to ensure that a procedure is drawn up to cover those exceptional circumstances where they have to decide whether or not disclosure is justified in the public interest.

Draft legislation was introduced into the 1995–6 Parliamentary session but was not enacted. Many of the principles were incorporated in the DH's NHS Code of Practice on confidentiality.

Department of Health Code of Practice on confidentiality[33]

This was published in November 2003, replaces previous guidance[34] and is available on the DH website. It covers the following topics:

- Introduction and Glossary
- Confidentiality
- What is Confidential Patient Information?
- Disclosing and Using Confidential Patient Information
- Patient Consent to Disclosing
- Obligations on Individuals Working in the NHS
- Providing a Confidential Service
- The Confidentiality Model
- Using and Disclosing Confidential Patient Information
- Legal Considerations
- Key Questions for Confidentiality Decisions
- Annex A – Providing a Confidential Service: Detailed Requirements
  - A1 Protect Patient Information
  - A2 Inform Patients Effectively – No Surprises
  - A3 Provide Choice to Patients
  - A4 Improve Wherever Possible
- Annex B – Confidentiality Decisions
- Disclosure Models
- Is it Confidential?
- Health Records are for Healthcare
- Consent Issues
- Informing Patients
- Common Law and the Public Interest
- Administrative Law
- Data Protection Considerations
- Human Rights Act 1998
- Health & Social Care Act 2001: Section 60
- Legal Restrictions on Disclosure
- Legally Required to Disclose
- Legally Permitted to Disclose
- Annex C – index of confidentiality decisions in practice
- Model B1: Healthcare Purposes
- Model B2: Medical Purposes other than Healthcare
- Model B3: Non-medical Purposes

The NHS Code of Practice was endorsed by the Information Commissioner, the President of the General Medical Council and the Chairman of the Medical Ethics Committee of the BMA. The DH has also published an NHS Care Record Guarantee, which promises to use personal health records in ways that respect patients' rights and promote their health and wellbeing.[35]

Access to anonymous data is discussed in Chapter 9.

Implications for the physiotherapist

The CSP in its guidance on Rule 3 on confidentiality gives examples of practical situations which the physiotherapist might encounter.

- If a telephone call is received in a physiotherapy department, unless the physiotherapist is confident that they recognise the voice of an anxious relative, the caller must be informed that no information about the patient can be divulged.
- Messages from the physiotherapist should not be left on a patient's unscreened answer phone without permission.
- Information relating to confirmation of an appointment and/or notification of attendance for physiotherapy must be treated as confidential.
- If a patient is proposing to undertake an activity, which because of their clinical and/or other condition could be harmful to themselves and/or others (e.g. driving or operating potentially dangerous machinery) the physiotherapist must try to persuade the patient not to undertake this activity, usually by informing the patient of the possible consequences of doing so. However, if the physiotherapist is unsuccessful, he/she should inform the patient's doctor or other relevant authority, having first informed the patient of the action proposed.

Julius Sims[36] discussed the duty of confidentiality in relation to the question whether a physiotherapist needed to know the HIV status of the patient. He concluded that except when progression to AIDS has occurred (in which case the diagnosis will be known to the therapist) a physiotherapist does not need to know a patient's HIV status. The reasons he gave are that:

- a patient's HIV status does not determine the choice or effectiveness of therapy;
- the adoption of universal precautions provides optimum protection against transmission of HIV and does not depend upon a knowledge of who is or is not seropositive;
- nor could it be argued that the patient should know of the therapist's status since the chance of contracting HIV from an infected physiotherapist is so remote as to be virtually no risk.

A procedure is necessary for the physiotherapist to ensure that he/she preserves the confidential nature of information about the patient. This would also include safe storage of the records that he/she keeps and should also cover any sharing of records on a multidisciplinary team basis. In addition, the exceptions to the duty should be clarified so that the physiotherapist can be confident that he/she is acting within the law and retains the trust of the patient (see Chapter 12 on record keeping).

Figure 8.8 shows a checklist for ensuring that precautions are taken against any unauthorised disclosure.

Link with ethical issues

This chapter has been concerned with the legal basis for the duty of confidentiality and the legal justifications for breaching that duty in specific situations. It has not been concerned with the moral or ethical dimensions. These are discussed in an article by Julius Sims.[37] He considered that it is rarely permissible to breach confidentiality in the client's own interests and cited an example of a therapist learning that a person wished to commit suicide. In such circumstances it is essential for an assessment to be made of the competence of the patient. If, for example, the patient is suffering from mental disorder and

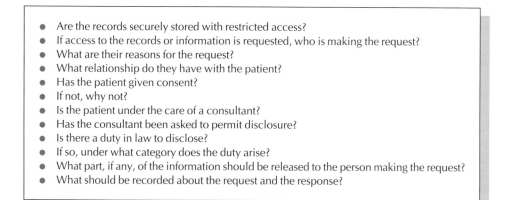

- Are the records securely stored with restricted access?
- If access to the records or information is requested, who is making the request?
- What are their reasons for the request?
- What relationship do they have with the patient?
- Has the patient given consent?
- If not, why not?
- Is the patient under the care of a consultant?
- Has the consultant been asked to permit disclosure?
- Is there a duty in law to disclose?
- If so, under what category does the duty arise?
- What part, if any, of the information should be released to the person making the request?
- What should be recorded about the request and the response?

Figure 8.8   Checklist for good practice in maintaining confidentiality

the physiotherapist failed to take action to protect the patient against these suicidal wishes, the physiotherapist would be failing in his/her duty of care to that patient. It is essential that an understanding of the legal situation should accompany any consideration of the ethical issues. References to books on ethical issues in health care can be found in Further Reading.

Conclusions

The European Directive on Data Protection[38] requires member states to establish a set of principles with which users of personal information must comply, gives individuals the right to gain access to information held about them and provides for a supervisory authority to oversee and enforce the law (see also Chapter 9 on access to health records). The Information Commissioner is taking a pro-active role in ensuring that the principles of confidentiality are respected and stronger criminal sanctions have been called for as a result of recent losses of unencrypted data by the Child Support Agency, the Driving Standards Agency, the Revenue and Customs, the Ministry of Works and Pensions and the Ministry of Defence in 2007 and 2008. A cross-party Commons Justice Committee called for stronger criminal sanctions where personal data are lost.[39]

Questions and exercises

1 Examine your practice in relation to passing on confidential information. What faults would you see in it?
2 To what extent can an employer enforce the duty of confidentiality among employees? Prepare a procedure for this.
3 What exceptions have you relied upon in passing on confidential information?

References

1 Health Professions Council (2003 revised 2008) *Standards of Conduct, Performance and Ethics*. HPC, London.
2 www.hpc-uk.or/aboutus/consultations/closed / index
3 Chartered Society of Physiotherapy (2002) *Rules of Professional Conduct*, 2nd edn. CSP. London.
4 *Furniss* v. *Fitchett* [1958] NZLR 396.
5 *X* v. *Y* [1988] 2 All ER 648.
6 *Murray* v. *Express Newspapers PLC and another*. The Times Law Report, 12 May 2008.
7 *Campbell* v. *MGN Ltd* [2004] UKHL 22, [2004] 2 A.C. 457 HL.
8 Kennedy, D, (2008) E-mails from Mosley to madam held missing key to orgy case. *The Times*, 25 July; *Moseley* v. *News Group Newspapers* [2008] EWHC 1777.

9   *Liberty and others* v. *United Kingdom*. The Times Law Report, 11 July 2008. [2008] ECHR 568.

10 *Attorney General* v. *Guardian Newspaper Ltd (No 2)* [1988] 3 All ER 545.

11 *Stephens* v. *Avery and others* [1988] 2 All ER 477.

12 Leigh-Pollitt, P., Mullock, J. (2000) *The Data Protection Act Explained*, 2nd edn. The Stationery Office, London.

13 European Directive on Data Protection adopted by the Council of the European Union in October 1995.

14 NHS Executive, Data Protection Act 1998 HSC 2000/009 and supporting information: DH and NHS Executive, Data Protection Act 1998 Protection and Use of Patient Information; www.dh.gov.uk/en/index/htm

15 www.connectingforhealth.nhs.uk

16 http://www.ico.gov.uk

17 www.ico.gov.uk

18 *R (on the application of the Secretary of State for the Home Department)* v. *Information Tribunal (Information Commissioner, interested party)* [2006] EWHC 2958 Admin, [2007] 2 All ER 703.

19 Information Commission. The Data Protection Act: Your rights and how to enforce them. http://www.ico.gov.uk/for_organisations/data _protection_guide.aspx

20 *S. and Marper* v. *UK* [2008] ECHR 1581.

21 O'Neill, S. (2008) DNA Database Under Threat from the EUROPEAN Court, Warns Police Chief. *The Times*, 7 June, p. 34

22 Ford, R. (2008) Ruling Could Wipe out Criminal Records. *The Times*, 22 July, 5

23 NHS Executive, HSC 1999/012, Caldicott Guardians, 31 January 1999

24 dh.gov.uk/en/managingyourorganisation/ informationpolicy/patientconfidentiality

25 HSC 2002/3 Implementing the Caldicott principles in social care, appointment of Caldicott guardians.

26 Department of Health Information Governance toolkit 2003.

27 *Waugh* v. *British Railways Board* [1980] AC 521.

28 *Lask* v. *Gloucester Health Authority*. The Times Law Report, 13 December 1985.

29 *Expandable Ltd and others v Rubin*. The Times Law Report, 10 March 2008

30 www.justice.gov.uk/civil/procrules_fin

31 *W.* v. *Egdell* [1989] 1 All ER 1089; (CA) [1990] 1 All ER 835.

32 Multi-disciplinary Professional Working Group (1994) *An Explanatory Handbook of Guidance Governing Use and Disclosure of Personal Health Information*. British Medical Association, London.

33 Department of Health (2003) *NHS Confidentiality Code of Practice*. DH. Available from www.dh.gov.uk/ipu/confiden/protect (superseding HSG(96) 18 LASSL (96)5)

34 HSG (96)18/LASSL (96) 5 – The Protection and Use of Patient Information.

35 Department of Health 2007 NHS Care Record Guarantee.

36 Sims, J. (1997) Confidentiality and HIV Status. *Physiotherapy* **83**, 2, 90–96.

37 Sims, J. (1996) Client confidentiality: ethical issues in occupational therapy. *British Journal of Occupational Therapy* **59**, 2, 56–61.

38 European Directive on Data Protection Adopted by the Council of the European Union in October 1995.

39 Hurst, G. (2008) Whitehall should be prosecuted over data loss, say MPs in call for new law. *The Times*, 3 January.

9 Access to Records and Information

Patients have a statutory right to see their health records, whether they are held in computer or manual form. This is subject to only a few exceptions. The definition of health records is any record of information relating to someone's physical or mental health that has been made by (or on behalf of) a health professional. This definition would include all patient personal information kept by the physiotherapist, whether electronically or manually. The only limitation on the manually held records is that they must be held in a relevant filing system. The statutory right of access also applies to records held by those health professionals working in private practice, but here access might also be subject to conditions agreed in the contract between therapist and private patient. The contractual conditions cannot limit the statutory right. Separate statutory provisions cover the records held by those who work for social services departments (SSDs). The right of access is not absolute and, as will be seen, there are restrictions both by statute and by common law on the patient's right of access.

A physiotherapist's records may also become relevant to reports written by the patient's doctor for insurance or employment purposes and therefore come under the rules relating to disclosure of such reports under the Access to Medical Reports Act 1988 (see below).

In addition to the statutory rights of access to health records and personal files kept by SSDs, there is also a right at common law for the patient to receive, as part of the duty of care owed by the health professional to the patient, information that is relevant to decisions which the patient may be required to consider in relation to his/her treatment and care. The rights at common law of the patient to obtain information are set out in the leading case of Sidaway,[1] considered in Chapter 7. The rights at common law are not unlimited however, as was seen in the case of Martin[2] where the Court of Appeal held there is no absolute right to access personal health records.

This chapter also considers the right to access information under the Freedom of Information Act 2000.

The following topics are considered in this chapter:

- Statutory rights
- Non-statutory access
- Access and the physiotherapist
- Access by others
- Freedom of Information Act 2000

Statutory rights

The legislation giving statutory rights is as follows:

- Data Protection Act 1998 Act
- Access to Medical Reports Act 1988
- Access to Health Records Act 1990 (for the records of deceased persons)
- Data Protection (Subject Access Modification) (Health) Order 2000
- Data Protection (Subject Access Modification) (Social Work) Order 2000
- Data Protection (Subject Access Modification) (Education) Order 2000
- Education (Pupil Information) (England) Regulations 2005
- Freedom of Information Act 2000.

The Data Protection Act 1998

The Data Protection Act 1998 was passed in accordance with the EC Directive (see Chapter 8) and replaces the 1984 Act. The basic principles are similar to the 1984 Act but there are subtle differences of emphasis and terminology. The Registrar (now known as the Information Commissioner) published a document entitled *The Data Protection Act 1998: An Introduction*, which is available from the Office of the Data Protection Registrar.[3]

The Data Protection Act 1998 gives rights of access to automated processed personal health information and to manual records if they form part of a relevant filing system subject to the conditions laid down by statutory instrument.[4] Clarification is given of the statutory provisions by the Department of Health, which can be accessed from the Connecting for Health site (www.connectingforhealth.nhs.uk).

The Act covers only those records which consist of information relating to a living individual who can be identified from that information (or from other information in the possession of the data user), including any expression of opinion (see Chapter 8).

Principles

The Data Protection Act 1998 regulates the collection, processing and storage of information in automated form from which an individual can be identified. Data users are required to register with the Information Commissioner their recording and use of personal data and must comply with the Data Protection Act principles. These are shown below in Figure 9.1.

Provisions on access by data subject

The data subject, i.e. the person about whom the information is recorded, has a right of access under the 1998 Act. He/she has the right to be informed by the data user whether any personal identifiable information about him/her is being held and if so he/she has the right to be supplied with a copy of that information.

Children have the right of access if they have the maturity to make a valid application. The concept of being 'Gillick Competent' would apply (see Chapter 23).

The Act provided for regulations to be made to enable those who are responsible for the management of the affairs of an incompetent adult to have access, but no regulations have been passed. Regulations may be passed under the 1998 Act (see below) as a result of the Mental Capacity Act 2005.

Exceptions

Under a statutory instrument, the access provisions are modified in the case of access to personal health records. This applies to data held by a health professional or data held by a person other than a health professional where the information constituting the data was first recorded by or on behalf of a health professional. The appropriate health professional is defined in the Statutory Instrument as:

(a) The health professional who is currently or was most recently responsible for the clinical care of the data subject in

Personal data shall:

(1) be collected and processed fairly and lawfully and shall not be processed unless one of the conditions in Schedule 2 is met, and in the case of sensitive personal data, one of the conditions in Schedule 3;

(2) only be obtained for specified, lawful registered purposes and shall not be further processed in any manner incompatible with that purpose;

(3) be adequate and relevant and not excessive to the purpose for which they are held;

(4) be accurate and, where necessary, kept up to date;

(5) be held no longer than is necessary for the stated purpose;

(6) shall be processed in accordance with the rights of data subjects under this Act;

(7) appropriate technical and organisational measures shall be taken against unauthorised or unlawful processing of personal data and against accidental loss or destruction or damage to personal data;

(8) personal data shall not be transferred to a country outside the European Economic Area unless that country ensures an adequate level of protection for the rights and freedom of data subjects in relation to the processing of personal data.

Figure 9.1   Data Protection Act principles

connection with the matters to which the information which is the subject of the request relates, or

(b) Where there is more than one such health professional, the health professional who is the most suitable to advise on the matters to which the information which is the subject of the request relates; or

(c) Where:

(i) there is no health professional available falling within paragraph a. or b., or

(ii) The data controller is the Secretary of State and data relates to the Child Support Act, of his functions in relation to social security or pensions.

A health professional who has the necessary experience and qualifications to advise on the matters to which the information which is the subject of the request relates.

Figure 9.2 sets out the health professionals who would be concerned with access to health records.

- registered medical practitioner
- registered dental practitioner
- registered chemist
- registered optician
- registered pharmaceutical chemist
- registered nurse, midwife or health visitor
- registered chiropodist
- dietician
- music therapist employed by a health authority
- scientist employed by a health authority as head of department
- occupational therapist
- orthoptist
- physiotherapist
- clinical psychologist
- child psychotherapist
- speech therapist
- osteopath
- chiropractor

Figure 9.2   Definition of health professional

Access is not permitted where disclosure:

- would be likely to cause serious harm to the physical or mental health of the data subject, or any other person;
- would be likely to reveal to the data subject the identity of another individual (who has not consented to the disclosure of the information);
- where any person is enabled by or under any enactment or rule of law to make a request on behalf of a data subject (who is a child and the applicant has parental responsibility or the data subject lacks mental capacity and the applicant has been appointed by the court to have responsibility) and has made such a request, personal data are exempt from disclosure in any case to the extent to which the application of that section would disclose information:
  - (a) provided by the data subject in the expectation that it would not be disclosed to the person making the request;
  - (b) obtained as a result of any examination or investigation to which the data subject consented in the expectation that the information would not be so disclosed;
  - (c) which the data subject has expressly indicated should not be so disclosed;
- provided that sub-paragraphs (a) and (b) shall not prevent disclosure where the data subject has expressly indicated that he no longer has the expectation referred to therein;
- personal data processed by a court and consisting of information supplied in a report or other evidence given to the court by a local authority, Health and Social Services Board, Health and Social Services Trust, probation officer or other person in the course of any proceedings to which the Family Proceedings Courts (Children Act 1989) Rules 1991,[5] the Magistrates' Courts (Children and Young Persons) Rules 1992 and other legislation apply where the court has the power to withhold the information.

The data user, who is not a health professional, is required to consult the appropriate health professional before permitting or refusing access. The appropriate health professional is defined as:

- the medical practitioner or dental practitioner who is currently or was most recently responsible for the clinical care of the data subject in connection with the matters to which the information which is the subject of the request relates;
- where there is more than one such practitioner, the practitioner who is the most suitable to advise on the matters to which the information which is the subject of the request relates;
- where there is no practitioner available falling within subparagraph a. or b., a health professional who has the necessary experience and qualifications to advise on the matters to which the information which is the subject of the request relates.

If the exclusion provisions apply, the data user does not have to notify the applicant that information is being withheld. It is sufficient for the data user to notify the applicant that there is no information being held which has to be revealed to the data subject.

Procedure for application

The application is made in writing to the data controller, i.e. the person who holds the personal data, giving sufficient information for the relevant data and the subject user to be identified, together with the appropriate fee (at the present time £10 for computerised records and £50 for records held in manual form or a mix of manual and computerised records). The data controller has 40 days in which to respond.

Rights of the data subject

- Unless the exclusion provisions discussed above apply, the data subject is entitled to be supplied with a copy of the information requested within 40 days of the date on which the application, giving all the necessary information is received.

- The applicant would receive information on the following: a description of the data; why the data is held; who the data may have been given to; a copy of the data with any technical terms explained; any information available on the source of the data; an explanation as to how any automated decision taken about them has been made.
- If the information supplied to the data subject is inaccurate he or she can request that the information is rectified or erased and has the right to enforce this in the Court.
- If the inaccuracy causes distress to the data subject, then the data subject has the right to claim compensation for the harm suffered. The data user has a defence if the inaccurate information was received from the patient or a third person or if the data user took such care as was reasonably required in the circumstances to ensure the accuracy of the data at the material time.
- If the data subject is refused the information, he or she can either make an application to the County or High Court or to the Information Commissioner for the enforcement of the statutory rights.

The Access to Medical Reports Act 1988

Basic principles

This Act enables a patient to see and if necessary suggest corrections where an insurance company or employer requests a medical report from the patient's own doctor for insurance or employment purposes. The records to which the doctor might refer may include information received from physiotherapists.

The right of access can be withheld in similar circumstances to those stated above. Therefore if, in the unlikely circumstances that the physiotherapist is concerned that any information is likely to cause serious harm to the physical or mental health of the patient or identify a third person who has requested not to be identified, then he/she should ensure that the information

which he/she passes to the doctor is suitably annotated. The British Medical Association has provided guidance on access to medical reports, which was revised in June 2007.[6]

Situation: what comes under the Access to Medical Reports Act 1988?

Do physiotherapy reports to insurance companies come under the Access to Medical Reports Act? Although the Act refers only to medical reports, information from the physiotherapist could be included or referred to in the medical report in which case that information would come within the Act. It would be wise practice for a physiotherapist who is asked to give information to an insurance company about a patient to ensure that he/she has the patient's consent, and to assume that his/her report comes within the Act. Technically this may not be so, but the Chartered Society of Physiotherapy has recommended to the Association of Chartered Physiotherapists in Occupational Health and Ergonomics (ACPOHE) that they should act in the spirit of the law. It states:

> The options you give your patients to see, and if necessary amend, their reports, is right and proper and the timescales (21 days given by the ACPOHE) are indicative of the requirements in law.

Access to Health Records Act 1990: deceased persons

The Access to Health Records Act 1990 came into force on 1 November 1991 to give a right of access to manual records since the Data Protection Act 1984 only applied to automated records. However the Data Protection Act 1998 covers both computerised and manually held records in a filing system and therefore most of the Access to Health Records Act 1990 has been repealed and only those sections relating to the records of deceased persons remains in force. Under Section 3(1)(f) of the Access to Health Records Act 1990 where a person has died, the patient's personal representative and any person who may have a claim arising out of the patient's death may apply for access to the deceased patient's health records. Where such an application is made, access shall not be given if the record includes a note, made at the patient's request, that he/she did not wish access to be given on such an application. Nor will access be given by the record holder to any part of the record, if he/she is of the opinion that it would disclose information which was not relevant to any claim which may arise out of the patient's death.

A life insurance company may seek information in order to decide whether to make a payment under a life assurance policy and require doctors to give information about the cause of death. Doctors could release information in accordance with the Access to Health Records Act 1990.

The Information Tribunal ruled that a dead woman's medical records should not be released because a duty of confidentiality survives her death and this was challenged by the mother of the deceased.[7] The case of *Bluck* v. *Information Commissioner* is discussed in this chapter.

The Access to Personal Files Act 1987, which enabled access to housing and social services records, has now been repealed by the Data Protection Act 1998 and regulations have been made under the 1998 Act, including the Data Protection (Subject Access Modification) (Health Records) Order 2000, the Data Protection (Subject Access Modification) (Social Work) Order 2000[8] and the Data Protection (Subject Access Modification) (Social Work) Order 2005.[9]

Education (Pupil Information) (England) Regulations 2005[10]

These regulations, which revoke and re-enact with modifications the Regulations of 2000, enable education records on pupils held by maintained and special schools to be open to access on specified conditions.

Under Regulation 5(3), the governing body must provide a copy of a pupil's educational record to the parent, on payment of a specified fee, within 15 days of receipt of the parent's written request for access to that record. This regulation is subject to the conditions, that the record may not be made available for inspection or a copy provided if:

(a) it could not lawfully be disclosed to the pupil himself under the Data Protection Act 1998;

(b) if the pupil would have no right of access to it under the Data Protection Act 1998 or under any regulations made under the Act.

Regulations under the Data Protection Act[11] set out similar exclusions from the right of access to those under the Access to Health Records, including those cases where access would be likely to cause serious harm to the physical or mental health or condition of the data subject or any other person. There is also an exclusion from access where the data subject is or may be at risk of child abuse and access would not be in the best interests of the data subject. This latter exemption from access applies where the data subject is a child and the applicant has parental responsibility for the data subject or the data subject is incapable of managing his/her own affairs. Child abuse includes physical injury (other than accidental injury) to, and physical and emotional neglect, ill-treatment and sexual abuse of a child.

Non-statutory access

There appear to be few formal applications made under the statutory provisions, which suggests that health professionals are disclosing the records without requiring the patient to make a formal application. It should be remembered that the existence of statutory rights of access for the patient does not mean that the patient necessarily has to apply formally for access. There may be many reasons why the health professional agrees to informal access of the patient to his/her records and this could then be arranged. There is the possibility that greater openness with the patient over access to records and information may make the patient less suspicious and there will be even fewer formal applications for access under the statutory provisions.

It has, however, been established that, if the statutory provisions do not apply, the patient does not have an absolute right of access at common law.[12] The Court of Appeal in the case brought by Martin against Mid Glamorgan Family Health Services Authority[2] stated that a doctor or health authority was entitled to deny access to the records by the patient on the ground that their disclosure would be detrimental to him/her.

Access and the physiotherapist

It is seldom that secrecy of information from the patient can be justified in the case of the treatment provided by the physiotherapist. There are very few situations where the physiotherapist would feel that serious harm could arise to the physical or mental health of the patient if access were to be permitted. However, the physiotherapist should be aware of the statutory limitations on the right of access and advise the patient if appropriate.

Orders to withhold information

Sometimes however the problems that can arise are not of the physiotherapist's making as the following situation illustrates.

Situation: orders to withhold information

A consultant physician treating a patient has diagnosed multiple sclerosis. It is his view that the patient could not yet cope with this diagnosis and he therefore instructs the multidisciplinary team caring for the patient that she should not be told. The physiotherapist takes part in a pre-discharge assessment of the patient and accompanies her home to decide if she could cope with living on her own. During the visit the patient raises with the physiotherapist her concerns about her illness and asks the physiotherapist directly if she has multiple sclerosis. What is the legal situation?

Although the physiotherapist is a personally accountable registered professional who should use her own discretion in making health decisions, she may also be part of the multidisciplinary team usually headed by the consultant responsible for the care and treatment of the patient. In this case her concerns about openness and disclosure to the patient should have been raised as soon as she was aware of the restrictions ordered by the consultant and she should have taken up this with him then. However, in the situation which occurs she has the following options:

- to refuse to say and suggest that the patient should have an appointment to discuss with the consultant her diagnosis and treatment;
- to answer the patient honestly and ignore the consultant's orders;
- to lie to the patient.

It would be hoped that the third option would be unacceptable to all health and social services professionals. The first option would probably be appropriate in most cases. The second option may be justified in exceptional circumstances. However, if the physiotherapist follows this line, then he/she must be prepared to justify his/her actions:

- before disciplinary proceedings should the consultant report the physiotherapist to his/her managers and they decide to take such action;
- in civil litigation, if the patient reacts to this information by attempting to take (or succeeding in taking) his/her own life and the employer of the physiotherapist is sued for its vicarious liability for the harm caused by him/her;
- in professional conduct proceedings if it is decided that his/her fitness to practice is impaired by reason of misconduct.

It may be that before all three forms of hearings, the physiotherapist is able to justify his/her actions as being in the best interests of the patient. The physiotherapist should ensure that his/her records are comprehensive and explain clearly why the decisions that he/she made. In deciding whether it is appropriate to ignore the consultant's direction the physiotherapist should be mindful of the fact that there is no absolute duty to disclose everything to the patient. Under the statutory provisions there is a right of exclusion from access which the holder of the records can exercise on the basis of the advice of the health professional concerned and at common law. The House of Lords in the *Sidaway* case recognised the right of therapeutic privilege, i.e. to withhold information from the patient in exceptional circumstances when it is justified as being in the best interests of that patient (see Chapter 7).

Nevertheless, the General Medical Council (GMC) has advised registered medical practitioners that they should ensure that patients are given full information about their condition and that those who fail to tell patients the truth about their treatment risk being struck off. The new guidelines were issued in the updated *Good Medical Practice* booklet issued by the GMC (revised again in 2006).[13] These follow a Court of Appeal decision in a case brought by the father of a boy suffering from Addison's disease, who claimed that doctors should have informed him about his son's condition. The Court of Appeal held that doctors were not under a legal obligation to tell the truth and therefore could not be sued for concealing the failures that led to the child's death. The health authority accepted liability for the failure to diagnose the condition. The father, Will Powell, took his case to the European Court that the medical records had been falsified and this was a breach of Article 2 of the European Convention of Human Rights and no remedy had been provided for that breach. The Court held that the UK was not in breach of its protective duty since it had made adequate provision for health professionals to meet high standards. As far as the state's

investigative duty was concerned, the court said that the UK had discharged that duty since the parents had settled civil proceedings against the health authority: they were not therefore victims and their application was therefore inadmissible.[14]

A distinction may also have to be made between those physiotherapists who work for social services, where the patient may not be directly under a consultant and the general practitioner is therefore the lead medical practitioner responsible for the clinical care of the patient, and those physiotherapists who work in health care, where there would usually be an identifiable consultant in charge of the patient's care.

Truth telling

'Truth telling in occupational therapy'[15] by Rosemary Barnitt is an excellent analysis of the ethical issues which arise in deciding whether or not the patient should be given the full information. The principles also apply to physiotherapy. The article shows the difficulties that can arise in a multidisciplinary team over who controls the truth telling. She concluded that there was a clear need for simple policies and procedures to be established around truth telling in healthcare settings, and for these to be made available to all participants in the treatment transaction. Her research was based on a postal questionnaire across England and Wales. As shown above, there is a right recognised both by statute and at common law for information to be withheld from the patient in exceptional circumstances if it would cause serious harm to the mental or physical condition of the patient.

Situation: telling the patient

A physiotherapist received a referral form for a patient whose diagnosis was Parkinson's disease. She told the patient that she was visiting to assist him following his diagnosis of Parkinson's disease. He stated bluntly that he did not have Parkinson's.

In this situation, the physiotherapist was wrong-footed because she assumed that the patient had been told and had accepted the diagnosis. She could only attempt to retrieve the situation by glossing over the diagnosis and concentrating on any weaknesses that the patient had.

Diagnosis not given to the physiotherapist

A variant of the above situation would be where the physiotherapist is not him/herself told of the patient's diagnosis. Problems can then arise for the physiotherapist when he/she does not know the medical condition of a referral – how for example can he/she decide on priorities? Can the doctor be forced to disclose? What happens if the patient does not want the physiotherapist to get in touch with the doctor?

In such a situation each case would have to be treated on its merits and many different legal principles apply. The duty in relation to confidentiality is discussed in Chapter 8, where it is noted that providing personal patient information to the multidisciplinary team caring for the patient is a justifiable exception to the duty of confidentiality since it would be in the interests of the patient.

Another issue which arises in the situation where the doctor is refusing to give the physiotherapist patient information is that of the standard of care to be provided by the physiotherapist. If he/she is kept in ignorance of certain information about the patient's condition, he/she may make some grave errors of judgment which could cause harm to the patient. His/her right to have the relevant information to care appropriately for the patient is clear and he/she should bring up any such issue with the multidisciplinary team. It is more difficult in the community, where a physiotherapist working for social services may not be a member of such a team and it may be the GP who is refusing to give the necessary information. It might have to be explained to the GP by senior management that, unless specific information is made available, priorities cannot be set reasonably nor the appropriate care given.

Situation: a matter of opinion

A physiotherapist is concerned that a patient is malingering and would be capable of walking if she wished to do so. She noted this in her records. A few months later, she was notified that the patient was exercising her right of subject access and wished to see these records. She considered that access should be refused on the grounds that seeing her opinion could cause grievous harm to the mental state of the patient. What is the law?

In such a situation it is extremely doubtful if the exemption of the right of access on the grounds that serious harm to the physical or mental health or condition of the patient would be caused would apply. Certainly seeing the physiotherapist's opinion, if this had never been made clear to the patient, might well upset her, but for the exemption to apply, 'serious harm' must be shown.

The Information Commissioner's Office has issued a good practice note on how the Data Protection Act applies to professional opinion.[16] It gives several examples where patients have disagreed with the opinion expressed by the health professional and as a result of a request by the patient, a comment to the effect that the patient did not agree with the opinion is added to the notes. The advice is considered in Chapter 12.

Access by others

Statutory rights of persons other than the patient under the 1990 Act are discussed above. Other rights of access including those of the courts and where certain statutes require information to be disclosed are considered in Chapter 8 on confidentiality.

Anonymous data

The Department of Health challenged a data-collecting company that was using information provided by GPs and pharmacists about pre-scribing habits.[17] The company believed the information would be useful to drug companies and would provide useful data for those interested in monitoring prescribing patterns. Even though the information would be anonymous, the Department of Health challenged the use of this information as a breach of the guidelines put forward by the Department of Health[18] in 1996. It succeeded before the High Court but the Court of Appeal[19] reversed this decision. It held that GPs and pharmacists providing prescription information that did not identify the patient was not a breach of confidence. Anonymous data did not involve a risk to the patient's privacy, even if, with effort, the patient could be identified.

In 2008 the House of Lords held that data on childhood leukaemia could be released if it was anonymised.

Case: *Common Services Agency* v. *Scottish Information Commissioner Times 2008*[20]

A researcher acting on behalf of a member of the Scottish Parliament asked the Common Services Agency which collected and disseminated epidemiological information for details of all incidents of childhood leukaemia for all the Dumfries and Galloway postal areas by census ward. The agency refused the researcher's request. There was a danger of indirect identification of living individuals because of the low numbers involved. The data were personal data within the meaning of the 1998 Act and were exempt from disclosure under the Freedom of Information (Scotland) Act 2002. The researcher appealed to the Scottish Information Commissioner who decided that the information could be disclosed if it had undergone a process known as Barnardisation, which rendered the data anonymous and more difficult to identify individuals. The effect of this process could mean that the data were no longer 'personal'. The House of Lords declared that the researcher should reapply to the Commissioner so that he could consider whether the process of Barnardisation had resulted in the data being anonymised and therefore no longer personal data, or whether disclosure by the Agency would be in accordance with Schedules 1, 2 and 3 of the Data Protection Act 1998.

Freedom of Information Act 2000

As a consequence of the Freedom of Information Act 2000, some of the information retained in physiotherapy departments may be accessible to the general public. The Act gives a general right of access to information held by public authorities, but this right is subject to significant exceptions. The main exemptions from the duty are set out in Part 2 of the Act. Some of the exemptions are subject to a public interest test and these are shown in Box 9.1. Others are absolute exemptions and these are shown in Box 9.2. In addition to these exemptions, under Section 14 a request that is vexatious or that the public authority has already complied with does not have to be complied with. For the exemptions listed in Box 9.1, a public interest test applies. This means that a public authority

---

Box 9.1   Exempt information where the public interest test applies.

Information intended for future publication
National security
Defence
International relations
Relations within the UK
The economy
Investigations and proceedings conducted by
    public authorities
Law enforcement
Audit functions
Formulation of government policy
Prejudice to effective conduct of public affairs
Communication with Her Majesty, etc., and
    honours
Health and safety
Environmental information
Personal information
Legal professional privilege
Commercial interests

Box 9.2   Absolute exemptions from the Act.

Information accessible to the applicant by other means

Information supplied by or relating to bodies dealing with security matters

Court records

Parliamentary privilege

Prejudice to effective conduct of public affairs

Personal information where the applicant is the subject of the information

Information provided in confidence

Prohibitions on disclosure where a disclosure is prohibited by an enactment or would constitute contempt of court

---

must consider whether the public interest in withholding the exempt information outweighs the public interest in releasing it. The majority of exemptions fall into this category. For those exemptions listed in Box 9.2, there is no requirement for the public authority to consider the public interest.

Data protection and freedom of information legislation

From Box 9.2 it will be noted that personal information where the applicant is the subject of the information is absolutely exempt from the Freedom of Information Act. Section 40 states that:

> [A]ny information to which a request for information relates is exempt information if it constitutes personal data of which the applicant is the data subject.

If a data subject wants access to personal information, then the route for that application is the Data Protection Act 1998 and in general the Freedom of Information Act 2000 tries to prevent an overlap between the two Acts.

Restriction on freedom of information

Mother of deceased woman refused access to her daughter's records

The mother of a girl who had died in hospital appealed against the decision of the Information Commissioner to refuse her access to her daughter's records.[21] The trust was unwilling to release the records without the consent of the daughter's husband as her next of kin. The hospital had admitted liability for the daughter's death and had reached a settlement with the husband involving payment of substantial compensation. The mother contended that the records did not fall within the exception for confidential information under the Freedom of Information Act 2000 Section 41, since the trust would have the following defences to any breach of confidence claim arising from the disclosure: (1) the public interest in the disclosure of information in cases where a hospital had been negligent in its treatment of a patient, leading to the patient's death, outweighed the public interest in maintaining confidence; (2) neither the daughter nor her estate would suffer any detriment as a result of the disclosure; (3) a cause of action in breach of confidence could not survive the death of the person to whom the duty of confidence was owed; and (4) even if the cause of action did survive, the deceased's personal representative would not be entitled to bring an action to enforce the deceased's right to confidentiality in relation to medical records.

The Judge refused the application:

(1)   The public interest ensuring that patients retained trust in confidentiality of information they gave to doctors outweighed, by some way, the countervailing public interest in disclosure of a deceased's medical records.

(2)   If disclosure would be contrary to an individual's reasonable expectation of maintaining the confidentiality of his or her private information, then the absence of detriment in the sense contemplated by the mother was not a necessary ingredient of the cause of action.

(3) The duty of confidence was capable of surviving the death of the confider
(4) The trust would be in breach of confidence owed to the daughter if it disclosed her medical records other than under the terms of the Act, and the breach would be actionable by the daughter's personal representatives. Her records were exempt information under Section 41 and should not be disclosed.
(5) The rights of the next-of-kin had to prevail where the rights and wishes of family members differed.

Codes of practice

Codes of practice giving practical guidance to public authorities on the discharge of their duties under the Act has been issued by the Lord Chancellor as required under Section 45 of the Act[22] (referred to as the Section 45 Code of Practice). In December 2003 a model action plan for preparation for the implementation of the Freedom of Information Act 2000 was published.[23] Although this model action plan is not compulsory, it is intended as a tool to disseminate ideas and best practice and to assist public authorities in creating a structured path towards full implementation of the Act in 2005.

Freedom of Information Act Awareness Guidance leaflets are available from the Information Commissioner's website.[3]

Conclusion

The impact of statutory rights of access has led to greater openness between patient and health professional. Informal sharing of information is important and the practice by some NHS Trusts, as an income generation method, that the patient should be compelled to take the formal statutory route in order to obtain access is unsupportable. A Health Records and Data Protection Review Group was set up in 2002 to represent patient groups, health and social professionals and regulatory bodies in advising the government on charges for access to records, screening of records by doctors prior to patient access, issues relating to family and family history and any conditions over the use of the NHS number. Concerns relating to the new IT system for electronic patient records are considered in Chapter 12.

Questions and exercises

1   A client asks for sight of the clinical records you are keeping on her. What action do you take and what considerations do you take into account?
2   Explain to a colleague the legal procedure under the Data Protection Act 1998 that enables a patient to have sight of her records.
3   In what circumstances do you consider that it would cause serious harm to the physical or mental health of the patient to see her records?
4   What is the significance of the Freedom of Information Act 2000 for information held in your physiotherapy department?

References

1   *Sidaway* v. *Bethlem Royal Hospital Governors* [1985] 2 WLR 480.
2   *R* v. *Mid Glamorgan Family Health Services Authority, ex parte Martin* [1995] 1 All ER 356.
3   www.ico.gov.uk
4   Data Protection (Subject Access Modification) (Health) Order 2000 SI No. 413.
5   www.opsi.gov.uk
6   British Medical Association (2007) *Guidelines on Access to Medical Reports*. BMA, London.
7   *Bluck* v. *Information Commissioner* (2007) 98 B.M.L.R. 1.
8   SI 2000/415.
9   SI 2005/467.
10 Education (Pupil Information) (England) Regulations 2005 SI No. 1437.
11 The Data Protection (Subject Access Modification) (Education) Order 2000 (SI 2000/414).

12   *R* v. *Mid Glamorgan Family Health Services Author-ity, ex parte Martin* [1993] 137 SJ 153; (QBD) The Times Law Report 2 June 1993; upheld by (CA) The Times Law Report, 16 August 1994; [1994] 5 Med LR 383.

13   General Medical Council (1998 revised 2006) *Good Medical Practice*. GMC, London.

14   *Powell* v. *UK* Application 45305/99 unreported 4 May 1999.

15   Barnitt, R. (1994) Truth Telling in Occupational Therapy. *British Journal of Occupational Therapy* **57**, 334–40.

16   Information Commissioner's Office (2006) *Data Protection Good Practice Note. How Does the Data Protection Act Apply to Professional Opinions*? ICO, London.

17   *R* v. *Department of Health ex parte Source Informatics Ltd* [1999] Lloyd's Rep Med 264, [1999] 4 All ER 185.

18   Department of Health HSG (1996) 18, *Protection and Use of Patient Information*, DH circular, March 1996 (superseded by Department of Health, NHS Confidentiality Code of Practice, DH, 2003. Available from www.dh.gov.uk/ipu/confiden/protect

19   *R* v. *Department of Health ex parte Source Informatics Ltd* [2000] TLR 17, [2000] 1 All ER 786 CA.

20   *Common Services Agency* v. *Scottish Information Commissioner*. Times Law Report, 14 July 2008 HL.

21   *Bluck* v. *Information Commissioner* (2007) 98 B.M.L.R. 1.

22   Lord Chancellor, Code of Practice on the Discharge of Public Authorities' Functions under Part 1 of the Freedom of Information Act 2000; Lord Chancellor, Code of Practice on the Management of Records (Section 46 Code of Practice); www.dataprotection.gov.uk

23   www.dca.gov.uk/foi/map/modactplan.htm

Section C

Accountability in the Civil and Criminal Courts

10 Negligence

Litigation is increasing as the expectations of clients in relation to health care grow and the publicity about awards of compensation raises hopes of vast settlements. In September 2007 it was revealed that current claims against the NHS for negligence handled by the NHS Litigation Authority amounted to almost £4.5 billion, of which £3.3 billion related to incidents alleging oxygen starvation at birth. In the decade ending in 2008 there were 1179 clinical negligence claims relating to cancer treatment leading to £47 million paid out in compensation and claims of £50 million still outstanding.[1] At present there are few reported cases of negligence involving physiotherapy services, but this does not mean that the physiotherapist can ignore the implications of civil actions being brought.

The employed physiotherapist is unlikely him/herself to be sued personally. This is because employers are indirectly responsible in law for the wrongful acts of their employees while an employee is acting in course of employment. This is known as the vicarious liability of the employer and is explained further below. However, the private practitioner who does not have an employer must ensure that he/she has the necessary insurance cover to pay out any compensation claims brought against him/her.

Even if the physiotherapist is an employee he/she still needs to have an understanding of the law relating to negligence so that he/she is appropriately prepared to defend any allegations against him/her.

This chapter covers the following topics:

- Civil actions
- Principles of negligence
- Vicarious and personal liability distinguished
- Defences to an action
- Calculating compensation (quantum)
- Examples of situations involving physiotherapists
- Liability for students and unqualified assistants
- Care of property
- Documentation
- NHS Redress Scheme
- Future developments

Civil actions

These include those actions which are brought in the civil courts by an individual or organisation, usually with the aim of obtaining compensation or other remedy that the court is able to order. The main group of civil actions affecting health professionals are called torts, i.e. civil wrongs excluding breach of contract. Within the group various causes of action are included – negligence, trespass, breach of statutory duty, defamation, nuisance and others. In each case the burden will usually be upon the person bringing the action [known as the claimant (formerly known as the plaintiff)] to establish on a balance of probabilities the existence of each of the elements which make up each cause of action. Thus, in an action for trespass to the person (see Chapter 7) the claimant must show that there was a direct interference or touching of his/her person and that it was without his/her consent or other lawful justification.

Principles of negligence

This is the most common tort, being actions brought in situations where the claimant [the word replacing plaintiff following the Woolf Reforms (see Chapter 2)] alleges that there has been personal injury or death, or damage or loss of property caused by another. Compensation is sought for the loss which has occurred. To succeed in the action the claimant has to show the following elements:

- that the defendant owed to the person harmed a duty of care;
- that the defendant was in breach of that duty;
- that the breach of duty caused reasonably foreseeable
- harm to the claimant.

These four elements – duty, breach, causation and harm are discussed below.

Duty of care

The law recognises that a duty of care will exist where one person can reasonably foresee that his or her actions and omissions could cause

reasonably foreseeable harm to another person. A duty of care will always exist between the health professional and the client, but it might not always be easy to identify to which people such a duty extends. For example, would a physiotherapist have a duty of care to report that the neighbour of a client appears to be requiring the assistance of the community team?

Situation: a duty of care?

A physiotherapist is visiting a client who has just been discharged from hospital and is told that the neighbour has not been seen for a few days and there are concerns about her health. Could the physiotherapist say 'that person is not my client and so I am not going to take any further action'? It could happen, that the neighbour dies and the relatives, on hearing that the physiotherapist had been told of possible problems, commence a civil action for failure to fulfil the duty of care. Would the allegation that a duty of care existed be upheld?

There is no decided case on the point, but it is likely that the courts would recognise a duty of care on the part of a health professional as existing in such circumstances. However, this then gives rise to other such questions as whether the physiotherapist has a duty of care when he/she is on holiday and discovers that a person nearby is in need of help. The usual legal principle is that there is no duty to volunteer services unless a pre-existing duty exists. It is likely that the courts would not recognise a duty as arising in a holiday situation. There may however be a professional duty recognised by the registration body (see Chapter 4) and the Health Professions Council (HPC) might have to decide if the physiotherapist is guilty of unprofessional conduct.

In the case of *Donoghue* v. *Stevenson*[2] the House of Lords defined the duty of care owed at common law (i.e. judge-made law):

You must take reasonable care to avoid acts or omissions which you can reasonably foresee would be likely to injure your neighbour. Who then in law is my neighbour? The answer seems to be persons who are so closely and directly affected by my act that I ought reasonably to have them in contemplation as being so affected when I am directing my mind to the acts or omissions which are called in question.

Despite there being such a straightforward definition laid down by the House of Lords there is often a difficulty in deciding how far and to whom, precisely, the duty of care extends. Cases are decided on their particular facts.

In a case involving the escape of borstal boys who caused serious damage to a yacht,[3] the House of Lords held that a duty of care was owed by the Home Office to any persons who were injured or whose property was damaged as a result of the institution's failure to keep the boys under proper control. A footballer owes a duty of care to other players and a tackle that was judged an intentional foul and caused an injury to another player was held to be a breach of that duty of care.[4]

In a case in 1998,[5] the Court of Appeal held that although the ambulance service owed no duty to the public at large to respond to a telephone call for help, once a 999 call had been accepted, it was arguable that the ambulance service did have an obligation to provide the service for a named individual at a specified address. Subsequently, the Court of Appeal dismissed an appeal by the London Ambulance Authority that it should pay the victim £362 377. The facts of the case are shown below.

Case: *Kent* v. *Griffiths and Others*[6]

A doctor called an ambulance for a woman who was asthmatic at 4.27 p.m. on 16 February 1991. The standards recommended were that the ambulance should come within 14 minutes. The husband phoned again at 4.39 p.m. and was told they would be there within 7 to 8 minutes. The doctor phoned at 4.55 p.m. and was told it would be a couple of minutes. The ambulance arrived at 5.05 p.m., 38 minutes after the first call. (A record prepared by a member of the crew indicated that it had

arrived after 22 minutes.) During the journey, the claimant was given oxygen, but on the way suffered a respiratory arrest with tragic consequences, including serious memory impairment, change of personality and miscarriage. The judge found that the record of the ambulance's arrival had been falsified. The Court of Appeal refused to strike out the case as disclosing no reasonable cause of action for negligence, but held that the case should continue to trial.

The Court of Appeal held that a duty of care could be owed by the ambulance service which was comparable to hospital services rather than to the police or fire services.

In the second appeal, the Court of Appeal held that the acceptance of the call in the present case established the duty of care. It was delay that caused the further injuries. If wrong information had not been given about the arrival of the ambulance, other means of transport could have been used.

In the case of *Phelps* v. *Hillingdon London Borough Council*,[7] the Court of Appeal held that an educational psychologist, employed by a local education authority to give advice to it in respect of children in its schools suffering from learning difficulties, did not owe a duty of care to such a child, unless he or she had assumed responsibility for that child. The House of Lords, however, allowed the appeal.[8] It held that a local education authority is liable for the negligent actions of a teacher or educational psychologist and can be sued for a failure to provide an education commensurate with a child's needs. The House of Lords gave a judgment on four cases: the Phelps case against London Borough of Hillingdon; Marcus Jarvis against Hampshire County Council (failing to diagnose dyslexia); G against Bromley (failure to provide him with computer technology and suitable training to help him deal with a muscular problem); and Rhiannon Anderton against Clwyd County Council (she sought pre-action disclosure of educational records: to succeed she had to show that she was suffering from personal injury). It held that a failure to improve a condition from which a child suffered could count as personal injury. It rejected the argument that providing psychological advice was part of a multidisciplinary approach that, in the past, has justified immunity from negligence in care claims.

In the case of *X(1) and Y(2)* v. *London Borough of Hounslow* the High Court[9] held that a duty of care is owed by a local authority when a couple with learning disabilities were being assaulted and victimised by a gang of youths. The case is discussed in Chapter 22.

Duty of care and economic loss

In an interesting case the London Borough of Islington tried to recover the costs of the care they were providing to a person who had been injured as a result of the negligence of University College London Hospital NHS Trust.

London Borough of Islington v. *University College London Hospital NHS Trust*[10]

Mrs J was due to be admitted to hospital for a mitral valve replacement and was told to stop taking the warfarin she had been prescribed a week before the operation. The operation was cancelled and she was told not to restart the warfarin. However, she started having pains in her legs and checked with the hospital who stated that the pains were not connected with the lack of warfarin and she should continue not taking it. She then suffered a stroke and became severely dependent on others. She sued University College Hospital Trust, which admitted liability. A settlement was reached under which Mrs J's daughter was able to buy a house in which to care for her plus £40 000 a year so long as she remained in the care of her daughter. All the sums payable under the settlement were paid in to the Court of Protection. The total cost of the local authority caring for Mrs J was over £80 000 per year and they could not recover their costs from her settlement, since they were bound to disregard the compensation she had received for the purposes of calculating her liability to pay. Mrs J could not recover the care costs from the defendants because she was not liable to pay

them. The local authority therefore brought an action against the defendants claiming from them the costs of the care provided to Mrs J as a result of the duty of care they owed to the local authority in the law of negligence. The defendants held that there was no duty of care owed to the local authority. The trial judge held that there was no duty of care owed, and the Court of Appeal dismissed the appeal holding that no duty of care was owed by the hospital to the local authority. Policy considerations such as proximity, fairness, justice and reasonableness were limiting factors in deciding the extent to which reasonable foreseeability of loss from an action should give rise to a duty of care owed to the person suffering from the loss. The Court of Appeal applied the ruling of the House of Lords in the Alcock case (see below).[11]

The issue may be of importance to physiotherapists in the context of referrals – at what point does the physiotherapist owe a duty of care to a client? Immediately after a referral or only after the referral has been accepted? Negligence relating to referrals and priority setting is discussed below.

Specific situations where the disputes over the existence of a duty of care might arise include:

- Conflict between different health professionals and social services staff, e.g. the boundaries between nurses and physiotherapists on discharge of patients from continuing care. This is considered in Chapter 18 on community care.
- What is the duty of care to a person who refuses to leave hospital? Can he be compelled to leave a hospital bed
  - if the hospital is being closed;
  - if he no longer needs NHS help;
  - if relatives refuse to move him?
  This is also considered in Chapter 18.
- What is the duty of care if people wish to take their own discharge? Can health professionals refuse to let people take their own discharge when they could cause harm to themselves at home? This is considered in Chapter 7 on consent.

- In what circumstances does the physiotherapist have a duty of care to the carer? This would be answered in law on the basis of the principles set out in the *Donoghue* v. *Stevenson* case quoted above. (See also Chapter 18 and accountability for a carer paid from direct payments.)

  When does the duty of care arise following a referral?

  Following a referral, whether self-referral or from another clinician, a physiotherapist would have a duty of care to assess the priority and suitability of the referral. If the physiotherapist has insufficient information, he/she would have to take steps to obtain the information necessary to make the assessment of priority, notifying the referror or the patient (if a self-referral) in the meantime. Once he/she decides that the referral is appropriate the duty of care to provide the reasonable standard of care would commence.

- Who is liable if a patient is discharged from one service and referred to another, but the latter refuses to accept the referral? Who has the responsibility for patient care?

  The duty of care to the patient would continue until the transfer of the patient to another service had been appropriately completed or the patient notified that the treatment had now ended. If the physiotherapist is notified that a suggested transfer is not acceptable, it would be the duty of the physiotherapist to continue to care for that patient until the patient is either discharged from her care, or is transferred to another service which accepts the patient.

- Does a physiotherapist who works in occupational health have a duty of care to report to the employers if he/she becomes aware of a pattern of repetitive strain injury (RSI) type symptoms arising from a particular new task in the workplace, even if such a duty is not specifically set out in his/her job description.

  It is probable that the answer to the question in this last situation is 'yes'. The job description is not a contractual term and can be changed by the employer within the contract of employment. An implied term in the contract of employment requires the employee to act with reasonable care and skill in fulfilling his/her duty of care. In the circumstances described here the duty of care could include a responsibility to report.

Breach of duty

Determining the standard of care

In order to determine whether there has been a breach of the duty of care, it will first be necessary to establish the required standard. The courts have used what has become known as the 'Bolam test' to determine the standard of care required by a professional. In the case from which the test took its name[12] the court laid down the following principle to determine the standard of care which should be followed:

> The test is the standard of the ordinary skilled man exercising and professing to have that special skill. (McNair, Ref. 12, p. 121)

The Bolam test was applied by the House of Lords in a case[13] where negligence by an obstetrician in delivering a child by forceps was alleged:

> When you get a situation which involves the use of some special skill or competence, then the test as to whether there has been negligence or not . . . is the standard of the ordinary skilled man exercising and professing to have that special skill. If a surgeon failed to measure up to that in any respect (clinical judgement or otherwise) he had been negligent and should be so adjudged.

The House of Lords found that the surgeon was not liable in negligence and held that an error of judgment may or may not be negligence. It depends upon the circumstances.

This standard of the reasonable professional man following the accepted approved standard of care can be used to apply to any professional person – architect, lawyer or accountant, as well as any health professional. The standard of care that a physiotherapist should have provided would be judged in this way. Expert witnesses would give evidence to the court on the standard of care they would expect to have found in the circumstances giving rise to the claim. These experts would be respected members of the profession of physiotherapists, possibly head of a physiotherapy department or training college (see Chapter 13).

In a civil action, the judge would decide, in the light of the evidence which has been given to the court, what standard should have been followed.

Experts can, of course, differ and a case may arise where the expert giving evidence for the claimant states that the accepted approved standard of care was not followed by the defendant or its employees, whereas in contrast the expert evidence for the defendant states that a reasonable standard of care was followed. Where such a conflict arises the House of Lords in the case of *Maynard* v. *West Midlands Regional Health Authority*[14] has laid down the following principle:

> It was not sufficient to establish negligence for the plaintiff [claimant] to show that there is a body of competent professional opinion that considered the decision was wrong, if there was also a body of equally competent professional opinion that supports the decision as having been reasonable in the circumstances.

The determination of the reasonable standard of care has been more recently considered by the House of Lords in the case of *Bolitho* v. *City Hospital Hackney*.[15] In this case the House of Lords stated that:

> The use of these adjectives – responsible, reasonable and respectable – [in the Bolam case] all show that the court has to be satisfied that the exponents of the body of opinion relied upon can demonstrate that such opinion has a logical basis . . . [T]he judge before accepting a body of opinion as being responsible, reasonable or respectable, will need to be satisfied

that, in forming their views, the experts had directed their minds to the question of comparative risks and benefits and had reached a defensible conclusion on the matter.

> [I]t will very seldom be right for a judge to reach the conclusion that views genuinely held by a competent medical expert are unreasonable.

Setting standards in physiotherapy practice

The Chartered Society of Physiotherapy (CSP) has published guidance on standards for physiotherapy practice. The central documents, which support the *Rules of professional Conduct*, are *Core Standards of Physiotherapy Practice*, 2005, and *Service Standards of Physiotherapy Practice*, 2005. These two documents should be seen as supporting each other. The former covers Patient Partnership, Asessment and Treatment Cycle, Communication, Documentation, Promoting a Safe Working/Treatment Environment and Continuing Professional Development. The latter covers Clinical Governance, Human Resourses and Service Provision.

The White Paper[16] that is discussed in Chapter 17 has led to increasing emphasis on standard setting. The establishment of the National Institute for Health and Clinical Excellence (NICE), the Healthcare Commission (now replaced by the Care Quality Commission) and the National Service Frameworks (NSF) provide guidance on standards to be achieved in all sectors of hospital and community care. The NHS Litigation Authority (NHSLA) has set risk management standards for acute trusts, which were revised in 2008.[17] These replace the general clinical risk management standards prepared by the Clinical Negligence Scheme for Trusts (CNST). Physiotherapists will be expected to follow the results of clinical effectiveness research in their treatment and care of the patients. Patients will be able to use these national guidelines to argue that inadequate care has been provided.

Guidance on standards is available from a variety of sources including voluntary organisations and professional associations. For example

Diabetes UK (London)[18] published in March 2003 guidance on physical activity and diabetes which is available from its website. The Cystic Fibrosis Trust published in June 2007 guidance on physiotherapy treatment for airway clearance techniques and in May 2007 physiotherapy treatment for babies and toddlers with cystic fibrosis and other fact sheets that are available from its website.[19]

Standards for stroke victims can be found in the NSF for older people (what makes a good stroke service and how do we get there). The NSF for older people planned that everyone who had a stroke would have access to a specialist stroke service by 2004. In addition, a second edition of the National Clinical Guidelines for stroke were published in 2004 by the Royal College of Physicians. This was followed in 2006 by the Physiotherapy Concise Guide for Stroke published by the CSP and the Royal College of Physicians. NICE Clinical guideline for Parkinson's Disease was published in June 2006.

Physiotherapists should be aware of the relevant specialist guidelines set by many organisations in developing their practice.

The CSP has laid down two sets of standards: Core Standards[20] pertaining to the individual practice of the physiotherapist and Service Standards.[21] The latter are described as follows:

The service standards describe components of the physiotherapy service for which the organisation is responsible, in order to maintain the safety and quality of services for patients, and provide an environment conducive to the safety of staff. The standards provide a benchmark against which the service can be measured, and a framework for an organisation to review and improve its service provision. By contrast, the core standards are the responsibility of individual physiotherapists. The service standards are intended to apply to all physiotherapy services, including those in NHS, independent and voluntary sectors, both large and small, and in all settings. However, there will be some standards that do not apply to certain services, for example parts of standard nine, on workforce, will not apply to single-handed practitioners. Similarly, the standards on hydrotherapy (17, 18) will only apply to services with a hydrotherapy pool.

As with the core standards, the service standards are not minimum, nor standards of excellence, but they are considered to be achievable.

Has there been a breach of the duty of care?

Once it has been established in court what the reasonable standard of care should have been, the next stage is to decide whether what took place was in accordance with the reasonable standard, i.e. has there been a breach of the duty of care. Evidence will be given by witnesses of fact as to what actually took place. The role of such witnesses is considered in Chapter 13.

Difficulties can arise in establishing the standard of care, especially in circumstances where the technique gives rise to complications. It is in such circumstances that the internet discussion within the CIOGs of best practice in a given clinical situation can be of considerable assistance in determining the recommended practice. (See the case of Maynard above for the situation where there is a responsible body of opinion in favour of and another responsible body against a procedure.) It would also be necessary to show that the patient was informed of the significant risks of substantial harm before the treatment commenced (see Chapter 7).

Standards, guidelines, procedures and protocols

Various names are given to guidance material issued for healthcare professionals. The term 'standards' is probably best kept to statements of practice that can be used as a measure of quality. Guidelines, procedures and protocols may be issued by professional bodies, employers or other organisations and their weight will vary according to their source. For example, failure to follow guidance issued by employers could result in disciplinary action. However, whatever term is used, the professional judgment of the healthcare professional is never ousted. NICE has made it clear that its guidelines are subject to the professional discretion of the healthcare profession in their implementation. Clearly, however, in deciding that the guidance is inappropriate for the particular circumstances of that individual patient, the practitioner must ensure that the reasons are explicitly and carefully recorded. A book by Brian Hurwitz is useful on this topic.[22] The CSP has carried out a Guideline Programme Review and is implementing this in a project known as Supporting Knowledge in Physiotherapy Practice. Further information is available on the CSP website. The CSP itself has issued several guidelines, such as those issued in 2006 for the physiotherapy management of persistent low back pain. It is hoped that such guidelines are based on clinical research and there would therefore be a presumption in favour of following them. However, where the professional judgment is that they are contrary to the individual needs of a particular patient, then the physiotherapist should be able to show that reasonable practice according to the Bolam test would be contrary to following them. Thus, the ruling in the Maynard case (see above) would apply.[14]

Causation

The claimant must show that not only was there a breach of the duty of care, but that this breach of duty caused actual and reasonably foreseeable harm to the claimant. This requires

- factual causation to be shown;
- evidence that the type of harm which occurred was reasonably foreseeable;
- that there was no break in the chain of causation (i.e. *novus actus inerveniens* – a new action intervening).

Factual causation

There may be a breach of the duty of care and harm but there may be no link between them.

The following is the classic case[23] illustrating an absence of factual causation.

Case: *Barnett* v. *Chelsea* HMC

Three nightwatchmen drank tea that made them vomit. They went to the casualty department of the local hospital. The casualty officer, on being told of the complaints by a nurse, did not see the men, but told them to go home and call in their own doctors. Some hours later one of them died from arsenical poisoning. The court held that

- the casualty department officers owed a duty of care in the circumstances; and
- the casualty doctor had been negligent in not seeing them; but
- even if he had, it was improbable that the only effective antidote could have been administered in time to save the deceased.

Therefore, the defendants were not liable. The patient would have died anyway.

The onus is on the claimant to establish that there is this causation link between the breach of the duty of care and the harm that occurred. In the following case,[24] the claimant failed initially to establish causation although ultimately the House of Lords ordered a new hearing on the issue and at the end of the day, faced with more protracted litigation, the parties agreed to a settlement.

Case: *Wilsher* v. *Essex Area Health Authority*

A premature baby was being treated with oxygen therapy. A junior doctor mistakenly inserted the catheter to monitor the oxygen intake into the vein rather than an artery. A senior registrar when being asked to check what had been done failed to notice the error. The baby was given excess oxygen. The parents claimed compensation for the retrolentalfibroplasia that the baby suffered, but failed to prove that it was the excess oxygen which had caused the harm. They therefore failed in their claim.

It was agreed that there were several different factors that could have caused the child to become blind and the negligence in question was only one of them. It could not be presumed that it was the defendant's negligence that had caused the harm.

It has also been difficult for claimants to establish causation when suing for compensation for harm that it is claimed has resulted from vaccine damage. In the case of *Loveday* v. *Renton and another*[25] a claim was brought against the Wellcome Foundation, who had made vaccine against whooping cough, and against the doctor who had administered it, seeking compensation for brain damage which was alleged to have been caused by the vaccine. The case failed because the judge held that the claimant had not established on a balance of probabilities that the pertussis vaccine had caused the brain damage.

Subsequently, however, in an Irish case brought against the Wellcome Foundation and others for vaccine damage[26] it has been held that causation as well as breach was established. The High Court had dismissed the claimant's claim because of the lack of proof of causation, but on appeal the Irish Supreme Court held that the Wellcome Foundation was liable for the negligent manufacture and release of a particular batch of triple vaccine and that the brain damage was caused as a result. It referred the case back to the High Court on the amount of compensation and in 1993 the court approved an award of £2.75 million as compensation for the brain damage sustained in September 1969. The award was so high because it included the cost of care for the 24 years since the injury occurred and also the cost of future care which, in cases of brain damage, can be very high.

Reasonably foreseeable harm

The harm that might arise may not be within the reasonable contemplation of the defendant so that, even though there is a breach of duty and there is harm, the defendant is not liable. For example, a physiotherapist may have ordered the wrong equipment for a person at home and therefore be in breach of the duty of care, but the client may have suffered harm because he/she used the equipment in an inappropriate way.

Case: *Jolley* v. *Sutton London Borough Council*[27]

Some children found a boat abandoned on grass beside council housing. The local authority had a duty under the Occupier's Liability Act 1957 (see Chapter 11) to any visitor to ensure the area was safe. In the High Court the claimant was awarded £633 770 (taking into account contributory negligence of 25%) for the injuries he sustained when the boat, which some children had propped up with a car jack so that they could repair it, collapsed on top of him crushing his back.

However, the Court of Appeal found in favour of the defendant council and the award was withdrawn. This was because, although it was reasonably foreseeable that injuries could have occurred in the event of children playing on the boat, the injuries sustained by the claimant were not reasonably foreseeable and therefore the defendants were not liable for them. The Council had not disputed that it was negligent, but simply claimed it was not liable because the accident was of a different kind from anything which it could have reasonably foreseen. The claimant appealed to the House of Lords, which upheld the appeal.[28] The House of Lords held that the ingenuity of children in finding unexpected ways of doing mischief to themselves and others should not be underestimated. Reasonable foreseeability was not a fixed point on the scale of probability. The Council was liable under the Occupiers' Liability Act 1957 and under Section 2(3) had to take into account the fact that children would be less careful than adults (see Chapter 11). The Council had admitted that it should have removed the boat and the risk that it should have taken into account was that children would meddle with the boat and injuries would thereby occur.

Section 2(3) states that:

The circumstances relevant for the present purpose include the degree of care, and of want of care, which would ordinarily be looked for in such a visitor, so that (for example) in proper cases: an occupier must be prepared for children to be less careful than adults.

New intervening cause (*novus actus interveniens*)

It may also happen that any causal link between the claimant's breach of duty and the harm suffered by the client is interrupted by an intervening event.

Situation: intervening act

> A physiotherapist failed to make an appropriate assessment for the discharge of the patient from the department, but the patient was injured in a road accident as a result of another person's negligence and died from her injuries.

In this situation the negligence of the physiotherapist has not caused the death of the patient so her employer would not be vicariously liable.

Harm

To succeed in an action for negligence claimants or their representatives must establish that they have suffered harm that the court recognises as being subject to compensation. Thus, personal injury, death and loss or damage to property are the main areas of recognisable harm. In addition, the courts have ruled that nervous shock (now known as post-traumatic stress syndrome) can be the subject of compensation within strict limits of liability (and where an identifiable medical condition exists). A test of proximity to the defendant's negligent action or omission has been set by the House of Lords in the case of *Alcock* v. *Chief Constable of South Yorkshire* 1992.[11] This test of proximity can be used to argue that the harm is not subject to compensation or that no duty of care is owed in the circumstances (see cases above under Duty of care).

In one case[29] where a mother claimed compensation for post-traumatic stress the defendants argued that since the events took place over a period of time it was not simply one horrifying event.

Case: *North Glamorgan NHS Trust* v. *Walters* 2003

A 10-month-old boy was admitted to hospital suspected of suffering from hepatitis. The doctors failed to diagnose that this was acute and accepted that had it been properly diagnosed and treated by means of a liver transplant, he may have lived. During the night he suffered a fit and the mother was told by the nurse that it was unlikely that he had suffered any brain damage. In fact, there had been a major epileptic seizure that led to a coma and irreparable brain damage. A scan was carried out and the mother was told incorrectly that it showed no brain damage. He was transferred to a London hospital where he was placed on a life support machine. A further scan showed that he had suffered severe brain damage and the parents agreed that it was in the boy's best interests for the life support to be turned off. He died in his mother's arms. She was subsequently told that had he been transferred earlier he would have had a far better chance of survival.

It was agreed that the mother was suffering from a pathological grief reaction, which was a result of witnessing, experiencing and participating in the events described. The judge found that the mother was a secondary victim and her psychiatric injury was caused by sight and sound of a horrifying event that had covered a period of time. The defendants appealed to the Court of Appeal on the grounds that the 36-hour period could not be regarded in law as one horrifying event, but the claimant's appreciation was not sudden. The Court of Appeal held that the 36-hour period could be viewed as a single horrifying event and the judge was correct to find that the claimant's appreciation of the events was sudden as opposed to an accumulation of gradual assaults on her mind.

A similar decision is seen in another Court of Appeal case[30] where the claimant suffered post-traumatic stress syndrome after her daughter was killed in a road accident when a car mounted the pavement. The claimant rushed to the scene of the accident, which was cordoned off, and she was prevented from crossing the tape. She was told that her daughter was dead and she screamed hysterically and collapsed to the ground. Subsequently at the mortuary, although the worst of the injuries on the girl's lower part were covered by a blanket, the mother saw that the daughter's face and head were disfigured. She cradled the daughter saying she was cold. She lost her case on the grounds that the judge could not accept that what happened in the mortuary could be said to be part of the aftermath. The shock from which she suffered was a result of what she had been told by the police. The Court of Appeal allowed the claimant's appeal holding that the immediate aftermath extended from the moment of the accident until the moment that the claimant left the mortuary. The judge had artificially separated out the mortuary visit from what was an uninterrupted sequence of events.

A victim of the Ladbroke Grove rail crash who suffered depression which led to his killing someone was able to recover damages for the loss of his earnings after the manslaughter from the defendant's who admitted liability for negligence up to the date of the manslaughter.[31] Although his physical injuries were minor the accident had a major psychological impact on him. He suffered post-traumatic stress disorder with a marked depressive component and a significant personality change. In August 2001 he stabbed a stranger to death. The Court held that his claim was not founded on an illegal act. The manslaughter was not inextricably bound up with the claim for loss of earnings before and after the manslaughter, which resulted from the defendant's negligence. It was for the court to determine to what extent the manslaughter was the claimant's fault and therefore could be viewed as contributory negligence under the 1945 Act (see below).

Some of the types of harm covered by the effect of personal injury are illustrated below in the section showing how compensation is calculated.

Vicarious and personal liability distinguished

As stated above it is unlikely that an employed physiotherapist will be sued personally since the employer would be vicariously liable for his/her actions.

To establish the vicarious liability of the employer the claimant must show:

- the employee
- was negligent or was guilty of another wrong
- while acting in course of employment.

An independent practitioner would have to accept personal and professional liability for his/her actions but he/she may also be vicariously liable for the harm, caused during the course of employment, by anyone he/she herself employs.

Each of the elements shown above must be established. It follows that:

- the employer is not liable for the acts of his/her independent contractors (i.e. self-employed persons who are working for him/her on a contract for services) unless he/she is at fault in selecting or instructing them; and
- the employer may challenge whether the actions were performed in the course of employment.

The definition of 'in the course of employment' was widened in a decision by the House of Lords. In the following case, the House of Lords held that school owners were vicariously liable for acts of sexual abuse committed by the school warden against pupils – the abusive acts were sufficiently connected with his work as to be in the course of employment.

Case: *Lister* v. *Hesley Hall*[32]

The Board of Governors was sued by the victims of abuse by the warden at Hesley Hall, a children's home, because of its vicarious liability for his actions. The home denied liability on the grounds that the abuse was not committed in the course of his employment. The House of Lords held that it was vicariously liable for the acts of the warden in abusing the claimants: the home had undertaken the care of the children and entrusted the performance of that duty to the warden and there was therefore sufficiently close connection between his employment and the acts committed by him.

The House of Lords stated that the approach which was best when determining whether a wrongful act was to be deemed to be done by the employee in the course of his employment, was to concentrate on the relative closeness of the connection between the nature of the employment and the particular wrong doing. The defendant undertook to care for the claimants through the services of a warden so there was a very close connection between the torts of the warden and the defendant. The torts were also committed at a time and place when the warden was busy caring for the claimants. The warden was carrying out his duties though in an unauthorised and improper mode.

In a recent case, the Court of Appeal had to decide whether throwing a punch in a rugby match could be considered to be in the course of employment so as to make the club vicariously liable.[33] The case is considered in Chapter 20.

Issues relating to vicarious liability can occur with complementary therapies. For example, a physiotherapist may have undertaken training in a complementary medicine such as aromatherapy. If he/she decided to use these new skills while at work without the agreement, express or implied, of the employer and through his/her use of the remedies caused harm to the client, his/her employer might refuse to accept vicarious liability on the grounds that he/she was not acting in the course of employment. To claim that he/she was covered by vicarious liability he/she would have to show that there was such a close connection between the aromatherapy and his/her normal work as a physiotherapist that the employer should be held vicariously liable for his/her negligence. (See Chapter 27 on complementary therapies.)

The physiotherapist may also undertake extracurricular activities with patients such as horse riding or going to a commercial gym. Would these activities be considered to be in the course of employment so that if the physiotherapist were negligent, the employer would be vicariously liable for this negligence? It is not possible to generalise since it all depends upon the circumstances. Thus a physiotherapist who in his/her own time returned to work to give his/her clients assistance with horse riding might be considered by the employer to be doing this on his/her own account and not on its behalf. However, it would be different, if this activity were included in the client's treatment plan and there was an expectation that the physiotherapist would provide attendance. Similarly, if it is agreed that the physiotherapist should accompany the client on a day trip, even though it is his/her day off, it may still be considered to be in the course of employment.

Where such uncertainties are likely to arise it is wise to clarify such issues in advance with the employer, so that the physiotherapist knows whether he/she ought to obtain private insurance cover for such activities or notify his/her existing insurer about their taking place. An independent physiotherapist in private practice should ensure that he/she notifies his/her insurers of the exact content of his/her work and whether it involves possibly risky activities (see Chapter 19 on the private practitioner).

Defences to an action

The main defences to an action for negligence are listed below:

- Allegations of fact are disputed.
- It is denied that all elements of negligence are established.
- The defendant alleges contributory negligence on the part of the claimant.
- The defendant claims exemption from liability.

- The time set in law for bringing a claim has expired.
- The defendant alleges the claimant voluntarily assumed the risk.

Disputed allegations of fact

Many cases will be resolved entirely on what facts can be shown to exist. Thus the effectiveness of the witnesses for both parties in establishing the facts of what did or did not occur will be the determining factor in who wins the case. Reference should be made to Chapter 12 on record keeping and Chapter 13 on witnesses in court for further discussion on the nature of evidence and the role of the witnesses. In theory, it might appear before the court hearing that one party has a particularly strong case but, unless the facts on which that case rests can be proved in court, the actual outcome of the case might be that the opponent wins.

Basically every case depends on proper hard evidence and whether the witnesses of fact (either about the event or about the extent of the injuries), including the parties themselves, can be believed. In a civil case of negligence, the judge determines both the facts of the case and whether there is liability by the defendant and, if so, what amount of compensation (i.e. quantum) should be paid (unless either liability or quantum are agreed by the parties).

Elements of negligence not established

The claimant must establish that all elements required to prove negligence are present, i.e. duty, breach, causation and harm. If one or more of these cannot be established then the defendant will win the case.

Contributory negligence

If the client is partly to blame for the harm that has occurred then there may still be liability on the part of the professional but the compensation payable might be reduced in proportion to the client's fault. In extreme cases such a claim may be a complete defence if 100% contributory negligence is claimed. In determining the level of contributory negligence, the physical and mental health and the age of the client would be taken into account.

Situation: Contributory negligence

> A physiotherapist made a negligent assessment of a person's needs but, in addition, the client failed to give the physiotherapist vital information relevant to those needs. Harm subsequently befell the client as a result of the assessment being inaccurate.
>
> In an action brought by the client the client's contribution to that harm is taken into account.

The Law Reform (Contributory Negligence) Act 1945 enables an apportionment of responsibility for the harm that has been caused which may result in a reduction of damages payable. The Court can reduce the damages 'to such extent as it thinks just and equitable having regard to the claimant's share in the responsibility for the damage' (Section 1(1)).

One of the most frequent examples of contributory negligence being taken into account is in road traffic accidents where the injuries sustained by the claimant are greater because he or she was not wearing a seat belt. (For contributory negligence by a child see Chapter 23.)

The defences of contributory negligence, *volenti non fit injuria* (see below) and *novus actus interveniens* (see above), were all used by the defendant in a case brought against the Commissioner for the Metropolitan police.[34] The administratrix of L, who had committed suicide while in police custody, sued the police for breach of their duty of care to the prisoner, who was known to be a suicide risk. The trial judge found that there was a breach of the duty of care by the police since they had left the hatch of his cell door open and it had been used in the suicide. However, he held that this breach of duty had not caused the death on the basis of either *volenti non fit injuria* or *novus actus interveniens*, the sole cause of death was L's deliberate act in killing himself. The Court of Appeal allowed the claimant's appeal holding that neither *volenti non fit injuria* nor *novus actus interveniens* applied where the act which caused the death was the act which the defendant was under a duty to prevent. It awarded £8690 compensation. The defendant appealed and the House of Lords held that there was a duty of care owed to L and it was self-contradictory to say that breach of that duty could not have been a cause of harm because the victim had caused it to himself. The police were in breach of their duty of care and caused the death, but so did L cause his own death. However, L was in sound mind and therefore he must be considered to have some responsibility for his death. Applying the 1945 Act compensation was reduced by 50% to allow for L's responsibility for the death.

No duty of care of police and fire service

In contrast, the Court of Appeal decided that the police did not owe a duty of care to the victims of crime in deciding whether or not to prosecute a suspected offender, even where the decision took into account the interests of the victim.[35] V and her sisters alleged that the police had failed to investigate allegations of indecent assault and cruelty and to prosecute. The Court of Appeal held

that there were policy reasons for the general rule that the police owed no duty of care to investigate allegations of crime victims, in particular the diversion of resources and that police investigations might be carried out defensively. Their claim was struck out. The ruling in the cases of *Hill* v. *Chief Constable of West Yorkshire Police*[36] and the case of *Brooks* v. *Commissioner of Police of the Metropolis*[37] was applied. The Court of Appeal held that a fire brigade did not owe a duty of care to an owner or occupier merely by attending a fire.[38]

Exemption from liability

It is possible for people to exempt themselves from liability for harm arising from their negligence but the effects of the Unfair Contract Terms Act 1977 means that this exemption can only apply to loss or damage to property. A defendant cannot exclude liability for negligence that results in personal damage or death, either by contract or by a notice.

Where exemption from liability for loss or damage to property is claimed by the defendant, it must be shown by the defendant that it is reasonable to rely upon the term or notice which purported to exclude liability. The relevant provisions of the Unfair Contract Terms Act 1977 are shown in Figure 10.1.

2(1)   A person cannot by reference to any contract term or to a notice given to persons generally or to particular persons exclude or restrict his liability for death or personal injury resulting from negligence.

2(2)   In the case of other loss or damage, a person cannot so exclude or restrict his liability for negligence except in so far as the term or notice satisfies the requirement of reasonableness.

[The 'reasonableness' test is explained in Section 11]

11(3)   In relation to a notice (not being a notice having contractual effect) . . . it should be fair and reasonable to allow reliance on it, having regard to all the circumstances obtaining when the liability arose or (but for the notice) would have arisen.

11(5)   It is for those claiming that a contract term or notice satisfies the requirements of reasonableness to show that it does.

Figure 10.1   Unfair Contract Terms Act 1977: Sections 2 and 11 (extracts)

- Those suffering from a disability:

  - Children under 18 years – the time does not start to run until the child is 18 years.
  - Those suffering from a mental disability – time does not start to run until the disability ends. In the case of those who are suffering from severe learning disabilities or brain damage this may not be until death.

- Discretion of the judge. The judge has a statutory power to extend the time within which a claimant can bring an action for personal injuries or death if it is just and equitable to do so.

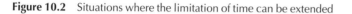

Figure 10.2   Situations where the limitation of time can be extended

Limitation of time

Actions for personal injury or death should normally be commenced within 3 years of the date of the event which gave rise to the harm or 3 years from the date on which the person had the necessary knowledge of the harm and the fact that it arose from the defendant's actions or omissions. The Court of Appeal held that the cause of action accrues when the injury is suffered.[39]

Exceptions

There are however some major qualifications to this general principle and these are shown in Figure 10.2.

The implications of the rules relating to limitation of time are that in those cases that might come under one of the exceptions to the 3-year time limit, records should be kept and not destroyed. This is particularly important in the case of children and those with learning disabilities. For example in the case of *Bull* v. *Wakeham*[40] the case was brought 18 years after the claimant's birth. In a news item report in 1995,[41] a man then 33 years old obtained compensation of £1.25 million because of a failure to diagnose severe dehydration a few weeks after his birth.

Knowledge

Claimants are assumed to have the necessary knowledge (and so the 'clock' starts running) when they know or it is reasonable to expect them to know the following facts:

- that the injury in question was significant;
- that the injury was attributable in whole or in part to the act or omission which is alleged to constitute the negligence, nuisance or breach of duty;
- the identity of the defendant;
- (if it is alleged that the act or omission was that of a person other than the defendant) the identity of that person and the additional facts supporting the bringing of an action against them.

Knowledge that any acts or omissions did or did not, as a matter of law, involve negligence, nuisance or breach of duty is irrelevant. The claimant cannot bring an action out of time if he/she knew all the facts more than 3 years ago but has only just found out they could give rise to a claim.

A person is not fixed with knowledge of a fact ascertainable only with the help of expert advice so long as he/she has taken all reasonable steps to obtain and, where appropriate, to act on that advice.

In a significant decision, the House of Lords[42] ruled in January 2008 that claims could be brought by the victims of rape and sexual assault outside the time limit, if the judge ruled that the personal characteristics of the claimant might have prevented him or her acting as a reasonable person. Three of the cases were remitted to High Court for reconsideration in the light of the House of Lords ruling. It overruled its previous decision in the case of *Stubbings* v. *Webb*[43] and allowed time-barred appeals in cases which involved a rape victim whose rapist had subsequently won the lottery, and several victims of sexual assault by council employees in council run schools or residential homes. The consequence of the decision is that many thousands of victims of indecent assault may pursue claims against the councils and churches.

Judge's discretion

Even where the claimant is unable to establish that he/she did not have the requisite knowledge within the time period, the judge has a discretion under Section 33 of the Limitation Act to permit the case to proceed if it is equitable to do so. For example, in the case of *Amanda Godfrey* v. *Gloucester Royal Infirmary NHS Trust*,[44] the claimant argued that although she had been told following an ultrasound scan that her baby (who was born in 1995) had severe abnormalities, she did not have sufficient information to make a decision about a termination until she read the medical report in 2001, the judge did not accept this argument but was still prepared to exercise his discretion under Section 33 of the Limitation Act 1980 and held that it was equitable to allow the case to proceed.

The evidence of the physiotherapist was relevant in a case where the claimant had suffered a Colles fracture to her wrist and claimed negligence by the hospital in failing to X-ray at her second appointment, undertaking a negligent remanipulation and negligently applying plaster of Paris.[45] The defendant argued that the claimant was out of time because more than 3 years elapsed from the date of her knowledge that the injury was significant and the judge should not have used his discretion under Section 33. The Court of Appeal allowed the defendant's appeal holding that the case was statute barred, because a reasonable person in the claimant's position would have appreciated that she had a significant injury, and the judge's exercise of his discretion was seriously flawed. The full facts of the case can be seen on the bailii website.[46]

Voluntary assumption of risk

Volenti non fit injuria is the latin tag for the defence that a person willingly undertook the risk of being harmed.

In a case[47] where a rugby player was injured following a tackle which he alleged threw him against a concrete wall it was held that, even if there had been any liability under the Occupier's Liability Act 1957 (which the court did not find – see Chapter 11), the player must be taken to have willingly accepted the risk of playing on the field, which complied with the regulations.

It is unlikely to succeed as a defence in an action for professional negligence since the professional cannot contract out of liability where harm occurs as a result of his/her negligence (see the Unfair Contract Terms Act considered above). However, it may be relevant to the physiotherapist who undertakes potentially risky activities with a client, such as horse riding, gymnastics or certain types of dance. Such activities may have an element of danger about them and, if the risks are explained to the client and the client has the competence to assume the risk of harm arising, then this may be a successful defence to a claim against the physiotherapist that he/she was negligent in proposing a risky activity. However, where the client lacks the mental competence to make such a decision, then there is a duty of care placed upon the physiotherapist to take all reasonable care, according to the Bolam test, that harm would not occur. This may entail not undertaking such an activity (see Chapter 24 for risks in the care of older people). It is unlikely that the courts would hold that a mentally incompetent adult voluntarily assumed the risk of being harmed as a result of the negligence of the physiotherapist.

Calculating compensation (quantum)

In some cases of negligence, liability might be accepted by the defendant, but there might still be disagreement between the parties over quantum, i.e. the amount of compensation.

Alternatively, there might be agreement over the amount of compensation and liability alone might be disputed. In others, both liability and quantum might be in dispute.

Physiotherapists are sometimes called as expert witnesses to give evidence of assessment in cases, where there is a dispute over quantum. This is further discussed in Chapter 13.

An example of a case giving details of a compensation calculation is shown below.

Case: brain damage at birth *Webster v. Hammersmith Hospital NHS trust* 2002[48]

The girl, aged 7 at the date of hearing, suffered brain injury at birth. Liability was admitted by the defendants. The birth injury resulted in dyskinetic choreoathetoid cerebral palsy producing severe physical disability in all four limbs, but leaving her awareness and intelligence intact. She was likely to live to the age of 65 years. She could not walk unaided and would always be dependent on a wheelchair, with the assistance of one (and in many circumstances two) carers for any venture taking her out of her home. She had good sight and hearing but her speech was dysarthric and difficult to understand. She was a gifted child with high verbal ability. She was very determined in her attitude to life. She would be likely to have had a university education and to have pursued some form of professional career. General damages of £180 000 were awarded within a total award of £4 186 221 made up as follows:

Past losses: travel (£394); incidental (£2195); aids (£3144); past care (£45 000); property (£70 000); interest (£120 733)

Future loss: loss of earnings £407 000; aids (£416 257); care up to age 19 (£546 601); care 19+ (£1 946 185); IT equipment (£75 000); physiotherapy (£37 000); property (£400 000); investment (£18 780); pain, suffering and loss of amenity (£180 000); interest (£5 500)

Total £4 186 221

The court in its calculation of compensation takes into account the fact that the award is being made at once and therefore the claimant is benefiting from the ability to obtain interest on the lump sum. Calculations are made as to what interest can be expected. It is difficult to balance matters fairly but in a recent case the House of Lords has ruled that, in the award of compensation, victims should not be expected to speculate on the stock market and therefore lower levels of return based on index-linked government securities can be used as the basis of calculation.[49] The effect of this ruling will be to increase the capital amount awarded to victims. In the case itself James Thomas, a cerebral palsy victim as a result of negligence at birth, was awarded £1 285 000 by the High Court judge, but in a very controversial decision this was reduced by the Court of Appeal by £300 000 on the basis that the capital could be invested in higher return (but more risky) equities. The House of Lords restored the original amount.

The Court of Appeal held in January 2008 that where compensation was being awarded in the case of catastrophic injury, then in calculating the future cost of the wages of carers, the court should use the annual earnings survey published for care assistants and home carers rather than the retail price index.[50]

The difficulties of assessing compensation for loss of future earnings can be seen in the case of *Brown* v. *Ministry of Defence*.[51] In the case, the Court of Appeal heard an appeal against the assessment of compensation where the claimant had suffered a serious fracture of her left ankle in the course of basic training in the army. She was unable to complete her training and left the army and after a period of convalescence and a variety of temporary jobs she began training as a physiotherapist. She claimed damages for personal injury resulting from the MOD's negligent failure to properly manage and supervise her training. Her claim included compensation for loss of pension rights in the sum of £148 856.31 calculated on the assumption that she would have remained in the Army for the full service term of 22 years that would have qualified her for an immediate pension, compensation for disadvantage in the labour market in the sum of £107 028 and compensation for loss of congenial employment in the sum of £12 000. The MOD admitted liability but contested the amount of her claim. The Court of Appeal held that there was evidence that the claimant would have probably remained in the service for 22 years and would therefore have been entitled to a pension taking into account the probability of promotion. In addition there was evidence that there was a more than insignificant risk that Miss Brown would develop osteoarthritis in her injured ankle of sufficient severity to force her to give up practice as an active physiotherapist and require her to accept a more sedentary type of employment and would therefore find herself looking for a new job in about 25 years' time.

Requirements for ongoing physiotherapy treatment can be included in the compensation claim and, if they are disputed, it will be essential for a physiotherapist to give expert evidence on the matter (see Chapter 13). In a case where the claimant, a senior psychiatric registrar, suffered a cardiac arrest and irreparable brain damage following a minor gynaecological operation the High Court awarded £249 239. This sum included the costs of one full-time and two part-time physiotherapists five times per week. The Court of Appeal did not overturn the award.[52] The physiotherapist may also give evidence as a witness of fact on his/her assessment of the future physiotherapy needs of a patient. Clearly, if the assessment is to be based on a high standard of quality of life, then the cost of independent supported living must be assessed for the purposes of the claim. Any physiotherapist involved in such assessments, either as a witness of fact or as an expert witness must ensure that all his/her calculations are based on evidence and can be defended. He/she may be cross-examined in court (see Chapter 13).

Compensation following death

Where a claim is brought under the Fatal Accidents Acts in respect of a death caused by negligence, the statutory payment for bereavement for deaths after 1 January 2008 is £11 800.[53] Dependants of the deceased can sue for the income and support which the deceased provided and which they have lost as a consequence of the death.

Under the Law Reform Miscellaneous Provisions Act 1934, the estate of the dead person is able to continue certain legal actions as though the person were still alive. The personal representative acts on behalf of the estate and can continue actions that have already commenced or begin those which the deceased was entitled to bring but died before being able to do so. This includes the right to sue those responsible for bringing about the death of the deceased.

Examples of situations involving physiotherapists

Failures in assessment

Assessment of the client's needs is the first step for a physiotherapist in developing a treatment plan. It is clear that the physiotherapist would have a duty to use his/her own professional judgment in determining the client's clinical situation and what physiotherapy treatments were indicated. If the expressed reason for referral by a doctor differed from the physiotherapist's assessment, the latter would have a duty to notify the doctor that in his/her judgment different treatments were required. He/she should not professionally undertake treatment which in his/her view is not clinically indicated: a defence of obeying orders would not suffice if harm were caused to the client as a consequence of this.

The CSP has included in its *Standards of Physiotherapy Practice* standards for assessment. It defines the assessment/treatment cycle as:

A cyclical process describing the thought processes of clinicians from information gathering to analysis and assessment, planning implementation, evaluation and transfer of care/discharge.

Standard 5 covers the collection of information relating to the patient and his/her presenting problem. The criteria for standard 5 compliance include:

(1) Written evidence on a compilation of data consisting of:
   - the patient's perception of their needs
   - the patient's expectations
   - the patient's demographic details
   - presenting condition/problems
   - past medical history
   - current medication/treatment
   - contra-indications/precautions/allergies
   - social and family history/lifestyle
   - relevant investigations.
(2) There is written evidence of a physical examination carried out to obtain measurable data with which to analyse the patient's physiotherapeutic need. This includes:
   - observation
   - use of specific assessment tools/ techniques
   - palpation/handling.
(3) The findings of the clinical assessment are explained to the patient.

If any of the required information is missing or unavailable, reasons for this are documented.

Failures in communication

Failures in communication can also give rise to liability should the physiotherapist fail to pass on information or if he/she has failed to communicate appropriately with other health professionals or the client and carers. An understanding of practitioner–client and practitioner–practitioner interaction is therefore essential to ensure real communication. An essential part of the evidence in one case involving a failure to identify that the patient had a deep vein thrombosis (DVT) was the communication between physiotherapist and doctor after her examination of the patient.

Case: *Starcevic* v. *West Hertfordshire Health Authority* 2001[54]

A young man of 37 died of a massive pulmonary embolism, the source of which was a DVT in his left leg. Ten years earlier he had injured his left knee while playing football. He had treatment in hospital and physiotherapy but the knee never completely recovered. Some weakness remained but it was not such as to prevent him from leading a normal and active life. Then on 17 September 1993 he was at work when, in the course of bending down, his left knee suddenly locked. The knee had locked several times before but on those occasions he had been able to straighten it himself. One of his colleagues took him to Hemel Hempstead Hospital, where the leg was manipulated and straightened and put into a thigh to ankle plaster cast tube. He was given painkillers and crutches, discharged and told to report to the fracture clinic in 5 days' time. That he did and the plaster cast was removed. The registrar or surgeon who examined him, noticed a moderate effusion in the left knee and advised an operation to remove what he considered to be a damaged portion of the meniscus. The operation, termed an arthroscopy, was arranged for the following Saturday, 25 September, at St Albans. The operation was performed, but subsequently the patient was transferred to intensive treatment unit and died.

The widow complained and eventually sued the hospital. The judge found that there was no negligence by the doctors. The Court of Appeal however found that there was failure by the physiotherapist to advise the doctors of the patient's swollen calf muscle. The physiotherapy records documented the pre-operative advice and exercises (including the insert sheet) but there was no reference to his swollen calf muscle. The physiotherapist told the customer services manager that she did recall the patient mentioning a tight left calf muscle but at the time she felt that the swelling and tightness was consistent with the knee injury, the leg having been in plaster and his having been non weight-bearing. The physiotherapist subsequently made a statement to the customer services manager that included the following:

During the pre-operative conversation and examination I found that he could not fully straighten his knee. He said that the muscles behind the knee felt tight. I felt that this could be due to the fact that he had been in plaster (which may have been slightly flexed at the knee to allow safe mobility) for a week. It is not uncommon, in my experience, for these tendons to tighten even in this time. It is also not uncommon for swelling to occur in the lower leg after plaster removal. I advised Mr Starcevic on stretching exercises, to do post operatively, to help relieve this situation.

The trial judge found that there was no negligence on the part of the doctor treating the deceased since it was accepted that there was nothing to alert the doctor to the problem and therefore no duty to investigate. The widow appealed on the ground that there was negligence on the part of the physiotherapist and a nurse who had noticed that the patient's leg was a funny colour and had failed to take appropriate action. The Court of Appeal found that the judge had failed to consider the conflict between the evidence of the widow and that of the physiotherapist and held the widow to be obviously articulate and literate and professed to have a clear recollection of what had been said by her husband to the physiotherapist. It accepted her evidence as to what had been said and what she recalled was entirely consistent with what is now known to have been her husband's condition and, indeed, typical of the symptoms which present themselves following a deep vein thrombosis. The appeal was allowed and judgment was entered for the claimant. Damages were awarded as agreed between the parties in the sum of £175 000.

Communication and trust

It would be difficult to overestimate the importance of the communication between patient and healthcare professional in developing a trust relationship. If the patient trusts the physiotherapist, then the patient is more likely to follow instructions on exercise and ongoing care, the patient is more likely to attend for appointments and more likely to disclose all the facts of their condition to the physiotherapist. If the physiotherapist is open with the patient and able to disclose the full details of their diagnosis and prognosis, it is probable that the patient will be less likely to have recourse to litigation.[55]

Unknown contra-indications

For example, it is now increasingly the practice for metal staples to be used in the repair of hernias. Physiotherapists who use short-wave diathermy (SWD) over a hip should be aware if metal staples have been used since metal within the magnetic field is a contra-indication. Therefore, if a physiotherapist, in ignorance of the metal staples inside the patient, used SWD and caused the staples to heat and harm the patient, the patient would have grounds for an action. The fact that the physiotherapist was not aware of the staples would not be an adequate defence if any reasonable physiotherapist, in following the Bolam test, would have discovered this information prior to using such a treatment.

Bad news

Policies are necessary to ensure that 'bad news' is communicated in an appropriate way.

Case: *AB and Others* v. *Tameside & Glossop Health Authority*[56]

This case involved notifying persons that they had been treated by an HIV-positive health worker. It was alleged by 114 of the patients who had been so notified that the two defendant health authorities were negligent in choosing to inform patients by letter as opposed to face to face, and moreover that the facilities offered by the letter were not properly provided. The High Court judge found in favour of the claimant on the grounds:
- that the health authorities did not exercise due care in that they should have realised that the best method of communicating such news was face to face;

- that there was a foreseeable risk that some vulnerable individuals might suffer psychiatric injury going beyond shock and distress.

The health authorities appealed. The Court of Appeal found for the defendants on the facts of this particular case, but confirmed that in law there was a duty on the defendants to take such steps as were reasonable to inform patients of such news, having regard to the possibility of psychiatric injury. Subsequently policy has changed and the Department of Health has updated its guidance on the management of infected healthcare workers and patient notification.[57] It states that it is no longer necessary to notify every patient who has undergone an exposure prone procedure by an HIV-infected heathcare worker because of the low risk of transmission and the anxiety caused to patients and the wider public.

Overhearing

Patients (and relatives) overhearing careless or insensitive discussion is an issue throughout health care.

A stroke patient has described how he heard doctors writing him off as a hopeless case as he lay in hospital unable to respond.[58]

In this case the patient made a partial recovery with some movement in his left hand and, computer-aided, has written an account of his experience. There would be the possibility of legal action if he were able to show that harm has occurred as a result of this lack of thought by the doctors.

Many physiotherapists may forget that their unconscious patients may be able to hear and they therefore need to beware of what they say to their colleagues and to relatives.

Rationing and setting priorities

Rationing in physiotherapy services

In a paper published in 1997 the CSP provided information on the rationing of physiotherapy services.[59] It noted that physiotherapy has always been rationed by lack of referral, lack of resources or lack of available expertise. Among the issues that it asked physiotherapists to consider were:

- the duty of care to patients (see above)
- rules of professional conduct (see Chapter 4)
- efficacy of treatment (see below)
- delegation of physiotherapy tasks (see below)
- prioritising of services (see below).

Prioritising

Prioritising of services will always be an unenviable task in every physiotherapy department within the NHS. The CSP information leaflet on rationing considered a number of options in reviewing working practices to make the most effective use of existing resources. It recognised however that it may be necessary to reduce the breadth of service offered.

> This then ensures that those patients who are accepted for treatment receive a safe, optimum service. Often it is necessary to withdraw the service to one section or category of patient.

The CSP recommended that management should be notified about the decisions that have had to be made. It is also essential that those commissioning the services should be aware of the limitations on the services and the implications of any decisions over priorities which are set.

The determination of priorities is as much a part of the duty of care owed by a physiotherapist as is the assessment and the provision of care. Thus if a physiotherapist was at fault in failing to recognise the priority which should be given to a client following a carefully carried out assessment, and no reasonable physiotherapist following the accepted standard of care (i.e. the Bolam test) would have made a similar decision, the physiotherapist or his/her employer may be liable in negligence should harm befall the client as a consequence.

Referrals and information

The proper determination of priorities cannot be done unless there is full information about a referral. Failure to obtain the full information about a referral can cause many problems for the physiotherapist. Sometimes it may not be possible to make a judgment on priorities unless the patient has been seen.

● What is the situation if a physiotherapist is unable to follow these standards?

Situation: referrals

A physiotherapist receives referrals regularly from doctors with little information about the patient's diagnosis. There is a waiting list for physiotherapy services. What should the physiotherapist do?

In this situation it is impossible for the physiotherapist to make any determination on priorities without adequate information from the person referring. This should be made clear to those referring and a referral form should be designed and the necessary information obtained before an assessment of priorities is made. When the physiotherapist actually sees the patient he/she would, of course, have to make his/her own examination and take a case history and determine the treatment plan and the priority which is assigned to that patient.

● What is the situation in the case of a self-referral, where the client is not prepared to allow the physiotherapist to make contact with his/her doctor?

In such circumstances, the physiotherapist should make it clear to the client that, unless he/she has contact with the client's doctor over pre-existing medical conditions and existing treatment, he/she cannot fulfil her duty of care to the client according to the approved standard of care. Ultimately the physiotherapist could advise that it would be hazardous to treat the client without the full information and therefore may have to refuse the referral. He/she should of course make every effort to discover what are the reasons for the client's objection to the information being passed on.

Inadequate time to see patient

● Where does the physiotherapist stand legally if he/she has only time to see an inpatient for 5 minutes in a day when he/she believes professionally that he should be seen for 30 minutes?

The physiotherapist has a duty to provide a reasonable standard of care to each individual patient. If the 5 minutes is too short to ensure that the patient is appropriately treated, then the physiotherapist has a duty to inform his/her manager that, because of pressure of work, he/she is not providing a reasonable standard of care. It may be that there is a need to reassess priorities and some patients may have to be omitted entirely from the service. Similar problems occur in out-patients where a physiotherapist could consider that a patient should be seen three times per week but in practice can only offer an appointment once a week. Again the allocation of resources to patients must be made according to the reasonable standards of care as set out in the Bolam test. The physiotherapist would have a professional duty to ensure that any concerns about the availability of resources are taken up with management.

Situation: reduced service

A physiotherapist is only able to see an out-patient once a week instead of a preferred frequency of three times per week. Five years later the patient declares an intention of suing the NHS trust for failures to provide adequate physiotherapy, which he alleges has delayed his full recovery.

On these facts it would firstly be important to check if the time limits set by law for bringing an action have been breached (see above). If an action is brought the physiotherapist would have to show that the patient received a reasonable standard of care, even though ideally additional sessions would have been of benefit. There may be evidence that the treatment plan included exercises for the patient to undertake at home to offset the reduced number of sessions and failure on the client's part do to so could reduce any liability on the part of the health authority or Trust (see contributory negligence above). Clearly, the records kept by the physiotherapist will be of vital importance in determining the facts and whether the reasonable standard of care was followed.

Where a patient is given instructions for after-care treatment including exercises to be undertaken, there is considerable advantage in ensuring that this is in writing. For example in the case brought by Frank Cunningham[60] (see Chapter 13), there was a dispute whether he was given written instructions following application of plaster about the circumstances in which he should return to hospital. The hospital said he was, but Mr Cunningham denied this. A tear-off slip signed by the patient may be useful in such disputes.

Resourcing

It is important that resources are used effectively. An announcement by the Department of Health[61] stated that patients failed to turn up for 5.5 million appointments out of a total of 40 million between 1996 and 1997. On average this results in a waste of £275 million. More effective methods of making appointments in a physiotherapy department might improve the rate of non-attenders and hence the use of physiotherapy resources.

In determining the standard of care that should be followed in resourcing a department, reference could be made to such works as that by Joyce Williams[62] on staffing levels. This mentions the duty of care in the context of negligence and setting staffing levels: workload levels should be monitored regularly and unacceptable levels defined. The action to be taken in dealing with unmet needs at that point should also be stated, e.g. to refer back, to prioritise and to record in the patient's notes that treatment was not given or reduced and the reason for this.

> As a basic principle therapists should not accept responsibility for a workload or an individual patient if they are unable to fulfil their duty of care by providing adequate effective treatment in a reasonable time period.[62]

Physiotherapists must clearly distinguish between services which are reduced as a result of pressure from resources and those where any increase would not benefit the patient's condition. For example, in one case[63] concerning special needs, the local authority and health authority gave evidence that, although the child was receiving the maximum physiotherapy treatment which they were able to provide, there was no guarantee that increased physiotherapy would actually improve L's physical condition.

Interprofessional practice

Communication between health and social services professionals is essential in ensuring that the client receives the appropriate standard of care. This is particularly important where one person is designated as the key worker on behalf of the multidisciplinary team (see below). However, the Court of Appeal[64] has stated that the courts do not recognise a concept of team liability and it is therefore for each individual professional to ensure that his/her practice is according to the approved standard of care. Nor should a professional take instructions from another professional which he/she knows would be contrary to the standard of care which his/her profession would require. The physiotherapist is entitled to refuse to act contrary to his/her professional judgment and this would include refusing to take instructions from the patient where these are inappropriate as the case of *R. (on the application of Burke) v. GMC*[65] shows (see Chapter 6).

The sharing of records is considered in Chapter 12.

- Where the physiotherapist has strongly advised a certain course of action what is the situation if his/her advice is then ignored?

He/she should ensure that his/her recommendations are in writing and that a copy is kept. He/she would still have a duty to take all reasonable precautions to prevent the client suffering harm. This would include consultation with his/her managers. If it is clear, that the client is in danger, steps may have to be taken to ameliorate this. It would be professionally unacceptable for the physiotherapist to deny responsibility for the case just because his/her advice was ignored. A client who has the requisite mental capacity has in law the right to refuse any treatment. However, where a client lacks the requisite mental capacity, action may have to be taken in his or her best interests under the Mental Capacity Act 2005 (see Chapter 7).

Home visits

Physiotherapists are confronted with many potential legal situations arising from a home visit, such as:

- What if the client refuses to return to hospital, against the advice of the physiotherapist?
- What if the physiotherapist advised against the immediate discharge of the client but his/her advice is not followed?
- Can the physiotherapist enter private accommodation without the owner or client being present?
- In what circumstances could the physiotherapist insist upon having an escort when accompanying a client on a home visit?

These questions are considered in Chapter 7 on consent, Chapter 11 on health and safety and rights of occupation and Chapter 18 on community care.

Key worker system

The physiotherapist may be appointed as the key worker for an individual patient/client and work with other members of the multidisciplinary team in the care of the patient. In such a situation, he/she should ensure that he/she works within his/her sphere of competence and knows his/her own limitations, bringing the other members of the team into the direct care of the patient where their professional expertise is required. As is discussed above, the courts do not recognise any concept of team liability. The scope of professional practice of the physiotherapist is discussed in Chapter 4.

Negligent advice

There can be liability for negligence in giving advice but the claimant would have to show that it was clear to the defendant that he or she would rely upon the advice and in so doing had suffered reasonably foreseeable loss or harm.[66] An example can be seen from the following situation.

Situation: failure to give clinical advice

A physiotherapist did not warn a patient that until his condition improved he should avoid contact sports. He later returned to the department with further injury and stated that he was holding the physiotherapist responsible for not warning him to avoid such sporting activity.

In a situation like this the advice given to the patient by the physiotherapist would be judged by the reasonable standard of the profession in those circumstances, which would include the knowledge he/she had of the patient's activities, how thoroughly he/she had taken note of such background information, and any general warning given which could be deemed to include specific warnings. In addition there may be an element of contributory negligence if it would have been reasonable to expect the patient to refrain from activities which could obviously worsen his condition.

Situation: advice ignored

> The physiotherapist gives appropriate advice relating to the post-operative care of a patient, but the patient ignores this. Is the physiotherapist responsible for any harm which occurs?

The answer is that, provided that the information was given and understood by the patient, then the physiotherapist would not be liable. The patient would be 100% responsible for the harm. If however the patient was mentally incapacitated, then this fact should be taken into account by the physiotherapist in giving the information, and it may be necessary to communicate with a relative or carer as well, the need to act in the best interests of the patient overriding issues of confidentiality.

In circumstances where the same information is frequently given it may be of help if the information is put in writing in a simple leaflet for the patient. The physiotherapist should note in his/her records that the leaflet has been given out and in certain circumstances could obtain the signature of the patient that the leaflet has been received.

References

If a negligently written reference is provided liability can arise, either to the recipient of the reference (if in reliance upon that reference he has suffered harm[66]) or to the person who is the subject of the reference.

Situation: providing a reference

> A physiotherapist is asked to provide a reference for a patient who has a mental health problem. The patient asks the physiotherapist not to refer to the history of mental illness. What is the position if the physiotherapist gives the reference without

mentioning the mental illness, the patient obtains the post, and then the employer blames the physiotherapist for an inaccurate reference which has led to harm?

If the mental health of the patient was relevant to the use the recipient would make of the reference, then it should have been mentioned in a reference and, if it is omitted, the physiotherapist could be liable for negligent advice. In such circumstances the physiotherapist should have told the patient that, if he/she gave a reference, it would have to include a mention of the mental illness. This is a difficult area, since many persons who have suffered mental ill health may find that they are discriminated against without justification. The physiotherapist should, if uncertain, consider consulting his/her line manager for advice on whether the job in question requires mental health information and the physiotherapist should also look very carefully at the person specification and job description which should come with the request for a reference or which the patient him/herself should have or could ask for.

There can also be liability to the person on whose behalf the reference is given if the reference is written without reasonable care and if 'harm' or pecuniary loss occurs to the subject of the reference as a result of potential employers relying upon an inaccurate and misleading reference.[67]

Every care should be taken to ensure that any reference is written accurately in the light of the facts available.

Volunteering help

Many physiotherapists volunteer to use their skills to assist in a great variety of situations on an unpaid basis and outside the course of their employment (for example many will volunteer to assist disabled persons to ride horses) but this can in itself lead to difficulties. Unfortunately it does not follow that, because the help has been volunteered, the recipients, in their gratitude, will ignore any harm which arises from negligence. In recent years there have been successful cases brought against a referee in a rugby match[68] and against a mountain rescue guide.

Case: *Cattley v. St John Ambulance Brigade*[69]

The St John Ambulance Brigade were sued by a person helped by two of their members on the grounds that these volunteers had caused the victim further harm. The person claiming compensation was 15 at the time of the accident. He had been competing in a motor cycle scramble for school boys. He came off his bike and was treated at the track by two brigade members. He suffered from cracked ribs and also compression fractures of the sixth and seventh dorsal vertebrae, which had damaged the spinal cord and caused incomplete paraplegia. He claimed that the spinal injury was aggravated by the negligent examination and treatment offered him by the St John Ambulance personnel in the period immediately after the fall. It was alleged that he had been lifted to his feet causing further damage to his already injured spinal cord.

The question arose, was there a duty of care owed and if so what was the standard? The judge found no difficulty in holding that there was a duty of care and he held that the standard should be an adaptation of the Bolam test. Did the first-aider act in accordance with the standards of the ordinary skilled first-aider exercising and professing to have the special skills of a first-aider?

In applying this test the judge rejected the version of events given by the boy and his father and held that all the evidence pointed to the fact that at all times the first-aiders had acted in accordance with the ordinary skill to be expected of a properly trained first-aider, i.e. not to move a victim of suspected fracture. The claim was therefore rejected but the legal principle was established that even a volunteer has to act in accordance with a certain standard of care.

Situation: holidays for terminally ill children

A physiotherapist belonged to an association which raised moneys for holidays for terminally ill children. She used two weeks of her holiday to accompany the children with friends and other health professionals. She is concerned that she does not have any insurance cover for this work. What is her situation?

Anyone volunteering help should ensure that they do have insurance cover for their actions. In volunteering help outside the physiotherapist would probably not be covered in law by the vicarious liability of his/her employer (see above) and, therefore, were any harm to arise as a result of his/her negligence, the physiotherapist could then face litigation and, if the claimant succeeded, damages would be awarded against him/her personally. It is essential that such volunteers check with the CSP that they have insurance cover for the voluntary activities which they undertake, making expressly clear the nature of their voluntary help and any associated risks.

In the light of decided cases and situations such as discussed above, the following would appear to be essential requirements for any physiotherapist volunteering help. The physiotherapist should:

- determine his/her competence to assist;
- identify the standard of care required;
- ensure that this standard of care is followed;
- check that he/she has the appropriate insurance cover;
- ensure that any necessary records are kept of the activity.

Instructing clients

Physiotherapists, even those who are not tutors, may find that they are expected to take classes. Often they may have had no training in teaching and instructing others. However, they would still be expected to follow a reasonable standard in explaining treatments and exercises to clients. If they are negligent in this and as a result of that negligence harm occurs then their employer could be vicariously liable.

Situation: taking classes

A physiotherapist takes classes in the following topics: shoulder, back, neck, and ankle. She instructs from five to ten people at a time and finds that it is an effective use of her time. Unfortunately, during one of the ankle classes, one of the patients in attempting to carry out the instructions, tripped very badly and now requires further surgery. She is blaming the physiotherapist and threatening to sue the trust.

In this situation, the procedure followed by the physiotherapist and the instructions which she gave will be compared with the reasonable, safe and competent practice which could be expected from a physiotherapist in that situation, given the reasonably foreseeable risks relating to each client.

Liability for students and unqualified assistants

Exactly the same principles apply to the delegation and supervision of tasks as to the carrying out of professional activities. The professional delegating a task should only do so if he/she is reasonably sure that the person to whom he/she is delegating is reasonably competent and sufficiently experienced to undertake that activity safely in the care of the patient. At the same time the professional must ensure that the person to whom the activity has been delegated has a sufficient level of supervision to ensure that the person is reasonably safe in carrying out that delegated activity.

Should harm befall a client because an activity was carried out by a junior member of staff, a student or a physiotherapy assistant, it is no defence to the client's claim to argue that the

harm occurred because that person did not have the ability, competence or experience to carry out that task reasonably safely.[70]

Situation: too inexperienced

A physiotherapist, recently qualified, was attending a patient on the ward. The patient was on IV antibiotics. The physiotherapist agreed to take the patient for a walk in the grounds. He disconnected the IVs and went with the patient for 10 minutes in the sunshine. On his return he reconnected the drip. Unfortunately, he set it at the wrong speed so that the patient received 4 hours of the drug in half an hour.

In this situation there is no doubt that the physiotherapist has been negligent and therefore, if the patient has suffered harm, the Trust will be vicariously liable for the actions of the physiotherapist. The fact that he was only recently qualified cannot be used as a defence. Clearly senior staff also have a responsibility that junior staff do not act outside their experience and competence.

The CSP assistants list

The CSP has prepared a code of conduct for physiotherapy assistants.[71] The code covers the topics shown in Figure 10.3.

The Chartered Society of Physiotherapy keeps a register of assistants but this does not confer membership of the CSP. Assistants who fail to conform to the Code of Conduct can nevertheless be disciplined by the CSP. Examples of conduct that could lead to disciplinary action by the CSP include:

- criminal convictions;
- disciplinary proceedings by an employer (dismissal by an employer will be automatically followed by the assistant being removed from the CSP assistants list);
- abuse of occupational privilege or skills; and
- personal conduct derogatory to the reputation of the CSP.

Rule 1   Scope of practice
Rule 2   Relationships with physiotherapists
Rule 3   Relationships with patients
Rule 4   Confidentiality
Rule 5   Relationships with professionals, staff and carers
Rule 6   Duty to report
Rule 7   Advertising
Rule 8   Sale of services and goods
Rule 9   Standards of conduct

Figure 10.3   Code of conduct for physiotherapy assistants

Delegation criteria

Advice is also given by the CSP on when to delegate tasks.[72] It suggests that the principles shown in Figure 10.4 should be followed when delegating. *Supervision, Accountability and Delegation of Activities to Support Workers*[73] was published jointly by the CSP, RCN, Royal College of Speech and Language Therapists and the British Dietitic Association in 2006 for registered practitioner and support workers. The Department of Health has also published a consultation document on the registration of healthcare assistants.[74] The timetable envisaged that regulatory provisions would be in place by early 2007. This has not been met.

Rule 1 of the assistant's code of conduct states that:

Physiotherapists assistants shall only practice to the extent that they have established, maintained and developed their ability to work safely and competently to the tasks delegated to them by Chartered physiotherapists.

Concern over the use of unregistered assistants is likely to grow as the skill mix of qualified registered staff and support staff changes and more work is undertaken by persons who are not registered practitioners. Physiotherapists have a responsibility to ensure that the activities which they delegate are appropriate for that person and that the person is given proper supervision. Assistants in turn have a responsibility to

ensure that they 'confine themselves to tasks delegated to them by the physiotherapists for which they have established and maintained their competence'.[75]

Liz Saunders carried out an audit of physiotherapy services in an out-patient department 3 years after the implementation of a change in skill mix and increased delegation to assistants.[76] It was found that the systematic approach to delegation had succeeded in terms of costs and patient satisfaction with no loss of quality of service. In her paper she suggests a seven-point strategy for delegation:

- ensure competence of assistant
- give formal instructions to assistant
- give explanation to patient
- arrange appointments
- supervise assistant
- ensure communication links are understood
- inform assistant of outcome of episode of care.

Liability for harm

- If the physiotherapist ensures that there is appropriate delegation, what is the situation if the unqualified person causes harm to the client?

If the physiotherapist has acted reasonably in following the approved standard of professional practice according to the Bolam test, the physiotherapist would not be liable in negligence.

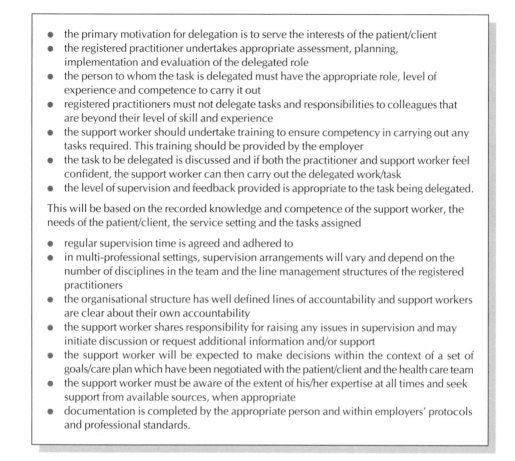

- the primary motivation for delegation is to serve the interests of the patient/client
- the registered practitioner undertakes appropriate assessment, planning, implementation and evaluation of the delegated role
- the person to whom the task is delegated must have the appropriate role, level of experience and competence to carry it out
- registered practitioners must not delegate tasks and responsibilities to colleagues that are beyond their level of skill and experience
- the support worker should undertake training to ensure competency in carrying out any tasks required. This training should be provided by the employer
- the task to be delegated is discussed and if both the practitioner and support worker feel confident, the support worker can then carry out the delegated work/task
- the level of supervision and feedback provided is appropriate to the task being delegated.

This will be based on the recorded knowledge and competence of the support worker, the needs of the patient/client, the service setting and the tasks assigned

- regular supervision time is agreed and adhered to
- in multi-professional settings, supervision arrangements will vary and depend on the number of disciplines in the team and the line management structures of the registered practitioners
- the organisational structure has well defined lines of accountability and support workers are clear about their own accountability
- the support worker shares responsibility for raising any issues in supervision and may initiate discussion or request additional information and/or support
- the support worker will be expected to make decisions within the context of a set of goals/care plan which have been negotiated with the patient/client and the health care team
- the support worker must be aware of the extent of his/her expertise at all times and seek support from available sources, when appropriate
- documentation is completed by the appropriate person and within employers' protocols and professional standards.

Figure 10.4   Principles for delegation[91]

However, the person undertaking the delegated activity would be liable and the employer would be vicariously liable for this individual's negligence, subject, of course, to the harm occurring as a reasonably foreseeable result of the negligent act or omission (see above).

Non-registered junior staff in the multidisciplinary team

There is a danger that the real contribution which can be made to care planning and multidisciplinary decision making by persons such as physiotherapy assistants, technicians and support workers may not be recognised or may be treated dismissively. Many support workers develop a close rapport with clients and it is essential that any relevant information that they possess should be made known to the team and listened to.

Chapter 4 of the inquiry report about the homicide committed by Jason Mitchell,[77] a mentally disordered person, is concerned with assessments on Jason made by professional staff in disciplines other than psychiatry and nursing and points out:

They contained observations and insights into Jason Mitchell's thoughts and feelings which were rarely recorded in the medical and nursing notes and which could present a different perspective on his case. They tended to be recorded in detail, but were marginalised.

Attention is drawn in the report to the contribution of a technical instructor in the occupational therapy department at West Park Hospital whose report on Jason Mitchell is given in full as an addendum to the chapter. The Inquiry noted that her report was not included in the Mental Health Review Tribunal papers. In general, her report had been ignored or discounted by the doctors central to the care and treatment of Jason Mitchell but in the Inquiry's view, 'the material in her report ought to have prompted at least an assessment, if not a further therapeutic involvement, with a qualified and experienced clinician, possibly a psychologist'. The Inquiry concluded:

> Jason Mitchell's case illustrates how contributions from an unqualified member of staff were disregarded, and consequently how important data were put out of sight and mind. Nothing relevant to the assessment and treatment of a patient should be ignored, whatever its origins.

Generic or specific assistants?

Jane Langley[78] in an article in *Physiotherapy* discusses the moves to include physiotherapy assistants with a core body of non-professional workers in order to provide a flexible, cost-effective workforce able to help a range of professionals. She stresses the importance of considering the needs of the patients and the importance of using the resources available to a physiotherapy service to the best effect. It is of course essential, whether general or specific assistants are used, to ensure that they are capable of performing the tasks delegated to them and the appropriate level of supervision is provided to meet their needs. Clearly, the more specialist the tasks to be delegated, the more useful it is to have specific assistants.

Analysis of task delegation

The management of delegation to physiotherapy assistants is discussed by Liz Saunders[79] who suggested a functional analysis model to determine issues arising in delegation: tasks are analysed to determine whether sub-tasks are knowledge, rule or skill based and thus suitable or not for delegation. The four stages which are identified are:

- examination of the current system
- identification of the level of delegation
- establishment of the new procedure for delegation
- monitoring the new system.

As a result of a systematic analysis of task delegation, management can adjust physiotherapist–assistant ratios to create appropriate skill mix for the area. Saunders also considers the training implications of delegation following the task analysis.

It is essential that delegation is on a personal basis and takes into account the individual assistant's personal knowledge, experience, skill and training.

Care of property

Failure to look after another person's property could lead to criminal prosecution, e.g. theft, or a civil action for trespass to goods, or negligence in causing loss or damage to property.

In an action for negligence, the person who has suffered the loss or damage to property must establish the same four elements that must be shown in a claim for compensation for personal injury, i.e. duty, breach, causation and harm.

Situation: breaking china

> A physiotherapist, visiting a patient at home, knocked a piece of china off a dresser. The carer stated that it was a very valuable piece of Spode and would have to be replaced. Where does the physiotherapist stand?

Clearly the physiotherapist has a duty of care in relation to the property of the patient. However, it may not be entirely her fault that the accident occurred. Was the china in a sufficiently safe place in relation to its value? Would it have been possible for a person taking care still to have knocked it? If the answers are affirmative then this may amount to contributory negligence by the patient. The employer of the physiotherapist would be vicariously liable for the loss since she was acting in the course of employment.

Where, however, property is left in the care of a person (the bailee) then, should the property be lost or damaged, the burden would be on the bailee to establish how that occurred without fault on his or her part. It should be noted that liability for loss or damage to property can be excluded if such an exclusion is reasonable (see the Unfair Contract Terms Act above).

Receipt of gifts from clients is discussed in Chapter 4 on professional conduct.

Documentation

In every area of professional practice, it is essential to ensure that comprehensive clear records are kept in the interests of patient care and also for the defence of the practitioner in the event of any dispute or complaint. In a case in 1994,[80] the claimant claimed that, during a physiotherapy treatment session, he felt something go wrong with the lower part of his spine and alleged negligence on the part of the physiotherapist. The judge and Court of Appeal both found that he was, first, exaggerating his claims and, second, had not proved the necessary causal link. However, the defendants' case was not helped by the paucity of notes of the physiotherapists and they were fortunate that this did not affect the findings of the judge. Reference should be made to Chapter 12 on record keeping.

Woolf Reforms

Considerable criticisms were made of the civil litigation procedures and Lord Woolf was appointed to recommend reforms. His final report was published in July 1996 and was accompanied by a draft of the general rules that would form the core of a single, simpler procedural code to apply to civil litigation in the High Court and county courts. He recommended three tracks for civil litigation: a small claims track; a fast track and a multiclaim track. His specific proposals on medical negligence included:

- training health professionals in negligence claims;
- the GMC and other regulatory bodies to consider the need to clarify their professional conduct responsibilities in relation to negligence actions;
- improvement of record systems to trace former staff;
- the use of alternative dispute mechanisms;
- a separate medical negligence list for the High Court and county courts;
- specially designated court centres outside London for handling medical negligence cases;
- reducing delays by improving arrangements for case listing;
- investigation of improved training in medical negligence for judges;
- standard tables to be used where possible to determine quantum;
- practice guidance on the new case management;
- a pilot study to consider medical negligence claims below £10 000.

The Woolf Reforms were implemented in 1999 in new Civil Procedure Rules. They can be accessed at the Ministry of Justice's website.[81]

The NHS litigation authority

The NHSLA[82] is a special health authority, i.e. a statutory body, set up in 1995 to oversee the Clinical Negligence Scheme for Trusts (CNST) in the handling of claims. The NHSLA uses an approved list of solicitors to handle litigation. It exercises functions in connection with the establishment and the administration of the scheme for meeting liabilities of health service bodies to third parties for loss, damage or injury arising out of the exercise of their functions. Guidance on NHS indemnity for clinical negligence claims has been issued by the NHS Executive.[83]

The Law Commission recommended changes to the present system relating to the quantifying of damages for personal injury[84] in 1996 and suggested, among other recommendations, that the NHS should be able to recover the costs arising from the treatment of road traffic and other accident victims. It was estimated that this might bring in £120 million to the NHS but more radical measures would be necessary to make any serious reduction in the present costs of the NHS. The charges levied against those involved in road traffic accidents have continued to increase to meet in-patient and out-patient costs, on the assumption that they will be recovered from the insurance company covering the driver. Other possibilities of recouping NHS costs which are debated include contributions from drinks companies to cover the cost of drink-related conditions, from tobacco companies for smoking-related disorders, food companies for obesity-related disorders and from insurance companies for those activities for which insurance cover is purchased, e.g. sports injuries, travel accidents, accidents at home.

Clinical Negligence Scheme for Trusts

The CNST was established in 1996[85] to administer a scheme where trusts and other NHS bodies take part in a voluntary scheme whereby compensation is met from a pooling system. The payment into the pool depends on an assessment of the risk presented by that particular trust and amounts over a specified minimum will be met from the pool. The CNST visits organisations that belong or wish to belong to the scheme in order to assess their risk: they examine, in particular, the standard of risk assessment and management in the organisation, and the standards of record keeping. In the light of their assessment, premiums payable into the scheme are assessed. Over 95% of NHS trusts are members of CNST. Liabilities prior to April 1995 are covered by the Existing Liabilities Scheme (ELS), which is centrally funded.

NHS redress scheme

The costs of compensation resulting from clinical negligence in the NHS has been constantly growing. The Department of Health announced in July 2001[86] that it was setting up a committee under the chairmanship of the Chief Medical Officer of Health to consider a new scheme for compensation for clinical negligence. A consultation paper was published in July 2001.[86] This was followed, on 30 June 2003, by a further consultation document *Making Amends*.[87] *Making Amends* provided a comprehensive account of the background to the present situation. It looked at the present system of medical negligence litigation and its costs. It analysed public attitudes and concerns and the earlier reviews of the negligence system by the Pearson Commission,[88] the Woolf Report on Access to Justice[89] and the National Audit Office Report in 2001.[90] It considered recent action taken to reform civil court procedures, claims handling by the NHSLA and the use of alternative dispute resolution. It analysed systems of no-fault liability in Denmark, Finland, France, New Zealand, Norway and Sweden and discussed no-fault liability as an option along with continued reform of the present tort process, a tariff-based national tribunal or a composite option drawing on all three. The scheme eventually recommended in *Making Amends* was a composite package of reform drawing on the best elements of these three options. It included suggestions for the care and compensation for severely neurologically impaired babies; for the NHS redress scheme to be part of the system for handling complaints; for the retention of right to pursue litigation through the courts and changes to existing scheme for civil proceedings; and for a duty of candour to be placed on healthcare professionals and managers to inform patients where they become aware of a possible negligent action or omission.

NHS Redress Act 2006

The NHS Redress Act that was eventually agreed was a very much less radical scheme than that proposed in the consultation paper *Making Amends*. It gives power to the Secretary of State to establish a scheme for the purpose of enabling redress to be provided without recourse to civil proceedings. Regulations are to be drawn up giving the details. The scheme can cover services provided by the Secretary of State, a Primary Care Trust or a designated Strategic Health Authority or an organisation or person providing services under an arrangement with these bodies. Excluded from the redress scheme are primary dental services, primary medical services, general ophthalmic services and pharmaceutical services. A scheme does not apply in relation to a liability that is or has been the subject of civil proceedings (S.2(2)). Ordinarily the scheme will provide for the following redress:

- an offer of compensation in satisfaction of any right to bring civil proceedings;
- giving an explanation;
- giving an apology;
- giving a report on the action which has been or will be taken to prevent similar cases arising.

The scheme may make provision for compensation to take the form of entry into a contract to provide care or treatment or of financial compensation or both. It can also detail the circumstances in which different forms of compensation may be offered. The scheme can set the upper limit on the amount of financial compensation to be offered and if it does not do so, it must specify an upper limit on the amount of financial compensation that may be included in such an offer in respect of pain and suffering. The scheme may not specify any other limit on what may be included in such an offer by way of financial compensation. The scheme can detail the following provisions relating to the commencement of proceedings:

- who may commence proceedings;
- how proceedings are commenced;
- time limits for commencing;
- circumstances precluding proceedings being commenced;
- proceedings being commenced in specified circumstances;
- notification of the commencement of proceedings in specified circumstances.

The scheme may also make provision for proceedings under the scheme including details of the investigation of cases, decisions about the application of the scheme, the time limits within which an offer can be accepted, certain settlements in specified cases to be subject to approval by the court and the termination of proceedings under the scheme.

The scheme must make provision for the findings of an investigation of a case to be recorded in a report and make provision for a copy of the report to be provided on request to the individual seeking redress. However, no copy of an investigation report need be provided before an offer is made under the scheme or proceedings are terminated or in other specified circumstances. A settlement agreement must include a waiver of the right to bring civil proceedings in respect of the liability to which the settlement relates and the scheme must also provide for the termination of proceedings under the scheme if the liability to which the proceedings related becomes the subject of civil proceedings. The scheme must also provide for the suspension of the limitation period under the Limitation Act 1980.

The provision of legal advice (from a specified list of persons) without charge to individuals seeking redress may be specified under the scheme. The scheme may also include the provision of other services including the services of medical experts who must be instructed jointly by the scheme authority and the individual seeking redress. The Secretary of State also has a duty to arrange, to such extent as he considers necessary to meet all reasonable requirements, for the provision of assistance (by way of representation or otherwise) to those seeking redress (S.9(1)). Payments may be made to any person under these arrangements, who should be independent of any person to whose conduct the case related or who is involved in dealing with the case. The Secretary of State can make provision about the membership of the scheme and the functions of members. Section 10 sets out the members responsibilities, including the duty to publish an annual report. The Secretary of State may also make provision for the scheme authority, i.e. the special health authority to have specified functions. The scheme must include provision requiring the scheme authority and the members of the scheme, in carrying out their functions under the scheme, to have regard in particular to the desirability of redress being provided without recourse to civil proceedings (S.12). Section 13 specifies a general duty of cooperation between the scheme authority and the Commission for Healthcare Audit and Inspection, and between the scheme authority and the National Patient Safety Agency. Regulations may determine provisions about complaints on the handling and consideration of complaints relating to the scheme (S.14) and the remit of the Health Service Commissioner is extended to include complaints about the exercise of functions under a scheme established under the NHS Redress Act 2006.

Conclusions

Even after the implementation of the Woolf Reforms, civil action in respect of negligence by health professionals is still slow and costly. The implications of the NHS Redress Act 2006 are still to be seen. It may be that, together with an improved system for complaints handling (see Chapter 14) that redress compensation schemes become a speedy and effective method of resolving disputes in the NHS. There are however no signs that litigation is decreasing and physiotherapists must therefore bear in mind the possibility that they may be drawn into a dispute and their records become essential evidence (see Chapter 12). In addition physiotherapists are often caring for patients whose progress is delayed because of their emotional involvement in a compensation claim which seems to require them to prove their pain and suffering and hold on to their disabilities. Speedy dispute resolution of compensation claims is in the interests of all.

Questions and exercises

1   Explain the difference between vicarious liability and personal liability.
2   Take any situation where harm nearly occurred to a client, and work out what the client would have had to prove to obtain compensation if he/she had suffered an injury.
3   How would you define the reasonable standard of care in relation to any chosen treatment provided by yourself?
4   Prepare a protocol to ensure safe delegation to and supervision of a physiotherapy assistant.
5   What would you take into account in determining your liability in relation to voluntary activities?
6   Examine the provisions of the NHS Redress Act 2006 and consider the extent to which it could impact upon your practice.

References

1   Rose, D. (2008) £100 million payouts for cancer negligence. *The Times*, 10 March.
2   *Donoghue* v. *Stevenson* [1932] AC 562.
3   *Home Office* v. *Dorset Yacht Co Ltd* (HL) [1970] 2 All ER 294.
4   *McCord* v. *Swansea City AFC Ltd* (1997) *The Times*, 11 February 1997; CL 1997 3780.
5   *Kent* v. *Griffiths and Others*, The Times Law Report, 23 December 1998.
6   *Kent* v. *Griffiths and Others* (No. 2), The Times Law Report, 10 February 2000; [2000] 2 All ER 474.
7   *Phelps* v. *Hillingdon London Borough Council* [1998] 1 All ER 421.

8   Phelps v. Hillingdon London Borough Council; Anderton v. Clwyd CC; Jarvis v. Hampshire CC; Re G (A Minor) [2000] 4 All ER 504; [2001] 2 AC 619.

9   *X and Y v. London Borough of Hounslow* [2008] EWHC 1168 (QB) 23 June 2008.

10 *London Borough of Islington v. University College London Hospital NHS Trust* [2005] EWCA Civ 596.

11 *Alcock v. Chief Constable of South Yorkshire* (HL) [1992] 1 AC 310.

12 *Bolam v. Friern Hospital Management Committee* [1957] 1 WLR 582.

13 *Whitehouse v. Jordan* [1981] 1 All ER 267.

14 *Maynard v. West Midlands Regional Health Authority* (HL) [1985] 1 All ER 635.

15 *Bolitho v. City and Hackney Health Authority* [1997] 3 WLR 1151; [1997] 4 All ER 771.

16 DoH (1997) White Paper. *The New NHS – Modern, Dependable* HMSO, London.

17 www.nhsla.com/RiskManagement

18 www.diabetes.org.uk

19 www.cftrust.org.uk/aboutcf/publications/factsheets

20 Chartered Society of Physiotherapy (2005) *Core Standards of Physiotherapy Practice.* CSP, London.

21 Chartered Society of Physiotherapy (2005) *Service Standards of Physiotherapy Practice.* CSP London.

22 Hurwitz, B. (1998) *Clinical Guidelines and the Law.* Radcliffe Medical Press, Abingdon.

23 *Barnett v. Chelsea Hospital Management Committee* [1968] 1 All ER 1068.

24 *Wilsher v. Essex Area Health Authority* (CA) [1986] 3 All ER 801; (HL) [1988] 1 871.

25 *Loveday v. Renton and another* (1998) *The Times*, 31 March.

26 *Best v. Wellcome Foundation and others* [1994] 5 Med LR 81; discussed in *Medico Legal Journal* **61**, 3, 178.

27 *Jolley v. Sutton London Borough Council* (CA) The Times Law Report, 23 June 1998.

28 *Jolley v. Sutton London Borough Council,* The Times Law Report, 24 May 2000; [2000] 3 All ER 409.

29 *North Glamorgan NHS Trust v. Walters,* Lloyd's Rep Med 2 [2003] 49 CA.

30 *Giullietta Galli-Atkinson v. Sudhaker Seghal,* Lloyd's Rep Med 6 [2003] 285.

31 *Gray v. Thames Trains Ltd and another* The Times Law Report, 9 July 2008 CA.

32 *Lister & Others v. Hesley Hall Ltd, [2001] UKHL 22 [2002] 1 AC 215;* The Times Law Report, 10 May 2001; [2001] 2 WLR 1311.

33 *Gravil v. Carroll and Another* The Times Law Report, 22 July 2008.

34 *Reeves v. Commissioner of Police for the Metropolis* [1999] ll ER (D) 793.

35 *Victoria v. Commissioner of Police of the Metropolis* [2007] EWCA Civ 1361; The Times Law Report, 4 January 2008 CA.

36 *Hill v. Chief Constable of West Yorkshire Police* [1989] AC 53.

37 *Brooks v. Commissioner of Police of the Metropolis* [2005] 1 WLR 1495.

38 *Capital & Countries plc v. Hampshire County Council* (CA) [1997] WLR 331.

39 *Spencer v. Secretary of State for Work and Pensions; Moore v. Secretary of State for Transport and Another* The Times Law Report, 24 July 2008.

40 *Bull v. Wakeham 2 February 1989 Lexis Transcript.*

41 Laurance, J. (1995) Man Handicapped as a Baby 33 Years Ago Wins £1.25m. *The Times* 15 November p. 5.

42 *A. v. Hoare; X and Another v. Wandsworth LBC; C. v. Middlesborough Council; H. v. Suffolk CC; Young v. Catholic Care (Diocese of Leeds) and Another.* The Times Law Report, 31 January 2008.

43 *Stubbings v. Webb* 1993 AC 498.

44 *Amanda Godfrey v. Gloucester Royal Infirmary NHS Trust* Lloyd's Rep Med 8 [2003] 398.

45 *Berry v. Calderdale Health Authority* [1998] EWCA Civ 248.

46 www.bailii.org

47 *Simms v. Leigh Rugby Football Club Ltd* [1969] 2 All ER 923.

48 *Webster (A Child) v. Hammersmith Hospital NHS Trust,* February 2002 (taken from *Quantum of Damages,* Vol. 3, Kemp, Kemp, and Sweet, Maxwell, pp. 51507–51508 and 51565–51575).

49 *Wells v. Wells; Thomas v. Brighton HA; Page v. Sheerness Steel Co Plc* (HL) [1998] 3 All ER 481.

50 *Thompstone v. Tameside and Glossop Acute Services NHS Trust* (and other cases). The Times Law Report, 30 January 2008 CA.

51 *Brown v. Ministry of Defence* EWCA [2006] 546.

52 *Lim Poh Choo v. Camden and Islington Health Authority* [1979] 1 All ER 332.

53 Damages for bereavement (Variation of Sum) (England and Wales) SI 2007 No 3489.

54 *Starcevic v. West Hertfordshire Health Authority* [2001] EWCA Civ 192.

55 Thom *et al.* (2004) Health Affairs, **23**, 4, 124–132.

56 *AB and Others v. Tameside & Glossop Health Authority* [1997] 8 Med LR 91.

57 Department of Health (1999 updated July 2005) AIDS/HIV *Infected Health Care Workers: Guidance on the Management of Infected Health Care Workers and Patient Notification.* DH, London.

58 Hawkes, N. (1996) 'Hopeless' Patient Overheard Prognosis. *The Times,* 5 April.

59 CSP Professional Affairs Department (1997) *Rationing of Physiotherapy Services.* No. PA 30. CSP, London.

60 *Cunningham* v. *North Manchester Health Authority* (CA) [1997] 8 Med LR 135.

61 Landale, J. (1998) No-Show Patients cost NHS £275 Million. *The Times* 15 September.

62 Williams, J. (undated) *Calculating Staffing Levels in Physiotherapy Services.* PAMPAS, Rotherham.

63 *Hereford County Council* v. *L* 4 September 1997 (QBD) Lexis Transcript.

64 *Wilsher* v. *Essex Area Health Authority* (CA) [1986] 3 All ER 801.

65 *R. (on the application of Burke)* v. *General Medical Council and Disability Rights Commission and Official Solicitor to the Supreme Court* [2004] EWHC 1879; [2004] Lloyd's Rep. Med 451; [2005] EWCA Civ 1003, 28 July 2005.

66 *Hedley Byrne and Co Ltd* v. *Heller and Partners Ltd* (HL) [1963] 2 All ER 575.

67 *Spring* v. *Guardian Assurance PLC and others* Times Law Report, 8 July 1994.

68 *Smolden* v. *Whitworth* (1996) *The Times,* 23 April 1996; CL 1996 4534; (CA) *The Times,* 18 December 1996.

69 *Cattley* v. *St John's Ambulance Brigade* (QBD) 25 November 1989 (unreported but see Griffiths, G. (1990) in: *Modern Law Review* **53**, 255).

70 *Wilsher* v. *Essex Area Health Authority* (CA) [1986] 3 All ER 801.

71 Chartered Society of Physiotherapy (2002) *Physiotherapy Assistants Code of Conduct.* CSP, London.

72 CSP Professional Affairs Department (no date) No. PA 6. *Criteria for the Delegation of Tasks to Assistants.* CSP, London.

73 RCN, CSP, and others (2006) *Supervision, Accountability and Delegation of Activities to Support Workers – a Guide for Registered Practitioner and Support Workers.* RCN, London.

74 Department of Health (2004) *Regulation of Healthcare Staff in England and Wales: Consultation.* DH, London.

75 Chartered Society of Physiotherapy (1995) *Rules of Professional Conduct of the CSP: Code of Conduct of Physiotherapy Assistants.* CSP, London.

76 Saunders, E. (1998) Improving the Practice of Delegation in Physiotherapy. *Physiotherapy* **84** 5, 207–15.

77 Blom-Cooper, E. *et al.* (1996) *The Case of Jason Mitchell: Report of the Independent Panel of Inquiry* Duckworth, London.

78 Langley, J. (1996) General or Specific Assistants. *Physiotherapy* **82**, 605.

79 Saunders, E. (1996) Managing Delegation to Physiotherapy Assistants: Application of a Functional Analysis Model. *Physiotherapy* **82** 4, 246–252.

80 *Jago* v. *Torbay Health Authority* 23 May 1994 (CA) Lexis Transcript.

81 www.justice.gov.uk/civil/procrules_fin

82 National Health Service Litigation Authority (Establishment and Constitution) Order 1995 SI No. 2800 of 1995.

83 HSG(96)48 NHS Indemnity: Arrangements for Clinical Negligence claims in the NHS.

84 Law Commission (1996) *Damages for Personal Injury: Medical, Nursing and Other Expenses* HMSO, London.

85 National Health Service (Clinical Negligence Scheme) Regulations XI 1996 No. 251; amendment regulations SI 2002 No. 1073.

86 Department of Health press release 2001/0313, New clinical compensation scheme for the NHS, 20 July 2001.

87 Department of Health (2003) *Making Amends.* Consultation paper setting out proposals for reforming the approach to clinical negligence in the NHS. CMO, London.

88 Royal Commission on Civil Liability and Compensation for Personal Injury (1978) *Pearson Report.* HMSO, London.

89 Lord Woolf (1996) *Final Report: Access to Justice.* HMSO, London.

90 National Audit Office, Handling Clinical Negligence Claims in England, Report of the Comptroller and Auditor General, HC 403 Session 2000–2001, 3 May 2001.

91 RCN, CSP, and others (2006) *Supervision, Accountability and Delegation of Activities to Support Workers – a Guide for Registered Practitioners and Support Workers.*

11 Health and Safety

The physiotherapist works in a potentially dangerous environment, whether in a domestic setting or in hospital therapy centres and workshops. This chapter covers the basic principles of law relating to the health and safety at work, taking examples from physiotherapy practice. The topics to be covered are as follows:

- Health and Safety at Work etc. Act 1974
- Risk assessment
- Manual handling
- Reporting risks, injuries, etc.
- Control of Infection
- Occupier's liability and consumer protection
- Employment matters
- Special areas

Many of these areas are covered in the health and safety information prepared by the Industrial Relations Department of the Chartered Society of Physiotherapy (CSP). Issues relating to insurance are considered in Chapter 15. Many of the *Rules of Professional Conduct, the Core and Service Standards of Physiotherapy Practice* relate to health and safety laws and the CSP has also published an information paper on patient/client health and safety.[1] This illustrates how the *Rules of Professional Conduct* underpin patient/client health and safety. The CSP core standards of practice build on the principles (especially Core Standards 2 and 4) and Service 13 applies to patient information. Core standards 6, 9, 10 and 16 and Service Standard 16 are applicable to treatment delivery, evaluation and environment. Core Standards 18 refers to equipment. Service Standards 1, 2, 3, 4, 5, 9, and 12 are applicable to quality assurance/clinical governance, including risk management. The document also considers the health and safety implications in manual handling, hydrotherapy, exercise therapy, injection therapy and acupuncture.[2] The CSP regularly updates its health and safety publications for members.

Health and Safety at Work etc. Act 1974

Enforcement

The Health and Safety at Work etc. Act 1974 (HASAW) is enforced through the criminal courts by the Health and Safety Inspectorate, which has the power to prosecute for offences under the Act and under the Regulations and which also has powers of inspection and can issue enforcement or prohibition notices. Inspectors are not liable for any economic loss suffered by the organisation as a result of their issuing a notice.[3]

Since the abolition of the Crown's immunity in relation to the health and safety laws (by the National Health Service Amendment Act 1986) prosecutions and notices can be brought against the health authorities. Trusts do not enjoy any immunity from health and safety legislation. Social services departments can also be prosecuted.

Basic employer/employee duties

The basic duty of the employer is set out in Figure 11.1.

Section 2(2) of the 1974 Act gives examples of the various duties which must be carried out, but these do not detract from the width and comprehensiveness of the general duty.

The Act also places a specific responsibility upon the employee. This is shown in Figure 11.2.

It is also a criminal offence for any person to interfere with health and safety measures (see Figure 11.3).

General health and safety duty of employer to non-employees

Under Section 3 of the 1974 Act the employer has a general duty of care to persons not in his employment (see Figure 11.4). This duty would therefore cover patients, visitors and the general public.

Section 2(1). It shall be the duty of every employer to ensure, so far as is reasonably practicable, the health, safety and welfare at work of all his employees.

Figure 11.1   Duty under the Health and Safety at Work etc. Act 1974

It shall be the duty of every employee while at work:

(a)   to take reasonable care for the health and safety of himself and of other persons who may be affected by his acts or omissions at work; and

(b)   as regards any duty or requirements imposed on his employer or any other person ... , to co-operate with him so far as is necessary to enable that duty or requirement to be performed or complied with.

Figure 11.2   Employer's statutory duty under Section 7 of The Health and Safety at Work etc. Act 1974

No person shall intentionally or recklessly interfere with or misuse anything provided in the interests of health, safety or welfare in pursuance of any of the relevant statutory provisions.

Figure 11.3   The Health and Safety at Work etc. Act 1974 – Section 8

> The employer has a duty to conduct his undertaking in such a way as to ensure, so far as is reasonably practicable, that persons not in his employment who may be affected thereby are not thereby exposed to risks to their health and safety.

Figure 11.4   The Health and Safety at Work etc. Act 1974 – Section 3

The Court of Appeal has held[4] that the employer was not guilty of an offence under Section 3 if an employee was negligent and caused harm to others, provided the employer had taken all reasonable care in laying down safe systems of work and ensuring that the employees had the necessary skill and instruction and were subject to proper supervision, with safe premises, plant and equipment. However, if a civil claim were brought, the employer would be liable to pay any compensation found to be due under the principle of vicarious liability (see Glossary and Chapter 10). In the following case the Court of Appeal had to determine whether a particular risk was part of everyday life or an offence under Section 3 of HASAW.

Case: *R v. Porter* 2008[5]

The headmaster of a private school was prosecuted under Section 3 following an accident to a child of 3 years. The boy jumped down some steps in the playground. He fell and suffered a head injury. He was taken to hospital and subsequently died after contracting MRSA. In the crown court the headmaster was convicted of failing to ensure the health and safety of persons not in his employment contrary to Section 3(1) of the Health and Safety at Work Act 1974. His appeal to the Court of Appeal succeeded. The Court of Appeal held that the risk which the prosecution had to prove was a real risk as opposed to a fanciful or hypothetical risk. The fact that risk was a part of everyday life went to the issue of whether the injured person was exposed to that risk by the conduct of the operation in question. The evidence suggested that there was no real risk of the kind statutorily contemplated.

Unless it could be said that the child was exposed to a real risk by the conduct of the school, no question as to the reasonably practicable measures taken to meet risk arose.

Safety Representatives and Safety Committees Regulations 1977

The Safety Representatives and Safety Committees Regulations 1977 (SRSC) brought into force the requirement in HASAW that employers should permit safety representatives appointed by the recognised trade union to inspect the workplace, get information held by the employer relating to health, safety or welfare and have paid time off for training and carrying out their functions. Each employer is required to set up a health and safety committee to consider matters relating to health and safety. Further information on the powers and responsibilities of safety representatives and the role of the committees is set out in the information manual prepared for safety representatives by the Industrial Relations Department of the CSP.[6] In addition the CSP has a national health and safety officer who is a member of the TUC's union safety specialists group and a TUC nominee to the health and safety committee's health service advisory committee. The CSP has over 700 safety representatives who should be the first point of contact if a member has concerns about health and safety which are not being addressed by management. A CSP publication in 2007 provides guidance for union safety representatives in assisting their members in preparing for health and safety assessments.[7] The CSP has also

- Management of Health and Safety at Work Regulations 1992 (SI No. 2051) (updated 1999)
- Provision and Use of Work Equipment Regulations 1992 (SI No. 2932) (updated 1998)
- Manual Handling Operations Regulations 1992 (SI No. 2793) (amended 2002)
- Workplace (Health, Safety and Welfare) Regulations 1992 (SI No. 3004) (updated 1999)
- Personal Protective Equipment at Work Regulations 1992 (SI No. 2966) (updated 1999)
- Health and Safety (Display Screen Equipment) Regulations 1992 (SI No. 2792) (updated 1999)

Figure 11.5   Health and Safety Regulations

prepared a checklist for safety representatives as part of its guidance on the 1999 Regulations (see below).

For those workplaces which are not covered by SRSC the Health and Safety (Consultation with Employees) Regulations 1996 require employers to consult with workers or their representatives on all matters relating to employees' health and safety.

Regulations under Health and Safety at Work

Regulations came into force on 1 January 1993 as a result of European Directives and most have been revised since that time. They are shown in Figure 11.5.

Figure 11.6 shows the areas covered by these regulations relating to the management of health and safety at work.

The Management of Health and Safety at Work Regulations 1992 (revised 1999)

Of the regulations that came into force in 1993, the Management of Health and Safety at Work Regulations are the most far reaching in that they apply to all work environments and both employers and the self-employed. They were updated in 1999 and a code of practice and guidance on the regulations was issued in 2000.[8] Figure 11.6 shows the areas covered by these regulations.

The Code of Practice

A Code of Practice has been approved in conjunction with these regulations.[8] This Code does not have legal force in itself but as the preface states:

> The Code has special legal status. If you are prosecuted for breach of health and safety law, and it is proved that you did not follow the relevant provisions of the Code, you will need to show that you have complied with the law in some other way or a court will find you at fault. . . .
>
> Following the guidance is not compulsory and you are free to take other action. But if you do follow the guidance you will normally be doing enough to comply with the law. Health and safety inspectors seek to secure compliance with the law and may refer to this guidance as illustrating good practice.

Risk assessment

Not all the provisions in the Management of Health and Safety at Work Regulations can be covered in detail in a book like this, but Regulation 3 on risk assessment will be looked at in detail.

The law

Figure 11.7 sets out the basic requirement as specified in Regulation 3(1).

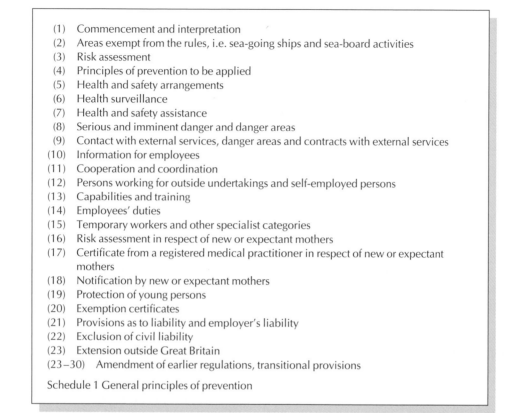

(1)   Commencement and interpretation
(2)   Areas exempt from the rules, i.e. sea-going ships and sea-board activities
(3)   Risk assessment
(4)   Principles of prevention to be applied
(5)   Health and safety arrangements
(6)   Health surveillance
(7)   Health and safety assistance
(8)   Serious and imminent danger and danger areas
(9)   Contact with external services, danger areas and contracts with external services
(10) Information for employees
(11) Cooperation and coordination
(12) Persons working for outside undertakings and self-employed persons
(13) Capabilities and training
(14) Employees' duties
(15) Temporary workers and other specialist categories
(16) Risk assessment in respect of new or expectant mothers
(17) Certificate from a registered medical practitioner in respect of new or expectant mothers
(18) Notification by new or expectant mothers
(19) Protection of young persons
(20) Exemption certificates
(21) Provisions as to liability and employer's liability
(22) Exclusion of civil liability
(23) Extension outside Great Britain
(23–30) Amendment of earlier regulations, transitional provisions

Schedule 1 General principles of prevention

Figure 11.6   Management of Health and Safety at Work Regulations 1999

Every employer shall make a suitable and sufficient assessment of:

(a)   the risks to the health and safety of his employees to which they are exposed whilst they are at work; and
(b)   the risks to the health and safety of persons not in his employment arising out of or in connection with the conduct by him of his undertaking,

for the purpose of identifying the measures he needs to take to comply with the requirements and prohibitions imposed upon him by or under the relevant statutory provisions.

Figure 11.7   Regulation 3(1). Management of Health and Safety At Work 1999

The duty also applies to physiotherapists in private practice. Figure 11.8 sets out Regulation 3(2).

There is a duty under Regulation 3(3) to review the assessment when there is reason to suspect that it is no longer valid or there has been significant change in the matters to which it relates.

Regulation 3(4) introduces a new limitation on an employer employing a young person (i.e. a person under 18 years) unless they had made an assessment in relation to risks to the health

Every self-employed person shall make a suitable and sufficient assessment of:

(a)   the risks to his own health and safety to which he is exposed whilst he is at work; and
(b)   the risks to the health and safety of persons not in his employment arising out of or in connection with the conduct by him of his undertaking,

for the purposes of identifying the measures he needs to take to comply with the requirements and prohibitions imposed upon him by or under the relevant statutory provisions.

Figure 11.8   Regulation 3(2). Management of Health and Safety At Work 1999

and safety of a young person. Regulation 3(5) sets out particular factors which must be taken into account in such an assessment.

Under Regulation 3(6) where more than five people are employed there must be a record of the findings of the assessment and any group of employees identified as being especially at risk.

The guidance

The guidance in the Code of Practice emphasises that risk assessment must be a systematic general examination of work activity, with a recording of significant findings, rather than a reactive procedure.

Definition of risk and aims of assessment

The definition of risk includes both the likelihood that harm will occur and its severity and the number of people who may be exposed to that risk. The aim of risk assessment is to help the employer or self-employed person determine what measures should be taken to comply with their statutory obligations laid down under HASAW and its regulations and the fire regulations.

The key words 'suitable' and 'sufficient' are defined in the guidance as being a risk assessment that:

(a)   should identify the significant risks arising from or in connection with work. The level of detail in a risk assessment should be proportionate to the risk . . .

(b)   should enable the employer or the self-employed person to take reasonable steps to identify the measures that need to be taken to comply with the relevant statutory provisions

(c)   should be appropriate to the nature of the work and should identify the period of time for which it is likely to remain valid.

How the risk assessment is to be carried out

Figure 11.9 sets out the requirements of a valid risk assessment set out in Paragraph 18 of the Code.

It may be possible for several employers engaged in the same activity to share model risk assessments.

Recording (Paragraph 23)

The record should represent an effective statement of hazards and risks, which then leads management to take the relevant action to protect health and safety. It should be in writing unless in computerised form and should be easily retrievable. It should include:

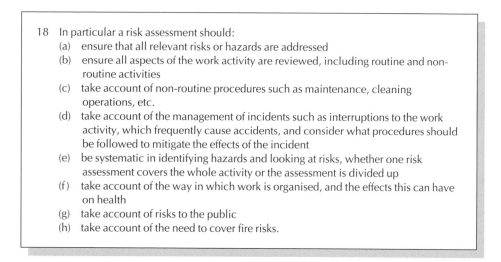

18   In particular a risk assessment should:
  (a)   ensure that all relevant risks or hazards are addressed
  (b)   ensure all aspects of the work activity are reviewed, including routine and non-routine activities
  (c)   take account of non-routine procedures such as maintenance, cleaning operations, etc.
  (d)   take account of the management of incidents such as interruptions to the work activity, which frequently cause accidents, and consider what procedures should be followed to mitigate the effects of the incident
  (e)   be systematic in identifying hazards and looking at risks, whether one risk assessment covers the whole activity or the assessment is divided up
  (f)   take account of the way in which work is organised, and the effects this can have on health
  (g)   take account of risks to the public
  (h)   take account of the need to cover fire risks.

Figure 11.9   Requirements of valid risk assessment (Guidance paragraph 18)

- the significant hazards;
- a record of the preventive and protection measures in place to control the risk;
- what further action, if any, needs to be taken to reduce the risk sufficiently;
- proof that a suitable and sufficient assessment has been made.

Preventive and protective measures (Regulation 4 and Schedule 1)

The following principles apply:

- avoid risks;
- evaluate risks that cannot be avoided;
- combat risks at source;
- adapt work to the individual;
- adapt to technical progress;
- replace the dangerous by the non-dangerous or the less dangerous;
- develop a coherent overall policy that covers technology, organisation or work, working conditions, social relationships and the influence of factors relating to the working environment;
- give collective protective measures priority over individual protective measures; and
- give appropriate instructions to employees.

New or expectant mothers and young employees

The 1999 Regulations include new provisions on the health and safety of new and expectant mothers and young people. Specified factors must be taken into account in undertaking risk assessments and preventive measures in relation to their health and safety. The employer may be required to alter her working conditions or hours of work or offer her suitable alternative work or suspend her from work (when she would be entitled to full pay under the Employment Rights Act 1996). Young people should not be employed for work which is beyond their physical or psychological capacity or in other specified circumstances (unless it is necessary for training, where they are supervised and any risk is reduced to the lowest level that is reasonably practicable.)

The Court of Appeal[9] held that the duty of the employer to provide a suitable and sufficient risk assessment under Regulation 3 of the Management of Health and Safety at Work Regulations 1999[10] and training for its employees under Regulation 9 of the Provisions and Use of Work Equipment Regulations 1998[11] imposed a higher standard that the common law duty which incorporated reasonable foreseeability. The claimant worked for London Underground first as a guard and then as a driver and developed tenosynovitis in her shoulder due to the strain from the prolonged use of the traction brake controller, known as the dead man's handle. The employer had a duty to provide adequate training, which included a duty to investigate the risks inherent in its operations taking professional advice where necessary. The right approach to deciding whether the training was adequate for health and safety purposes was to examine whether the risk assessment was suitable and sufficient.

In another case on the Provisions and Use of Work Equipment Regulations 1998 Regulation 4 and 5, the Court of Appeal[12] held that an employer was not liable for a slip on another's ramp. The facts were that Mrs Smith was employed by the council as carer/driver and collected a client in a wheelchair from her home. When pushing the chair down the ramp, which had been installed by the NHS, she stepped on the edge and it gave way.

The trial judge had held that Regulation 5 imposed strict liability on the council for maintaining the ramp as work equipment for use at work and found in favour of Mrs Smith. The Court of Appeal however allowed the council's appeal and held that strict liability should only be imposed by clear language. For someone to have an obligation to maintain something it would normally have to be within his/her power to do so without obtaining someone else's consent. Strict liability should not flow out of a position in which there was no right and no responsibility to do that thing or insist on doing that thing for which strict liability was being imposed.

The House of Lords[13] held that a door-closing device could be work equipment for the purposes of Regulation 2 of the Provision and Use of Work Equipment Regulations,[14] so that a mechanic who was injured while repairing such a device could bring proceedings against his employer.

Risk management and the physiotherapist

The CSP published in April 2008 an updated briefing paper on risk assessment.[15] It covers guidance on the 1999 Regulations, risk assessment and risk prevention, the roles of risk assessors, the role of safety representatives and organising risk assessments. It also has a checklist for safety representatives.

For the most part, the physiotherapist would share common health and safety hazards with other hospital-, community- or social services-based employees and thus models of risk assessment and management which applied to other health professionals would also apply to physiotherapy. Thus hazards relating to the safety of equipment, cross-infection risks, safe working practices or to violence at work would all apply to physiotherapists, who should be involved in the system of the assessment of risk. The CSP has provided guidance on risk assessment in the form of a health and safety checklist.[16]

Moreover, the nature of physiotherapy involves the physiotherapist regularly weighing risk against benefit as clients are pushed to the limits of what they can achieve in the restorative process. Each physiotherapist should therefore be able to carry out a risk assessment of health and safety hazards in relation to clients as well as for colleagues, carers and the general public.

Manual handling

More than a third of over-3-day injuries reported each year to the NHS and local authorities are caused by manual handling.[17] Back injuries have been recognised as a major reason for sickness and staff retiring early on grounds of ill health. Physiotherapists are vulnerable to the possibility of back injury because of the work that they undertake in the movement of clients and the lifting of equipment. It is essential therefore that they should have a good understanding of the regulations relating to manual handling and the duties of the employer and of themselves.

The CSP has recently published guidance on manual handling, which is discussed below.[18] It has also provided guidance for physiotherapists in relation to musculoskeletal injuries.[19] This maps out hazardous areas in the workplace.

Legal duties are placed upon employers in relation to manual handling by the Manual Handling Regulations and also as a result of the duty of the employer under the contract of employment to take reasonable care of the health and safety of an employee. A duty of care is also owed to employees and the general public under the laws of negligence (see Chapter 10).

Manual handling regulations and guidance

Regulations were introduced in 1992 as a result of an EC directive[20] (see Figure 11.5) and amended in 2002.[21] Figure 11.10 sets out the content of the regulations. The list shown in Figure 11.10 constitutes the regulations which have been enacted under HASAW. In addition guidance on manual handling is offered by the Health and Safety Executive.[22] The guidelines are not themselves the law and the booklet advises that they

should not be regarded as precise recommendations. They should be applied with caution. Where doubt remains a more detailed assessment should be made.

A working group set up by the Health and Safety Commission produced a booklet on *Guidance on Manual Handling of Loads in the Health Services*.[23] Part of this health services-specific guidance material relates to staff working in the community. Subsequently the Health and Safety Executive has provided a short guide for employers called *Getting to Grips with Manual Handling*.[17] The guide includes a table on making an assessment that looks at the problems to be considered in making an assessment and the corresponding ways of reducing the risk of injury. It lists the factors to be taken into account in good handling technique for lifting and for pushing and pulling.

The CSP published guidance in manual handling in 2008[18] which provides a comprehensive account of the professional and legal framework, risk management in treatment handling, a review of the special circumstances and settings, delegation, guidance and advice and education and continuous professional

(1) Commencement
(2) Interpretation
(3) Disapplication of the regulations
(4) Duties of employers
　　　(1) (a) Avoidance of manual handling
　　　　　　(b) (i)   Assessment of risk
　　　　　　　　　(ii)   Reducing the risk of injury
　　　　　　　　　(iii) The load – additional information
　　　(2) Reviewing the assessment
(5) Duty of employees
(6) Exemption certificates
(7) Extension outside Great Britain
(8) Repeals and revocations

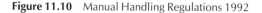

Figure 11.10   Manual Handling Regulations 1992

development. Useful appendices provide further information on assessment and other areas relevant to the physiotherapist. In addition, a joint publication between BackCare, the RCN, and the National Back Exchange provides practical guidance on handling people.[24]

Content of the regulations

The duty under the regulations can be summed up as follows:

- If reasonably practicable avoid the hazardous manual handling.
- Make a suitable and sufficient assessment of any hazardous manual handling which cannot be avoided.
- Reduce the risk of injury from this handling so far as is reasonably practicable.
- Give both general indications of risk and precise information on the weight of each load, and indicate the heaviest side of any load, where the centre of gravity is not positioned centrally.
- Review the assessment.

Avoiding the risk

By Regulation 4(1)(a) each employer *shall*

> so far as is reasonably practicable, avoid the need for his employees to undertake any manual handling operations at work which involve a risk of their being injured.

The guidance asks the question, as an example of this, whether a treatment can be brought to a patient rather than taking the patient to the treatment. It may be that in the case of physiotherapy it would be very difficult to remove the risk of injury entirely without reducing patient choice to unacceptable levels or denying the patient any therapeutic handling (see below).

Carrying out the assessment

By Regulation 4(1)(b) Each employer *shall*

> where it is not reasonably practicable to avoid the need for his employees to undertake any manual handling operations at work which involve a risk of their being injured . . . make a suitable and sufficient assessment of all such manual handling operations to be undertaken by them, having regard to the factors which are specified in column 1 of Schedule 1 to these Regulations and considering the questions which are specified in the corresponding entry in column 2 of that Schedule.

Schedule 1 is set out in Figure 11.11.

Appendix 2 of the Regulations gives an example of an assessment check list:

- Section A covering the preliminary stage;
- Section B the more detailed assessment where necessary; and
- Section C identifying the remedial action which should be taken.

Taking appropriate steps to reduce the risk

By Regulation 4(1)(b)(ii), where it is not reasonably practicable to avoid manual handling operations involving a risk of employees being injured each employer *shall*

> take appropriate steps to reduce the risk of injury to those employees arising out of their undertaking any such manual handling operations to the lowest level reasonably practicable.

For example, in carrying out the assessment of risk and deciding how to minimise the risk, it could be decided, in the circumstances of that particular case, to install a hoist. This may include the possibility of installing a hoist for a domiciliary confinement, even though only temporarily.

Situation: Oswestry frame

A patient needs to be lifted into an Oswestry frame but this would involve the physiotherapist in manual handling. On its own the frame would cost about £500, but if it is fitted with a mechanised

Factors to which the employer must have regard and questions he must consider when making an assessment of manual handling operations

Factors	Questions
(1) The tasks	e.g. do they involve holding or manipulating loads at a distance from the trunk?
(2) The loads	e.g. are they heavy, bulky or unwieldy etc.?
(3) The working environment	e.g. are there space constraints preventing good posture, uneven slippery or unstable floors etc.?
(4) Individual capability	does the job require unusual strength, height etc.?
(5) Other factors	e.g. is movement or posture hindered by personal protective equipment or by clothing?

Figure 11.11 Schedule 1 of Manual Handling Regulations 1992

hoist attachment it could cost over £3000. Can the physiotherapist refuse to use the frame if it is not fitted with a hoist?

The risk assessment in these circumstances should take account of the reasonable possibility of avoiding any manual handling. The requirement imposed by the regulations is not absolute, but rather a matter of what is reasonably practicable. All the circumstances must be taken into account. It may be possible that in some cases the patient can move into the standing frame without involving the physiotherapist in manual handling. The additional cost involved in purchasing the hoist would have to be judged against other priorities as part of the assessment.

Giving general and specific information

By Regulation 4(1)(b)(iii) where it is not practicable to avoid the need to undertake manual handling:

Each employer shall . . . [T]ake appropriate steps to provide any of those employees who are undertaking any such manual handling operations . . . , where it is reasonably practicable to do so, precise information on:
(aa)   the weight of each load, and
(bb)   the heaviest side of any load whose centre of gravity is not positioned centrally.

Review

Regulation 4(2) requires the employer to review the assessment:

(a)   if there is reason to suspect that it is no longer valid; or
(b)   there has been a significant change in the manual handling operations to which it relates;
(c)   and where as a result of any such review changes to an assessment are required, the relevant employer shall make them.

It is in the interests of all physiotherapists to ensure that the employer is reminded when a review becomes necessary under the above provisions.

Temporary staff

The duty which is owed by the employer is owed not only to employees but also to temporary staff such as agency or bank staff who are called in to assist. All such persons are entitled to be included in the risk assessment process, since, as has been seen, the assessment must take into account the individual characteristics of each employee. Physiotherapists who are unusually small in height or not so strong as the average might require special provisions in relation to manual handling.

Physiotherapists in private practice

Independent physiotherapists are not employees and as self-employed persons would be responsible for carrying out the assessments and taking the necessary precautions for themselves and any staff whom they employ. Where they work alongside employed physiotherapists, they should ensure that the NHS Trust takes into account hazards to their health and safety and that the agreement which they have with the NHS Trust reflects this duty. Appendix 6 of the CSP guidance (2008)[18] provides a self-assessment pro forma for use in private practice.

Enforcement

- What action can be taken if the employer ignores these regulations?

The regulations are part of the health and safety provisions which form part of the criminal law. Infringement of the regulations can lead to prosecution by the Health and Safety Inspectorate. The Inspectorate has the power to issue enforcement or prohibition notices against any corporate body or individual. A health authority no longer enjoys the immunity from the criminal sanctions that it once did as a crown authority and therefore these enforcement provisions are available against it. Similarly, an NHS Trust is subject to the full force of the criminal law.

- What if the carer or client refuses to use a hoist?

If a risk management assessment for manual handling in a patient's home indicates that a hoist is necessary to prevent harm to any carer/professional, then the professional can insist that when he/she visits the home the hoist will be used. If the patient refuses to be placed in a hoist, the professional can advise the patient that the only way of safely moving her/him is by a hoist, and if the patient continues to refuse, then the patient can be told that support and assistance will not be provided if it endangers the health and safety of the professionals. The professional can also advise the carer on the reasons why a hoist is necessary, but of course the use of the hoist by the carer cannot be enforced. If the carer ignores the instructions, fails to use the hoist and injures his/her back, then there should be no liability on the staff, who gave the correct guidance.

A dispute between paid carers and clients over the use of hoists was considered in the following case.

Case: East Sussex human rights and manual handling 2003[25]

In February 2003 the High Court gave judgment on a case, where the claimants raised the issue of their human rights not to be hoisted. A and B were sisters born in 1976 and 1980 who suffered from profound physical and learning disabilities. They lived in the family home which had been specially adapted and equipped for them and were looked after on a full-time basis by their mother X and their stepfather Y. A dispute arose between the claimants and East Sussex County Council (ESCC), which provided community care services over the extent to which moving and lifting should be done manually. ESCC's policy on manual handling did not permit care staff to lift A or B manually. The claimants, supported by the Disability Rights Commission, argued that ESCC's manual handling policies, as applied to A and B, were unlawful and unjustifiable, on the basis that they improperly failed to take into account the needs of the disabled people involved. Its policy was subsequently amended to make it clear that ESCC did not operate a blanket no lifting policy. The claimants argued that the application of the policy to the specific circumstances of A and B's care and the draft protocols prepared by the independent handling adviser were unlawful.

The judge considered the effect of Sections 2 and 3 of the Health and Safety at Work Act 1974, the

Manual Handling Operations Regulations 1992 and the Management of Health and Safety at Work Regulations 1999, and cases already decided on manual handling and the implications of the European Convention for Human Rights and the Charter of Fundamental Rights of the European Union. He emphasised that one must guard against jumping too readily to the conclusion that manual handling is necessarily more dignified than the use of equipment. Hoisting is not inherently undignified, let alone inherently inhuman or degrading. He identified the principles which applied and stated that, ultimately, the employer must balance the impact of the assessment on both carer and disabled person.

This balancing exercise is to be resolved in the context of Article 8 of the European Convention on Human Rights (see Appendix 1) by enquiring of each claimant whether the interference with his/her right to be respected is such as to be 'necessary in a democratic society'. Once the balance has been struck, if it comes down in favour of manual handling, then the employer must make the appropriate assessment and take all appropriate steps to minimise the risks that exist. The assessment must be properly documented and lead to clear protocols which cover all situations, including foreseeable emergencies and, in the case of patients such as A and B, events such as episodes of spasm and distress that might arise. The judge accepted that protocols developed by the employer cannot be too prescriptive. He emphasised that it was for ESCC to formulate its manual handling policy and to make the appropriate assessment in relation to A and B. Neither of those is a matter for the court. The making and drafting of the kind of assessments called for in a case such as this was outside the competence and expertise of the court. What the court could and should do was to assist ESCC by identifying the relevant legal principles.

The outcome of the case was that ESCC was required to complete with the assistance of the independent manual handling adviser the appropriate assessments and protocols. If these were not acceptable to the claimants, they could challenge them by way of judicial review.

- What remedies exist for compensation?

Section 47 of HASAW prevents breach of certain duties under the Act being used as the basis for a claim in the civil courts. Breach of the regulations can however be the basis of a civil claim for compensation unless the regulations provide to the contrary. Nevertheless, even where what is alleged is a breach of the basic duties, a physiotherapist who suffered harm as a result of the failure of the employer to take reasonable steps to safeguard his/her health and safety could sue in the civil courts on the basis of the employer's duty at common law (see below).

The statutory duty to ensure the Act is implemented is paralleled by a duty at common law placed upon the employer to take reasonable steps to ensure the employee's health and safety. Contracts of employment should state clearly the duty upon the employer to take reasonable care of the employee's safety and also the employee's duty to cooperate with the employer in carrying out health and safety duties under the Act, the Regulations and at common law. It is, of course, in the long-term interests of the employer to prevent back injuries thereby reducing the incidence of sickness and absenteeism and also avoiding payment of substantial compensation to his injured employees.

Training

This is essential to ensure that staff have the understanding to carry out the assessments and to advise on lifting and the appropriate equipment. Regular monitoring should take place to ensure that the training is effective and the policies for review are in place. There is also a duty on the employer to ensure that staff who are not expected to be regularly involved in manual handling are aware of the risks of so doing.

An example is a case where a social worker succeeded in a claim against the County Council that employed her.[26]

Case: *Colclough* v. *Staffordshire County Council*

The plaintiff [claimant] was employed as a social worker in the elderly care team. Her duties consisted largely of assessing clients for residential placement and other needs. She was called out to an elderly man's home after referral from his GP. When she arrived she gained access with a neighbour, only to find the man halfway out of his bed. He was in a very distressed state and she felt it was important for him to be lifted back into the bed as she was worried about him being injured. The neighbour, who had some nursing experience, told the social worker how to lift the man. As both of them attempted to lift the man, who weighed around 15 stone, the social worker sustained a lumbar spine injury. She sued on the grounds that the employers had failed to provide her with any training and/or instruction in lifting techniques. The employers denied liability on the ground that it was not a normal part of a social worker's duties to undertake any lifting tasks. They alleged that she should have summoned some assistance from the emergency services.

The judge held that it was reasonably foreseeable that the plaintiff would be confronted with emergency situations when working as a social worker in the elderly care team. Although the situation which arose was most unusual, the employers were under a duty to warn her that she should not lift in such circumstances. This duty did not go so far as to impose upon the employer in these circumstances a duty to provide a long training course but certainly to bring to the notice of social workers the risks of lifting. Her claim succeeded without a finding of contributory negligence (see Glossary and Chapter 7).

The implications of this decision are that even staff who are not expected to be involved in manual handling as part of their work must be trained in risk awareness in order to protect them should they ever be in the situation where they could be endangered through manual handling.

Lifting and instructing others

Physiotherapists may be asked to instruct others such as carers, clients or other health or social service employees in operations involving manual handling and compliance with the regulations. Before they instruct others they should be sure that they receive the necessary additional training to undertake the task of instruction, since failure to instruct competently could in itself give rise to an action in negligence if harm should occur as a result of negligent instructions (see Chapter 10 on negligent advice). The CSP guidance on manual handling also provides advice to physiotherapists who become back care advisers/coordinators or manual handling advisers/coordinators to ensure that they develop the specialist skills necessary as set out in the requirements of National Back Exchange, multidisciplinary association.

As in all situations where there is the potential for litigation full records should be kept and the information which the CSP recommends should be recorded is set out in Figure 11.12.

- the names of trainees, their qualifications and job titles
- the sessions attended by each
- the length of each session
- a full and accurate note of contents of each session
- a record and copy of any handouts
- the signature of each participant countersigned by trainer
- a note of those who failed to attend

Figure 11.12   Documentation and manual handling training

Failures to instruct by agencies

Sometimes physiotherapists become aware that agency staff have not been instructed in manual handling techniques. It would be reasonable practice in this situation for the physiotherapist to ensure that senior management of the agency were informed so that steps could be taken to provide formal training for agency staff.

Therapeutic handling

It is sometimes argued that therapeutic lifting, e.g. in orthopaedic wards to facilitate early mobilisation does not come under the manual handling regulations. There are however no grounds for this assertion. The definition of manual handling is

> any transporting or supporting of a load (including the lifting, putting down, pushing, pulling, carrying or moving thereof) by hand or by bodily force.

This would therefore include therapeutic situations.

'No lifting policy' and therapeutic handling

The first requirement of any manual handling policy is to avoid any manual handling where it is reasonably practicable to do so. Clearly, if this were to be implemented in the therapeutic regime, patients would never get mobilised following strokes and orthopaedic or other trauma. The physiotherapist should ensure that a risk assessment is carried out which takes into account both the needs of the patient to become mobile and also dangers that staff face in promoting this mobilisation. Guidance is provided by the CSP on treatment involving manual handling.[18] It emphasises that therapeutic handling may involve the taking of calculated risks but that it is appropriate and essential if the patient's prompt progress towards optimal function is not to be impeded or stopped. The

wide statutory definition of manual handling means that breaking the fall of a person would come within that definition. The ethical dilemmas of such a situation are considered by Mike Betts[27] but there are also clear legal implications in deciding what action to take.

Lifting extremely heavy persons

This is of considerable concern to physiotherapists. The National Institute for Health and Clinical Excellence (NICE) defined morbid obesity as having a body mass index of more than $40 \text{ kg}/\text{m}^2$ or between $35 \text{ k}/\text{m}^2$ and $40 \text{ k}/\text{m}^2$ with comorbidities.[28] Section 38 of the 2008 manual handling guidance from the CSP considers the challenges presented by bariatric patients who increase the risk of work-related musculoskeletal disorders to physiotherapists, as they will exceed the guideline weights set by the Health and Safety Executive in 1998.[29] A review of methods of dealing with obese patients is provided by Graham Clews.[30] An article on support for bariatric employees includes the case study of a nurse who weighed 27 stone but was assessed as medically fit for practice by the occupational health consultant.[31]

The legal issues arising are significant. Staff cannot cease to provide services for such persons, but the consequences in terms of costs and effort in minimising the risk of harm are considerable. Delegates at the CSP conference in 2008 backed a motion calling on the CSP to provide information resources to members, safety reps and managers and to help employers to be more pro-active in dealing with bariatric patients, many of whom face inequality of care. It was reported that special equipment for moving heavier patients was not always available when required.

Physiotherapists, manual handling and the courts

(See also Chapter 13 on these issues.)

Recent years have seen an increase in litigation in respect of back injuries when failures in fulfilling health and safety duties in respect of manual handling are alleged. The physiotherapist may be a witness of fact or expert witness (see Chapter 13). As a witness of fact he/she may have to give evidence in respect of the physiotherapist's involvement in training the individual concerned (see above), or in carrying out a risk assessment or as a witness to the alleged incident.

The records of a physiotherapist concerning the patient who is involved in a manual handling situation may be relevant in determining the risks to any staff involved in manual handling. Thus in *Bowfield v. South Sefton (Merseyside) Health Authority*,[32] (in respect of a manual handling incident) records taken by physiotherapists during multidisciplinary rounds were important in determining the extent to which the claimant employee would have been aware of any limitations on the patient's part. (A decision in favour of the employee was overturned by the Court of Appeal.) The recently published guidance on manual handling from the CSP covers special circumstances and settings of the physiotherapist including: neurological rehabilitation, paediatrics, hydrotherapy, oncology and palliative care, learning disabilities, therapeutic riding, bariatric rehabilitation and private practice. Reference can also be made to publications by the BackCare (formerly the National Back Pain Association) including *Safer Handling of People in the Community*.[33] In the following case the court ordered arrangements to be made for a client to be moved from a wheelchair.

Case: Wolstenholme

Lorraine Wolstenholme, a disabled woman of 50 in Milton Keynes had slept in a wheelchair for 17 months after nurses stopped lifting her in case they were injured. A High Court judge ordered that arrangements for moving her should be made by 19 December 2003.[34]

Case: carrying by ambulance men

The Court of Appeal[35] held that the employers were not in breach of the directive or regulations on manual handling where King, an ambulance technician, suffered serious injuries carrying an elderly patient down the stairway of his home. King and his colleague had taken the patient down the stairway, which was narrow and steep, in a carry chair. He had been injured when forced for a brief moment to bear the full weight of the chair. The trial judge found in favour of the ambulance technician holding that the employers were in breach of Council Directive (90/269 Article 3(2)) and the Manual Handling Regulations and that the employers had acted negligently by discouraging employees in circumstances such as those in this particular case from calling the fire brigade to take patients from their homes.

Sussex Ambulance NHS Trust appealed against the finding. The Court of Appeal held that the NHS Trust was not liable either under the directive or under the Manual Handling Regulations. There was nothing to suggest that calling the fire brigade would have been appropriate in the case. The evidence showed that such an option was rarely used because it had to be carefully planned, took a long time and caused distress to the patient. There might be cases where calling the fire brigade would be appropriate, but that would depend on the seriousness of the problem, the urgency of the case and the actual or likely response of the patient or his/her carers and the fire brigade. King had failed to show that given that possibility, more emphasis in training would have avoided his injuries. The ambulance service owed the same duty of care to its employees as did any other employer. However, the question of what was reasonable for it to do might have to be judged in the light of its duties to the public and the resources available to it when performing those duties. While the risks to King had not been negligible, the task that he had been carrying out was of considerable social utility.

Furthermore, Sussex Ambulance NHS Trust had limited resources so far as equipment was concerned. There was no evidence of any steps that the trust could have taken to prevent the risk and the only suggestion made was that it should have called on a third party to perform the task for it. Since calling the fire brigade was not appropriate or reasonably practicable for the purpose of the directive and the regulations, the Sussex Ambulance NHS Trust had not shown a lack of reasonable care. Accordingly, it had not acted negligently.

Reporting risks, injuries, etc.

Reporting of Injuries, Diseases and Dangerous Occurrences Regulations 1995

RIDDOR 1995 came into force on 1 April 1996 replacing earlier statutory instruments. The lists of reportable diseases and occurrences were updated. It is legally possible for reports to be made by telephone. A new accident book (known as B1510) has been designed by the Department of Work and Pensions to take account of the Data Protection Act 1998 and the Human Rights Act 1998 Guidance on RIDDOR is provided by the Health and Safety Executive (HSE) and available from its website.[36]

Encouraging others to report accidents

Situation: failure to report

A physiotherapist is visited by a patient for treatment and is told that the injury occurred in an accident at work. The physiotherapist asks if the patient reported it and is told that she did not. Should the physiotherapist take any action?

In the above situation, unless the physiotherapist worked with the patient or had some responsibilities for the accident, it is not the duty of the physiotherapist to report the incident. However, she should make every effort to persuade the patient to report it herself, wherever it took place.

In a case heard in 1987[37] the claimant gave evidence that she had to go into hospital because of her back for in-patient treatment, and that the physiotherapist there asked her whether she had reported the accident and told her that she was silly not to have done so. She (i.e. the claimant) said of that

I didn't really know who to report it to, and the physiotherapist said I'd have to go to court. I'd seen a lot of doctors who knew about the fall, none of them had ever advised me to make a claim.

It is important that the physiotherapist should give clear information to clients about the need for them to report industrial accidents to their employers. Physiotherapists should also know to whom clients can be referred to obtain information on criminal injury compensation.

Whistle-blowing

The additional protection against dismissal of employees who report health and safety hazards given by the Trade Union Reform and Employment Rights Act 1993 was consolidated in the Employment Rights Act 1996. In addition, the Public Interest Disclosure Act 1998 is intended to strengthen further protection given to employees who report health and safety hazards. This is considered in Chapter 17.

National Patient Safety Agency

The National Patient Safety Agency (NPSA) was established as a special health authority following a report, *An Organisation with a Memory*,[38] written by an expert group chaired by Professor Liam Donaldson, Chief Medical Officer, which had recommended the establishment of a national reporting system. All health organisations, including since 2003 primary care trusts, are required to report patient safety incidents and it in turn issues safety alerts. In its annual report for 2006/7 NPSA stated in the year ending in March 2007 1 406 416 patient safety incidents had been reported. It had initiated a project to evaluate and identify ways to improve reporting and learning. Following a successful pilot since May 2006, all reporting organisations had been able to access their incident data and compare their profile with similar NHS organisations. The first patient safety alert of the NPSA was issued on 23 July 2002 and was about preventing accidental overdose with intravenous potassium.[39] The alert notice refers to the possible risks from treatment with concentrated potassium and the need for additional safety precautions in the way potassium solutions are stored and prepared in hospital. Details of all the NPSA's alerts are available on its website.[40] A recent alert issued in March 2007 is concerned with safe practice with epidural injections and infusions.[41] The remit of the NPSA was extended in 2005 to include safety aspects of hospital design, cleanliness and food. It was also given the task of ensuring research is carried out safely through its responsibility for the National Research Ethics Service (NRES) [formerly the Central Office for Research Ethics Committees (COREC)]. It is also responsible for the National Clinical Assessment Service (NCAS), which is concerned with the performance of individual doctors and dentists and has taken over from NICE (see Chapters 10 and 17) responsibility for the three confidential enquiries: into Maternal Death and Child Health; Patient Outcome and Death; and Suicide and Homicide by Persons with Mental Illness. In July 2007 the NPSA published a study which investigated the circumstances in a sample of deaths of patients admitted with acute illnesses. It stated that in 2005 1804 serious incidents were reported as resulting in death, and of these 576 were avoidable. It set out a series of recommendations including improvements in communication, training and the provision of appropriate equipment. The NPSA report came at the same time as new guidelines issued by NICE on how health professionals should manage sudden declines in patients' health.

Control of Infection

Deaths resulting from failures to control cross-infection in the NHS have accelerated in recent years. The Department of Health (DH) published a strategy for tackling MRSA in November 2006. It was announced in June 2007 that the Healthcare Commission was to make unannounced spot checks on NHS trusts to cut rates of hospital-acquired infection.[42] The NHS trusts' performance would be measured against the DH hygiene code, which sets out 11 compulsory duties to prevent and cope with hospital superbugs. Sanctions for failure to comply with the Code could lead to a trust being placed under special measures. Further information on the DH strategy to reduce hospital-acquired infections can be found on the DH website.[43]

The Healthcare Commission published in May 2008 the results of its annual survey on patient satisfaction and found that there was an increasing number of concerns about cleanliness. The new powers under the Corporate Manslaughter and Corporate Homicide Act may be used against NHS trusts that fail to control hospital acquired infections. (See below and Chapter 2.)

It was reported on 17 January 2007 that Leslie Ash, an actress, received a £5 million settlement after she caught MRSA at the Chelsea and Westminster Hospital. It caused her devastating disabilities and meant that she would never again be able to play active roles as an actress. The case was due to be heard at the High Court in April 2008 but the NHS Litigation Authority settled it out of court.

In May 2008 it was reported that Elizabeth Miller, a 71-year-old woman, had been given approval to bring a test case against the NHS for allegedly giving her MRSA. She contracted the superbug while recovering from a heart operation at the Glasgow Royal Infirmary. She is claiming £30 000 compensation because she can no longer play with her great-grandchildren because she is so ill. The defendants argued that she may have had MRSA before she was admitted.

In Winchester it was suggested that new rules on the use of intravenous fluids had cut the incidence of MRSA. The use of cannulae has to be authorised by a specialist and once in place tubes are flushed with a saline solution and inspected daily.[44]

A Risk and Regulatory Advisory Council is being set up to review regulations on health and safety. Its first project is to look at the Government initiatives in relation to MRSA to assess their effectiveness.[45]

Concerns also surround the increasing incidence of *Clostridium difficile*. The Secretary of State, Alan Johnson, when appointed in 2007 was given £50 million to tackle MRSA and clostridium by doubling the size of the DH's infection improvement team who advise NHS trusts on developing plans to cut infections. In July 2007 the Healthcare Commission published a national study into healthcare-associated infection. In order to reduce the risk of infections the report recommended that trusts should develop a culture of safety, have a good system of corporate and clinical governance, review performance, manage risk and communicate with patients and the public. A report by the Healthcare Commission in October 2007 into Maidstone and Tunbridge Wells Trust revealed that up to 90 patients had died between 2004 and 2006 after being infected with *Clostridium difficile*. The Minister of Health responded by announcing plans for a new super-regulator to be established in April 2009, combining the Healthcare Commission, Mental Health Act Commission and the Commission for Social Care Inspection with powers to close NHS and private hospitals and residential care homes (see Chapter 17).

Implications for physiotherapists

Physiotherapists have a key role to play in maintaining high standards of cross-infection control and observing hospital policies on control of infection across the hospital and within their own departments. It is a duty placed on physiotherapists individually and upon their managers. The possibility that compensation may be payable as a result of negligence leading to incidents of infection and the likelihood that the Corporate Manslaughter and Corporate Homicide Act could be used where deaths occur as a consequence of organisational failures to control infection should lead to higher standards being set and implemented.

There could also be personal liability of a physiotherapist if he/she was negligent in allowing another person to be infected.

Criminal sanctions have been imposed on those spreading HIV. A man who infected his two lovers with HIV and exposed 13 others to the risk was jailed for 14 years. He was charged with exposing others to danger as well as having sex with under-aged girls.

National Institute for Health and Clinical Excellence Guidance

As part of its remit NICE has had the responsibility of producing public health guidance since 2005. It is producing guidance for employers to create a healthier workplace for the wellbeing of its staff. The Chief Executive of NICE explained this guidance in an article for the *British Journal of Healthcare Management*.[46] He stated that the guidance recommends that employers:

> Developed a plan to encourage employees to be physically active
>
> Encouraged employees to walk or cycle etc., to travel part or all of the way to and from work
>
> Help employees to be physically active during the working day, for example by providing information about walking or cycling routes or putting up signs to encourage them to use the stairs.

NICE issued guidance for employers on how to support staff who want to stop smoking before the ban in July 2007.[47]

Physiotherapists by reason of their expertise could play a major role in implementing the NICE workplace health guidelines within their organisations.

Occupier's liability and consumer protection

Occupier's Liability Act 1957

This Act places a duty of care upon the occupier (of whom there may be several) to take reasonable care of his visitors to ensure that they are safe for the purposes for which they are permitted to be on the premises. The Act is enforceable in the civil courts if harm has occurred.

Occupier

The occupier would be the person in control of the premises. This would normally be the NHS Trust in respect of hospital property and the ward sister would be acting as the agent of the occupier in respect of the safety of her ward. The Physiotherapist Manager could be deemed the occupier of the physiotherapy department. There can however be several occupiers. For example if painters employed by independent contractors come on to the premises they may also be in occupation of the premises and could be responsible for harm which occurs as a result of their lack of care.

Visitor

A visitor is a person on the premises with the express or implied consent of the occupier. In the context of hospitals the term would therefore include patients, staff, visitors, tradesmen or any one else with a *bona fide* reason to be there and who is not excluded by the occupier (see below).

The nature of the duty owed

The duty is set out in Section 2(2) of the Act and Section 2(3) clarifies the duty further in relation to specific circumstances as shown in Figure 11.13.

The Occupier's Liability Act 1957 and children is considered in Chapter 23.

The physiotherapist and premises in the community

Where a physiotherapist is visiting private homes, the occupier may be the owner of the house who is also in occupation, or the occupier may be a tenant. If the physiotherapist is injured on the premises it will depend upon how the injury occurred as to who would be liable: thus if he/she is injured as the result of a frayed rug, the

---

2(2)   The common duty of care is a duty to take such care as in all the circumstances of the case is reasonable to see that the visitor will be reasonably safe in using the premises for the purposes for which he is invited or permitted by the occupier to be there.

2(3)   The circumstances relevant for the present purpose include the degree of care, and of want of care, which would ordinarily be looked for in such a visitor, so that (for example) in proper cases:
(a)   an occupier must be prepared for children to be less careful than adults; and
(b)   an occupier may expect that a person, in the exercise of his calling, will appreciate and guard against any special risks ordinarily incident to it, so far as the occupier leaves him free to do so.

Figure 11.13   The Occupier's Liability Act 1957 Sections 2(2) and (3)

> (a) [if the occupier] is aware of the danger or has reasonable grounds to believe that it exists;
>
> (b) [if the occupier] knows or has reasonable grounds to believe that the other is in the vicinity of the danger concerned or that he may come into the vicinity of the danger (in either case, whether the other has lawful authority for being in that vicinity or not); and
>
> (c) the risk is one against which, in all the circumstances of the case, [the occupier] may reasonably be expected to offer the other some protection.

Figure 11.14   The Occupier's Liability Act 1984 – Section 1(3)

person in occupation (whether tenant or owner) would be liable; if he/she were injured as a result of a structural defect then the owner or landlord would be liable depending upon the nature of the tenancy agreement.

The occupier has the right to ask any visitor to leave the premises. Should the visitor fail to leave, then he/she becomes a trespasser and the occupier can use reasonable force to evict him/her. If, therefore, the physiotherapist should be asked by a client or carer to leave he/she should go. Should the physiotherapist be concerned for the wellbeing of the client, he/she should ensure that social services are notified so that appropriate action can be taken. Where there is a clash between carer and client and the former asks the physiotherapist to leave but the latter wants him/her to stay, the physiotherapist has to decide on the basis of the specific circumstances: the rights of the client to occupation compared with those of the carer, and the specific needs of the client. Where the physiotherapist considers it prudent to leave the premises he/she must discuss with his/her manager how best the client's needs can be met.

The Occupier's Liability Act 1984

The 1957 Act does not cover the situation relating to trespassers. Until the 1984 Act was passed the law relating to the nature of the duty owed to a trespasser was according to the common law (i.e. the decisions of judges or case law – see Chapter 2).

Whether or not a duty is owed by the occupier to trespassers, in relation to risks on the premises, depends upon the following factors set out in Section 1(3) and shown in Figure 11.14.

In applying these factors to decide whether a duty is owed to a trespasser, it would be rare for a duty to be owed to a mentally competent adult. It is, however, more likely that a duty will be owed to a child trespasser. Thus, for example, if a child on hospital premises is expressly told that he/she cannot go through a particular door or into another section of the hospital and he/she disobeys those instructions, then he/she becomes a trespasser for the purposes of the Occupier's Liability Acts. Although not protected by the 1957 Act, it is likely that a duty to the child would then arise under the 1984 Act depending on the child's age and understanding.

The nature of the duty owed to trespassers

Once it is held that a duty of care is owed to a trespasser, the 1984 Act by Section 1(4) defines the duty as follows:

> The duty is to take such care as is reasonable in all the circumstances of the case to see that he does not suffer injury on the premises by reason of the danger concerned.

The duty can be discharged by giving warnings, but in the case of children this may have limited effect – it would depend upon the age of the child.

(1)   Work out what hazardous substances are used in your workplace and find out the risks from using these substances to people's health.
(2)   Decide what precautions are needed before starting work with hazardous substances.
(3)   Prevent people being exposed to hazardous substances, but where this is not reasonably practicable, control the exposure.
(4)   Make sure control measures are used and maintained properly and that safety procedures are followed.
(5)   If required, monitor exposure of employees to hazardous substances.
(6)   Carry out health surveillance where your assessment has shown that this is necessary or where COSHH makes specific requirements.
(7)   If required, prepare plans and procedures to deal with accidents, incidents and emergencies.
(8)   Make sure employees are properly informed, trained and supervised.

Figure 11.15   Stages in Control of Substances Hazardous to Health (COSHH) assessment

The Consumer Protection Act 1987

This enables a claim to be brought where harm has occurred as a result of a defect in a product. It is a form of strict liability in that negligence by the supplier or manufacturer does not have to be established. The claimant will however have to show that there was a defect. These issues are considered further in Chapter 15 on the law relating to equipment. See also PA 4 *Equipment Safety and Product Liability* produced by the CSP.[48] The work of the Medical Devices Agency (which was been absorbed into the Medicine and Healthcare Products Regulatory Agency (MHRA) in 2003) is also relevant and is considered in detail in Chapter 15. The new Consumer Protection Regulations covering personal services are considered in Chapter 19.

The Control of Substances Hazardous to Health Regulations 2002

The Control of Substances Hazardous to Health (COSHH) Regulations 1988 came into effect in 1989 and were replaced by amended regulations in 1996. New regulations came into force in November 2002[49] replacing earlier Regulations in order to comply with the EC Chemical Agents Directive, which set more detailed rules of compliance. The HSE has set up a COSHH website to provide guidance for employers[50] and has provided a brief guide to the Regulations.[51] This guide sets out the eight stages of a COSHH assessment, which are shown in Figure 11.15.

All health workers have responsibilities under the COSHH Regulations. The physiotherapist who uses different substances in his/her work should be specifically alert to the need to ensure that the regulations are implemented. The CSP has provided guidance on the dangers of latex.[52] This information paper discusses the problems surrounding the use of latex and also includes information on the laws that apply and action points for safety representatives and also the contents of a policy on latex. It was reported that a former trainee nurse, who had to give up her job after developing a potentially fatal allergy to latex, won a six-figure compensation payout. Tanya Dod, who worked at Scarborough General Hospital, was threatened with disciplinary action if she was caught using latex-free gloves.[53]

There must be clarity over who has the responsibility for carrying out the assessment, but the guidance emphasises the importance of involving all employees in the task.

All potentially hazardous substances must be identified. These will include domestic materials such as bleach, toilet cleaner, window cleaner and polishes, and office materials such as correction fluids, as well as the medicinal products in the treatment room and materials and substances used in physiotherapy.

An assessment has to be made as to whether each substance could be inhaled, swallowed, absorbed or introduced through the skin, or injected into the body (as with needles). The effects of each route of entry or contact and the potential harm must then be identified. There must then be an identification of the persons who could be exposed and how. The stages to be followed in a COSHH assessment are set out in Figure 11.15.

Once this assessment is complete, decisions must be made on the necessary measures to be taken to comply with the Regulations and on who should undertake the different tasks. In certain cases, health surveillance of the employees is required if there is a reasonable likelihood that the disease or ill effect associated with exposure will occur in the workplace or hospital environment concerned. Physiotherapists should be particularly vigilant about any substances used in their activities and cleaning fluids and ensure that a risk assessment is undertaken and its results implemented.

Mangers should ensure that the employees are given information, instruction and training. Records should show what the results of the assessment are, what action has been taken and by whom, and regular monitoring and review of the situation.

Corporate manslaughter and corporate homicide

As a consequence of the Corporate Manslaughter and Corporate Homicide Act 2007, it is possible for an organisation to which the Act applies to be prosecuted in the case of a death under Health and Safety Legislation and the 2007 Act. The jury can be instructed to find the accused organisation guilty of both offences. An organisation can be found guilty of an offence under the 2007 Act only if the way in which its

activities are managed or organised by its senior management is a substantial element in the breach of duty of care owed by the organisation. Senior management means the persons who play significant roles in (i) the making of decisions about how the whole or a substantial part of its activities are to be managed or organised, or (ii) the actual managing or organising of the whole or a substantial part of those activities. The Act is further considered in Chapter 2.

Employment issues

Common law duty implied in the contract of employment

Some of the terms in the contract of employment are implied by the law. These include the obligation of the employer to safeguard the health and safety of the employee by

- employing competent staff
- setting up a safe system of work
- maintaining safe premises, equipment and plant.

The employee needs to obey the reasonable instructions of the employer and must take reasonable care in carrying out the work. Thus, as has been seen in the discussion on manual handling above, the employee may have a claim for breach of contract by the employer if back injuries result from failure on the employer's part in not providing appropriate training or equipment. To obtain compensation from the employer, the employee must show that the employer was in breach of the duty of care owed by the employer and as a reasonably foreseeable consequence of that breach the employee has suffered harm. In a recent case the House of Lords held that a widow was entitled to damages in respect of her husband's suicide where that had been the direct result of a depressive illness from which he had suffered as the direct and foreseeable consequences of an accident for which his employer had been responsible.[54]

Statutory requirements

The employer's duty at common law to take reasonable care to safeguard the employees against the reasonable foreseeable possibility of harm arising from work-related disorders is paralleled by the duties laid down in the Health and Safety at Work etc. Act 1974, and under the Regulations relating to Manual Handling (see above), the Management of Health and Safety at Work, Display Screen Equipment and the other regulations listed in Figure 11.5.

The Employer's Liability (Defective Equipment) Act 1969

Where

- the employee suffers personal injury in the course of employment as a consequence of a defect in equipment, and
- the equipment is provided by the employer for the purposes of his business, and
- the defect is attributable wholly or partly to the fault of a third party,

then the employee can recover compensation from the employer on the grounds that the injury is deemed to be also attributable to the employer. The employer can raise any contributory negligence by the employee as a defence in the action and can recover a contribution or indemnity from the third party.

The advantage of the Act is that it saves the employee from having to ascertain the identity of the third party and bringing an action directly against them.

Employers' Liability (Compulsory Insurance) Act 1969

This requires all non-Crown employers to be covered by an approved policy of insurance against liability for bodily injury or disease sustained by an employee and arising out of and in course of employment. Despite the abolition of crown immunity, Schedule 8 of the NHS and Community Care Act 1990 preserves the immunity of health authorities and trusts from this Act, but local authorities are bound by it, as are private hospitals. The employers of a physiotherapist working in the private sector or GPs employing a physiotherapist are, also, bound by the Act.

Effect of failure by the employer

The employer's failure to take reasonable care of the health, safety or welfare of the employee could result in the following actions by the employee:

- action for breach of contract of employment; and/or
- action for negligence, where the employee has suffered harm (the employee could also use as evidence any breach of specific health and safety regulations); and/or
- application to the employment tribunal claiming constructive dismissal (see Glossary and Chapter 17) if it can be shown that the employer is in fundamental breach of the contract of employment.

Examples of cases brought in relation to the employer's duty of care at common law are the manual handling cases above and the stress cases outlined below.

Special areas

Animals

A physiotherapist may be concerned with danger from dogs kept by clients and carers and needs to know what his/her rights are in this respect.

- Could he/she refuse to attend a client because there is an aggressive animal in the house?
- What are the physiotherapist's rights if he/she is injured?

If a client or carer has an animal which the owner does not have under control and, as a consequence, a visiting physiotherapist is injured, then the physiotherapist may be able to claim compensation under the Occupier's Liability Act 1957 above. The physiotherapist would need to establish that the owner as occupier of the premises failed to take reasonable care to ensure that he/she was safe. The fact that it was known that the animal could be aggressive would place upon the occupier a clear duty to protect visitors from it. Where it is known that an aggressive animal is on the premises then the owner can be warned that, unless the animal is kept under control, the physiotherapy department cannot provide a service to the client in that home. This would of course be an extreme situation, but the employer has a duty to take reasonable care of its employees and cannot therefore force the employee to enter a dangerous situation or take unreasonable risks. Under the Dangerous Dogs Act 1991 persons are prohibited from having in their possession or custody dogs belonging to types bred for fighting and other specially dangerous dogs. The Act also makes further provision for securing that dogs are kept under proper control. Under the Dogs Act 1871 as amended by the Dangerous Dogs Act 1989 magistrates can give orders for a dog to be destroyed.

Violence

The level of violence from patients, visitors and the general public on health professionals has been growing at an alarming rate. A survey by the Healthcare Commission in 2007 revealed that one in three NHS staff experienced violence or abuse in 2006.[55] In 2000 the DH adopted a policy of zero tolerance to violence within health care. Guidance is available from the DH website and from the Health and Safety Executive on how to prevent and deal with aggression and the action which can be taken subsequently. The National Audit Office[56] reported in March 2003 that reports of violence against NHS staff had risen by 13% over 2 years, costing the service at least £69 million annually. It estimated that about 40% of incidents were not being reported. In the light of this report, the Secretary of State for Health announced[57] that if the Department of

Public Prosecutions failed to take action against those attacking health workers, the victims could call on a new legal protection unit within the DH to support private legal action against the attackers. The NHS Security Management Service was established in April 2003 to take responsibility for all security management issues in the NHS, including violence to staff. It has published a strategy placing violence against staff as a top priority and has established mandatory reporting of incidents of violence. It is now incorporated into the NHS Counter Fraud and Security Management Service Division of the NHS Business Services Authority and has developed a programme of work from the Zero Tolerance Campaign.[58] The NHS Security Management Service reported that there were 58 695 physical assaults on NHS staff in England in 2005–6.

Remedies following violent attacks

If a member of staff is injured as a result of violence the following actions could be taken:

- a public prosecution of the offender;
- a private prosecution of the offender;
- a civil action for compensation against the offender;
- a civil action for compensation against the employer on the grounds that it has failed in its duty of care towards an employee as consequence of which the employee has been harmed;
- a claim under the criminal injury compensation scheme;
- social security benefits for injuries.

More than one of these courses of action could be taken.

The Court of Appeal held in 2006 that the NHS trust had failed in its duty of care to six nursing staff who were assaulted by a patient in Rampton Hospital. The Hospital had failed to carry out a risk assessment in accordance with the recommendations of the Tilt Report into security in high security hospitals and as a consequence the staff were injured.[59]

In theory a health professional injured by a patient could sue the patient, but difficulties arise if the patient was suffering from a mental disorder. In such circumstances a preferable course of action would be for the injured employee to sue his/her employer if it can be established that there were failures in the risk assessment or the action taken to manage the risk of harm to the employee. In Wales the Welsh Assembly Government has launched the All Wales NHS Violence and Aggression Training Passport and Information Scheme and in Scotland the Scottish Executive is coordinating a Zero Tolerance Campaign. In September 2007 funding of £97 million was announced for further protection of NHS staff from violence. Of this sum, £29 million is to be used for safety alarms for lone workers and the remainder for training, additional local security management specialists, more prosecutions and a centralised reporting system to the NHS Security Management Service.[60]

Situation: fear of violence

A physiotherapist visited a patient in his home following a stroke. She felt threatened by his attitude but found difficulty in defining exactly the reason for her fears. Should she record her concerns?

This is a situation with which many physiotherapists could identify. The feeling of fear is almost intuitive, but the physiotherapist would have a duty to ensure that her colleagues were warned of potential dangers. She might therefore record in her notes that it may be advisable for a second person to accompany the physiotherapist for the next house call. The duty of confidentiality owed to the patient (see Chapter 8) would be subject to an exception in the public interest where a physiotherapist needed to warn colleagues about a fear of violence from a particular patient. This might give rise to something of a dilemma since the patient has access as of right to the healthcare notes. However, in extreme cases access to this section of the notes could be withheld on the ground of the risk of causing

serious harm to the patient or another (see Chapter 8).

Conclusion on violence

Unfortunately the possibility of violence at work is a reasonable foreseeability for the physiotherapist. The HSE in its guidance on workplace violence[61] notes that the main factors that can create a risk of violence are impatience, frustration, anxiety, resentment and drink, drugs or inherent aggression/mental instability. Every employer has a responsibility to ensure that a risk assessment is undertaken and take the appropriate action to protect health staff and others. Much guidance is now available from the DH (and in particular the NHS Counterfraud and Security Management Service in England and the All Wales NHD Violence and Aggression Training Passport and Information Scheme) and from the HSE websites. Guidance is also available from the CSP and in particular its publication in 2004.[62]

Domestic violence

Physiotherapists may become aware especially in their community work, of domestic violence taking place. They should remember that such aggression is a criminal offence and under the Domestic Violence Crime and Victims Act 2004 more powers are available against the aggressor. Advice should be taken from senior management on the reporting of such incidents which would be a justifiable exception to the duty of confidentiality on the grounds of public safety.

Stress

Like violence, stress is also a reasonably foreseeable possibility for the health service professional. The first successful case brought by a public sector employee against his employer on grounds of harm resulting from stress follows.

Case: stress at work *Walker* v. *Northumberland County Council* 1994[63]

A social worker obtained compensation when his employer failed to provide the necessary support in a stressful work situation when he returned to work following an earlier absence due to stress. The employer was not liable for the initial absence, but that put the employer on notice that the employee was vulnerable, and its failure to provide the assistance he needed was a breach of its duty to provide reasonable care for his health and safety as required under the contract of employment.

In order to establish grounds for compensation for stress induced by work, an employee would have to show:

- that he/she was under an unacceptable level of stress at work
- that the employer was aware of this situation
- that there was reasonable action that the employer could have taken to relieve this pressure
- that the employer failed to take that action
- that as a result the employee has suffered a serious mental condition.

The Court of Appeal[64] has clarified the law relating to compensation for stress at work in four appeals which were heard together. In each one the employer appealed against a finding of liability for an employee's psychiatric illness caused by stress at work. Two of the claimants were teachers in public sector comprehensive schools, the third an administrative assistant at a local authority training centre and the fourth a raw material operative in a factory.

The Court of Appeal held that the ordinary principles of employer's liability applied to an allegation of psychiatric illness caused by stress at work. The threshold question was whether the particular kind of harm – an injury to health (as distinct to occupational health) that was attributable to stress at work (as distinct from other factors) – to the employee was reasonably foreseeable. Foreseeability depended on what the employer knew or ought reasonably to have known about the individual employee. Because of the nature of mental disorder, it was harder to foresee than physical injury, but might be easier to foresee in a known individual than in the population at large. An employer was usually entitled to assume that the employee could withstand the normal pressures of his/her job unless he/she knew of some particular problem or vulnerability. The test was the same whatever the employment: there were no occupations that should be regarded as intrinsically dangerous to mental health.

The relevant factors identified by the Court of Appeal in determining the reasonable foreseeability of stress were:

- nature and extent of the work done by the employee;
- signs from the employee of impending harm to his/her health.

The employer was entitled to take at face value what he/she was told by an employee; the employer did not have to make searching enquiries of the employee or seek to make further enquiries of the employee's medical advisers.

If there were indications of impending harm to health arising from stress at work and these indications were plain enough for any reasonable employer to realise that he/she should do something about it, the duty of the employer to take steps would be triggered. The employer could only be in breach of duty if he/she failed to take the steps which were reasonable in the circumstances, bearing in mind the magnitude of the risk of harm occurring, the gravity of the harm which might occur, the costs and practicability of preventing it and the justifications for running the risk. The factors to be taken into account in determining what was reasonable action by the employer included:

- size and scope of the employer's operation, its resources, and the demands it faced;
- interests of other employees;
- need to treat other employees fairly (for example, in any redistribution of duties).

An employer could reasonably be expected to take steps that were likely to do some good, and the court was likely to need expert evidence on that.

An employer who offered a confidential advice service, with referral to appropriate counselling or treatment services, was unlikely to be found in breach of duty. If the only reasonable and effective step would have been to dismiss or demote the employee, the employer would not be in breach of duty in allowing a willing employee to continue in the job.

In all cases, therefore, it was necessary to identify the steps that the employer both could and should have taken before finding him/her in breach of his/her duty of care. The claimant had to show that the breach of duty had caused or materially contributed to the harm suffered. It was not enough to show that the occupational stress had caused the harm. Where the harm suffered had more than one cause, the employer should only pay for that proportion of the harm suffered that was attributable to his/her wrongdoing, unless the harm was truly indivisible. It was for the defendant to raise the question of apportionment. The assessment of damages would take account of any pre-existing disorder or vulnerability and of the chance that the claimant would have succumbed to a stress-related disorder in any event.

Subsequently, the House of Lords (in a majority decision) allowed an appeal from one of the employees,[65] holding on the facts of the case the school's senior management team should have taken the initiative in making sympathetic enquiries about Mr Barber, head of the maths department, when he returned to work in June 1996 and in making some reduction in his workload to ease his return. In addition, his condition should have been monitored and, had it not improved, some more drastic action would have had to be taken.

In a subsequent case it was held that the mere fact that the employers had provided counselling services did not relieve them of the duty to take reasonable care of an employee who was being subjected to considerable stress because of overwork and lack of clear management controls. The Court of Appeal dismissed the employer's appeal against the finding of a breach of the duty of care and the award of £134 000.[66]

Prevention of stress in health care is firmly on the agenda of the HSE, which issued its first enforcement notice for failure to protect staff from stress in August 2003.[67] The West Dorset Hospitals NHS Trust was given 6 months to assess stress levels among its 1100 staff and introduce a new programme to reduce it. Stress reduction is one of eight key targets set by the HSE, which has set up a stress website[68] covering the reasons why stress must be tackled, management standards, advice for individuals and good practice. It has also provided a guide on improving efficiency, which shows how tackling stress at work can improve an organisation's efficiency.

The CSP has provided guidance on stress at work.[69]

Sexual and other harassment

Balancing privacy and protection

It is essential that physiotherapists are sensitive to the dangers of sexual harassment and make every effort to avoid potentially difficult situations. On the one hand they must preserve the patient's privacy and dignity (see below) but on the other hand they must ensure that they are chaperoned in any situation which could lead to accusations of harassment or impropriety by the physiotherapist or where the physiotherapist is herself (or himself) at risk.

The criteria for standard 1 of the CSP's core standards require the patient's privacy and dignity to be respected at all times.

Situation: sexual harassment

To his embarrassment a male physiotherapist discovered that a female patient appeared to have a 'crush' on him and sent him affectionate letters. He did not wish to appear rude to her, but found it difficult to maintain his professional distance.

In the above situation, the male physiotherapist should ask his senior to remove him from being involved in the treatment of that patient. The patient may well be upset by the move but it should be explained to her that the physiotherapist could not continue to care for her and fulfil his professional obligations.

The Protection from Harassment Act 1997

The Protection from Harassment Act 1997 can also provide some protection in the workplace if an individual considers that they are subject to unreasonable unwanted attention.

The Act creates the following:

- A criminal offence of harassment (Section 1) which is defined as a person pursuing a course of conduct which amounts to harassment of another and which he knows or ought to know amounts to harassment of the other [the reasonable person test (see Glossary) is applied].
- A civil wrong whereby a person who fears an actual or future breach of Section 1 may claim compensation including damages for anxiety and financial loss.
- The right to claim an injunction (see Glossary) to restrain the defendant from pursuing any conduct which amounts to harassment.
- The right to apply for a warrant for the arrest of the defendant if the injunction has not been obeyed.
- An offence of putting people in fear of violence, where a person on at least two occasions causes by his conduct another person to fear that violence will be used against them.
- Restraining orders made by the court for the purpose of protecting the victim of the offence or any other person from further conduct amounting to harassment or to fear violence.

Certain defences are permitted in the Act including that an individual is preventing or detecting crime.

Bullying at work

The Healthcare Commission, following a survey, estimated in February 2008 that 1 in 12 NHS staff are bullied by their managers. Only two out of five staff felt that their NHS Trust was taking effective action to deal with bullying. NHS Employers has issued guidance on how trusts can combat workplace bullying. Guidance is also provided by the Industrial Relations Department of the CSP[70] on bullying at work. It defines bullying as:

> Offensive, abusive, intimidating, malicious or insulting behaviour or abuse of power, which makes the recipient feel upset, threatened, humiliated or vulnerable, undermines their self-confidence and may cause them stress.

It discusses the different types of bullying and its causes and quotes the case of Janet Ballantyne. In June 1996 Unison negotiated for her an out-of-court settlement of £66 000 as compensation for the stress that she had suffered as a residential social worker. Bullying issues were central to her stress and compensation was paid for the anxiety, depression and panic attacks that were caused by the style of her abusive manager. The CSP briefing note suggests ways of negotiation to prevent bullying at work. It is hoped that any member of the CSP who is reported to be a bully would be subject to professional conduct proceedings. Subsequent guidance from the CSP[71] recommends that bullying and harassment are best dealt with under specific local policies and procedures for the prevention of bullying.

A teacher who alleged that he had been bullied by the head teacher and other staff when he was teaching in a school in Pembrokeshire accepted £100 000 in an out-of-court settlement.[72] Dyfed County Council denied negligence. He suffered a minor breakdown in October 1996 and was returned to the same school, although he had asked for a transfer. He claimed that he was isolated, ignored and subjected to a series of practical jokes. He then suffered a second nervous breakdown. It was claimed that a support plan worked out for him by the council had not been properly implemented. The lessons for managers from this case are obvious.

A review of the literature on bullying at work from the Health and Safety Laboratory is available from the HSE website.[73] The aim of the project is to enable the HSE to develop guidance for organisations on primary interventions in relation to bullying.

Repetitive strain injury

This condition is also now known as occupational overuse syndrome (OOS). Physiotherapists should be aware both for themselves and their clients of the legal implications of repetitive strain injury (RSI). The CSP published guidance on RSI in 1999.[74]

Repetitive strain injury and the courts

Even though in an early case a judge was quoted out of context as declaring that RSI had no place in medical books,[75] RSI has been recognised for the purpose of compensation in health and safety cases. Thus in the case of *Bettany* v. *Royal Doulton UK Ltd*[76] the High Court found that repetitive work causing only pain with no other associated symptoms could be classed as an overuse injury caused by the claimant's work (although on the actual facts of the case the employers were not found to be in breach of the duty of care owed to the plaintiff – they had warned her of the dangers, had introduced a system of reporting problems and had moved her to lighter work). Likewise £40 000 was awarded by the court to a legal secretary on the grounds that she had sustained physical injury, even though there was an absence of objective clinical signs.[77] In a case in May 1998 it was reported[78] that five women workers at the Midland Bank were awarded a total of £50 000 after a judge ruled that their part-time jobs processing cheques at high speed were responsible for giving them RSI. This was another case of 'diffuse' RSI, where the victims suffer disabling pains but no specific injuries can be diagnosed. The women said that even though they were part time they had to work under intense pressure processing cheques and other information into computers against strict time limits. Workers who achieved four keystrokes per second earned gold stars and more payment.

Reversing the trend

A decision of the House of Lords in 1998, however, has made it more difficult to obtain compensation for RSI. On 25 June 1998 the House of Lords[79] rejected claims that a secretary who was sacked after she developed a form of RSI should be able to sue her employers. It overruled the Court of Appeal decision that Ann Pickford should be allowed to make a claim against ICI. The Court of Appeal (reversing the High Court decision) had found that ICI was negligent in failing to warn her of the need to take breaks during her work using a word processor and gave her the right to take her case back to the High Court for an assessment of damages, which she estimated at £175 000. In a majority judgment (four to one) the House of Lords decided that ICI did not need to warn her about the dangers of repetitive strain injury because typing took up at a maximum only 75% of her workload. To impose a warning which might cause more harm than good would be undesirable since it might be counterproductive. The House of Lords also questioned whether she had proved that the pain was organic in origin. She had been sacked in 1990 after taking long periods off work because of pain in both hands. She claimed that the injury had been caused by the very large amount of typing at speed for long periods without breaks or rest periods. The House of Lords said that it could reasonably have been expected that a person of her intelligence and experience would take rest pauses without being told.

The House of Lords held that the Court of Appeal should not have overruled the findings of the High Court Judge, since he had ample evidence before him to justify his decision that in the plaintiff's case the giving of warnings was unnecessary even though typists in another department had been given warnings.

It also held that RSI as a medical term was unhelpful. It covered so many conditions that it was of no diagnostic value as a description of disease. On the other hand PDA4 (prescribed disease A4) had a recognised place in the DH and Social Security's list for the purposes of industrial injury, meaning a cramp of the hand or forearm due to repetitive movements such as those used in any occupation involving prolonged periods of handwriting or typing.

One of the lessons from this case, therefore, is that the physiotherapist should be wary of using such terms as RSI about a patient's condition unless there is clear medical evidence for it.

Physiotherapists, repetitive strain injury and giving evidence

Physiotherapists may become involved in the legal situation in several ways. They may be caring for clients suffering from this disability and so be asked to be witness of fact in terms of any litigation in which the client may be involved.

Alternatively, a physiotherapist may be asked to provide an independent expert opinion on an RSI case not involving one of his/her patients. The physiotherapist should be careful to act within the scope of his/her competence in giving an opinion about whether a patient is suffering from RSI. There may for example be a value in witnessing the function that was carried out by the patient within the work situation, seeing the actions which were involved, the speed, position and movements of the patient. The physiotherapist should be aware that if he/she gives negligent advice to a patient and to a solicitor or provides a report which is inaccurate the physiotherapist could be liable for that negligence. (See Chapter 10 on negligent advice and Chapter 13 on giving evidence in court for discussion on this topic.)

Other areas of concern

There is insufficient space to cover all hazardous areas in the work place, but the CSP employment relations department provides guidance across a wide area. The CSP has provided a guide to the workplace regulations.[80] In addition the CSP has provided a briefing note on the benefits available in the case of industrial injuries.[81] This paper sets out the definitions, benefits following industrial injury and assessment of disablement. It points out that NHS Industrial Injuries (II) scheme can be claimed at the same time as Department for Work and Pensions benefits but any NHS benefit will be offset against any social security benefit. There are two benefits available under the NHS II scheme: temporary injury allowance and permanent injury benefit. The briefing notes provided by the CSP form an excellent resource for many areas of health and safety laws. Since 1999 the NHS Litigation Authority has managed two schemes for non-clinical risks: liabilities to third parties (LTPS) and property expenses scheme (PES). They are known collectively as Risk Pooling Schemes for Trusts (RPST) and are considered in Chapter 15.

Conclusions

A risk management strategy is at the heart of any policy relating to health and safety, not just for employees but also for the clients and general public. Regular monitoring of the implementation of a risk management policy should ensure that harm is avoided and that a quality service is maintained for the public. This should be accompanied by clear, comprehensive documentation. There is now a wide range of information available on health and safety from the DH, the HSE, the National Patient Safety Agency and many professional organisations including the CSP which can assist the employer, the physiotherapy manager and the individual practitioner in securing the health and safety of him/herself and others in the workplace. The National Audit Office in April 2003 criticised the gap between the best and worst performing trusts in managing health and safety risks[82] and made recommendations for improving risk management, preventing under reporting of accidents and introducing procedures to assess the cost and impact of accidents. Its recommendations are still relevant and valid 5 years on.

The Health and Safety Commission and the HSE were originally established as part of the Health and Safety at Work etc. Act 1974 as two separate non-departmental public bodies. From 1 April 2008[83] the HSC and the HSE were abolished and replaced by a single national regulatory body responsible for promoting the cause of better health and safety at work. Further information on the strategy and structure of the new body can be found on its website.[84] In 2000 the HSE launched jointly with the government and Health and Safety Commission a 10-year strategy to improve health and safety at work. It contains three elements: a set of improvement targets, a 10-point strategy and 44 action points to improve health and safety. It remains to be seen whether the creation of a single statutory organisation will ensure improvements in the

standards of health and safety and the meeting of the targets.

Legal issues relating to smoking are considered in Chapter 20.

Questions and exercises

1 Undertake a risk assessment of your department.

2 Show the differences between the implementation of the Health and Safety at Work etc. Act by the Health and Safety Inspectorate and a case brought by an employee for compensation because of breach of the duty to care for the health and safety of an employee by the employer.

3 A physiotherapist reports that a house she visits is in a dangerous condition. What should her employer do?

4 A client complains that a hoist recently provided has broken. What actions lie against the manufacturers? (Refer also to Chapter 15 on equipment.)

5 What are the responsibilities of the independent practitioner in relation to health and safety?

6 A physiotherapy manager is notified that a senior physiotherapist has a reputation for bullying in the department. What action should she take?

References

1 Chartered Society of Physiotherapy (2005) *Information Paper on Patient/client Health and Safety for Physiotherapists*. Information Paper PA 62. CSP, London.

2 Chartered Society of Physiotherapy (Revised 2004) *AACP Safety Standards*. CSP, London.

3 *Harris* v. *Evans and another* (CA) The Times Law Report, 5 May 1998.

4 *R* v. *Nelson Group Services (Maintenance) Ltd* (CA) The Times Law Report, 17 September 1998.

5 *R.* v. *Porter* The Times Law Report, 9 July 2008.

6 Chartered Society of Physiotherapy (2002) *CSP Information Manual for Safety Representatives*. CSP, London.

7 Chartered Society of Physiotherapy (2007) *Mapping for Health and Safety*. ERUS, H&S, CSP, London.

8 Health and Safety Commission (2000) *Management of Health and Safety at Work. Approved Code of Practice and Guidance*. HMSO, London.

9 *Allison* v. *London* Underground Ltd. The Times Law Report, 29 February 2008.

10 Management of Health and Safety at Work Regulations 1999 SI No 3242.

11 Provisions and Use of Work Equipment Regulations 1998 SI No 2306.

12 *Smith (Joan)* v. *Northamptonshire County Council*. The Times Law Report, 24 March 2008.

13 *Spencer-Franks* v. *Kellog Brown and Root Ltd and Another*. The Times Law Report, 3 July 2008 HL.

14 Provision and Use of Work Equipment Regulations SI 1998 No 2306.

15 Chartered Society of Physiotherapy (2008) *Health and Safety Information Paper Number 3: Risk Assessment*. CSP, London.

16 Chartered Society of Physiotherapy (2007) *Health and Safety Checklist. Employment Relations and Union Services*. H&S No 15. CSP, London.

17 Health and Safety Executive (2007) *Getting to Grips with Manual Handling*. HSE London.

18 Chartered Society of Physiotherapy (2008) *Guidance on Manual Handling*. CSP London.

19   Chartered Society of Physiotherapy (2007) *Mapping for Health and Safety. A resource for CSP Safety Reps*. CSP, London. Gives guidance on drawing up workplace hazard maps + body mapping to identify the potential for work-related musculoskeletal disorders

20   EC Directive 90/269/EEC (on the minimum health and safety requirements for the manual handling of loads – fourth individual directive within the meaning of Article 16(1) of Directive 89/391/EEC).

21   Health and Safety (Miscellaneous Amendments) Regulations SI 2002 No 2174

22   Health and Safety Executive (2004) *Manual Handling: Guidance on Regulations*, 3rd edn. HSE, London.

23   Health and Safety Executive (1992) *Manual Handling: Guidance on Regulations*. HMSO, London.

24   Smith, J. (ed.) (2005) *The Guide to the Handling of People*, 5th edn. BackCare,Teddington.

25   *R (on the application of A and B, X and Y) v. East Sussex County Council (The Disability Rights Commission: an interested party)* Case No. CO/4843/2001 10 February 2003.

26   *Colclough v. Staffordshire County Council* June 30 1994, reported in *Current Law* No. 208 October 1994.

27   Betts, M. (2006) Catching, Supporting or Letting Go. *The Column* **18**, 3 12–15.

28   National Institute for Health and Clinical Excellence (2002) *Guidance on Surgery for Morbid Obesity*. NICE, London.

29   Health and Safety Executive (1998) *Getting to Grips with Manual Handling: a Short Guide for Employers*. London, HSE.; www.hse.gov.uk

30   Clews, G. (2008) Under Pressure. *Frontline* **14**, 2, 12–14.

31   Charlton, J., Pearce, M.J. (2007) Supporting Bariatric Employees. *The Column* **191**, 12–16.

32   *Bowfield v. South Sefton (Merseyside) Health Authority* (CA) 20 March 1991, Lexis Transcript.

33   BackCare (1999) *Safer Handling of People in the Community*. BackCare. Teddington

34   News item, *The Times*, 19 November 2003

35   *King v. Sussex Ambulance NHS Trust* [2002] EWCA 953, [2002] ICR 1413

36   www.hse.gov.uk/riddor

37   *Beer v. London Borough of Waltham* (QBD) 16 December 1987, Lexis Transcript.

38   Department of Health. *An Organisation with a Memory*: report of an expert group chaired by Professor Liam Donaldson, Chief Medical Officer, DH; http://www.dh.gov.uk

39   National Patient Safety Agency, Patient Safety Alert PSA 01, London, NPSA, 2002.

40   www.npsa.nhs.uk

41   National Patient Safety Agency Patient Safety alert No 21: Safer Practice with epidural injections and infusions March 2007.

42   Rose, D. (2007) Hit Squads to Stamp out Hospital Superbugs. *The Times*, 4 June p. 18.

43   www.dh.gov.uk/en/Policyandguidance/Healthandsocialcare

44   News Item. *The Times* 9 May 2008

45   Bennett, R. (2008) Risk Assessment Watchdog Set up to Halt March of the Nanny State. *The Times*, 16 January

46   Dillon, A. (2008) NICE Guidance for Healthy Workplaces. *British Journal of Healthcare Management* **14**, 6, 249.

47   www.nice.org.uk/phi005

48   CSP (1995) No. PA 4 (1995), *Equipment Safety and Product Liability*. CSP, London.

49   Control of Substances Hazardous to Health (COSHH) Regulations 2002 SI 2002 No. 2677.

50   www.coshh-essentials.org.uk

51   HSE COSHH: A brief guide to the Regulations INDG136 revised April 2005.

52   CSP (October 2003) Latex and Latex allergy ERUS Information paper

53   News item. *The Times*, 14 March 2008

54   *Corr v. IBC Vehicles Ltd*. The Times Law Report, 28 February 2008 HL

55   Healthcare Commission (2007) Annual NHS Staff survey. www.healthcarecommission.org.uk

56   National Audit Office, A Safer Place to Work: protecting NHS hospital and ambulance staff from violence and aggression, NAO, 2003; www.nao.gov.uk/publications

57   Lister, S. (2003) Ministers to fund action on abusive patients, *The Times*, 15 April.

58   www.cfsms.nhs.uk. Free phoneline 0800 028 40 60.

59   *Buck and others v. Nottinghamshire Healthcare NHS Trust* [2006] EWCA Civ 1576.

60   Department of Health press release 25 September 2007.

61   www.hse.gov.uk/healthservices/violence/index.htm

62   Chartered Society of Physiotherapy (2004) *Violence at Work*. ERUS H&S 02. CSP, London.

63   *Walker v. Northumberland County Council*, The Times Law Report, 24 November 1994 QBD.

64 *Hatton* v. *Sutherland; Barber* v. *Somerset County Council; Jones* v. *Sandwell Metropolitan Borough Council; Baker* v. *Baker Refractories Ltd*, The Times Law Report, 12 February 2002; [2002] EWCA 76 [2002] 2 All ER 1.

65 *Barber* v. *Somerset County Council.* The Times Law Report, 5 April 2004 HL.

66 *Daw* v. *Intel Corp (UK) Ltd* [2007] EWCA Civ 70; [2007] 2 All ER 126, (2007) 104(8) L.S.G 36.

67 de Bruxelles, S., Wright, O., Rumbelow, H. (2003) Bosses Will be Fined for Workers' Stress. *The Times*, 5 August.

68 www.hse.gov.uk/stress/

69 Chartered Society of Physiotherapy (2004) *Stress at Work.* ERUS H&S 01. CSP, London.

70 CSP Industrial Relations Department (1997) *Health and Safety Briefing Pack No. 5 (July 1997) Bullying At Work.* CSP, London.

71 Chartered Society of Physiotherapy (2000) *Bullying and Harassment Cases.* ERUS IP19. CSP, London.

72 Fletcher, V. (1998) Teacher 'bullied by staff' wins £100 000. *The Times*, 17 July.

73 Johanna Beswick *et al.* (2006) Bullying at work: a review of the literature WPS/06/04 Health and Safety Laboratory.

74 Chartered Society of Physiotherapy (1999) *Repetitive Strain Injury.* ERUS 08. CSP, London.

75 *Mughal* v. *Reuters Ltd* [1993] IRLR 571.

76 *Bettany* v. *Royal Doulton UK Ltd* reported in Health and Safety Information Bulletin (1994) Unidentifiable ULD/RSI can be occupationally caused HSIB (219) 20.

77 Jones, T. (1994) Strain Gains. *Law Society Gazette* **91**, 30, 20–1.

78 Frean, A. (1998) Bank Workers Win Claim for RSI. *The Times*, 23 May.

79 *Pickford* v. *Imperial Chemical Industries Plc* (HL) The Times Law Report, 30 June 1998.

80 The CSP Workplace (health and safety and welfare) Regulations Guidance 1992.

81 Chartered Society of Physiotherapy (August 2005) ERUS IP 12. *Industrial Injuries.* CSP, London.

82 National Audit Office (2003) *A Safer Place to Work: Improving the Management of Health and Safety Risks to Staff in NHS Trusts.* HC 623 2002–3. Stationery Office, London.

83 Legislative Reform (Health and Safety Executive) Order 2008 SI 960.

84 http://www.hse.gov.uk/aboutus/structure.htm

12 Record Keeping

Record keeping is considered in this section because the standard of record keeping is most likely to come to the fore when litigation commences, a prosecution is initiated or a complaint is made. However, it should not be ignored that the principal purpose of record keeping is to ensure the quality of care provided for the patient, to facilitate communication between professionals and maintain a record of the diagnosis, treatment and future plans for the patient. A good standard for documentation would be that if any health professional were to be called away in an emergency, his or her colleagues would be able to provide continuity of care on the basis of full comprehensive clear records. This chapter looks at the following issues:

- Principles of record keeping and standards of practice
- Transmitting records
- Storage of records and safe keeping
- Destruction of records
- Ownership and control of records
- Computerised records
- Litigation

Reference should also be made to Chapter 13 on giving evidence in court and statement writing, to Chapter 8 on confidentiality and to Chapter 9 on access by the patient and others to personal and health records.

Principles of record keeping and standards of practice

Standards

Standard 10 of the Health Professions Council (HPC) *Standards of Conduct, Performance and Ethics*[1] requires the registrant to keep accurate patient, client and user records and explains that:

> making and keeping records is an essential part of care and you must keep records for everyone you treat or who asks for professional advice or services. All records must be complete and legible, and you should write, sign and date all entries.

The Chartered Society of Physiotherapy (CSP) *Rules of Professional Conduct* set out the duty to ensure high standards of record keeping are maintained.

Rule 2 Paragraph 2.3 on the relationship with patients states that:[2]

> One of the rights every patient expects is that their medical records are full, clear and held securely. The duty of the physiotherapist, as part of their scope of practice and to comply with the patient's right, is to ensure that a full physiotherapeutic record is maintained. Core Standards 14 and 15[3] and Service Standard 19[4] provide further details. Further Information is available in the form of a PA information paper PA47 General Principles of Record Keeping and Access to Health Records.

Core Standard 14 requires patient records to conform to the following requirements:

- concise
- legible
- logical sequence
- dated
- accurate
- provide adequate detail of the intervention given
- signed after each entry/attendance
- name is printed after each entry/attendance
- no correction fluid is used
- written in permanent ink that will remain legible with photocopying
- any errors are crossed with a single line and initialled
- each side of each page of the record is numbered
- patient's name and either date of birth, hospital number or NHS number are recorded on each page of the record
- acronyms are used only within the context of a locally agreed abbreviations glossary
- records are appropriately countersigned
- if dictaphones are used to store information, the transcriptions of such records must include a date/time reference and a clinician/typist reference. Dictated notes must cover the same details as would a written record or manuscript.

Standard 15 relates to the retention and storage of records. There is also a guidance on computer-generated records.

The Department of Health (DH) in its *Code of Practice on Confidentiality* published in November 2003 sets out principles for good standards of record keeping which can be found in Figure 12.1. Reference should also be made to the *NHS Code of Practice on Records Management.*[5]

It should be clear from the Chapter 10 on negligence and Chapter 13 on evidence that the documentation can play a significant part in any court hearing and it is essential therefore that clear principles on the content, style, clarity, comprehensiveness and accuracy of records should be followed. Many civil cases may be contested several years after the events to which they relate and the records made at the time are therefore extremely important. Often a civil case will involve a dispute over the facts and a patient may challenge what has been documented in the records.

For example in one case (*Hardisty* v. *Aubrey* 2006) various entries in the medical records were put to the claimant. In particular, the physiotherapist who had treated her in 2002 had recorded in the notes on 8 August 2002 (at the end of the second series of sessions) that the claimant was much better, had full movements of the cervical spine and no headaches. The special pillow had helped tremendously. As to that the claimant said that she could not understand why the physiotherapist should have said that, as she, the claimant, was not completely better at that time. She could not answer for what had been written in the notes. She said that what had actually happened was that the physiotherapist had discharged her, but advised that she should return if her symptoms worsened as she was not completely pain free. And indeed they did worsen in the September and she had returned for another series of sessions from October to November 2002.[6] In this case the claimant appealed against an award of £4686 for whiplash injury following a road accident, holding that the effects of the injury were being felt long after November 2002, the date taken by the Recorder as the end of the effects of the accident. He had concluded that because the claimant had not sought any physiotherapy treatment between November 2002 and August 2003, she had made

Patient records should:

Be factual, consistent and accurate

- be written as soon as possible after an event has occurred, providing current information on the care and condition of the patient;
- be written clearly, legibly and in such a manner that they cannot be erased;
- be written in such a manner that any alterations or additions are dated, timed and signed in such a way that the original entry can still be read clearly;
- be accurately dated, timed and signed or otherwise identified, with the name of the author being printed alongside the first entry;
- be readable on any photocopies;
- be written, wherever applicable, with the involvement of the patient or carer;
- be clear, unambiguous, (preferably concise) and written in terms that the patient can understand. Abbreviations, if used, should follow common conventions;
- be consecutive;
- (for electronic records) use standard coding techniques and protocols;
- be written so as to be compliant with the Race Relations Act and the Disability Discrimination Act.

Be relevant and useful

- identify problems that have arisen and the action taken to rectify them;
- provide evidence of the care planned, the decisions made, the care delivered and the information shared;
- provide evidence of actions agreed with the patient (including consent to treatment and/or consent to disclose information).

And include

- medical observations: examinations, tests, diagnoses, prognoses, prescriptions and other treatments;
- relevant disclosures by the patient – pertinent to understanding cause or effecting cure/treatment;
- facts presented to the patient;
- correspondence from the patient or other parties.

Patient records should not include

- unnecessary abbreviations or jargon;
- meaningless phrases, irrelevant speculation or offensive subjective statements;
- irrelevant personal opinions regarding the patient.

Figure 12.1   Record keeping best practice[28]

a substantial recovery from the effects of the accident. The Court of Appeal allowed the claimant's appeal and remitted the case to a new judge to determine the issues of acceleration of pre-existing degenerative changes of the cervicial spine and the calculation of compensation. The Court of Appeal accepted the claimant's evidence that her symptoms continued during the time that she was not receiving physiotherapy.

Guidelines on actual recording

Figure 12.2 sets out some of the basic points to remember in writing the actual records. It is preferable if records document the facts of a situation, or where an opinion, such as a diagnosis is required, that the opinion is supported by the facts on which it is based. Clearly, no derogatory personal opinions of the patient should be

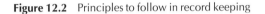

(1)   Records should be made as soon as possible after the events that are recorded
(2)   They should be accurate, comprehensive and clear
(3)   They should be written legibly and be jargon free
(4)   They should avoid opinion and record the facts of what is observed
(5)   They should be signed and dated by the maker
(6)   They should not include abbreviations
(7)   They should not be altered, unless the changes are made so that the original entry is
       clearly crossed out, but still readable
(8)   Any change should be signed and dated

Figure 12.2   Principles to follow in record keeping

recorded. It is also worth noting the dangers of failing to hang up after leaving a phone message on an answer phone. This occurred when a hospital left a message for a patient re-arranging an appointment, but the machine also recorded the slanderous statements subsequently made by the operator about the patient.[7]

Recording non-events and 'no change'

- What if there is no change in the care of the patient?

Physiotherapists often ask about what should be recorded when there is no change in the patient's condition and they simply continue the usual treatment. Many may write 'as above' to indicate that treatment has continued to plan. Is this sufficient? It is important that it is clear from the records what interaction there has been between patient and physiotherapist, what questions asked and what replies given and whether or not there are any changes in the patient's condition or the treatment plan. If the physiotherapist is able to follow the SOAP system of record keeping each time a patient is seen, then if the records are ever subject to scrutiny in a court case, the physiotherapist should be able to give a full explanation of the nature of his/her contact with the patient. It is important that a record should be made each time the physiotherapist sees the patient.

SOAP stands for 'subjective', 'objective', 'assessment' and 'plan', and covers:

- how patients are feeling;
- what they say about themselves;
- the objective examination by the physiotherapist;
- the physiotherapist's assessment following that assessment and whether to continue or to change the treatment plan.

Often there may be no change in any of these dimensions, but it is essential that the physiotherapist records the date when he/she saw the patient and that there was no change. Increasingly there is a tendency to interpret an absence of a record as meaning that there was no activity or interaction: if it's not written down, it didn't happen. This is not in fact an inexorable rule of the courts, but clearly a witness is in a much stronger position in giving evidence if there is a comprehensive record. A useful guide to writing SOAP notes is provided by Ginge Kettenbach.[8]

Situation: no record

A baby in neonatal care suffered scarring and a foot drop possibly as the result of an intravenous drip tissuing. The parents sued the Trust and there was no record that the drip site was regularly inspected by nurses. A physiotherapist who was involved in the chest treatment and movement of the baby gave evidence that she saw no evidence that the vein had tissued, but she had not recorded that fact.

Because of the absence of recorded information it will be difficult for the staff in this case to show that appropriate care was taken of the child and that the intravenous drip was regularly inspected. In such a case, the times on which the patient was seen and by whom could be very important.

The recording of the date of a treatment session may be extremely important if the patient is alleging that 'the physiotherapist only saw me twice', when the records of the physiotherapist may show far more frequent contact.

Illegibility

Several court cases have arisen as a result of illegible handwriting.

Case: *Prendergast v. Sam & Dee Ltd*[9]

The doctor prescribed amoxil (an antibiotic) for the patient which, because of bad handwriting, was misread as daonil (a drug used by diabetics) by the pharmacist. As a consequence of the wrong medication the patient suffered from severe hypoglycaemia and brain damage from oxygen shortage in the blood. The doctor was held 25% to blame and the pharmacist 75%. The latter should have been alerted to the misreading because of the dosage and the fact that the patient paid for the prescription.

More recently, in a coroner's inquest relating to the death of a woman following a routine hysterectomy, evidence was given that the junior doctor misread the consultant's prescription of 3 mg of diamorphine to be given by epidural as 30 mg.[10]

Abbreviations

It is preferable if the use of abbreviations can be avoided. However, realistically abbreviations and symbols can save time, but precautions must be taken to prevent mistakes. There are advantages in each NHS Trust or organisation agreeing a list of approved abbreviations with one specific meaning that can be used in that unit. A printed list of these abbreviations would then be provided in each set of records and accompany the records if they were sent to outside agencies. It could be made a disciplinary offence if abbreviations not on the approved list were used or if they were used for a different meaning. In this way the following ambiguities could be avoided:

PID	pelvic inflammatory disease or prolapsed intervertebral disc?
Pt.	patient or physiotherapist or part time?
CP	cerebral palsy or chartered physiotherapist?
BID	brought in dead or twice?
NAD	nothing abnormal discovered or not a drop (of urine)?
MS	multiple sclerosis or mitral stenosis?
NFR	not for resuscitation or neurophysiological facilitation of respiration?

and so on.

All that has been said about abbreviations also applies to the use of symbols and signs and other hieroglyphics. Their use can certainly assist record keeping, especially in spinal care, but there must be a clearly approved list available for both patients and health professionals to access.

Reference should also be made to the NHS code of Practice on record keeping standards which replaces earlier publications from the NHS Training Authority.[11] The NMC guidelines, *Standards for Records and Record Keeping*[12] are also of value to all health professionals.

Professional opinions

Records should contain the facts of what took place between patient and professional, the assessment, the diagnosis, treatment and care and outcome, together with details of what the patient has stated, the fact that consent was given and the information given to the patient about the risks of the recommended treatment. Sometimes however it is necessary to record the opinion of the professional. A Data Protection Good Practice Note has been provided by the Information Commissioner (ICO) on how the Data Protection Act applies to professional opinion.[13] The ICO suggests the following:

> When an opinion is recorded it is good practice to do the following:
> - make it clear that it is an opinion, showing who gave the opinion and when;
> - if possible, provide contact details;
> - structure the record so that if someone objects to its accuracy, their view or challenge can be included in such a way that it is given proper weight;
> - have a records policy that lays down the criteria that should be considered for continuing to keep the information or, where appropriate, specific retention periods for certain categories of information.

Changing records

Records should not be altered. If the writer discovers that the wrong information was recorded, it would be possible to put a line through that information and initial this and then write the correct information. Any attempt to cover what was previously written by correction fluid or heavy blocking out will arouse suspicions. What was erroneously recorded should still be legible.

It was reported in *The Times* newspaper[14] that a casualty nurse who told the parents of a sick baby that he probably had a sniffle and they should take him to the family doctor altered the notes when the baby died 1 hour later. She changed the words 'extremely pale' to 'quite pale' and added a pulse reading, although she had not taken his pulse. Even though an independent inquiry found that her actions probably had no bearing on the child's outcome, she faced internal disciplinary proceedings at which she was dismissed, and such circumstances could also lead to professional conduct proceedings with the possibility of her being struck off the register of the UKCC (now the NMC).

The reports of the HPC show that several of their registrants, including physiotherapists, have been found guilty of misconduct as a result of poor record keeping (see Chapter 4).

Transmitting records

The Consumers Association in its *Health Which* April 1998 noted that in the chains of walk-in surgeries opening in stations and shopping centres GPs are failing to keep records and are not passing on relevant information to the patient's local GP.[15] Passing client information from one health professional to another who needs to know it is not a breach of confidentiality (see Chapter 8) and, indeed, failure to ensure that relevant information is passed on can amount to a negligent breach of the duty of care with foreseeable harm as a result (see Chapter 10).

If personal information is to be communicated by fax machines it is essential that care must be taken to preserve the confidentiality of the information, and that steps are taken to ensure that a designated person is appointed to receive it and that they do so straight away. In 1997 it was reported that a girl died after a fax error at hospital.[16] She suffered from giant cell hepatitis and had fallen ill on a visit to Middlesbrough. Her records were faxed from her hospital in Crawley. Unfortunately, they were sent to a fax machine in a locked room to which no one had access over the weekend. Doctors, unaware of her medical history, gave her an overdose of drugs.

Use of emails

Correspondence between professionals and with patients is increasingly through the use of emails. This can give rise to some legal queries such as how is confidentiality protected? What record should be kept of any such correspondence? What information, if any, should not be sent by email? At present, there are no national guidelines for the use of email with patients and it is advisable for each NHS organisation or professional group to develop their own protocols.

The DH's *Records Management NHS Code of Practice*[11] suggests the use of 'Contact' for email within the NHS. Contact is a secure national email and directory service provided free of charge for NHS staff and developed specifically to meet the British Medical Association requirements for clinical emails between NHS organisations. The DH guidance suggests that contact can be used to replace paper communications for the following:

- patient referrals from GP to hospital
- hospital to hospital – or internal hospital referrals
- discharge letters
- clinical enquiries
- research links and
- clinical team communications.

The NHS Code of Practice recommends that local procedures need to be in place at the sending and receiving ends of communication. Clinical information should be clearly marked and properly addressed. It should be stored securely and added to patients' records when appropriate. Contact tracks what is received, by whom and when it is read.

Storage of records and safe-keeping

Records should be kept so that they are easily accessible to those who require to access them but at the same time with efficient controls to prevent unauthorised access and disclosure. The Audit Commission in its report on hospital records[17] considered that patients were being put at risk because their medical records are kept in a mess and sometimes lost. Failure to find records led to consultations being cancelled and to operations being postponed. It recommended that hospitals set up one main records library

with good security. The Clinical Negligence Scheme for Trusts standards and assessments, which include standards relating to record keeping, were withdrawn in March 2006 and replaced by the NHS Litigation Authority A Risk Management Standards for Acute Trusts. These are available from the NHSLA website together with the NHSLA *Risk Management Handbook*.

In its guidance on the criteria that records should be kept securely in lockable cupboards or rooms, Standard 15 of the *Core Standards of Physiotherapy Practice*[3] states:

> This relates to the individual's responsibility in relation to confidentiality. It applies to all patient related information; written, computer records, audiotape, emails, faxes, videotape, photographs and other electronic media. In a community setting, patient records should be taken with the physiotherapist and not left in any part of an unoccupied vehicle including the boot. Where whole caseloads need to be taken into patient's homes during the day's rounds, they should be stored in a locked container or suitable lockable document wallet.

- What if records are lost by the physiotherapist?

It may be that the physiotherapist has records in his/her car, which is stolen, or they are lost between hospital departments. Clearly, the failure to take reasonable care of records would be a disciplinable offence and could also be subject to proceedings by the HPC to determine fitness to practise. Once the records are lost there is little that can be done to retrieve them, although it may be possible to create a new patient file if parallel records are held by other departments. However, such duplicate record keeping is not necessarily good practice (see below).

As a general rule, records should not be left in a car. Even if the physiotherapist is visiting several patients in the community it is better for the physiotherapist to take all the records into each home (in a briefcase so that there is no breach of confidentiality) rather than risk them being stolen in the car.

Information security management

A Code of Practice on information security management has been prepared by the DH[18] and is available on its website. This Code of Practice is a guide to the methods and required standards of practice in the management of information security for those who work, or are under contract to or in business partnership with NHS organisations in England. It is based on current legal requirements, relevant standards and professional best practice. The Code of Practice replaces the manual published in 1996.

Destruction of records

Where litigation is being contemplated, reference should be made to the time limits within which action can be brought, which are discussed in Chapter 10, bearing in mind the extended limitation periods that apply to children and those with a mental disability. In such circumstances, where there is a possibility of litigation, it would be extremely unwise to destroy any records.

In other circumstances records could be destroyed according to the advice given by the DH in its *NHS Code of Practice on Records Management*[11] unless the records are so old as to amount to historical documents when the Public Records Act 1958 comes into play and legal advice should be taken.

Even though any critical time limits have been passed, most departments would prefer to transpose records on to microfilm rather than destroy them completely. However, this is expensive and time consuming and might not always be justifiable. If a decision is taken that records can be destroyed, it is important to prevent any breach of confidentiality during the destruction process.

Situation: destruction on request

A physiotherapist is treating a patient who is suffering from mental illness. In one session she became very aggressive and this was noted by the physiotherapist in the records. The next session she was very apologetic and asked if the physiotherapist would delete the record of her outburst since it was so uncharacteristic and she was extremely contrite. What is the legal situation?

The physiotherapist should be very clear that the records cannot be changed. There is a statutory process by which a patient can request under the Data Protection Act 1998 that records be amended if they are incorrect (see Chapter 9), but this does not apply here. Even though requested by the patient, deletion of the record would be a breach of professional practice. In July 1998 a GP who allowed a patient to destroy part of her records was found guilty of serious professional misconduct by the General Medical Council (GMC).[19] He had allowed the patient, who was involved in acrimonious property dispute with her children, to remove a letter in which she was described as 'bad tempered' and another document referring to her drinking.

Ownership and control of records

Ownership

NHS records are owned by the Secretary of State and responsibility is delegated to the statutory health organisations. This also applies to the NHS records kept by GPs as part of their terms of service. Primary Care Trusts (in Wales Local Health Boards) are responsible for arranging the transfer of the records to a new GP where patients have indicated their wish to transfer and for collecting the records from the GP when a patient has died.

For NHS Trusts the ultimate decision on disclosure to others rests with the chief executive officer of the Primary Care Trust or NHS Trust. Thus statutes such as the Data Protection Act 1998 give to the holder of the records the ultimate decision making on whether access should be permitted. The holder should however consult the health professional who cared for the patient (see Chapter 9) and any decision can be challenged in the Information Tribunal.

Records relating to private practice are owned by the health professional who made them. It can be agreed between the private practitioner and the patient before assessment and treatment commences as to what access is to be arranged and whether there should be patient held records. The patient receiving private care has the same statutory rights of access as the NHS patient (see Chapter 9).

Client held records

Many different professionals are increasingly allowing clients to hold their own records. There are considerable therapeutic advantages in physiotherapy practice if clients are encouraged to keep their own records and so become responsible and involved in their progress.

There are some fears associated with the patient acting as custodian of the records. Fears, however, that records could be lost if the health professional ceases to be in control of the care of the records are generally unfounded. The evidence from antenatal care with mothers holding their own records seems to indicate that they are less likely to go missing. Nevertheless, such fears could lead to the setting up of a second system of record keeping at a central point. The dangers of this dual system have been considered above, that neither set might be complete and there might be inconsistencies.

There is also the fear that if records in the custody of the client go missing and litigation is commenced then the professionals will be at a disadvantage in defending themselves. The burden is, however, on the claimant to establish negligence on a balance of probabilities and this may be difficult to do if the documentation is missing and it is the claimant who is responsible for that loss.

Legal effect of lost records

If records have been deliberately destroyed and are not therefore available as evidence in court, there is a presumption summarised in the Latin tag *omnia praesumuntur contra spoliatorem*, i.e. there is a presumption against those who caused the loss.[20] Where the records are lost accidentally then the judge can determine in the light of other evidence available any inferences that are appropriate.

Computerised records

The development of an electronic patient record has been on the agenda of the DH for many years and billions of pounds are being invested. Although the original timetable (press release by the DH on 4 February 2001) of an electronic health record for every patient by March 2005 has not been attained, the strategy to secure the computerisation of all patient health records is still in place. The strategy envisages that each patient will have an electronic health record. This is defined by the DH as a record holding summarised key data about patients, such as name address, NHS number, registered GP and contact details, previous treatments, ongoing conditions, current medication, allergies and the date of any next appointments. It is intended that it will be securely protected, created with patient consent, with individual changes made only by authorised staff. In addition, there is to be an individual patient record that will hold all the detailed information of the patient's treatment and care. Electronic transmissions of prescriptions is already taking place. There are two parts to the NHS care records service:

(1) Services that are common to all users nationally will be the responsibility of the national application service provider (NASP).
(2) Services delivered at a more local level will be the responsibility of five local service providers (LSPs). Together, they will ensure the integration of existing local systems and implement the new systems, if necessary.

The NASP and the LSPs will make IT work across the NHS to support the creation of the

NHS care records service. Further information is available on the dedicated website.[21]

The DH pledged guarantees in May 2005 relating to patients' control over access to their health records.[22] The Care Record Guarantee, drawn up by the Care Record Development Board, included the commitments that access to records by NHS staff will be strictly limited to those having a need to know to provide effective treatment to a patient; patients will be able to block off parts of their record to stop it being shared with anyone in the NHS, except in an emergency, and individuals will be able to stop their information being seen by anyone outside the organisation which created it.

The Information Governance toolkit can be downloaded from the NHS Connecting for Health website.[23]

The DH, the GMC and the Office of the ICO issued joint guidance on the use of IT equipment and access to patient data on 25 April 2007. It can be downloaded from the relevant websites. The joint statement was made to ensure that all those who have access to patient information in the course of their work are clear about what is expected of them. The DH strongly supported the call of the ICO for stronger penalties to apply where individuals obtain information unlawfully, and the law is to be changed to provide the possibility of a custodial sentence for those found guilty. In the case of the new NHS Information Management and Technology (IM&T) systems, authorised individuals will have to sign a statement to indicate their understanding and agreement to adhere to the standards set out in the joint guidance.

The ICO published his views on NHS electronic care records in January 2007 in response to the concerns of those made to the ICO that their health records would be available to everyone across the NHS. The ICO had been informed by NHS Connecting for Health that everyone, in the initial trial areas, whose Summary Care Record (current medication, known allergies and adverse reactions) is to be loaded onto the NHS Care Record Service will be contacted and given information about their options. Once the information is uploaded, patients can choose to remove some or even all of the information initially loaded or keep the uploaded information but make the Summary Care Record invisible. The ICO also referred to the range of access controls to be introduced by the NHS as the new systems develop. All access to the Summary Care Record will be logged and unusual access will be investigated by a member of staff in every NHS Trust (known as the Caldicott Guardian – see Chapter 8). NHS Connecting for Health had also informed the ICO that health information uploaded on to the NHS Care Records Service will not be accessible to any other organisations beyond the NHS without the patient's explicit consent, except where this is allowed or required by law. The ICO stated that the NHS must continue to comply with the Data Protection Act 1998 and this is vital to guarantee that public confidence is maintained. The ICO would monitor the implementation and operation of the NHS Care Records Service to ensure patients are provided with adequate information and choices and that their health data is maintained in a safe and secure way.

A National Audit Office (NAO) progress report published on 15 May 2008[24] on the national programme for electronic medical records stated that the Care Records Service is unlikely to be in place before 2014–5 at the earliest, because of serious delays in installing new software; the estimated total cost of the programme is broadly unchanged; some benefits from the programme are starting to emerge such as financial savings; trusts have experienced some technical problems in using the new care records system. The NAO made several recommendations including the fact that the DH and NHS should give priority to data protection, monitor levels of public confidence and review how the levels are being influenced by its communications about the protections in place to secure and manage access to care records. Separate recommendations are given for NHS trusts and for the DH and strategic health authorities.

Litigation

It will be apparent from Chapter 10 on accountability and the discussion on the extended times within which an action can be brought that in many cases witnesses would be unable to remember any details of the events in issue and, in giving evidence, will be completely dependent on the records that were kept at the time. There is considerable value in staff who have been involved in litigation, disciplinary proceedings and other hearings sharing the lessons which they have learnt with their colleagues and illustrating the significant role which documentation played in their giving evidence. In the case of *Starcevic* v. *West Hertfordshire HA*,[25] which is considered in detail in Chapter 10, crucial to the claimant's case were the records and statement of the physiotherapist. The claimant alleged that that there was negligence in the failure to diagnose her husband's deep vein thrombosis which led to his death. He had pointed out to the physiotherapist pain in his calf and a nurse had noticed that his leg was a funny colour.

This topic is further discussed in Chapter 13.

Records of fact and hearsay

It is important to distinguish between what the patient says caused an injury, what symptoms the patient complains about and what the physiotherapist personally observes. Records should clearly identify when it is the patient who is providing information, since this is hearsay. It does not, of course, follow that what the patient is reported as saying is factually correct. The patient may be proved wrong or, indeed, change his/her story. For example in one case,[26] the records showed that the patient said he had had a running accident, but this was denied by the patient in court.

This does not mean that the physiotherapist should not take full notes of what the patient says as well as his/her own observations. In another case,[27] the judge criticised the paucity of notes made by the physiotherapists, but these

criticisms did not, fortunately, affect the outcome of the case.

This topic is further discussed in Chapter 13.

Legal status of records and evidential value of records

When does a record become a legal record is a question often asked; and the answer is that any record, any information however recorded, can be ordered to be produced in a court of law if it is relevant to an issue which arises in the court proceedings and if it is not privileged from disclosure. (Reference should be made to Chapter 8 on confidentiality and the powers and limitations of the court in requiring the production of witnesses and documents.)

It does *not* follow that what is contained in any records is necessarily accurate or true. It is possible for a completely fictitious account to be recorded. If, for example, the casualty nurse referred to above had not immediately written up her notes so that rather than adding to the record she had put down a totally fictitious pulse rate and written 'quite pale' in the first instance, the deception would possibly not have been discovered and the false record taken at its face value on an initial enquiry into the baby's death. Therefore, in determining the weight to be attached to the records and to determine the evidential value, the judge would listen to the makers of the records being cross-examined and in the light of that oral evidence determine how much value could be placed upon the written records.

Conclusions

The importance of high standards of record keeping cannot be overemphasised as part of the professional duty of care to the patient. If this duty is met, then the records should also provide essential evidence in the event of litigation or other court hearing or inquiry. Regular audit is essential to ensure that high standards are maintained. The introduction of the electronic patient record, though much delayed and subject to much criticism in terms of the security of the system and the preservation of patient confidentiality, will have major implications for how records are kept. It should assist in obtaining and maintaining high standards of record keeping.

✐ Questions and exercises

1 With some colleagues carry out an audit of the standards of record keeping among yourselves. Imagine that you were having to answer questions on the records in 10 years time. How robust would the records be in protecting your practice?

2 What abbreviations do you consider could be usefully used in record keeping by physiotherapists? What steps would you take to ensure that there was no confusion arising from their use?

3 Consider ways in which the keeping of physiotherapy records could be made more efficient.

4 Consider the extent to which electronic patient records would impact upon your practice.

References

1   Health Professions Council (2004 reprinted 2007) *Standards of Conduct, Performance and Ethics*. HPC, London.

2   Chartered Society of Physiotherapy (2002) *Rules of Professional Conduct*, 2nd edn. CSP, London.

3   Chartered Society of Physiotherapy (2005) *Core Standards of Physiotherapy Practice*. CSP, London.

4   Chartered Society of Physiotherapy (2005) *Service Standards of Physiotherapy Practice*. CSP, London.

5   Department of Health Records Management (2006) *NHS Code of Practice on Records Management*. DH, London.

6   *Hardisty* v. *Aubrey* EWCA [2006] Civ 1196.

7   Malvern, J. (2008) Patient Bruised by Hospital's Blunt Message. *The Times*, 15 May, p. 23.

8   Kettenbach, G. (2003) *Writing SOAP Notes*. 3rd edn. F.A.Davis Company, Philadelphia, USA.

9   *Prendergast* v. *Sam & Dee Ltd* [1989] 1 Med LR 36.

10 Kennedy, D. (1996) Hospital Blamed in Report on Overdose Death. *The Times*, 3 July.

11 Department of Health (2006) *Records Management. NHS Code of Practice*. DH, London.

12 Nursing and Midwifery Council (2002) *NMC Guidelines for Records and Record Keeping* (reprint of UKCC 1998) (updated in 2005 to take account of legislative changes) NMC, London.

13 Information Commissioner's Office (2006) Data Protection Good Practice Note. *How Does the Data Protection Act Apply to Professional Opinions*? ICO, London.

14 Wilkinson, P. (1995) Notes on Dead Baby Altered by Nurse. *The Times*, 7 November.

15 Murray, I. (1998) Walk-in Surgeries Fail to Keep Records. *The Times*, 7 April.

16 News item. *The Times*, 16 December 1997.

17 Audit Commission (1995) *Setting the Records Straight: A Study of Hospital Medical Records*. HMSO, London.

18 Department of Health (2007) *Information Security Management: NHS Code of Practice*. DH, London.

19 Forster, P. (1998) GP Allowed Patient to Tamper with Records. *The Times*, 7 July.

20 *Malhotra* v. *Dhawan* [1997] 8 Med LR 319.

21 www.nhscarerecords.nhs.uk

22 Department of Health (2005) *Clear Rules Set for Patients' Electronic Records*. DH, London.

23 www.igt.connectingforhealth.nhs.uk

24 National Audit Office (2008) *The National Programme for IT in the NHS – Progress Since 2006*. HC 484-1 Session 2007–8. Stationery Office, London.

25 *Starcevic* v. *West Hertfordshire Health Authority* [2001] EWCA Civ 192.

26 *Peters* v. *Robinson*, 27 January 1997, Lexis transcript.

27 *Jago* v. *Torbay Health Authority* (CA) 23 May 1994, Lexis transcript.

28 Department of Health (2003) *NHS Code of Practice on Confidentiality*. DH, London.

13

Giving Evidence in Court

The increase in litigation where patients are seeking compensation for harm which has occurred makes it more likely that the physiotherapist may be called to give evidence in court on the alleged facts giving rise to the claim. In addition, many physiotherapists (especially those in private practice) are developing their role as expert witnesses.

This chapter covers both aspects and also looks at some of the rules of evidence and the terminology which is likely to be encountered. The following topics will be covered:

- Statement making
- Witness of fact
- Report writing
- Expert witness
- In court
- The future

Statement making

Witnesses can refer to any contemporaneous records and statements in giving evidence and, therefore, since it takes many years for some court hearings to take place, it is vital that comprehensive clear records have been kept and that statements are made at the earliest opportunity. If a physiotherapist is asked to prepare a statement he/she should ensure that he/she obtains advice from a senior colleague and, if possible, a lawyer. Many NHS Trusts now have solicitors who would provide assistance in the making of any statement. The physiotherapist's statement should be made with reference to the records that he/she has kept and the principles discussed in the previous chapter.

The statement should contain the elements shown in Figure 13.1.

The statement writer should ensure that the statement is:

accurate	relevant
factual	clear
concise	legible (usually typed).

Hearsay, i.e. repeating what another person has said, should be avoided. Other people could be asked to provide their own statements if they have relevant information relating to the subject. The statement maker should read it through, checking on its overall impact and whether all the relevant facts are included. A copy should be kept. Advice should be sought on its clarity and comprehensiveness and it should not be signed

- Full name, position, grade and location of maker
- Date and time the statement was made
- Date and time of the incident
- Full names of any persons involved, e.g. patient, visitor, other staff
- A full and detailed description of the events which occurred
- Signature
- (Any supporting statements or documents should be attached)

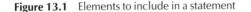

Figure 13.1   Elements to include in a statement

unless the maker is completely satisfied that it records an accurate, clear account of what took place. Many years later the statement could be used in evidence in court and it is an easy point for cross-examination (see below) if the witness is contradicting in court what she put in her statement.

Witness of fact

Anyone who can give evidence on a matter relevant to an issue before the court can be summoned to appear. The only grounds for refusing to attend and give evidence are if the evidence is protected against disclosure in court by legal professional privilege or if, on grounds of national security or other public interest, a minister of state has signed a public interest immunity certificate that the information should not be disclosed. (Legal professional privilege and public interest immunity are considered in Chapter 8 on confidentiality.)

Giving evidence: the witness of fact

As a witness of fact the physiotherapist may be required to give direct evidence over a matter with which he/she has been involved. In giving evidence the physiotherapist should ensure that he/she keeps to the facts and does not offer an opinion. In some cases the physiotherapist may be asked to pronounce upon the prognosis of the client: he/she should not magnify the extent of the disability and the poor prognosis in order to

obtain more compensation for the client. The practitioner has to ensure that his/her professional standards are maintained and he/she tells the court honestly the nature of the prognosis as he/she sees it. The physiotherapist may need guidance and training in how to withstand cross-examination. It is vital that the physiotherapist does not give facts which are outside his/her knowledge. Thus which ever party calls him/her as witness, the physiotherapist should not alter the facts or emphasis to support that party but should give his/her evidence according to professional standards of integrity. This is the best protection against hostile cross-examination (see below).

Physiotherapists who have not had any court experience may be surprised at the minutiae of detail that are considered in any court hearing. For example in one case[1] a physiotherapist and her senior manager were asked whether there were any steps under the traction couch as alleged by the plaintiff (now known as claimant). In another case,[2] a physiotherapist was required to give evidence of fact in a claim brought by a rugby football player against the club. He was the only person to have witnessed the accident and his failure to see any direct contact between the plaintiff's leg and a concrete post was a material fact in the judge finding against the claimant.

Cases other than negligence

Evidence from witnesses of fact could also be given at criminal court hearings and at civil proceedings for cases other than negligence. Thus in an action for 'passing off', the claimant company claimed that the defendant was marketing cushions for use in wheelchairs as though they were manufactured by the claimants, a well-known producer of such cushions.[3] Evidence was given by physiotherapists that these cushions were invariably bought at the instance of and fitted by healthcare professionals who would not be deceived by any passing off claim. The claimants lost the case. A physiotherapist also gave evidence in a libel action brought by John Williams, the Welsh Rugby player.[4]

Missing witnesses

Difficulties of course arise when a physiotherapist required to give evidence in court cannot be traced. Thus in a case heard in 1998[5] one of the problems was that

> the physiotherapist who had treated the plaintiff [claimant] and whose evidence might have been relevant to the allegations of contributory negligence, had disappeared without trace at an early stage.

If a witness is untraceable it may be possible for any statement prepared at the time to be placed before the court (although, of course, less weight will be given to it than would be the case if the witness were available to be cross-examined upon it).

Key points for witness of fact

Preparation

- Ensure that the records are available. Identify with stickers significant entries, but do not mark or staple or pin anything to the records. Read them through so that you are familiar with them.
- Try to obtain assistance from a lawyer or senior manager in preparation for the court hearing, so that you are prepared for giving

evidence in chief and answering questions under cross-examination.

- Try to visit the court in advance to familiarise yourself with its location, car parking, toilet facilities, etc.

At the court before the hearing

- Be prepared for a long wait and take work to do or something to occupy yourself with.
- Dress appropriately and comfortably but not too casually.
- Try to relax.

Giving evidence

- Keep calm.
- Give answers clearly and without exaggeration.
- Tell the truth.
- Do not feel that you are there to represent only one side; you must answer the questions honestly even though it might put the side cross-examining you in a good light.
- Take time over your answers and do not make up replies if you are unable to answer the question raised.
- Do not answer back or allow yourself to be flustered during the cross-examination.
- If you do not understand any legal jargon which is used, ask for an explanation.
- Keep to the facts and do not express an opinion.
- Ask for time to refer to the records if this is necessary.

Report writing

Expert witnesses will normally be asked to prepare a report by a solicitor representing one of the parties to the case. This report is vital since, if it is unfavourable to the party seeking it, the outcome may be that the case is settled or even withdrawn. On the other hand, if a party proceeds on the basis of a report that paints too rosy a picture of the case and where the expert witness fails to justify it under cross-examination, that party could lose the case or be awarded less compensation than had previously been offered in settlement and be heavily penalised in having to pay the other side's legal costs as well as their own. The first section in a book edited by Michael Foy and Philip Fagg called *Medicolegal Reporting in Orthopaedic Trauma* would be a useful resource for other conditions.[6] Appendix 1 to Chapter 1 sets out a medico-legal questionnaire that physiotherapists might find useful for their own assessments. Appendix 1 to Chapter 2 sets out the specimen format for a medico-legal report and Appendix 2 sets out Civil Procedure Rule (CPR) 35 on experts and assessors and the practice direction on experts and assessors which supplements Rule 35.

Principles to be followed in report writing

- Identify the purpose of the report (likely readership and the kind of language which can be used) and therefore the appropriate style to be used.
- Identify the main areas to be included.
- Decide the order to be followed: sometimes chronological order is appropriate, at other times subject order may be preferable.
- Identify the different kinds of information used in the report and state the source of the material, e.g.
  - hearsay evidence
  - factual evidence observed or heard by the author of the report
  - evidence of opinion of another person
  - statements by others
  - similar fact evidence.
- Sign and date it but only after reading it through and being 100% satisfied with it.

Common mistakes in report writing

- Lack of clarity
- too complex a style for reader
- use of inappropriate jargon

- use of misleading abbreviations
  - inconsistency
  - ambiguities
- inaccuracies
  - lack of dates within the report
  - wrong names included
- failure to follow a logical order
  - confusing account
  - mix of evidence and sources
  - opinion without facts
- failure to cite facts to support statements
- failure to give conclusions
- failure to base conclusions on the evidence
- lack of signature and/or date
- failure to ask someone else to read it through.

Good report writing

For most purposes the style likely to be of greatest use is one of simplicity – with short sentences, clear paragraphing and sub-paragraphing, and avoidance of jargon and meaningless clichés. The report should begin with the statement as to its purpose, the person(s) to whom it is addressed, and the name and status of the writer. If it is confidential this should be highlighted at the beginning. Other documents which are relevant should be carefully referenced.

The Chartered Society of Physiotherapy advice

The Chartered Society of Physiotherapy (CSP) published a legal work pack in March 2005[7] that contains information and general guidance on report writing and a suggested format for professional witness of fact report. The suggested format is shown in Figure 13.2.

- How binding is a report written by a chartered physiotherapist?

Every care must be taken to ensure that a report is written carefully. A person who has relied upon the accuracy of a negligently written report

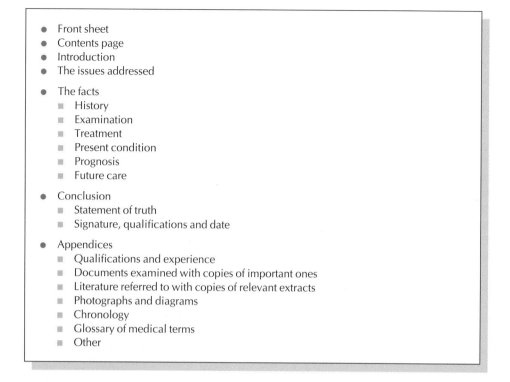

- Front sheet
- Contents page
- Introduction
- The issues addressed

- The facts
  - History
  - Examination
  - Treatment
  - Present condition
  - Prognosis
  - Future care

- Conclusion
  - Statement of truth
  - Signature, qualifications and date

- Appendices
  - Qualifications and experience
  - Documents examined with copies of important ones
  - Literature referred to with copies of relevant extracts
  - Photographs and diagrams
  - Chronology
  - Glossary of medical terms
  - Other

Figure 13.2 CSP advice on format of a report

to his/her detriment would have a prima facie case against the writer of the report. Where a report has been written by an expert witness for a party to litigation, then the expert witness would be cross-examined on that report and any inadequacies, ambiguities and other weaknesses brought out. At this stage it is extremely embarrassing for the expert to wish to change the report, unless of course other evidence emerges which was not available at the time the report was written.

Expert witness

Changes to the Civil Procedure Rules on expert witnesses following the Woolf Report were published in his final report, *Access to Justice*, in July 1996.[8] This is discussed in Chapter 10.

One of the consultation papers examined the use of expert evidence. Lord Woolf considered that the uncontrolled adversarial nature of the present system of civil litigation was the main cause of excessive cost, delay and complexity. He therefore recommended a new system in which the courts would have an active role in case management, including control over the use of expert evidence. He recommended a fast-track for cases below a certain financial limit where experts would normally be jointly appointed by the parties and would not be required to give oral evidence in court. Cases above this limit would be allocated to a multi-track, in which the court would have wide powers to define the scope of expert evidence and prescribe the way in which experts should be used in particular cases.

His proposals included the following:

- appointment of court experts and expert assessors;
- a clearer role for experts and guidance which emphasises their independence and their duty to the courts;
- appropriate choice and use of experts; and
- better arrangements for expert evidence at trial.

In *Access to Justice*, Lord Woolf stated that as a general principle single experts should be used. However, for medical negligence cases he had been advised by the Medical Negligence Working Group that there was no scope for the joint appointment of liability experts, except perhaps in the smallest and most straightforward cases. Lord Woolf regretted the polarisation of experts which so frequently took place and suggested that if joint instruction of experts was impossible, then it must be a prime objective to identify areas of agreement and disagreement between the experts as early as possible in the case.

The Civil Procedure Rules on Experts can be obtained via the website (see below).

The skills of physiotherapists in assessment mean that their evidence is relevant in a wide variety of court and tribunal hearings as expert witnesses. An expert witness is invited to give evidence of opinion on any issue which is subject to dispute. It might be what would be the appropriate standards of care which would have been expected according to the Bolam test (see Chapter 10). It may be an opinion on causation such as how long the effects of a road accident were felt by a claimant. It may be an opinion on the prognosis of the patient or the costs required to support a disabled patient, where the amount of compensation is disputed. In Chapter 18 the case of *Wright* v. *Sullivan*[9] is discussed. In this case the defendant, in a case concerned with the amount of compensation following a road accident, wished the clinical case manager to be given joint instructions and to be seen as an expert witness not a witness of fact. The Court of Appeal rejected that submission and saw the clinical case manager as a witness of fact with an ultimate responsibility of acting in the best interests of the patient.

The Civil Procedure Rule 35, which can be accessed on the Ministry of Justice website,[10] sets out the rules relating to experts and assessors. It states that there is a duty to restrict expert evidence to that which is reasonably required to resolve the proceedings (Rule 35(1) and covers the topics shown in Figure 13.3. The overriding duty of the expert to the court is discussed below. The Civil Justice Council prepared a protocol for the instruction of experts to give

- Interpretation
- Expert's overriding duty to court
- Court's power to restrict expert evidence
- General requirement for expert to give written report
- Written questions to expert
- Court's power to direct that evidence is to be given by a single joint expert
- Instructions to single joint expert
- Power of court to direct a party to provide information
- Contents of report
- Use by one party of expert's report disclosed by another
- Discussions between experts
- Consequences of failure to disclose expert's report
- Expert's right to ask court for directions
- Assessors

Figure 13.3   Civil Procedure Rules on Experts and Assessors Rule 35

evidence in civil claims in June 2005.[11] It is available on the Ministry of Justice website.

A directory of expert witnesses was drawn up by the CSP in 2004 and guidance on being an expert witness is included in its legal work pack.[7] The CSP provides training courses for those physiotherapists wishing to act as expert witnesses.

Reports and privilege

At present where an expert has prepared a report for a solicitor in anticipation or in the course of litigation, that report and any correspondence connected with it are protected by legal professional privilege and it cannot be ordered to be disclosed in court or the expert compelled to appear by the other side (see Chapter 8 on legal professional privilege). However, once the report is disclosed to the court it loses its professional privilege, although this continues to attach to any correspondence between the parties that has not been disclosed. For example, an expert may prepare a report on request but in the covering letter advise the solicitor that his client is likely to lose the case. Even if the solicitors do decide to disclose the report, the letter remains privileged. Under Rule 35(13) a party who fails to disclose an expert's report may not use the report at the trial or call the expert to give evidence orally, unless the court gives permission.

Impartiality and professional integrity

Under Rule 35(3) (see below) an expert witness has an overriding duty to the court. An expert witness should not change his/her views according to the side which calls him/her. The expert witness may be asked to edit his/her report to make it more favourable to the side asking for his/her opinion. The expert witness should only agree to any amendments if he/she is satisfied that the changed report accurately represents his/her opinion and the expert witness

is able to support it under cross-examination by oral evidence in court.

One useful rule for the practitioner to follow is to give an honest reasoned opinion whichever side calls him/her. The practitioner must not be partisan, nor should he/she exaggerate or belittle the amount of compensation. If the practitioner always gives an honest and professional view, he/she will be respected by the solicitors who will know that they will be able to trust him/her to withstand cross-examination as an expert witness and will know him/her to be reliable. The practitioner will not see the court battle personally as involving him/her and thus, whichever side wins, the practitioner will be able to feel that he/she has given an honest report to the court. A carefully prepared report, well substantiated, can reduce the length of a court hearing and enable many matters to be agreed by the parties, thus avoiding court time.

Duty of expert witness to the court

Rule 35(3) states that:

(1) It is the duty of an expert to help the court on the matters within his expertise.
(2) This duty overrides any obligation to the person from whom he has received instructions or by whom he is paid.

In a reported case[12] the court held that the expert witness had a responsibility to approach the task of giving evidence seriously and an expert should not be surprised if the court expressed strong disapproval if that was not done. In this case the expert in his report had stated that 'as far as I am aware no other previous seal manufacturer had used such a system'. In fact it became apparent not only that that system was used by others in the trade, but that the witness neither knew what systems were used by such others nor had made any effort to find out. More recently the House of Lords in the *Bolitho* case[13] has emphasised that expert witnesses must be able to show that the body of opinion which they are supporting has a logical basis (see Chapter 10).

The lesson from this is that an expert must not express an opinion unless it is clearly based on fact and where possible on established authorities or research.

A further lesson is that the expert should know and keep within his/her field of competence. Under Rule 35(4) no expert can be called or his/her report put in evidence without the permission of the court. A party must identify the field in which he/she wishes to rely upon expert evidence. There is a general requirement that expert evidence is to be given in a written report and if the claim is in the fast-track, the court will not direct an expert to attend a hearing unless it is necessary in the interests of justice.

Case: *Miles* v. *Cain*[14]

> Mrs Penelope Robinson, at that time from the professional affairs department at the Chartered Society of Physiotherapy, gave evidence about the treatments provided and the extent to which the removal of clothes would have been necessitated.

In this case where the plaintiff (now known as claimant) was suing an unregistered physiotherapist for assault, the judge commented:

> I accept her evidence. She was obviously being truthful and trying to help the court.

Conflicting expert evidence

What is the situation if there is a clash between the evidence given by different expert witnesses, who both purport to speak on behalf of a body of competent professional opinion. This was the situation which arose in the *Maynard* case,[15] which is mentioned in Chapter 10. The House of Lords held that where both sides were supported by equally competent professional opinion, then the claimant had not established the case.

Clearly there are advantages for experts to agree on the basic principles. Thus in one case[16] physiotherapy witnesses from the opposing sides, described by the judge as 'two impressive physiotherapists', agreed on the proposals for physiotherapy that the claimant would require in the future. In contrast, in a case in 1995[17] the two expert physiotherapists disagreed over the approach (the extent to which a physiotherapist was required rather than others providing physiotherapy under guidance) and also over the extent to which existing physiotherapy treatment was sufficient for the child's needs. Under the new CPR, the court can direct that evidence is to be given by a single joint expert (Rule 35(7)). Under this Rule where the parties cannot agree who should be the expert, the court may select the expert from a list prepared or identified by the instructing parties or direct that the expert be selected in such other manner as the court may direct.

The judge does not have to accept the evidence of any expert. Thus in *Miles* v. *Cain* described above (where an unregistered physiotherapist was sued for assault by a patient) two psychiatrists gave expert evidence whether the girl was telling the truth or not about the alleged trauma. The judge stated that the doctor for the claimant was

> unimpressive because I do not think he has sufficiently studied his brief . . . In my judgment it would be unsafe to utilise Dr Connell's views in formulating a judgment on the main issue as to whether the plaintiff [claimant] is a liar or is fantasising.

Of the other expert psychiatrist, the judge said 'I reject Dr Silverman also, distinguished though he is'.

It is essential that any expert opinion can be substantiated by the facts. In the light of the House of Lords ruling in the *Bolitho* case (see above and Chapter 10), judges are likely to look even more critically at the opinion of experts to ensure that it logically follows from the facts.

Opinions on quantum

As well as being required to give evidence on how the standards of care that were provided matched up with the reasonable standard which could have been expected, experts may also be required to give evidence on quantum, i.e. the amount of compensation which the claimant is seeking. The expert must have clear factual evidence as to how he/she arrives at the estimate of needs of the patient and the cost of meeting these. For example, in one case[18] a physiotherapist, Allison Sterling, was called to give evidence on the mobility problems of a client and stated that she had observed the patient using a walking frame, but

> when she pulls herself to her feet using the frame she is at risk of toppling backwards or sideways unless the frame is positioned in exactly the right position or if she fails to pull up strongly enough.

The judge decided in the light of this and other evidence that an electric wheelchair was required for outdoor use and included the cost of such a chair in the compensation awarded.

Exaggerated claims

Some physiotherapists find that clients place considerable pressure upon them to make assessments in their favour since a considerable sum of compensation may be dependent upon the outcome.

Situation: exaggerated claims

> A physiotherapist was asked to assess a client for the purposes of quantifying the compensation payable in a road traffic case. The physiotherapist formed the view that the client was exaggerating his symptoms and that he in fact had far greater movement than he was admitting to. She noticed in particular that he was able to bend down and pick up his tea cup and saucer from the floor as they spoke. She included this fact in her report and received an extremely abusive reply from the client contradicting her.

In such a situation the physiotherapist has a professional responsibility to undertake an honest and thorough assessment and should not omit aspects of her findings even though these might be unwelcome to the client. It might help if she points out at the time some of those features which she observes which the client might later disagree with. The client might not be aware that her observations of his mobility are of greater importance than what he himself says about it, particularly where the client appears to be exaggerating his symptoms.

Chartered Society of Physiotherapy guidelines

The CSP has laid down guidance for expert witnesses in its legal work pack[7] guidelines and criteria for the role of expert witness and has suggested that an expert, representing the profession by giving evidence as an expert, should:

- have been working within the specialty concerned for 5 years
- be a Senior I or higher
- have credibility with peers
- have published something
- have carried out a research project.

Points to remember

The expert witness:

- does not take sides;
- outlines his/her professional credentials (status, experience, appointments and academic qualifications);
- gives a professional, not personal, opinion;
- understands on what issues and topics he or she has expertise;
- provides a logical report (see above);
- always supports opinion with fact;
- avoids confusing technical language and jargon;
- avoids being verbose;
- gives concrete understandable examples and uses everyday analogies;

- keeps facts and opinions relevant to the issues before the court;
- ensures that he or she understands the purposes of the proceedings;
- dates and signs the report.

Dos and don'ts of the expert witness

- Do find out where the court is and turn up.
- Do make sure that the case has not been adjourned before travelling.
- Do not stand on your dignity.
- Do be acquainted with court procedure and the role of the judge, jury and counsel.
- Do know how to address the judge and others.
- Do dress appropriately.
- Do not get emotional or forget what to say.
- Do know your report and the facts contained in it.
- Do not deviate from the report or introduce new material.
- Do believe what you have written and what you are saying.
- Do be dispassionate about the outcome.
- Do not take an adversarial stance.
- Do prepare for cross-examination.
- Do remain calm under cross-examination.
- Do not exaggerate.
- Do keep to the facts.
- Do not try to hasten the case along.
- Do not try to be humorous.

Importance of records and other documentary evidence

Inevitably, the value of a physiotherapist as a witness will depend significantly upon the clarity and comprehensiveness of any records that he/she kept and/or any statement he/she prepared at the time. Documentary evidence may include reports from pathology, X-rays, and any other relevant information, in whatever form it is held. All this information would have been disclosed to the other side during the process known as 'discovery of documents'. It is important that this discovery has been carried out properly. In a case[19] brought by Frank Cunningham against North Manchester Health Authority, he alleged lack of care by medical staff as a result of which he lost his leg following a motorcycle accident. A retrial was ordered when it was discovered that the claimant's expert had only had access to miniaturised copies of the original X-rays and arteriograms, whereas the defendants' experts had seen the originals. Mr Cunningham subsequently accepted an offer of £325 000. He was a litigant in person. The changes to the CPR and greater openness between the parties should ensure that such situations are less likely to arise.

In court

Cross-examination

This is the term applied to the opportunity of the one side, **A**, to question the witnesses called by the other side, **B** (and *vice versa*). In the adversarial system (see Chapter 2) that is the basis of English court procedure each witness of fact or expert witness is subjected to detailed questioning on the oral evidence they have just given by the lawyers acting on behalf of the opposing side. Through this process, if the legal representatives are competent and the case adequately prepared so the barrister knows what questions to ask, it is usually possible for the true facts of a matter to be brought out before the court for the judge or jury to decide.

This is particularly important if claimants are bringing false or exaggerated claims. In *Jago* v. *Torbay Health Authority*[20] the judge ruled against the claimant (who was claiming compensation on the grounds that physiotherapy had been negligently undertaken), finding that he was guilty of self-deception, dishonesty and an element of fraud in what he said he could do and what he actually could do (neighbours had given evidence about his standing on a ladder and cutting a hedge). Both the claimant and the neighbours would have been subject to cross-examination and from this the judge could decide whom to believe.

It is for this reason that appeal courts rarely overturn the findings of fact made by first instance judges, since they are the ones who have had the benefit of assessing the demeanour of witnesses when giving evidence and under cross-examination which the appeal court has not.

There are two distinct objectives in cross-examination. The one is to discredit the witness or show that his or her evidence is irrelevant to the point being established. The other is to use this witness to strengthen the case of one's own side.

In pursuing the first aim, the cross-examiner will attempt to:

- undermine the confidence of the witness;
- show up inconsistencies and/or ambiguities in the evidence;
- show how the evidence being given is contradicted by other witnesses;
- show how the witness is unreliable and/or unintelligent.

In pursuing the second aim, the cross-examiner will attempt to ensure that the witness (for side **A**):

- gives evidence helpful to side **B**;
- praises side **B**;
- corroborates evidence being given by side **B**.

Attempts may also be made to use the witness to testify on professional/expert matters and express opinions useful to the other side.

Preparation and an unshakeable conviction in the accuracy of your evidence is essential to be able to handle cross-examination and most physiotherapists would now be able to obtain expert advice from the solicitors acting for their NHS Trust before attending court on behalf of the employer.

Procedure

The stages that are followed in criminal courts and civil courts are shown in Chapter 2, on the

legal system. The Civil Procedure Rules have been amended following Lord Woolf's review of the system for obtaining compensation in civil litigation. The changes are discussed in Chapter 10. The changes in relating to the use of expert witnesses are considered above.

Rules of evidence

This is a complex area and the rules depend upon the nature of the court hearing. For example, hearsay evidence (where a witness gives evidence about what was reported to him or her by an eye witness and of which he or she has no direct evidence) may be acceptable in some hearings, e.g. social security tribunals but not acceptable in civil or criminal hearings except in very specific circumstances.

Some of the issues that are covered by the rules include:

- rules on relevance, admissibility and hearsay
- weight of evidence
- burden of proof
- degrees (standard) of proof
- presumptions
- judicial notice
- competence of witness
- compellability of witness
- corroboration
- doctrine of privilege (see Chapter 8).

It is not possible in a work of this kind to give full details of the significance of the rules of evidence on the above topics and reference must be made to one of the specialist books listed for further reading.

Conclusion

There are considerable fears about giving evidence in court and it is vital that any witness, whether expert or witness of fact, should be properly prepared for the occasion. Even though they are not on trial themselves, their professional standing and integrity is being put to the test and it is therefore essential, that they follow the highest standard of professional practice. Witnesses of fact and expert witnesses will find that the Ministry of Justice website and the Civil Procedure Rules accessible on that site give helpful advice on preparation for the court hearing and the actual hearing.

✎ Questions and exercises

1 You have been asked to appear as a witness in a case. Draw up a list of your fears and try to work out ways in which these fears could be resolved.

2 Try to attend a court hearing and analyse the way in which it operates, the procedure followed and the actions of judge, jury (if present), barristers, solicitors, court clerk, court usher, witness, and any other person taking part in the court proceedings.

3 Prepare a protocol for the preparation of a report as an expert witness.

References

1   *McMenamin* v. *Lambeth Southwark and Lewisham Area Health Authority* (QBD) 28 October 1982, Lexis transcript.

2   *Simms* v. *Leigh Rugby Football Club Ltd* [1969] 2 All ER 923.

3   *Hodgkinson and Corby Ltd and Another* v. *Wards Mobility Services Ltd* [1994] 1 WLR 1564.

4   *Williams* v. *Reason and others* [1988] 1 WLR 96.

5   *Berry* v. *Calderdale Health Authority* (CA) 16 February 1998, Lexis transcript.

6   Foy, M., Fagg, P. (eds) (2003) *Medicolegal Reporting in Orthopaedic Trauma*, 3rd edn. Churchill Livingstone Edinburgh.

7   Chartered Society of Physiotherapy (2005) *Legal Work Pack*. CSP London.

8   Lord Woolf (July 1996) *Access to Justice Final Report*. HMSO, London.

9   *Wright* v. *Sullivan* [2005] EWCA Civ 656.

10 www.justice.gov.uk/civil/procrules_fin

11 Council of Justice (2005) *Protocol for the Instruction of Experts to give Evidence in Civil Claims*. Ministry of Justice, London.

12 *Autospin (Oil Seals) Ltd* v. *Beehive Spinning* (A firm) The Times Law Report, 9 August 1995.

13 *Bolitho* v. *City and Hackney Health Authority* [1997] 3 WLR 1151; [1997] 4 All ER 771.

14 *Miles* v. *Cain* 25 November 1988, Lexis transcript.

15 *Maynard* v. *West Midlands Regional Health Authority* [1985] 1 All ER 635.

16 *Simpson* v. *South East Hampshire Health Authority* (QBD) 16 July 1997, Lexis transcript.

17 *Stephens* v. *Doncaster Health Authority* (QBD) 16 June 1995, Lexis transcript.

18 *Havenhand* v. *Jeffrey* (QBD) 6 December 1996, Lexis transcript.

19 *Cunningham* v. *North Manchester Health Authority* (CA) [1997] 8 Med LR 135.

20 *Jago* v. *Torbay Health Authority* (CA) 23 May 1994, Lexis transcript.

14 Handling Complaints

It is a statutory requirement that every health care and social service organisation has an efficient procedure for handling complaints. Handling complaints should not be seen as a negative exercise since feedback through the complaints machinery can become an effective method of quality assurance and improving standards.

This chapter covers the following topics:

- Background to present complaints procedures
- The 2004 complaints procedure
- NHS and social services complaints: a unified procedure
- Patient representative organisations
- Complaints and the private sector
- Other quality assurance methods
- Future developments

Background to present complaints procedures

A statutory duty was established under the Hospital Complaints Act 1985 for each health authority to set up a complaints procedure. This was evaluated by the Wilson Committee in 1994,[1] which saw the system for dealing with complaints relating to health services to be confusing, bureaucratic, slow and inefficient. The report reviewed the current situation and set objectives for any effective complaints system. The principles it identified are set out in Figure 14.1.

A new complaints procedure came into effect on 1 April 1996 implementing the majority of recommendations contained in the Wilson Report. It established three levels of complaints handling: local level; independent review and the Health Service Commissioner. This complaints procedure was itself reviewed in 2003 when the Department of Health published the results of an investigation into the effectiveness of the complaints procedure established following the Wilson Report. The Department of Health (DH) publication, *NHS Complaints Reform: Making Things Right*[2] noted the following criticisms of the existing complaints procedure:

- It is unclear how, and also difficult, to pursue complaints and concerns.
- There is often delay in responding when concerns arise.

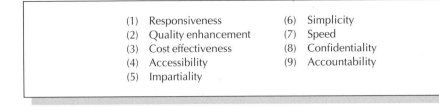

(1)	Responsiveness	(6)	Simplicity
(2)	Quality enhancement	(7)	Speed
(3)	Cost effectiveness	(8)	Confidentiality
(4)	Accessibility	(9)	Accountability
(5)	Impartiality		

Figure 14.1   Principles of an effective complaints system

- Too often there is a negative attitude to concerns expressed.
- Complaints seem not to get a fair hearing.
- Patients do not get the support they need when they want to complain.
- The independent review stage does not have the credibility it needs.
- The process does not provide the redress the patients want.
- There does not seem to be any systematic processes for using feedback from complaints to drive improvements in services.
- The aims of the 2003 reforms to the complaints procedure were to establish clear national standards and accountabilities, devolution to clinicians and managers backed up by independent scrutiny, flexibility and to ensure that patients can choose how they wish to pursue their concerns and have the support they need to help them do so.

The DH recommended that there should be:

- Increasing support and information for people who make complaints through local patient advice and liaison services and independent complaints and advice services (see below).
- Patient feedback and customer care and training for NHS staff, including board members, to improve the way people are dealt with to help resolve complaints quickly.
- Subject to legislation, placing responsibility for independent complaints review with the Commission for Healthcare Audit and Inspection (CHAI).

The complaints procedure established in 2004 (with minor revisions in 2006)

The new complaints procedure envisaged three similar stages to the procedure following the Wilson report: local, intermediate and Health Service Commissioner, but the intermediate stage was made more independent by its being placed upon the Healthcare Commission. Regulations were brought into force on 30 July 2004[3] on a new complaints system and amended in 2006.[4] Guidance is provided by the DH on both sets of regulations and is available on its website.

The regulations cover:

- nature and scope of arrangements for the handling and consideration of complaints;
- handling and consideration of complaints by NHS bodies;
- handling and consideration of complaints by the Healthcare Commission;
- publicity, monitoring and annual reports.

The regulations require each NHS body, CHAI and each primary care trust (PCT) to make arrangements for the handling of complaints in accordance with the regulations:

The arrangements must be accessible and such as to ensure that the complaints are dealt with speedily and efficiently, and that complainants are treated courteously and sympathetically and as far as possible involved in decisions about how their complaints are handled and considered.

The arrangements must be in writing with a copy given free of charge to any person who requests a copy.

Amendments were made to the Regulations in 2006[4] to facilitate the transfer of complaints which relate to social services, extending the persons who can be appointed as complaints managers (the complaints manager does not have to be an employee of the NHS body and can be appointed for more than one NHS body), changing the time limit for response to a complaint and broadening the remit of the Healthcare Commission in relation to complaints about NHS Foundation Trusts.

A primary care provider (and this includes pharmacists, ophthalmic opticians, dentists, GPs and PCTs) must ensure that a complaints procedure is in place. A complex complaint is one that relates to several different NHS bodies or local authority or primary care providers or is already subject to a concurrent investigation. If the NHS trust or PCT arranges for the provision of services through an independent provider, they are required to ensure that the independent provider has arrangements in place for the handling of complaints in accordance with the regulations.

Excluded from the complaints regulations are:

- Complaints made by an NHS body that relate to the exercise of its functions by another NHS body.
- Complaints by a primary care provider that relate either to the exercise of its functions by an NHS body or to the contract or arrangements under which it provides primary care services.
- Complaints made by an employee of an NHS body or primary care provider about any matter relating to his/her contract of employment.
- Complaints made by an independent provider about any matter relating to arrangements made by an NHS body with that independent provider.
- Complaints which relate to the provision of primary medical services in accordance with

arrangements made by a PCT with a Strategic Health Authority under S.28C of the NHS (Act 1977) or under a transitional agreement.
- Complaints that are being or have been investigated by the Health Service Commissioner.
- Complaints arising out of an NHS body's alleged failure to comply with a data subject request under the Data Protection Act 1998 or a request for information under the Freedom of Information Act 2000.
- A complaint about which the complainant has stated in writing that he/she intends to take legal proceedings
- A complaint about which an NHS body is taking or is proposing to take disciplinary proceedings in relation to the substance of the complaint against a person who is the subject of the complaint
- A complaint the subject matter of which has already been investigated under these Regulations
- A complaint relating to a scheme under the Superannuation Act 1972.

The regulations require a complaints manager to be appointed by each NHS body. This may include a person who is not an employee of the NHS body and a person who is appointed as a complaints manager for more than one NHS body.

A complaint can be made by a patient, or any person who is affected by or likely to be affected by the action, omission or decision of the NHS body that is the subject of the complaint. A complaint may also be made by the representative of a person who has died, is a child or is unable by reason of physical or mental incapacity to make the complaint him/herself or has asked the representative to act on his/her behalf.

Time limits for making a complaint are 6 months from the date on which the matter which is the subject of the complaint occurred or first came to the notice of the complainant, but the complaints manager can investigate complaints outside these time limits if he/she is of the opinion that having regard to all the circumstances, the complainant had good reasons for not making the complaint within that period and it is still possible to investigate the complaint effectively and efficiently.

Procedure

- The complaints manager must send to the complainant a written acknowledgement of the complaint within two working days of the date on which the complaint was made, together with details of the right to assistance from independent advocacy services.
- Where the complaint was made orally, the acknowledgement must be accompanied by the written record with an invitation to the complainant to sign and return it.
- The complaints manager must send a copy of the complaint and his acknowledgement to any person identified as the subject of the complaint

Investigation

The complaints manager must investigate the complaint to the extent necessary and in the manner that appears to him/her most appropriate to resolve it speedily and efficiently. Where the manager thinks it would be appropriate to do so he/she can, with the agreement of the complainant, make arrangements for conciliation, mediation or other assistance for the purpose of resolving the complaint. The NHS body must ensure that appropriate conciliation or mediation services are available. He/she must take such steps as are reasonably practicable to keep the complainant informed about the progress of his investigation.

Response

The complaints manager must prepare a written response to the complaint which:

- summarises the nature and substance of the complaint;
- describes the investigation under regulation 12;
- summarises its conclusions;
- the letter must be signed by the chief executive of the NHS body except in cases where for good reason the chief executive is not him/herself able to sign it, in which case it may be signed by a person acting on his/her behalf;
- the letter must be sent to the complainant within 25 days (amended from 20 by the 2006 Regulations) beginning with the date on which the complaint was made unless the complainant agrees to a longer period, in which case the response may be sent within that longer period;
- the letter must notify the complainant of his/her right to refer the complaint to the Healthcare Commission;
- copies of the response must be sent to any person who was the subject of the complaint and any other person to whom the complaint has been sent under the regulations.

Handling and considerations of complaints by CHAI (Healthcare Commission)

Part III of the regulations enable a complainant:

- who is not satisfied with the results of an investigation (except where the complaint relates to an NHS Bursary scheme);
- where the investigation has not been completed within 6 months of the date on which the complaint was made;
- where the complaints manager has decided not to investigate because it was out of time to request a consideration of the complaint by the Healthcare Commission within 6 months of the response being made (increased from 2 months by the 2006 Regulations).

The Healthcare Commission is then required to assess the nature and substance of the complaint and decide how it should be handled having regard to the views of the complainant, the views of the body complained about, the views of the Independent Regulator (where the complaint relates to a Foundation Trust), any investigation of the complaint and action taken as a result and any other relevant circumstances. The Healthcare Commission must notify the complainant as to whether it has decided to:

- take no further action;
- make recommendation to the body which is the subject of the complaint as to what action might be taken to resolve it;
- to investigate the complaint further, whether by establishing a panel to consider it or otherwise;
- to consider the subject matter of the complaint as part of or in conjunction with any other investigation or review;
- to refer the complaint to a health regulatory body;
- to refer the complaint to the Health Service Commissioner.

Where the Healthcare Commission proposes to investigate the complaint it must within 10 working days of the date on which it sent the notification send the complainant and any other person to whom the notice was sent its proposed terms of reference for its investigation.

The Regulations cover the investigation by the Healthcare Commission, including the use of an independent panel to hear and consider complaints and its powers to request the production of such information and documents as it considers necessary to enable a complaint to be considered properly. Members and employees of an NHS body and any person who is or was a healthcare professional or employee of a healthcare professional are excluded from being a member of a panel. Detailed procedural rules are laid down for the panels. The report of the Healthcare Commission's investigation must include the specified information and be completed as soon as reasonably practicable. The report must be sent to the complainant with a letter explaining to him his/her right to take his/her complaint to the Health Service

Commissioner (HSC); and also to the NHS body that was the subject of the complaint (and, in the case of a complaint involving a primary care provider, to the PCT), to any relevant strategic health authority and to the Independent Regulator for complaints about an NHS foundation trust, where he/she so requests. The Independent Regulator may make an individual request for a report or make a standing request that identifies a type of complaint for which he/she wishes to receive a report.

Part IV of the regulations requires each NHS body and the Healthcare Commission to ensure that there is effective publicity for its complaints arrangements. For monitoring purposes, each NHS body must prepare a quarterly report specifying the number of complaints received, the subject matter of the complaints, summarise how they were handled including the outcome and identify any complaints where the recommendations of the Healthcare Commission were not acted upon, giving the reasons. An annual report must be prepared on the handling and consideration of complaints and be sent to specified bodies including the Healthcare Commission, the strategic health authority and PCT, as appropriate.

Criticisms by the Healthcare Commission

In October 2007 the Healthcare Commission published its first audit (available on its website) on how the NHS trusts handled complaints.[5] It found considerable variation in how complaints were handled across the country. Its report highlighted the issues shown in Figure 14.2. The Healthcare Commission announced that it was working on a toolkit for complaints managers that should be available in 2008.

NHS and social services complaints: a single comprehensive procedure

Regulations relating to social services complaints[6] came into force on 1 September 2006. They

- More needs to be done to make the complaints systems open and accessible, especially for those with learning disabilities and from ethnic communities
- People who complain should be confident that their care will not suffer
- Trusts should use complaints data to inform decision making
- Whilst there is no one-size-fits-all approach to investigating complaints, a common approach would improve risk management of complaints and manage the expectations of complainants
- There are no nationally available standard tools and resources such as case studies, checklists and training aids for staff

Figure 14.2   Criticisms by the Healthcare Commission on the 2004 complaints system

impose time limits on making complaints, new timescales for handling stages of the process and provide greater independence at the final review panel stage. They can be downloaded from the Office of Public Sector Information.[7] The NHS complaints regulations have been amended[4] following the White Paper commitment to develop a single comprehensive complaints procedure across health and social care by 2009. The amendments are intended to make the system more responsive and give better links with the arrangements for responding to social care complaints.

Commission for Patient and Public Involvement in Health

In accordance with the strategy set out in the NHS Plan,[8] the Commission for Patient and Public Involvement in Health (CPIHH) was established under Section 20 of the NHS Reform and Health Care Professions Act 2002 in January 2003. Its functions, set out in Section 20(2) of the 2002 Act, included advising the Secretary of State about arrangements for public involvement in and consultation about matters relating to the health service in England and the provision of independent advocacy services. It was abolished in 2008, when the Local Government and Public Involvement in Health Act 2007, which set up Local Involvement Networks, came into force (see below).

Independent complaints and advice services

Under Section 12 of the Health and Social Care Act 2001, the Secretary of State has a responsibility to provide independent advocacy services to assist patients in making complaints against the NHS. The independent complaints advisory services (ICAS)[9] were available nationally from September 2003. A consultation paper, *Involving Patients and the Public in Healthcare*[10] was issued by the DH in September 2001 for consultation on proposals for greater public representation to replace the community health councils (CHCs).

ICAS focus on helping individuals to pursue complaints about NHS services. They aim to ensure complainants have access to the support they need to articulate their concerns and navigate the complaints system, maximising the chances of their complaint being resolved more quickly and effectively. ICAS work alongside the trust-based patients' forums and patient advocacy and liaison services. Information about ICAS and the current range of pilot services is available on the DH website.[11] It was announced in January 2006 that following a rigorous exercise, the DH awarded contracts to three organisations to deliver a new and improved Independent Complaints Advocacy Service from 1 April 2006. Community Health Councils were abolished in 2003 in England but retained in Wales.

Patient advice and liaison services

A significant proposal in the NHS Plan[12] (see Chapter 17) was the patient advocacy and liaison services (PALS). The Plan envisaged that by 2002 PALS will be established in every major hospital with an annual national budget of around £10 million. All NHS trusts were required to establish a PALS service by April 2002. Their core functions were:

- to provide on the spot help and speed resolution of problems;
- to act as a gateway to independent advice and advocacy services;
- to provide accurate information about the trust's services and other related services;
- as a key course of feedback to the trust, to act as a catalyst for change and improvement;
- to support staff in developing a responsive, listening culture.

Patients Forums

Under Section 15 of the NHS Reform and Health Care Professions Act, the Secretary of State has a duty to set up in every trust and primary care trust a body to be known as a Patients Forum. The members of each Patients Forum are appointed by the Commission for Patient and Public Involvement in Health. Statutory functions[13] were laid down in Section 15(3) of the 2002 NHS Reform and Health Care Professions Act. In 2006 the DH published its report *A Stronger Local Voice*, which announced that Patient Forums in England were to be abolished and replaced by local authority run Local Involvement Networks (LINKS) under the Local Government and Public Involvement in Health Act 2007.

Local Involvement Networks

Part 14 of the Local Government and Public Involvement in Health Act 2007 established local involvement networks for health and social services. Under Section 221 each local authority is required to make contractual arrangements for the purpose of ensuring that there are means by which specified activities can be carried on in the area. The activities specified include:

- Promoting and supporting the involvement of people in the commissioning, provision and scrutiny of local care services.
- Enabling people to monitor for the purposes of their consideration of specified matters (standard of provision of local care services, how they could be improved and whether and how they ought to be improved) and to review for those purposes the commissioning and provision of local care services.
- Obtaining the views of people about their needs for, and their experience of local care services.
- Making these views known and making reports and recommendations about how local care services could or ought to be improved, to persons responsible for commissioning, providing, managing or scrutinising local care services.

Local care services means services provided as part of the health services and services provided as part of the social services of a local authority. The local involvement network (LINK) that results from these arrangements cannot include a local authority or health services organisation. The service providers must allow entry by local involvement networks. The local involvement network must provide an annual report that contains matters to be specified by the Secretary of State and sent to the local authority and NHS organisations in the area.

Regulations on local involvement networks came into force on 1 April 2008.[14] As a consequence of this, the Patient Forums and the Commission for Public and Patient Involvement in Health are abolished. The Audit Commission and the Healthcare Commission reported in June 2008 that the reforms costing £1 billion to make the NHS more efficient and patient-friendly have failed to have much impact. They stated that services have improved as a result of central targets and extra money but the marketisation initiative has yet to contribute much.

Consultation with patients

Section 11 of the Health and Social Care Act 2001 (now Section 242 of the National Health Service Act 2006) places a duty on NHS trusts, PCTs and Strategic Health Authorities to make arrangements to involve and consult patients and the public in service planning and operation and in the development of proposals for changes. An action seeking judicial review of a decision to close twin in-patient wards without consultation in breach of Section 11 succeeded, the trust's defence of it being a decision taken in an emergency situation was not accepted.[15]

Complaints and the private sector

Individual hospitals and private practitioners can set up their own complaints procedures. There would be advantages, however, in their following the same principles as those accepted for the public sector. There would in particular be benefit to them in ensuring that at some stage in the procedure the complainant would be able to secure the assistance of an independent person or review panel. It may be that those working in independent practice could provide a panel from which independent persons could be chosen to investigate or mediate a complaint. Under the 2004 complaints procedure if an independent physiotherapist were to contract with an NHS organisation for the provision of services, it would be a requirement that the physiotherapist has in place a complaints procedure.

Complaints and litigation

Case: *R v. Canterbury and Thanet DHA and another, ex parte F and W*[16]

Complaints were made under the previous hospital complaints procedure by eight families that a doctor employed by the first defendants and seconded to the second defendants diagnosed sexual abuse when it should not have been so diagnosed and delayed in telling the parents of the diagnosis. A legal aid certificate was obtained by one of the complainants. The doctor withdrew her cooperation in view of the possibility of legal proceedings. The defendants subsequently considered that an inquiry was inappropriate. The complainants applied for judicial review contending *inter alia* that there was a duty to review their complaints.

The court held that the complaints procedure was not appropriate where litigation was likely because:

- the purpose of the inquiry was either to obtain a second opinion and a change of diagnosis or to enable the health authority to change its procedures in the light of matters brought to its attention during the investigation; and
- the procedure depends on the cooperation of the doctor concerned which obviously would not be forthcoming if legal proceedings were likely.

Complaints and the physiotherapist

Before a change in the bye-laws, members of the Chartered Society of Physiotherapy (CSP) were subject to a double complaints machinery: that of the CSP and also that of the Health Profession Council (HPC) (see Chapter 4). In April 2006 the decision was taken to change the bye-laws to bring an end to the dual prosecution of its members. The CSP role in providing defence representation for its members before the CSP continues.

Other quality assurance methods

Individuals who have complaints about the services provided in the NHS do not have any contractual right to bring an action before the court for breach of contract. If harm has been suffered as a result of a failure or omission, they may have a successful claim in the law of negligence (see Chapter 10) or if a service has not been provided they may in exceptional circumstances be able to bring a case of breach of statutory duty for failure to provide that service (see Chapter 6) or seek judicial review of administrative failures. Otherwise, they must rely upon the complaints procedures.

There are, however, many other mechanisms to ensure the maintenance of high standards of health care, although these cannot be directly implemented by the patient. The White Paper put forward a strategy for improving quality assurance and its mechanisms which included the establishment of a National Institute for Health and Clinical Effectiveness (NICE), a Commission for Health Improvement, which was replaced by the Commission for Health Audit and Inspection (CHAI) (now known as the Healthcare Commission) and National Service Frameworks for national standards. The statutory duty to ensure quality of services was the foundation for the establishment of Clinical Governance whereby chief executives and Trust Boards are held accountable for the clinical performance of their organisations. These initiatives are further considered in Chapter 17.

The CSP has been concerned to establish high standards of practice and has introduced many initiatives to improve the quality of services provided by its members. The Core Standards and the Service Standard are considered in Chapter 4 and its strategy for 2005–10[17] is considered in Chapter 1.

Conclusions

The fact that there have been three statutory complaints procedures since 1985 and that the present one has been subjected to significant criticisms is indicative of the difficulty of putting into place a mechanism which meets the requirements set out in Figure 14.1. It is however in the interests of all health professionals to ensure that any complaints by parents and children relating to the provision of health or social services are resolved as speedily as possible informally without requiring the complainant to make use of the formal procedure. Physiotherapists should have the confidence to realise:

- that complaints can be a useful way of monitoring and improving the services to clients,
- that it takes courage to make a complaint, especially where the client suffers from a chronic condition, and
- that improvements can be made if clients are prepared to discuss with the health professionals ways in which the services could be enhanced.

Every complaint should be dealt with objectively and no assumptions made about the genuineness or grounds for the complaint until it has been effectively and thoroughly investigated. Complaints should be seen as only a small part of the quality assurance mechanisms in every organisation. In April 2009 the Care Quality Commission replaced the Healthcare Commission and other bodies (see Chapter 17).

Questions and exercises

1　Draw a diagram showing how a complaint by a client of physiotherapy services would be processed.
2　A client tells you that he is not happy with the care provided by another health professional. What action do you take and what advice do you give?
3　In what way could the handling of informal complaints be improved?
4　As a private practitioner how would you deal with complaints to ensure that some independent review takes place?

References

1 Department of Health (1994) *Being Heard. The Report of a Review Committee on NHS Complaints Procedures*. (The Wilson Report) DH, London.

2 Department of Health (2003) *NHS Complaints Reform: Making Things Right*. DH, London.

3 The National Health Service (Complaints) Regulations 2004 SI 1768.

4 The National Health Service (Complaints) Amendment Regulations 2006 No 2084.

5 www.healthcarecommission.org.uk

6 The Local Authority Social Services Complaints (England) Regulations 2006 SI 2006 No 1681.

7 www.opsi.gov.uk

8 DH, NHS Plan Cm 4818, 1 July 2000 (Chapter 10).

9 Information on ICAS is available from the DH website www.dh.gov.uk/complaints

10 Department of Health (2001) *Involving Patients and the Public in Healthcare*. DH, London.

11 www.dh.gov.uk/en/ContactUs/Complaints Procedures/index.htm

12 Department of Health (2000) *The NHS Plan: a Plan for Investment, a Plan for Reform*. Cm 4818-1. DH, London, www.nhs.uk/uk

13 Section 15(3) NHS Reform and Health Care Professions Act 2002.

14 The Local Involvement Networks Regulations S.I. 2008 No 528.

15 *R (on the application of Morris)* v. *Trafford Healthcare NHS Trust* [2006] EWHC 2334.

16 *R* v. *Canterbury and Thanet District Health Authority and South East Thames Regional Health Authority, ex parte F and W* (QBD) [1994] 5 Med LR 132.

17 Chartered Society of Physiotherapy (2005) *Strategy for 2005–10*. CSP, London.

15 Equipment and Medicinal Products

Physiotherapists use equipment in the treatment of patients and may also be involved in work relating to the assessment for, provision of, installation of and maintenance of equipment. The Chartered Society of Physiotherapy (CSP) has provided contract details and product overview for a number of rehabilitation equipment suppliers.[1] See also works by Michael Mandelstam.[2] The CSP has also provided guidance on the clinical use of electrophysical agents.[3] It covers relationships and advice to third parties, maintenance of equipment, competence to practise, contraindications, precautions, safety and application issues, and specific guidance on individual agents such as laser therapy, ultrasound and high-frequency therapy. Increasingly too, physiotherapists have been trained to become supplementary prescribers, and this chapter therefore covers the legal issues relating to prescribing.

No easy line can be drawn between the role of the occupational therapist and that of the physiotherapist in relation to the ordering, supply and maintenance of equipment. Different local authorities, Primary Care Trusts and NHS Trusts have worked in different ways and often these differences are historical rather than planned. What is essential is that there is clarity and consensus

between the different professional groups in each area as to who is responsible for what and that the appropriate training is provided.

This chapter covers the following topics:

- Legal rights against the supplier
- The Consumer Protection Act 1987
- Medicines and HealthCare Products Regulatory Agency and Medical Devices
- Maintenance of equipment
- Exemption from liability and written instructions
- Equipment as a resource
- Choice of equipment and instruction by physiotherapists
- Prescribing of medicinal products

Legal rights against supplier

Common law action in negligence

The law of negligence enables an action to be brought against the manufacture of a defective product if harm has been caused to a consumer or third person. This principle was established in the leading case of *Donoghue* v. *Stevenson*.[4] This form of action is discussed in detail in Chapter 10 on negligence. It should be noted that, in order to succeed, the claimant must establish:

- that there was a duty of care owed to the claimant;
- that there has been a breach of this duty of care;
- that as a reasonably foreseeable result of that breach of duty, harm has been caused.

Contractual action against supplier

The supplier is under a contractual duty to provide goods in accordance with the contract terms. In addition, where the purchaser is a private individual purchasing from a person in course of business, he or she can rely on the legal rights given under the Sales of Goods and Services legislation, which, by implying certain terms (e.g. that the goods are fit for the purpose for which they are sold) in such a contract, provides additional protection over and above that contained in the contract documents.

Where the purchaser is a large consortium or organisation in its own right, the fact that it could threaten to remove the contract to other suppliers may assist both in enabling the purchaser to have terms that give it protection written into the contract at the outset and in enforcing the performance of the contract terms without any recourse to legal action.

The Consumer Protection Act 1987

The parts of the Act are set out in Figure 15.1. Part I on product liability covers the sections shown in Figure 15.2.

The provisions of this Act are discussed in this chapter but reference should be made to other legal rights of action in Chapter 11 on health and safety.

Basis of the Act

The Consumer Protection Act 1987 (CPA) enables a claim to be brought where harm has occurred

Part I	Product liability
Part II	Consumer safety
Part III	Misleading price indications
Part IV	Enforcement of Parts II and III
Part V	Miscellaneous and supplemental

Figure 15.1 Consumer Protection Act 1987

Section 1	Purpose and construction of Part I
Section 2	Liability for defective products
Section 3	Meaning of defect
Section 4	Defences
Section 5	Damage giving rise to liability
Section 6	Application of certain enactments
Section 7	Prohibition on exclusions from liability
Section 8	Power to modify Part I
Section 9	Applications of Part I to the Crown

Figure 15.2 Product liability under the Consumer Protection Act 1987

as a result of a defect in a product. It was enacted as a result of the EC Directive No. 85/374/EEC. It is a form of strict liability in that negligence by the supplier or manufacturer does not have to be established. The claimant will, however, have to show that there was a defect. The supplier can rely upon a defence colloquially known as 'state of the art', i.e. that the state of scientific and technical knowledge at the time the goods were supplied was not such that the producer should have discovered the defect (see below).

A product is defined as meaning any goods or electricity and includes a product which is comprised in another product, whether by virtue of being a component part or raw material or otherwise.

Who is liable under the Consumer Protection Act?

The producer

Section 2(1) states that 'where any damage is caused wholly or partly by a defect in a product, every person to whom Section (2) below applies shall be liable for the damage.'

Section 2(2) includes the following as being liable:

- the producer of the product;
- any person who by putting his name on the product or using a trademark or other distinguishing mark, has held himself out to be the producer of the product; and
- any person who has imported the product into the EC in the course of business.

The supplier

In addition to producers or original importers as set out under Section 2(2), Section 2(3) provides that any person who has supplied the product to the person who suffered the damage or to any other person shall be liable for the damage, if:

- the person who suffered the damage requests the supplier to identify one or more of the

persons who were producers (as set out above);
- that request is made within a reasonable period after the damage occurs and at a time when it is not reasonably practicable for the person making the request to identify all those persons;
- the supplier fails, within a reasonable period after receiving the request, either to comply with the request or to identify the person who supplied the product to him.

This provision makes it essential for the physiotherapist to keep records of the manufacturer/supplier of any goods (including both equipment and drugs) that he/she provides for the client. In the absence of the physiotherapist being able to cite the name and address of the manufacturer or the company that supplied the goods to him/her, the physiotherapist may become the supplier of the goods for the purposes of the Act and therefore have to defend any action alleging that there was a defect in the goods which caused harm. Harm includes both personal injury and death and loss or damage of property.

Where a social services authority or health service body supplies equipment for use in the community then that body can become the supplier for the purposes of the CPA. If harm results from a defect in the equipment the appropriate supplier must provide the client with the name and address of the firm from which the equipment was obtained otherwise it will become itself liable for the defects. Records of the sources of equipment are therefore essential in order that clients can be given this information.

What is meant by a defect?

This is defined in the Act as set out in Figure 15.3.

Defences

Certain defences are available under Section 4 and are shown in Figure 15.4.

(1)   Subject to the following provisions of this section, there is a defect in a product for the purposes of [Part 1 of the Act] if the safety of the product is not such as persons generally are entitled to expect; and for those purposes 'safety', in relation to a product, shall include safety with respect to products comprised in that product and safety in the context of risks of damage to property, as well as in the context of risks of death or personal injury.

(2)   In determining . . . what persons generally are entitled to expect in relation to a product all the circumstances shall be taken into account, including:

(a)   the manner in which, and purposes for which, the product has been marketed, its get-up, the use of any mark in relation to the product and any instructions for, or warnings with respect to, doing or refraining from doing anything with or in relation to the product;

(b)   what might reasonably be expected to be done with or in relation to the product; and

(c)   the time when the product was supplied by its producer to another.

Figure 15.3   Definition of defect: Consumer Protection Act 1987: Section 3

(a)   that the defect is attributable to compliance with any requirement imposed by or under any enactment or with any Community obligation; or

(b)   that the person proceeded against did not at any time supply the product to another; or

(c)   that the following conditions are satisfied, that is to say:

(i)   that the only supply of the product to another by the person proceeded against was otherwise than in the course of a business of that person's; and

(ii)   that section 2(2) above [that the person is the producer or importer] does not apply to that person or applies to him by virtue only of things done otherwise than with a view to profit; or

(d)   that the defect did not exist in the product at the relevant time; or

(e)   that the state of scientific and technical knowledge at the relevant time was not such that a producer of products of the same description as the product in question might be expected to have discovered the defect if it had existed in his products while they were under his control; or

(f)   that the defect:

(i)   constituted a defect in a product ('the subsequent product') in which the product in question had been comprised; and

(ii)   was wholly attributable to the design of the subsequent product or to compliance by the producer of the product in question with instructions given by the producer of the subsequent product.

Figure 15.4   Defences under the Consumer Protection Act 1987: Section 4(1).

What damage must the claimant establish?

Compensation is payable for death, personal injury or any loss of or damage to any property (including land) (Section 5(1)). The loss or damage shall be regarded as having occurred at the earliest time at which a person with an interest in the property had knowledge of the material facts about the loss or damage (Section 5(5)). Knowledge is further defined in subsections 5(6) and (7).

There have been few examples of actions being brought under the CPA in healthcare cases and only a handful of cases brought under it have been reported. One reported in March 1993[5] led to Simon Garratt being awarded £1400 against the manufacturers of a pair of surgical scissors which broke during an operation on his knee, with the blade being left embedded. A second operation was required to remove it. Had he relied upon the law of negligence to obtain compensation he would have had to show that the manufacturers were in breach of the duty of care that they owed to him. Under the CPA he had to show the harm, the defect and the fact that it was produced by the defendant. In one of the few cases[6] involving hospital treatment, a claimant brought an action against manufacturers of an artificial hip that sheared in two beneath the femoral head close to the radial base of the spigot region of the stern. A further operation was required, which led to less movement and mobility. At the trial it was agreed that the prosthesis fractured as a result of fatigue failure initiating from a defect in the titanium alloy from which it was made. The defendants argued that there was no defect in the product when it left them, and that the defect occurred at the time of implantation. The trial judge found in favour of the defendants. The claimant's appeal failed.

The meaning of 'defect' in the CPA was considered by the Court of Appeal in a case brought against Tesco Stores.[7] In this case the trial judge had found Tesco and the manufacturer of the bottle to be in breach of the CPA in that the fitting on a bottle of dishwasher powder was not child-proof. The mother had left her child of 13 months while she went to answer the phone and found the child sitting in the kitchen with the powder on his lips and his head right back. The mother was not found to be negligent. The Court of Appeal unanimously held that the definition of defect in the Act as 'if the safety of the produce is not such as persons generally are entitled to expect' could not be interpreted to imply that every producer of a product warrants that the product fulfils its design standards. The public would expect that the bottle was more difficult to open than an ordinary screw top, though not so

difficult as if the British Standard had been met. A requirement to meet British Standards could not be read into the CPA. There was therefore no breach of the CPA. In contrast in another case[8] brought under the CPA and the common law of negligence the Court of Appeal unanimously dismissed an appeal against an award of damages of almost £40 000 to a boy who at 12 years old was injured in the eye by the buckle on elastic straps attached to Cosytoes, a fleece lined sleeping bag, which he was helping his mother attach to a pushchair. He lost the central vision of his left eye. The Court of Appeal held that there was a defect in the product because of the risk of the elasticised strap springing back into the eye. The defendants' argument that at the time the scientific and technical knowledge of the defect was not available did not succeed. The safety of the product was not such as persons generally are entitled to expect. There was however no finding of negligence at common law. In a claim for damages in relation to a defect in vaccination, the Court of Appeal unanimously dismissed an appeal against the trial judge's permitting the substitution of Smith-Kline Beecham in place of Merck as defendant even after the expiry of 10 years referred to in Section 11A(3).[9]

Since the client is not an employee, she cannot use the provisions of the Employer's Liability (Defective Equipment) Act 1969 (see Chapter 11).

Chartered Society of Physiotherapists guidance on consumer protection

Professional Affairs paper No. 4 gives guidance on equipment safety and product liability.[10] It emphasises the importance of:

- record keeping
- procedure sheets
- equipment inventory
- the labelling of equipment
- clear procedures covering loan and issue of equipment
- procedures for the servicing of equipment.

Defining responsibility

It is essential when equipment is first supplied that the responsibility for it and the rights of action, if any defect be discovered, should be clearly defined. This is discussed below.

Situation: dangerous nebuliser

An NHS Trust has nebulisers which are used for patients suffering from chronic chest conditions and are given out by the physiotherapists to patients for home use. Unfortunately, the patient suffered a severe electric shock when using the nebuliser and is seeking compensation from the NHS Trust.

In this situation the possible defendants are:

- The NHS Trust if its employees failed to purchase safe equipment or if its employees fitted the equipment negligently.
- The suppliers or manufacturers if there was a defect in the nebuliser. They could be liable under the CPA. However, if it were to be shown that the reuse of the nebuliser and its maintenance was at fault, then they might be able to show that because of this intervention the NHS Trust had become the supplier of the equipment.
- Any person who tampered with the nebuliser.

The causes for the nebuliser causing an electric shock would have to be investigated in order to establish responsibility.

Care services efficiency delivery

In June 2006 the then Prime Minister announced the launch of a Transforming Community Equipment and Wheelchair Services Programme as part of the Care Services Efficiency Delivery (CSED) Programme (see Chapter 18).The new system changed the way that equipment is provided with accredited retailers exchanging equipment for a prescription. The aim is to give state-supported users the choice that they have

not previously enjoyed. They also have the option of topping up existing prescriptions to a different product within the same functional range to suit the user's lifestyle or preference. Further information can be obtained from the CSED website[11] and from the Department of Health (DH) community equipment services' site.[12] The Wheelchair services programme has, at the time of writing not been established and further evidence is being collated. Details of the objectives and content of the programme can be found on the CSED website.

Medicines and Healthcare products Regulatory Agency and Medical Devices Agency

The Medical Devices Agency (MDA) was established to promote the safe and effective use of devices. It was absorbed into the Medicines and Heathcare Products Regulatory Agency (MHRA) in 2003. In particular, its role is to ensure that whenever a medical device is used it is:

- suitable for its intended purpose;
- properly understood by the professional user; and
- maintained in a safe and reliable condition.

The MHPRA is a government-appointed body that has an advisory role in drafting regulations and issues publications on specific matters, 'device bulletins' (DBs) and 'safety notices' (SNs).

What is a medical device?

Annex B to safety notice 9801[13] gives examples of medical devices. It covers the following:

- equipment used in the diagnosis or treatment of disease, monitoring of patients (e.g. syringes and needles, dressings, catheters, beds, mattresses and covers, physiotherapy equipment);
- equipment used in life support (e.g. ventilators, defibrillators);

- *in vitro* diagnostic medical devices and accessories (e.g. blood gas analysers) including *in vitro* diagnostic devices;
- equipment used in the care of disabled people (e.g. orthotic and prosthetic appliances, wheel-chairs and special support seating, patient hoists, walking aids, pressure sore prevention equipment);
- aids to daily living (e.g. hearing aids, commodes, urine drainage systems, domiciliary oxygen therapy systems, incontinence pads, prescribable footwear);
- equipment used by ambulance services, but not the vehicles themselves (e.g. stretchers and trolleys, resuscitators);

Other examples of medical devices include condoms, contact lenses and care products and intrauterine devices. Bed rails also come within the definition of medical devices and the Health and Safety Executive (HSE) has issued a circular on bed rail risk management.[14] Between 2001 and 2005 RIDDOR (Reporting of Injuries, Diseases and Dangerous Occurrences Regulations) identified 10 fatal accidents and a number of major injury incidents in which the use of bed rails was implicated. The HSE circular sets out the major problems, legal considerations and risk management stages and strategy.

Essential requirements

Regulations[15] require that from 14 June 1998 all medical devices placed on the market (and made available for use or distribution even if no charge is made) must conform to 'the essential requirements' including safety as required by law, and bear a CE (Conformité Européenne) marking as a sign of that conformity. Although most of the obligations contained in the Regulations fall on manufacturers, purchasers who are positioned further down the supply chain may also be liable – for example, for supplying equipment which does not bear a CE marking or which carries a marking liable to mislead people.[16] This marking is the requirement of the EC Directive on medical

devices.[17] The manufacturer who can demonstrate conformity with the regulations is entitled to apply the CE marking to a medical device.

The essential requirements include the general principles that:

- a device must not harm patients or users, and any risks must be outweighed by benefits;
- design and construction must be inherently safe and, if there are residual risks, users must be informed about them;
- devices must perform as claimed and not fail due to the stresses of normal use;
- transport and storage must not have adverse effects;

Essential requirements also include prerequisites in relation to:

- the design and construction
- infection and microbial contamination
- mechanical construction
- measuring devices
- exposure to radiation
- built-in computer systems
- electrical and electronic design
- mechanical design
- delivery of fluids to a patient
- the function of controls and indicators.

Excepted devices

Exceptions to these regulations include the following:

- active implants (covered by the Active Implantable Medical Devices Regulations[18]);
- devices made specially for the individual patient ('custom made');
- devices undergoing clinical investigation;
- devices made by the organisation ('legal entity') using them.

Implementation of the regulations

In January 1998 the MDA issued a device bulletin[19] giving guidance to organisations on

- Strategies for deploying, monitoring, and controlling devices
- Purchasing medical products
- When a device is delivered
- Prescription of devices
- Record keeping
- Maintenance and repair
- Training
- Community issues

Figure 15.5   Device bulletin of the Medical Devices Agency January 1998

implementing the regulations. The Bulletin covers the sections shown in Figure 15.5.

The Medical and Healthcare products Regulatory Agency (MHRA) (formerly the MDA) has powers under the Consumer Protection Act 1987 to issue warnings or remove devices from the market.

Devices are divided into three classes according to possible hazards, Class 2 being further subdivided. Thus:

Class 1 – low risk, e.g. a bandage
Class 2a – medium risk, e.g. a simple breast pump
Class 2b – medium risk, e.g. a ventilator
Class 3 – high risk, e.g. an intraortic balloon.

Any warning about equipment issued by the MHRA should be acted upon immediately. Notices from the Agency are sent to Regional General Managers, chief executives of health authorities and NHS Trusts, directors of social services, managers of independent healthcare units and rehabilitation service managers. Failure to ensure that these notices are obtained and acted upon could be used as evidence of failure to provide a reasonable standard of care.

Adverse incident reporting procedures

In 1998 the MDA issued a safety notice[20] requiring healthcare managers, healthcare and social care professionals and other users of medical devices to establish systems to encourage the prompt reporting of adverse incidents relating to medical devices to the MDA. The procedures should be regularly reviewed, updated as necessary, and should ensure that adverse incident reports are submitted to MDA in accordance with the notice. The notice was revised in 2007 and can be accessed via the MHRA website.[21]

What is an adverse incident?

The safety notice defines this as

an event which gives rise to, or has the potential to produce, unexpected or unwanted effects involving the safety of patients, users or other persons.

Such incidents may be caused by shortcomings in:

- the device itself
- instructions for use, servicing and maintenance
- locally initiated modifications or adjustments
- user practices including
  - training
  - management procedures
  - the environment in which it is used or stored or
  - incorrect prescription.

The incident is 'adverse' where it has led to or could have led to the following:

- death
- life-threatening illness or injury
- deterioration in health

- temporary or permanent impairment of a body function or damage to a body structure
- the necessity for medical or surgical intervention to prevent permanent impairment of a body function or permanent damage to a body structure
- unreliable test results leading to inappropriate diagnosis or therapy.

Minor faults or discrepancies should also be reported to the MHRA and there should be regular links with the website to keep up to date with their warnings. The MHRA publishes a list of one-liners: examples of reported hazards. The One-Liner issue in January 2008 gives examples of incidents where things have gone wrong because of user faults. For example, a medical air hose attached to an intensive care ventilator ruptured because the hose had been melted by the heat from a reading light placed next to the ventilator. Another example involving physiotherapy was where a portable examination couch collapsed and folded up during treatment, injuring the patient and the physiotherapist. The couch had been overloaded and had not been regularly maintained. An MHRA warning published in 2008[22] related to the fact that Beatle wheelchairs in front-wheel drive configuration have tipped when travelling on slopes. Amended instructions for users were to be distributed. Warnings were issued in 2007 about Invacare Action wheelchairs fitted with a manual ratchet recliner mechanism[23] and Invacare Action 2000 wheelchairs (blue frame).[24]

Liaison officers

Organisations should appoint a liaison officer who would have the necessary authority to:

- ensure that procedures are in place for the reporting of adverse incidents involving medical devices to the MHRA;
- act as the point of receipt for MHRA publications;
- ensure dissemination within their own organisation of MHRA publications; and

- act as the contact point between MHRA and their organisation.

Medical devices and the community

The MDA device bulletin published in January 1998[19] gives specific guidance on equipment used in the community. It suggests that the delivery and collection of equipment procedures should include checks that:

- the correct equipment has been delivered in good order;
- the end-user has received training; or
- the end-user has been told not to use the device until trained; and
- the delivery and collection process does not risk cross-contamination.

The guidance emphasises that good device management is the same for hospitals and the community. It covers in particular:

- delivery and commissioning of loan equipment;
- collection of equipment when no longer needed;
- checking and testing returned equipment;
- adaptation of equipment;
- insurance;
- device safety for medical and dental surgeries.

Specific guidance on sterilisers, dental X-ray equipment and resuscitators is also provided. For resuscitators it suggests that the best practice is for the equipment to be checked daily including the pressure in the oxygen cylinder, whether the bag is working, that any drugs are still in date, and that any sterile materials are in date and the packaging is undamaged.

Medical Devices Regulations 2002

Additional regulations[25] came into force on 13 June 2002 that cover (a) active implantable medical devices and accessories to such devices and (b) *in vitro* diagnostic medical devices and accessories to such devices. They can be accessed on the Office of Public Sector Information website.[26]

Maintenance of equipment

It follows that as a result of the regulations relating to medical devices there should be clear procedures over the maintenance and servicing of any equipment. Often when equipment is installed or handed out for use at home, there is no clarity over who has the responsibility for ensuring that the equipment is regularly checked and, if necessary, serviced or maintained. It is essential that there should be procedures to determine this responsibility when the equipment is first supplied. Some equipment must by law be regularly serviced, for example lifts. When this equipment is installed, an agreement for the future inspection and servicing of the lift should be arranged.

Responsibility for the maintenance would normally reside with the owner of the equipment. If the Primary Care Trust (PCT), NHS Trust or the social services authority remains the owner and the equipment is merely loaned to the client then the Trust/authority should set up an appropriate system for inspection and maintenance. This system should also take into account the avoidance of cross-infection.

Medical and Healthcare products Regulatory Agency guidance

The guidance issued by the MDA (prior to its incorporation within the MHRA)[19] suggests the use of a computer system to identify equipment in terms of:

- whether it is simple
- whether it requires:
  - assembly
  - fixing
  - that a prescribing professional be present
  - special instructions for the end-user

- the time and personnel needed to ensure successful and safe delivery, installation and end-user training.

Client-owned equipment

Where the equipment is transferred into the ownership of the client or clients purchase it themselves, then the client would usually be the one responsible for inspection and maintenance. However, the authority would have a responsibility to ensure that all the necessary information was passed on to the client. Account would also have to be taken of the physical and mental capacity of the client to undertake this responsibility. Since the NHS is based on the principle that services are supplied free at the point of delivery, unless there is specific statutory provision (as there is in the case of prescriptions), it would be unlawful for an NHS Trust to supply equipment on loan to a patient and then expect the patient to arrange to pay the maintenance costs. For example, nebulisers provided by an NHS physiotherapy department must be serviced and maintained by the NHS.

Once the responsibility for ensuring inspection and maintenance is defined, then liability should be clear in the event that harm result from a failure to inspect and/or maintain.

Failure to ensure that the equipment is in working order could lead to litigation if harm occurs to a patient.

Inventory

Each physiotherapy department should ensure that they keep a list of equipment that is given out for use in the community and that information is kept on the dates for servicing. There should also be a regular review to ensure that the equipment is still in use or whether it should be recalled. The inventory should have details of:

- nature of the equipment
- date issued

- name of patient
- name of physiotherapist
- item/s issued
- manufacturer/model/number
- labelling of equipment
- date of service.

Situation: old equipment

A physiotherapist obtained from a client's home equipment used in treating enuresis. Unknown to her this was a very old model. She reissued it without ensuring that it was checked by the electrical maintenance department and was horrified to hear that a child had been burnt as the result of a fault in the equipment.

In the above situation there has been clear negligence by the physiotherapist in reissuing the equipment. She should have ensured that it was checked over before the equipment was passed to another client. Her employer would be vicariously liable for her negligence.

Adaptation of equipment

If equipment is modified for the specific uses of the client, every care should be taken to ensure that it remains safe. The following situation is taken from the Bulletin issued by the MDA in January 1998.

Situation: adapting a wheelchair

A physiotherapist inadvertently destabilised a wheelchair by changing the frame structure to accommodate a reclined backrest angle without considering stability effects, or consulting the manufacturer.

In so doing, she would have affected the safety properties of the wheelchair, and thus probably invalidated the CE marking which the manufacturer placed on the wheelchair as a sign that it conformed to the essential requirement of the Medical Devices Regulations.

As a result of the physiotherapist's adaptation, her employers may also have become in law liable as a supplier under the Consumer Protection Act 1987 and subject to a claim should any harm befall the patient or another person.

Maintenance of hospital equipment

There is a danger that, in these days of increasing pressure on resources, some of the equipment used within physiotherapy departments is not systematically serviced and maintained and unacceptable risks are taken.

Situation: on the blink

A physiotherapist was aware that an alarm clock was not completely reliable. She had applied for a replacement but in its absence continued to make use of the old one. She set up a patient for ultra-violet treatment setting the alarm. She was then called by an assistant to help with another patient. She forgot about the first patient. When she remembered, she discovered that the alarm had not sounded and the patient had probably suffered serious harm.

One cannot imagine any possible defence being offered in the above situation. There is clearly negligence on the part of the physiotherapist and her employer will be vicariously liable for the harm.

Assistive Technology Centre

The MHRA has established an Assistive Technology Centre in Blackpool. Its purpose is to take all reasonable steps to protect the public health and safeguard the interests of users by ensuring that all assistive technology equipment meets the appropriate standards of safety, quality and performance and complies with the relevant directives of the EU. Assistive technology includes mobility aids such as wheelchairs, powered scooters, walking frames and artificial limbs; environmental controls such as personal alarm systems; speech and hearing aids; posture and pressure management; moving and handling systems (hoists, bath lifts) and aids to daily living. The Centre provides technical advice and testing facilities and also investigates adverse incidents. The Centre can be accessed via the MHRA website.

The European Commission launched a public consultation on proposals to revise the medical devices directive to which at the time of writing the MHRA is preparing a response. The deadline for responses was 2 July 2008.

Exemption from liability and written instructions

Effect of exemption notices

Some authorities use a form that is signed by the client to exempt themselves from liability should harm occur. An example of such a form is shown in Figure 15.6.

The notice in Figure 15.6 would *not* be effective in removing liability from the NHS Trust or social services department if one of their staff had been negligent in carrying out their duties and responsibilities. This is because the provisions of the Unfair Contract Terms Act prohibit evasion of liability for negligence if personal injury or death occurs as a result. If there has

been negligence then the notice will be of no effect (see Chapter 10).

Sometimes, however, the notice is not to exempt from liability but to instruct the client on the use of the equipment and to ensure the client will be safe. To provide this kind of written instruction may well be a duty. However, any attempt to use it as an exemption notice will not be effective if personal injury occurs.

An exemption notice may, however, be effective if loss or damage to property occurs (see Chapter 10).

The limitations of the disclaimer notice must be noted. It cannot relieve the physiotherapist if he/she has been at fault. However, if he/she has taken all reasonable care, it could act as a reminder to the client that the advice must be followed and that failure to follow the advice will absolve the physiotherapist and his/her employer from liability for any harm that follows in consequence. The notice is not so much a disclaimer as a reminder of the effects of contributory negligence (see Glossary and Chapter 10).

Use of specialist equipment by a non-client

The same principles apply if it is feared that the equipment would be used by someone other than the client.

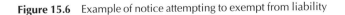

I . . . acknowledge that the following equipment has been provided to me by the . . . NHS Trust

(1)   . . .

(2)   . . .

(3)   . . .

and I agree to be responsible for the installation and maintenance of this equipment and not to hold the . . . NHS Trust liable for any loss, harm or injury caused by the said equipment.

Signature:

Witness:

Date:

Figure 15.6   Example of notice attempting to exempt from liability

Situation: loaning out equipment by the client

Walking aids were provided for the client who allowed a friend to use them. The friend suffered harm whilst using these aids when they broke under her weight. Is the physiotherapist liable?

If written instructions had been given when the equipment was delivered that the equipment should not be used by anyone else, then the NHS Trust should not be liable for that other person's harm, if the equipment was safe for the client. Again the written instructions act not as a disclaimer, but as information about the correct use of the equipment. If the physiotherapist has given all the necessary information and instruction according to the Bolam test, neither the physiotherapist nor his/her employer should be found liable in negligence.

Failure by the client to follow instructions

The same principles would apply where the client fails to follow instructions: the physiotherapist should not be regarded as negligent if he/she has used all reasonable care in instructing the client and warning of the dangers of ignoring this advice. However, the physiotherapist must take account of any disabilities of the client in giving this advice and in some situations would have to explain to a carer how the equipment should be used. Physiotherapists may say that they have no time to put instructions to the client or carer in writing but if this could be done it could prevent a lot of wasted time, make the instructions clearer for client and carer and also give them a document to which they could refer. In addition, of course, in the event of any dispute over what instructions were given, the physiotherapist could refer to the document.

Equipment as a resource

Determining priorities

Given the limitation on resources it is inevitable that there is often a waiting list for equipment for home use. Even if the equipment is available there might still be a delay in arranging installation. This is a major concern to those who have recommended equipment since there may be liability if harm should occur while the client is waiting for the equipment.

However, the determination of priorities is part of the duty of care owed by the professional to the client. If a professional fails to assess the urgency of a client's need for equipment and harm befalls the client, then there is likely to be an investigation as to the priority which had been attached to that client's needs in comparison with the needs of others.

In the case of *Deacon* v. *McVicar*[27] the judge ordered the disclosure of the records of the other patients on the ward at the same time as the claimant (formerly plaintiff) patient in order to assess whether sufficient regard had been given to the needs of the claimant patient in comparison with the needs of the other patients on the ward at the same time. This is an unusual step but it indicates that the determination of priorities is a legal duty and can be evidenced from the records.

Client demands

- When can a physiotherapist refuse to supply equipment or equipment of the patient's choice?

Often there may be no clinical need for the patient to have specific equipment, or equipment of the standard insisted upon by the patient. For example, the patient may request a more sophisticated walking aid (such as a shop trolley). The physiotherapist has to be responsible in the allocation of resources and providing a more sophisticated item for one patient may mean that the resources are not available for others. Similar problems arise with temporary residents, are they entitled to receive the equipment necessary for their short stay? The answer depends on all the circumstances. If the equipment is available and the duration short, then it might be reasonable to provide a temporary resident with the equipment. However, the costly installation of equipment may not be justified.

Some equipment is lent for the short term, but thereafter patients are expected to purchase it themselves, for example TENS (transcutaneous electrical nerve stimulation) machines.

If the equipment is properly described as medical equipment, provided under the NHS, then there will probably be a duty to provide this both in the short term and the long term since facilities under the NHS are free at the point of delivery, unless there is statutory provision for charging (e.g. prescriptions).

Where decisions have to be made over the priority in the allocation of equipment the physiotherapist should ensure that reasonable defensible decisions are made and are clearly recorded. The physiotherapist can never be compelled by a patient to provide equipment that is contrary to his/her professional judgment of the patients' needs. This principle established in relation to medical treatment was stated by the Court of Appeal in the case of *Burke* v. *General Medical Council*[28] (see Chapter 6).

Refusal of patient to return equipment

Where property is loaned to a patient there is a duty upon the patient or carer to return the equipment when there is no longer a medical need, e.g. after the death of the patient. It should be made clear when the equipment is initially supplied that it is only on loan, that it must be returned on any request by the hospital and that good care must be taken of it. This should also be put in writing. If the patient refuses to return the equipment legal proceedings could in theory be taken, although in practice the cost of such a step

is unlikely to be justified. If possible the equipment should be labelled as hospital equipment and speedy collection of the equipment when it is no longer needed should prevent it being passed on to friends, jumble sales or to a charity. Cooperation with community nursing services over what equipment has been supplied and the duty to retrieve it following a death should make it easier to recover the equipment. It may be worthwhile to have an amnesty day every so often, when the local residents are invited to return property to the hospital on a 'no questions asked' basis.

Responsibility for damage to the equipment

Who is responsible if equipment is loaned to a patient and is damaged? Normally, if there is no evidence of deliberate damage, the hospital would not pursue any claim against the patient. If however the equipment is deliberately broken or misused, or even damaged through carelessness, the NHS Trust as the owner of the equipment has a theoretical legal right against the bailee (see Glossary) of the equipment since it was loaned on the understanding that care would be taken. However, again it is unlikely that any hospital would wish to pursue this legal right except in extreme circumstances.

Insurance cover

At the same time that responsibility for the inspection and servicing of the equipment is decided, the liability for providing insurance cover should be agreed where this is deemed necessary. It may be that the NHS Trust or local authority has its own group policy for insurance cover that can be used to protect an individual client. It may be that the client is covered by his or her own house or personal insurance cover. The physiotherapist should ensure that this question is raised and answered. The MDA Bulletin points out that

Equipment loaned by the NHS or social services departments normally remains the property of those statutory services and users cannot be required to insure it. However where end-users are using equipment in public places (e.g. powered wheelchairs) it may be advisable for them to consider third party insurance against personal liability in case of accident.[19,29]

A survey carried out by the NHS executive between January and April 1998 concluded that over £55 million a year was being spent on commercial insurance premiums by NHS Trusts. This led to two schemes for non-clinical risks being set up under the NHS Litigation Authority (NHSLA): liabilities to third parties (LTPS) and property expenses scheme (PES). Both schemes commenced in April 1999, can be joined by NHS bodies and are known collectively as Risk Pooling Schemes for Trusts (RPST). The LTPS covers employers' liability claims from slips and trips in the work place to serious manual handling, bullying and stress claims. It also covers public and products liability claims, from personal injuries sustained by visitors to NHS premises to claims arising from breaches of the Human Rights Act, Data Protection Act and Defective Premises Act. Cover is also provided for defamation, professional negligence by employees and liabilities of directors. PES provides cover for 'first party' losses such as theft or damage to property. Further information on the two schemes can be found on the NHSLA website[30] together with details of the reporting criteria, the fees and the excesses.

Choice of equipment and instruction by physiotherapists

The physiotherapist has to make a determination of the nature of the equipment required by the client, the supplier and any other features in relation to the individual circumstances and physical and mental capabilities of the client. The individual circumstances will also require consideration of the carers and their capacities. Alternatives other than the provision of equipment are also important. For example, it may be that there is a danger in the client making use of the equipment on his/her own and additional visits by community staff are necessary instead. Even simple equipment such as a walking or support stick has to be prescribed and chosen with full professional judgment. It is important for a physiotherapist to ensure that the records show the reason for the non-traditional choice of aids, since it is likely that if litigation were to be brought several years later, when the memory of the reasons for the choice has gone, it may still seem a 'wrong' decision and therefore appear indefensible when in fact it was fully justified.

Failures by the physiotherapist in selecting equipment that no reasonable therapist would have selected for a specific client could lead to liability if harm is incurred. In addition, the physiotherapist must be aware of the cost implications of the equipment which he/she is recommending and have access to a value for money audit which is kept up to date. The physiotherapist can refer to the Assistive Technology Centre discussed above for technical advice and testing.

Situation: choice of walking frame

A physiotherapist recommends that a disabled person should be supplied with a particular walking frame. However, she failed to take into account the nature of the flooring in the house. The patient slips while using the frame at home. Who is responsible for the accident?

If the patient can show that any reasonable physiotherapist would not have provided that particular type of frame, then there is evidence of negligence by the physiotherapist. It may be however that the accident was not caused by the type of frame but there were inherent defects within the frame, in which case the patient may have a case under the Consumer Protection Act 1987.

Wheelchairs

The NHS wheelchair service

The NHS wheelchair services are run by local health authorities which are responsible for allocating funds to the wheelchair service and PCTs who provide the service. This may include contracting out the running of the service to an outside company. Eligibility criteria, the time-scales of provision and the types of chair offered vary between different areas. Four types of powered wheelchair are offered because a user cannot propel or use a manual wheelchair: electric indoor chair (user controlled); electric outdoor chair (attendant controlled); electrically powered indoor/outdoor chair (user controlled); and dual purpose chair – user controlled indoors, attendant controlled outdoors. Further information on the service, referrals, assessments, maintenance and repairs can be obtained from the direct government website.[31] Information on the voucher schemes for hiring or buying a wheelchair is available from the same site, which considers other options for obtaining a wheelchair. A new wheelchair service for Wales was announced in 2002 and information on it provided by the CSP Wales.[32]

Safety of wheelchairs

Many warnings have been issued by the MHRA in relation to wheelchairs – some have been noted above. A MHRA warning issued in 2005[33] noted that an incorrectly fitted or adjusted posture belt attached to a wheelchair can lead to death or serious injury to a wheelchair user. Were a physiotherapist to act in ignorance of these warning notices and harm were to be caused to a client or the person, there would be a prima facie case of negligence. If death occurred there could be criminal prosecution for manslaughter. There would also be disciplinary action by an employer and possibly fitness to practice proceedings before the Health Professions Council. The MHRA issued guidelines on wheelchair stability in 2004,[34] which

were followed by discussions with manufacturers to produce a simplified set of guidelines. These are available from the MHRA website.[35]

Instruction by physiotherapist

Many items of equipment will require instruction from the physiotherapist before the patient is able to use it safely. The physiotherapist should provide a reasonable standard of care in giving this instruction, where possible providing a written leaflet for the patient. (Reference should be made to Chapter 27 on the liability that can arise from instructing others. See also Chapter 10 on negligence.)

Refusal by client to use hoist

It may be that a hoist has been provided to reduce the risk in manual handling, but the client or carer refuses to use it. The physiotherapist can show them the reasons why a hoist is advisable and give them clear instructions in its use, but cannot prevent their ignoring such advice and instructions when they are on their own. The Trust would not be liable for any harm which client or carer thereby incurs. However, the client could not refuse to use a hoist if healthcare support workers or other health professionals were in attendance. Their health and safety should not be endangered by the refusal of the client and the client might have to be warned that it may not be possible to provide the service required if the health and safety of employees is put at risk. A court case[36] where the clients claimed that they had a human right not to be hoisted is considered in Chapter 11.

Rehabilitation Supplies and Services Association

The Rehabilitation Supplies and Services Association (RSSA) was a trade association for manufacturers, distributors and maintainers of 'active' (electrical and mechanical) rehabilitation equipment.[37] It was formed in response to the needs of the Organisation of Chartered Physiotherapists in Private Practice (OCPPP) (now Physio First), which wished to compile a list of 'approved suppliers' for its accredited members. It set basic minimum operating standards to which its members had to work in order to remain in the association. There were three categories of membership: sales, manufacture and service.

If a complaint was alleged against an RSSA member it could be made to the RSSA, which would consider the complaint, offering an independent point of view and the chance to mediate a satisfactory conclusion. If the complaint was upheld and the RSSA member failed to meet its obligations then it risked being removed from the register of members. The work of the RSSA is now largely covered by the MHRA and Assistive Technology Centre and the CE conformity marking standards.

Keeping up to date

All specialisms throughout the wide scope of physiotherapy practice are required by their professional rules of conduct and by the duty of care that they owe to their clients in the law of negligence to ensure that they keep up to date in relation to the developments within equipment and technology.

Professional warnings

Physiotherapists have a professional duty to be aware of any information that can affect their safe practice. The physiotherapist must be alert to any warnings issued by the MHRA and must in turn ensure that he/she completes the appropriate forms to feed back any dangers or hazards which come to her attention. The physiotherapist must also be aware of warnings issued by the CSP.

Community equipment services

The prime minister launched the transforming community equipment and wheelchair services (TCEWS) programme in June 2006. The aim of the programme was to develop a new model for community equipment and wheelchair services in England and to look at how to make the best use of the strengths of the third and private sector. The model is not mandatory but it effectively demonstrates a way to deliver a personalised service, for both self-funders and those supported by the state. Further information can be obtained from the DH website.[38]

Physiotherapist and medicinal products

The prescribing, dispensing and administration of medicinal products has been closely controlled by law. The principle laws are the Medicines Act 1968 and the Misuse of Drugs Act 1971 and regulations made under both Acts. Medicines are grouped in the following categories:

(1) *Pharmacy-only products*, (P) i.e. these can be sold or supplied retail only by someone conducting a retail pharmacy business when the product must be sold from a registered pharmacy by or under the supervision of a pharmacist.

(2) *General sales list*, (GSL) i.e. medicinal products that may be sold other than from a retail pharmacy, as long as provisions relating to Section 53 of the Medicines Act are complied with, i.e. the place of sale must be the premises where the business is carried out; they must be capable of excluding the public; the medicines must have been made up elsewhere and the contents must not have been opened since make-up.

(3) *Prescription-only list*, POM) i.e. these medicines are available only on prescription drawn up by an appropriate practitioner. Schedule 1 of the subsequent regulations lists the prescription-only products and Part II of the schedule lists the prescription-only

products that are covered by the Misuse of Drugs Act.

The next paragraphs set out the history of the extension of the prescribing, supply and administering of medicines to other professions. Physiotherapists are now able to prescribe medicines if they are supplementary prescribers. They have not yet achieved the status of being independent prescribers. They are able to supply and administer medicines under patient-specific directions (see below) and patient group directions (see below)

Groups protocols or patient group directions and patient-specific directions

There has over the last 20 years been an extension of prescribing powers from registered medical practitioners to other health professionals. Community nurses were the first group to be given the legal powers to prescribe certain medicines and medicinal products in the community. In hospitals, patient group directions (PGDs) or group protocols were being used to enable other professionals to prescribe medication for patients who had not been seen by a doctor. The Crown Committee was set up to consider the regulation of the prescribing of medicines. It first considered the arrangements for and legality of group protocols and reported in March 1998 and recommended legislation to ensure that their legal validity was clarified. It was followed by new regulations that came into force on 9 August 2000.[39] These provided for patient group directions to be drawn up to make provision for the sale or supply of a prescription-only medicine in hospitals in accordance with the written direction of a doctor or dentist or other independent prescriber. To be lawful, the patient group direction must cover the particulars that are set out in Part I of Schedule 7 of the Statutory Instrument. These particulars are shown in Figure 15.7. It will be noted from Figure 15.7 that a registered physiotherapist may be one of the professions recognised as able to prescribe under a specific or group patient

direction, if the other conditions set out in Figure 15.7 are satisfied.

Mixing of medicines in physiotherapy practice

The CSP has issued a position paper[40] warning that the MHRA has advised that the mixing of two licensed medicines such as a local anaesthetic and a corticosteroid constitutes 'manufacture' of a new unlicensed product and therefore cannot be subsequently administered under a PGD. Mixing is only allowed where one substance is an inert vehicle for the other, such as saline or water. This ruling does not apply where the physiotherapist is a supplementary prescriber working within a Clinical Management Plan (see below). Nor does it apply to Patient Specific Directions.

The CSP points out:

> It is however possible for a physiotherapist to administer mixed medicines under a Patient Specific Direction (PSD) for a named patient in accordance with a director's directions. In these situations, the administration is on the doctor's direct responsibility.

Clearly, however, if the physiotherapist has any reasonable doubts about the correctness and appropriateness of the PSD, he/she should check out the instructions with a pharmacist or senior doctor, rather than rely on the prescribing doctor's instructions.

The CSP also points out that since the supply and administration of medicines under a PGD cannot be delegated and the physiotherapist actually administering the injection of the patient must be named on the PGD, it follows that in a training situation, both the trainee injector and the supervisor must both be named on the PGD document. (At the time of writing the CSP is revising this document.)

Independent and supplementary prescribing

Following its report on PGDs, the Crown Committee considered the overall regulation of

Particulars for validity of a patient group direction:

- Period during which the direction shall have effect
- Description or class of prescription-only medicines to which the direction relates
- Whether there are any restrictions on the quantity of medicine which may be supplied on any one occasion and, if so, what restrictions
- Clinical situations that prescription-only medicines of that description or class may be used to treat
- Clinical criteria under which a person shall be eligible for treatment
- Whether any class of person is excluded from treatment under the direction and, if so, what class of person
- Whether there are circumstances in which further advice should be sought from a doctor or dentist and, if so, what circumstances
- Pharmaceutical form or forms in which prescription-only medicines of that description or class are to be administered
- Strength, or maximum strength, at which prescription-only medicines of that description or class are to be administered
- Applicable dosage or maximum dosage
- Route of administration
- Frequency of administration
- Any minimum or maximum period of administration applicable to prescription-only medicines of that description or class
- Whether there are any relevant warnings to note and, if so, what warnings
- Whether there is any follow-up action to be taken in any circumstances and, if so, what action and in what circumstances
- Arrangements for referral for medical advice
- Details of the records to be kept of the supply or the administration of medicines under the direction

The classes of individuals by whom supplies may be made are set out in Part III of Schedule 7 and include the following:

- ambulance paramedics (who are registered or hold a certificate of proficiency)
- pharmacists
- registered health visitors
- registered midwives
- registered nurses
- registered ophthalmic opticians
- state registered chiropodists
- state registered orthoptists
- state registered physiotherapists
- state registered radiographers

The person who is to supply or administer the medicine must be designated in writing on behalf of the authorising person (see below) for the purpose of the patient group direction. In addition to compliance with the particulars set out above, a patient group direction must be signed on behalf of the authorising person. This is defined as the Common Services Agency, the (special) health authority, the NHS trust or primary care trust. The Department of Health has developed PGDs for certain chemical and biological countermeasures in emergency situations, such as atropine and these can be downloaded from its website.[50] The Royal Pharmaceutical Society of Great Britain published in September 2007 a resource pack for pharmacists on patient group directions which would also be of interest to registered physiotherapists.

Figure 15.7   Regulations on group protocols or patient group directions

independent and supplementary prescribing. Its final report was published in 1999[41] and it was followed by Health and Social Care Act 2001, which amended Section 58 of the Medicines Act 1968 to enable new registered professional groups to be designated by order for the purpose of prescribing medicines for human use. Physiotherapists are not yet specified as independent prescribers but they are recognised as supplementary prescribers under Regulations which amend the Medicines Act 1968. In April 2002[42] the DH announced its intention of introducing supplementary prescribing by a nurse or pharmacist in 2003. The aim was to enable pharmacists and nurses to work in partnership with doctors and help treat such conditions as asthma, diabetes, high blood pressure and arthritis. The doctor would draw up a plan with the patient's agreement, laying out the range of medicines that may be prescribed and when to refer back to the doctor. This early announcement was followed by a press release in November 2002,[43] which gave further details of the patient conditions and the medicinal products that would be the subject of supplementary prescribing. In April 2005 chiropodists and podiatrists, physiotherapists and radiographers were added to the list of those who could become supplementary prescribers and restrictions on their prescribing controlled drugs or unlicensed medicines were removed.[44] The supplementary prescriber works within a clinical management plan (CMP) agreed with the independent prescriber. Physiotherapists have not yet been recognised in law as being eligible to become independent prescribers, where they are clinically responsible for the overall care of the patient and can prescribe without reference to another clinician.

In 2007 the HPC published changes to the approval process that education providers have to complete before a standalone POM programme is approved by the HPC.[45]

Implications for physiotherapists

The power to prescribe has developed the scope of professional practice of the physiotherapist

and at the same time opened up new challenges. As with direct access of the patient to the physiotherapist or self-referral considered in Chapter 4, it is essential to identify the boundaries within which the physiotherapist can safely and competently practice. An Information paper *Prescribing rights for Physiotherapists: an Update*[46] gave details of the Medicines Act 1968, the Cumberlege Report on Community Nursing (1989), and the Crown report (1999) and HSC 2000/026 (England only) WHC 2000/16 (Wales only) Patient group directions in England and Wales.[47] It identified the benefits to the patient and noted that the extension of prescribing rights will facilitate the transfer of models of physiotherapy service delivery across into other specialties.

At the time of writing this CSP paper has been withdrawn from publication pending its revision.

Bhanu Ramaswamy in a personal account of experience with supplementary prescribing provides guidance for other physiotherapists who would like to become supplementary prescribers.[48] The DH has provided guidance on prescribing, supply and administration of medicines.[49] Reference should be made to Chapter 4 and the discussion of the scope of professional practice.

Areas where supplementary prescribing by physiotherapists is already making its mark include respiratory care and rheumatology, and PGDs are being used in oncology and palliative care (hosiery is a prescribed item), neurology (antispasmodic drugs) burns and plastics (specific dressings and pain relief)). Eventually there is every likelihood that physiotherapists will be given the legal powers to become independent prescribers in certain specialties.

Standard of care for physiotherapists who are not supplementary prescribers

What are the implications of physiotherapy prescribing on the standard of care for those physiotherapists who are not recognised prescribers? Does the fact that a physiotherapist can now become a supplementary prescriber have an impact upon the basic role of the physiotherapist? For example, in taking a patient's history including the medicines, would a physiotherapist be expected to be able to identify any medicinal errors, e.g. wrong doses, likely drug interactions, etc.? Certainly this knowledge would be acquired by a physiotherapist who learnt to prescribe and therefore failure to recognise a significant error could be seen as negligent practice by a supplementary prescriber. However, if this knowledge is not considered to to be part of the basic understanding of the responsible physiotherapist following accepted approved practice, then there would probably be no liability. A decided case is necessary to determine the issue (I am grateful to Martin Hey for raising this concern).

Legal responsibilities of the supplementary prescriber

A physiotherapist is legally responsible for any harm that has been caused by his/her negligence in prescribing a medicine as a supplementary prescriber. The physiotherapist could face fitness to practice proceedings, criminal proceedings, if the patient has died or suffered, and disciplinary action. The physiotherapist would also have to give evidence in any civil litigation brought by the patient or his/her family if the patient has died against the employer who is vicariously liable for the negligence of the employee. It is essential that the physiotherapist works within the parameters of the powers delegated to him/her, that any concerns or doubts he/she has about the patient or the medicine, should be checked with the clinician identified as the independent prescriber and/or the pharmacist. If the patient asks the physiotherapist's advice about medicines, then it is essential that the physiotherapist remains within the scope of their competence. They may for example be able to suggest a medication that is available on the General Sales List (GSL) but only if they are aware of any other medications that the patient may be taking and from their knowledge and

training are sure that there are no contraindications. Nor should they advise a patient to stop or change any medication recommended by a doctor unless that advice is clearly within the scope of his/her knowledge and competence as a supplementary prescriber or the doctor has been consulted. The CSP Practice and Development Unit provides advice and guidance to members including concerns over medicines.

Can a physiotherapist in private practice sell GSL medicines?

Medicines which can be sold over the counter in any retail establishment, corner shop or supermarket could be sold by a physiotherapist in private practice, provided of course, that he/she conforms to the requirements set out in Section 53 of the Medicines Act (see above) and he/she complies with the Trade Descriptions Act and does not hold out him/herself as being able to give pharmaceutical advice. The physiotherapist must take care where he/she is treating the patient, that he/she follows the reasonable practice expected of a physiotherapist in supplying any medicines on the general sales list. It would be illegal for the physiotherapist to sell medicines which are pharmacy-only products.

Conclusions

Liability for the supply of equipment that causes harm has been clarified over recent years and the work of the MHRA makes clear the legal responsibilities of the physiotherapist. To keep up to date with technical developments in equipment and medicinal products is becoming a heavy burden for physiotherapists, but specialisation and clear allocation of responsibilities should ensure that the physiotherapist is supported in keeping up to date within his/her own specialist area and that the client is safe. The impact of devolution within the UK can be seen in the area of medicines and prescribing. Prescription charges of £7.10 per medicinal product are still being levied in England but were abolished in Wales in April 2007 and in Scotland the cost is reduced to £5 and all charges are to be removed by 2011. In Northern Ireland charges have been frozen for the time being. Divergences also exist in the area of independent and supplementary prescribing.

✎⟍ Questions and exercises

1 Review the procedure you follow in choosing equipment for a client.
2 Draw up a leaflet to give to the client about the supply of equipment in the home, and which covers instruction on use, maintenance, insurance and any other aspects you consider necessary.
3 A client is considering bringing a claim against manufacturers because of faulty equipment. What advice could you give her about her rights?
4 Your manager has asked if you would be prepared to become a supplementary prescriber. What are the implications of such a request?

Acknowledgement

I would like to acknowledge my gratitude for the assistance of Pip White, Professional Adviser CSP, in the section Physiotherapist and medicinal products.

References

1 Chartered Society of Physiotherapy (2005) *Rehabilitation Equipment Suppliers*, 2nd edn. CSP, London.
2 Mandelsam, M. (1996) *Equipment for Older or Disabled People and the Law.* Jessica Kingsley Publishers, London
3 Chartered Society of Physiotherapy (2006) *Guidance for the Clinical use of Electrophysical Agents.* CSP, London
4 *Donoghue* v. *Stevenson* [1932] AC 562.
5 Dimond, B.C. (1993) Protecting the Consumer. *Nursing Standard* **7**, 24, 18–19.
6 *Piper* v. *JRI (Manufacturing) Ltd* [2006] EWCA Civ 1344.
7 *Tesco Stores Ltd and another* v. *CFP (a minor by his litigation friend) and LAP* [2006] EWCA Civ 393.
8 *Abouzaid* v. *Mothercare (UK) Ltd* [2006] EWCA Civ 348.
9 *Smithkline Beecham* v. *Horne Roberts* [2001] EWCA Civ 2006.
10 CSP Professional Affairs Department (1996) No. PA 4. *Equipment Safety & Product Liability.* CSP, London.
11 www.csed.csip.org.uk/workstreams/transforming-community
12 www.dh.gov.uk/en/SocialCare/Socialcarereform
13 Medical Devices Agency (January 1998) SN 9801. *Reporting Adverse Incidents Relating to Medical Devices.* MDA, London.
14 www.hse.gov.uk/lau
15 Medical Devices Regulations 1994 SI No. 3017 of 1994 (came into force 1 January 1995; mandatory from 14 June 1998) Directive 93/42/EEC.
16 Medical Devices Agency (1998) DB 9801. *Medical Device and Equipment Management for Hospital and Community-based Organisations.* MDA, London.
17 Directive 93/42/EEC (concerning medical devices).
18 Directive 90/385/EEC (came into force 1 January 1993 and is mandatory from 1 January 1995).
19 Medical Devices Agency (January 1998) DB 9801 *Medical Device and Equipment Management for Hospital and Community-based Organisations.* MDA, London.
20 Medical Devices Agency (January 1998) SN 9801 *Reporting Adverse Incidents Relating to Medical Devices.* MDA, London.
21 MHRA (2007) *Reporting Medical Device Adverse Incidents and Disseminating Medical Device Alerts* MDA/2007/001. Available from www.mhra.gov.uk
22 Medical Healthcare Products Regulatory Agency MDA/2008/029 Beatle and Puma Battery powered wheelchairs manufactured by Movingpeople.net.
23 MDA/2007/075.
24 MDA/2007/074.
25 Consumer Protection Medical Devices Regulations SI 2002 No 618.
26 www.opsi.gov.uk/legislation

27 *Deacon* v. *McVicar and Another* (QBD) 7 January 1984, Lexis transcript.

28 *R (on the application of Burke)* v. *General Medical Council and Disability Rights Commission and Official Solicitor to the Supreme Court* [2004] EWHC 1879; [2004] Lloyd's Rep. Med 451; [2005] EWCA Civ 1003, 28 July 2005.

29 See also HSG(96)34 Powered indoor/outdoor Wheelchairs for severely disabled people.

30 www.nhsla.com/Claims/Schemes/RPST

31 www.direct.gov.uk/en/DisabledPeople/HealthAndSupport/Equipment.

32 CSP Wales 1st Floor Transport House 1 Cathedral Road Cardiff CF11 9SD, 02920 382 429.

33 MDA/2005/025 Posture belts fitted to wheelchairs and seating.

34 Medicines and Healthcare Products Regulatory Agency (2004) Stability of Wheelchairs DB 2004 (02).

35 www.mhra.gov.uk/Publications/Safetyguidance

36 *R (on the application of A and B, X and Y)* v. *East Sussex County Council (The Disability Rights Commission: an interested party)* Case No. CO/4843/2001 10 February 2003.

37 *In Touch* (1996/7) **82**, Winter, 29.

38 www.dh.gov.uk/en/SocialCare/Socialcarereform

39 Prescription-Only Medicines (Human Use) Amendment Order 2000 SI 2000 No. 1917.

40 Chartered Society for Physiotherapy (2008) *Position Paper on the Mixing of Medicines in Physiotherapy*. CSP, London.

41 Department of Health, Review of Prescribing, Supply and Administration of Medicines Final Report (Crown Report), Department of Health, London, March 1999.

42 Department of Health press release 2002/0189, Groundbreaking new consultation aims to extend prescribing powers for pharmacists and nurses, 16 April 2002.

43 Department of Health press release 2002/0488, Pharmacists to prescribe for the first time. Nurses will prescribe for chronic illness, 21 November 2002.

44 The National Health Service (Primary Medical Services) Miscellaneous Amendments) Regulations SI 2005 No 893; The Medicines for Human Use (Prescribing) Order SI 2005 No 765.

45 www.hpc-uk.org/aboutregistration/educationandtraining/pom

46 Chartered Society of Physiotherapy (2005) Information paper PA 58. *Prescribing Rights for Physiotherapists an Update*. CSP London.

47 Department of Health Patient group directions HSC 2000/026 (England) WHC 2000/16 (Wales).

48 Ramaswamy, B. (2006) An Experience of Supplementary Prescribing. *Agility* **2**, 9–10.

49 Department of Health (2006) *Medicines Matters: A Guide to Mechanisms for the Prescribing, Supply and Administration of Medicines*. DH, London.

50 www.dh.gov.uk

16 Transport Issues

Since many physiotherapists are required to drive a car as part of their duties and many legal problems can arise, devoting an entire chapter to this topic is justified. Issues relating to driving by disabled persons will also be considered. Concerns centre on the following areas:

- What is permitted in the course of employment
- Transporting other people and equipment
- Insurance issues
- Crown cars and lease cars
- Employer's responsibilities on transport and insurance
- Tax situation and private mileage
- Driving by disabled people

What is permitted in the course of employment

In Chapter 10 on negligence it was noted that an employer is only vicariously liable for the acts of the employee if the employee was acting in the course of employment. Many community professionals transport others as part of their work – clients, carers, colleagues and others.

Where this is clearly indicated in the job description then the employer would have to accept that it is vicariously liable for any harm caused by the employee while driving in the course of employment. The employee, if driving his/her own car, would have to ensure that all the necessary measures in terms of appropriate insurance cover have been taken.

Acting in the course of employment would cover all those journeys between the hospital, social services and clients' homes, but it would not necessarily cover the physiotherapist deviating from the route and going to a supermarket to do his/her shopping. This may be described in legal terms as 'a frolic of his/her own' and the employer is not vicariously liable for any harm that occurs during such a ride. However, this is subject to the implications of the decision by the House of Lords where it held that a Board of Governors was vicariously liable for the sexual assaults committed by a warden upon pupils since they were committed in the course of employment.[1] (See Chapter 10).

Giving lifts

It may be however that an employee is forbidden to give lifts to others and yet disobeys these instructions.

Situation: giving lifts

> A physiotherapist is aware that she is not permitted within her job description to give lifts to others. She visits an isolated cottage where the GP has called and left a prescription which the client has not been able to take to a chemist. She realises that the client has no transport and offers to take a carer to the chemist's shop and return with the medication. On the return journey she is involved in an accident. Her insurance company claims that it should not be liable for the injury to the passenger since she had not notified it that she took passengers as part of her job. Her employers claim that she was not acting in course of employment since she was forbidden to transport persons other than clients and she was employed as a physiotherapist not a chauffeur.

The fact that she was forbidden to take passengers will not necessarily take her actions outside the definition of 'in the course of employment' (see Chapter 10). However, she is likely to face disciplinary proceedings. In contrast, if she picked up hitch-hikers this would be unlikely to come within the course of employment. The employer would probably not be liable for any harm caused to the hitch-hikers.

It is of great benefit if employer and employee spell out exactly what use can be made of an employee's car for work purposes to prevent a dispute arising at a later time. It is also essential to clarify the use for insurance purposes (see below).

Any person injured in a road accident where the driver does not have insurance cover or cannot be traced may be able to recover compensation from the Motors Insurers' Bureau.

Transporting other people and equipment

People

Even where the employer expressly agrees that the physiotherapist can use her car for transporting clients, legal issues can arise if the client is injured or causes an accident.

- What if the passenger becomes disturbed?

Situation: Disturbed passenger

> A physiotherapist arranges to take an elderly mentally infirm patient to visit a leisure centre. On the journey the client becomes very disturbed and tries to get out of the car and succeeds in opening the back door and falls out. Is the physiotherapist liable?

This situation is of concern to many community physiotherapists. If the incident is reasonably foreseeable then it could be argued that the physiotherapist should have taken the precaution of arranging 'child locks' on the car so that this could not occur. Alternatively, the precautions may have involved taking an assistant with her. Her duty of care to the client would require her to take reasonable precautions against events which are reasonably foreseeable. Before embarking on the journey she should have made an assessment as to whether the client would be safe in the car and whether or not an assistant should have sat with the client. In making this decision she should be aware that she is responsible for taking precautions to meet all reasonably foreseeable risks of harm to the client or to others.

- What if the community professional took passengers on the basis that they were taken at their own risk?

Such an arrangement is prohibited under road traffic legislation and such a device could not be used to exempt the driver from liability for the passenger's safety.

Any notice purporting to exclude liability for death or personal injury arising from negligence is invalid (see Figure 10.1 for the provisions of the Unfair Contract Terms Act 1977). However, with mentally competent adults there may be contributory negligence (see Chapter 10) if they do not take all reasonable steps to ensure their own safety, such as using seat belts provided.

Case: *Eastman v. S.W. Thames Regional Health Authority*[2]

Damages were awarded against the health authority in respect of injuries which the plaintiff (claimant) sustained when travelling in an ambulance without a seat belt. Although the ambulance driver was acquitted of all blame for the accident it was held by the Court that a duty of care was owed to advise passengers to wear a seat belt. The defendants appealed to the Court of Appeal.

The appeal was allowed. It was held that adult passengers possessed of their faculties should not need telling what to do. The ambulance attendant was under no obligation to point out the existence of seat belts and a notice recommending their use. It should be noted that this case refers to the duty of care to adults possessed of their faculties. Where a health professional is transporting a client in his/her own car and the client is frail or mentally incompetent the courts would probably accept that a duty of care was owed to ensure that the client was reasonably safe. This might in exceptional circumstances require child proof locks or a person in attendance.

- What if a passenger causes damage to the physiotherapist's car?

It depends upon the circumstances as to whether there is likely to be any liability on the part of the employer. It would have to be established that the employer was aware that harm could occur and failed to take reasonable precautions against that harm arising. If such fault could not be found, then the employer would not be liable,

and the physiotherapist would be responsible for paying for the damage to be rectified.

- What if a client carried in the car is suffering from an infectious disease that another patient picks up while being transported in the same vehicle?

There would be a duty upon the physiotherapist, if he/she is aware that he/she is carrying in her car a person suffering from an infectious disease, to ensure that after this use the car is cleaned and disinfected to prevent any cross-infection. If the physiotherapist fails to do this to a reasonable standard then the physiotherapist and his/her employer could be liable. Similar provisions apply to any equipment that the physiotherapist removes from a client's home: the physiotherapist would have a responsibility to ensure that the equipment and his/her car was thoroughly cleaned to prevent the risk of cross-infection.

Equipment

It is also important that the physiotherapist is clear on his/her duties in relation to the transporting of equipment. To ensure that the client obtains equipment without delay he/she may be inclined to decide to take equipment him/herself rather than wait for a van to be provided by his/her employers. The physiotherapist should take special precautions to ensure that his/her visibility in the car is not impaired and that he/she does not suffer injury from manually handling equipment on his/her own. Should such injury occur, and the physiotherapist attempts to bring a claim, he/she may be met with the defence of contributory negligence (see Glossary) – that it was his/her own responsibility.

If the equipment is stolen his/her insurance company may not be prepared to pay compensation for the loss unless there is an express term covering such liability and the physiotherapist had made it clear in his/her application for insurance cover that the carrying of equipment for work purposes was part of his/her agreed activities. (See below on concerns about wheelchairs being used in vehicles when they are not designed for that purpose.)

Insurance issues

Absolute disclosure is required in any insurance contract and, therefore, if there is any likelihood that the employee will require to use the car during work, this and the reasons should be disclosed. Should the driver not inform the insurers of a significant fact, this could invalidate the cover even though that particular omission had no relevance to the claim in question. An interesting recent development has been the suggestion that if a driver uses his car for car boot sales without the consent of the insurance company this could invalidate his car insurance. This highlights the importance of ensuring that an insurance company is given full details of every use made of the car.

Crown cars and lease cars

Insurance and road tax

Crown cars

Where the employee has the use of a crown car, insurance is normally provided through the employer and the crown is exempt from the provisions of the road traffic legislation requiring payment of road tax.

Lease cars

Usually the company providing the car would ensure that the appropriate insurance cover is taken out. However, this is not always so and the driver must check that he/she has the correct insurance cover. The Chartered Society of Physiotherapy (CSP) has published an information paper on lease cars and mileage rates which sets out the information taken from *the Agenda for Change Terms and Conditions Handbook*, Section Annex L and M.[3]

Servicing

With both crown and lease cars there may be service agreements that enable the user to have the car serviced at regular intervals as part of the agreement. The responsibility would be upon the user to ensure that the car was regularly maintained and also to ensure that any faults were reported and rectified. Should an accident occur because the user has failed to take action to remedy a defect, the user could face disciplinary proceedings from the employer and in some cases also face criminal prosecution him/herself.

Permitted use

The definition of the permitted use of the crown car or lease car should also cover the use of the car outside the catchment area of the Trust, e.g. if the physiotherapist were to attend a conference or course. It should be made absolutely clear whether or not this is a permissible use of the car.

- What if a physiotherapist is required to have a car for work but is unable to afford to get the car repaired or to pay for its MOT?

If it is a requirement of the post that the physiotherapist uses his/her own car in the course of employment, then failure to have a car in working order could mean that the physiotherapist is unable to perform his/her job. This may justify dismissal or transfer to another post where driving a car is not necessary. It may be however that the physiotherapist is able to use a crown car or have one on lease. It depends upon local arrangements within the Trust or other employer.

Employer's responsibilities on transport and insurance

- What duties does an employer have in relation to transport by employee?

The following case illustrates the question.

Case: *Reid* v. *Rush and Tompkins Group plc*[4]

The plaintiff (claimant) suffered severe injuries while driving the defendant's Land Rover in Ethiopia in the course of his employment by the defendant. It collided with a lorry. The accident had been caused solely by the negligence of the lorry driver who could not be traced. The plaintiff contended that the defendant was in breach of its duty of care as employer in failing either to insure him so as to provide suitable benefits in the event of injury resulting from third party negligence or to advise him to obtain such insurance for himself; and that had he been so advised he would have obtained personal accident cover. The basis for these arguments was that there was an implied term in the contract of employment requiring such insurance cover or advice, or that there was a duty of care owed in the law of negligence by the employer to the employee; or that the employer had a duty of care because of the special relationship which existed between them.

None of these arguments succeeded. The Court of Appeal held that there was no duty on the employer to take all reasonable steps to protect the employee's economic welfare while acting in the course of employment even if loss was foreseeable. The Court of Appeal cited the case of *Edwards* v. *West Hertfordshire Hospital Management Committee*[5] in support of this decision. The duty of the employer was limited to the protection of the employee against physical harm or injury.

If therefore the employer fails to warn employees to take out insurance cover, that is the responsibility of the employee even if the car is used solely for work purposes. Where the employer assists the employee in the purchase of the car or provides the transport, the respective duties of employer and employee in relation to the transport should be made clear at the outset to prevent any misunderstanding or omissions.

Paying fines and fees

- If the physiotherapist incurs a parking fine when visiting a patient in the community, is he/she liable to pay that fine?

- Does it make any difference if the physiotherapist was driving a crown car?

The answer is that the employee would be personally responsible for the fine since he/she has broken the law by parking in a prohibited area. The fact that the physiotherapist was parking as part of his/her duties would be irrelevant since the commission of a criminal offence would normally not be regarded as being in the course of employment. (However, see the case of *Lister & Others* v. *Hesley Hall Ltd*[1] above and Chapter 10.) Similarly if the physiotherapist was in a hospital car, it would still be his/her personal responsibility.

Where parking fees are charged on a hospital site it is entirely a matter of discussion between employees and employers over the fees charged and the sanctions which can be used if an employee ignores the parking conditions. Employers may find however that the fact that certain staff are extremely difficult to recruit may influence the terms and conditions of service, and this may include offering more favourable parking terms to attract and retain staff.

If an employee refuses to use his/her car unless the employer is prepared to pay parking fines or parking fees, and if driving a car is a requirement of his/her contract of employment, then the dismissal of that employee may be reasonable and fair.

Tax situation and private mileage

It is impossible in a work of this kind to cover the details of the law relating to the taxation of the benefit obtained from the use of cars provided by employers and the way in which private mileage is treated by the Inland Revenue. However it is important that those employees who have the use of a car provided by the employer should keep accurate records of their use of the car for private purposes, as well as their use of the car for work. Records should be made as soon as possible after the journey.

Physiotherapists in private practice will also need to keep comprehensive records of all costs associated with the car in calculating their profit and income tax.

Driving by disabled people

Under the Road Traffic Acts it is an offence for an individual to drive a car if they are suffering from a physical or mental defect which impairs their driving safely. Physiotherapists may be confronted with patients very anxious to drive when it is medically contra-indicated.

Situation: insisting on driving

> A physiotherapist is treating a patient who has suffered a stroke. Movement on the left side is restricted but the patient is anxious to drive since he acts as the sole carer for his wife who has motor neurone disease. The physiotherapist suspects that he is driving contrary to clinical advice. What is the legal position of the physiotherapist?

This is not an uncommon situation since the inability to drive can be seen as a considerable hardship for many people who have suffered neurological damage or physical injuries. Many patients may therefore be tempted to commence driving before they are physically or mentally fit to do so. The physiotherapist can advise such patients that they are committing a criminal offence. In serious cases where the physiotherapist considers that there is a grave danger of serious harm to other people, it would probably be an exception to her duty of confidentiality to advise the DVLA or others of the dangers (see Chapter 8 on confidentiality). However, it would be preferable to attempt to persuade the driver to cease to drive or to notify the DVLA himself and show him any appropriate literature. Those suffering from diabetes which requires insulin are required to inform the DVLA. Those diabetics who take tablets but also have a complication such as retinopathy must also inform the DVLA. The charity Diabetes UK has called for the law to be changed following research in the USA that people with diabetes are unfairly being prevented from driving since the rate of road collisions is no higher among people with diabetes who controlled their condition with insulin than among non-diabetic people.[6]

Wheelchairs

An information sheet was issued by the Joint Committee on Mobility for Disabled People[7] stating that manufacturers were becoming increasingly worried that their products were being used as vehicle seats when they were never designed for such purposes. The Department of Transport was working with wheelchair manufacturers and restraint manufacturers in order to improve the situation. The safety of wheelchairs comes within the remit of the Medicines and Healthcare products Regulatory Agency, which took on the responsibilities of the Medical Devices Agency and its work in relation to wheelchairs is considered in Chapter 15.

Disabled parking and badges

The scheme

Physiotherapists may be involved in the assessment of the eligibility of a disabled person to have a badge which will entitle him/her to park in parking bays designated for the disabled. Each local authority has a duty to implement the provisions of the Chronically Sick and Disabled Persons Act 1970 and assist in travelling arrangements for disabled persons.

The Blue Badge scheme replaces the Orange Badge scheme and operates throughout the UK providing a range of parking concessions for people with severe mobility problems who have difficulty using public transport.

Concessions

The scheme applies to on-street parking and includes free use of parking meters and pay-and-display bays. Badge holders may also be exempt from limits on parking times imposed on others and can park for up to 3 hours on single and double yellow lines as long as they are not causing an obstruction and except where there is a ban on loading or unloading or other restrictions. The Blue Badge scheme does not apply to off-street car parks, private roads or at most airports. Therefore any complaint about misuse of a disabled parking bay in a shopping precinct should be made to the managers of that precinct. Blue badge holders also qualify for 100% exemption from the London Congestion Charge but applicants must register with Transport for London at least 10 days before the journey and pay a one-off £10 registration fee.

Entitlement

The following are automatically entitled to apply for a badge:

- Over 2 years old and either
  - receive the higher rate of the mobility component of the disability living allowance; or
  - are registered blind; or
  - receive a war pensioner's mobility supplement.

Others may be eligible for a badge if:

- Over 2 years old and either:
  - have a permanent and sustainable disability which means you cannot walk, or which makes walking very difficult; or
  - drive a motor vehicle regularly, have a severe disability in both arms, and are unable to operate all or some types of parking meter (or would find it very difficult to operate them).

The parent of a child who is less than 2 years old may apply for a badge for the child, if they have a specific medical condition which means that they either:

- must always be accompanied by bulky medical equipment which cannot be carried around without great difficulty; or
- need to be kept near a vehicle at all times, so that they can, if necessary, be treated in the

vehicle, or quickly driven to a place where they can be treated, such as a hospital.

The badges can be used throughout the UK and while travelling abroad through the EU. Further information on the use of the Blue Badge in EU countries can be obtained from the Institute of Advanced Motorists (IAM).[8]

Local authorities are responsible for issuing Blue Badge parking permits and applications should be addressed to them. It is an offence to park a vehicle that is not displaying a badge in a Blue Badge parking bay. It is also an offence to refuse or fail to produce a badge for inspection by police officers, traffic wardens, local authority parking attendants and civil enforcement officers.

Misuse of the Blue Badge

Local authorities can take away a badge if the badge holder misuses it such as by allowing other people to use it or if a disabled person's condition improves so that they are no longer eligible for the scheme. New measures are to be taken to prevent abuse of the disabled parking schemes.[9] The most frequent abuses are by friends and relatives misusing the badge. The Department of Transport is tightening eligibility criteria and making it harder to forge Blue Badges. Mobilise, a charity for disabled drivers and passengers, has urged the Government to tighten the procedure for issuing badges. The Commons Transport Select Committee in June 2008 found that some councils were ignoring the Department for Transport's guidelines and not ensuring that applicants for Blue Badges had an independent assessment of their mobility and instead taking recommendations from applicants' GPs which were given out under pressure from the patient. The parking concession is estimated to be worth up to £5000 per year.[10]

Wales and the Blue Badge scheme

Wales has its own Blue Badge scheme, which came into force in July 2000 replacing the Orange

Badge scheme. Blue badge holders qualify for free toll across the Severn Bridge. Eligibility is similar to the English scheme and applications should be made to the local authority in which the applicant lives. Further information can be obtained from the Welsh Assembly Government website.[11]

The Motability Scheme

Motability, an independent not-for-profit organisation, runs a scheme for disabled people to buy or lease an adapted car. Applications can be made by those who receive the war pensioner's mobility supplement or the higher rate of the mobility component of the disability living allowance. It is also possible for a person in receipt of either of those benefits to apply for a car as a passenger and nominate two other people as the driver. Through the car hire scheme a new car is supplied for lease by a Motability Accredited dealer for at least 3 years. Comprehensive insurance, routine servicing and breakdown assistance are included. Hire purchase can also be arranged. Motability also offers a hire purchase scheme for powered wheelchairs or scooters. Disabled people do not have to pay VAT on the cost of hiring a car through the Motability scheme. Further information is available on the Motability website.[12]

Public transport

The Accessibility Regulations under the Disability Discrimination Act apply to public transport under which improved accessibility to buses, coaches and trains must be provided. Taxis are also covered by similar regulations.

Giving Advice

Car driving is an area where physiotherapists can be expected to give advice to clients and patients. This could include the following situation:

> I have a patient with lower back pain exacerbated by prolonged driving in a car without lumbar support. He is about to ask for a new company car and wishes to know what make would be ergonomically good.

In giving advice in such a situation, the physiotherapist would be liable for any harm suffered by the patient if she gave negligent advice, knowing that it would be relied upon by the client, who did in fact rely upon it to his or her detriment (see Chapter 10). The physiotherapist could not exclude herself from liability for her negligent advice if personal injury or death resulted. (See Unfair Contract Terms Act 1977 and Chapter 10)

Conclusion

Whether a physiotherapist is provided with a car from his/her employer or a lease car, or whether his/her own transport is used, it is essential that the physiotherapist makes enquiries relating to any conditions laid down in relation to insurance cover and the exact terms on which he/she is allowed to use the car in connection with work. The physiotherapist should also be aware of any regulations that affect the rights of a disabled person in relation to transport. The Disabled Persons Transport Advisory Committee (DPTAC) was established as an independent body to advise the Government on the transport needs of all disabled people across the UK and further information can be accessed from its website.[13]

Questions and exercises

1   While giving a lift to a carer, contrary to the instructions of your employer, you are involved in an accident which leads to the carer being injured. What is the situation in law?

2   Draw up a procedure which can cover the use of crown, lease or employee-owned cars.

3   Advise a client on how to obtain a parking permit for disabled persons.

4   A client notifies you that he has had several blackouts, but since he always knows when they are about to occur, he does not intend to stop driving his car. What action, if any, would you take?

References

1   *Lister & Others* v. *Hesley Hall Ltd*, [2001] UKHL 22 [2002] 1 AC 215; The Times Law Report, 10 May 2001; [2001] 2 WLR 1311.

2   *Eastman* v. *S.W. Thames Regional Health Authority* CA The Times Law Report, 22 July 1991.

3   CSP Lease cars and mileage rates WX 320 CSP 2006

4   *Reid* v. *Rush and Tompkins Group plc CA* The Times Law Report, 11 April 1989.

5   *Edwards* v. *West Hertfordshire Hospital Management Committee* [1957] 1 WLR 1415.

6   News item (2008) *Road Ban for Diabetics 'Unfair'*. *The Times*, 12 May

7   Joint Committee on Mobility for Disabled People (1997) Travelling in Vehicles while in a Wheelchair. *Physiotherapy* **83**, 6, 305.

8   www.iam.org.uk

9   Webster, B. (2008) Clampdown on Blue Badge Parking Cheats. *The Times*, 24 January.

10   Webster, B. (2008) Disabled Badges Given too Easily, say MPs. *The Times*, 10 June p. 12.

11   http://new.wales.gov.uk/topics/Integrated Transport/BlueBadge

12   www.motability.co.uk

13   www.dptac.gov.uk

Section D

Management Areas

17 Employment and the Statutory Organisation of the NHS

This chapter sets out the basic principles of employment law and how they relate to the physiotherapist. It also considers the statutory organisation of the NHS and the physiotherapist as manager. Those in private practice should refer to Chapter 19. However the private practitioner may also be an employer of others in which case he/she should be aware of the principles of employment law in relation to those whom he/she employs.

The topics to be covered include:

- The employment contract
- Protection against unfair dismissal
- Employee protection and health and safety
- Local bargaining
- Rights of the pregnant employee
- Rights in relation to sickness
- Protection against discrimination
- Trade unions
- Whistle blowing
- Future changes in employment law
- Statutory framework of the NHS
- The White Paper on the new NHS
- The physiotherapist as manager

The employment contract

Formation of the contract

As soon as an unconditional offer of employment (by the employer) or to be employed (by the employee) has been accepted by the other party, a contract of employment comes into existence. This may be at the interview or it may be by letter from the prospective employee accepting an offer of a post. The contract may be subject to conditions, e.g. receipt of satisfactory references or a satisfactory medical examination. If these prove not to be satisfactory, then the contract will either not come into existence, or cease to exist.

Even though the contract has been agreed, the employee may not actually start working for several weeks. If the employee were to do anything incompatible with the contract prior to starting work, e.g. accepting a job from another employer, he/she would be in breach of the original contract. The remedies for breach of contract are, however, unlikely to be pursued by the aggrieved employer (see below).

Effect of the contract

As a result of the contract of employment both employer and employee have duties and rights. These duties and rights arise from:

- express terms, either agreed by the parties individually or resulting from collective bargaining procedures;
- implied terms;
- terms set by statute.

Express terms

Some duties arise by express agreement between the parties. These would include the basic terms of the contract – title of the post, starting date, salary, holidays, sickness, pensions, etc. Some of these terms may have already been part of collective bargaining within the work place. Thus health service employees may have agreed terms nationally through the Whitley Council bargaining and the Agenda for Change (see below) procedures (unless their Trust has negotiated contractual terms with its own employees) and if it is agreed that an employee is to commence at a specific level then all the other terms and the General Conditions of Service will flow from that.

The employee might also agree specific terms with the employer when commencing, e.g. that a previously booked holiday can be taken or that he/she can start the day an hour later than usual because of child commitments. Such terms are enforceable, but written evidence of the agreement that the term is part of the contract of employment would be of considerable assistance

to an employee who claimed that these terms were not being upheld.

Guidance is available from the Chartered Society of Physiotherapy (CSP) on aspects of contracts of employment within the NHS. For example, information on respiratory on-call working has been published.[1] This publication relates the core standards to on-call working with additional guidance standard. Its contents include (1) an individualised approach, (2) informed consent, (3) confidentiality, (4) assessment, (5) information collection, (6) outcome measure, (7) analysis, (8) treatment planning, (9) implementation, (11) transfer of care/discharge, (12) communication with patients and carers, (13) communication with other professionals, (17) physiotherapists working alone and (18) equipment safety. Appendix 1 covers Standard 2 on patient consent.

Implied terms

The law implies into a contract of employment certain terms that are binding upon both parties even though such terms were never expressly raised by the parties. Figure 17.1 lists the terms that would be implied by law as obligations upon the employer and Figure 17.2 lists the terms which would be implied by law as obligations upon the employee.

The basic principle is that where express terms cover the issue, terms will not have to be implied. Thus a contract would normally state the pay to be given to the employee. However, where this is not done, the court would imply that there is a duty for the employer to pay the employee a reasonable amount. Alternatively, where very

---

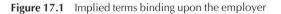

- A duty to take reasonable care for the health and safety of the employee, including the duty to ensure that the premises, plant and equipment are safe, that there is a safe system of work and that fellow staff are competent
- A duty to cooperate with the employee to enable him to fulfil his contract of employment
- An obligation to pay the employee

Figure 17.1   Implied terms binding upon the employer

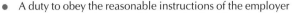

- A duty to obey the reasonable instructions of the employer
- A duty to act with reasonable regard to health and safety
- A duty to cooperate with the employer, including the duty to account for profits, to disclose misdeeds and not to compete with the employer
- A duty to maintain the confidentiality of information learnt during employment

Figure 17.2   Implied terms binding upon the employee

little has been agreed the court might hold that in the absence of agreement over significant terms there is no binding contract, i.e. the contract is void for uncertainty. The employee would be entitled to receive payment for any work performed, on a quasi-contractual basis.

In the case of a junior hospital doctor it was argued that there was an implied term that an employer would take care of its employees and not ask them to work an excessive amount of overtime.[2] In this case the junior doctor became ill as a result of the excessive amount of overtime he was asked to work. (The situation of excessive hours of work now comes under the Working Time Directives, see below.)

Statutory rights

The employer does not have complete discretion over what terms it can negotiate with the employee. Acts of Parliament require the employer to recognise certain rights, known as statutory rights, to which the employee is entitled. The employer could offer terms that improve upon these rights, but not reduce them. Certain qualifying conditions stipulate which employees are entitled to benefit from these statutory rights. Many rely upon a specified length of continuous service (see below).

Figure 17.3 sets out the principal rights given by statute.

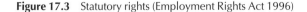

- Written statement of particulars
- Itemised statement of pay
- Time off provisions:

  - to take part in trade union (TU) duties and training
  - to take part in TU activities
  - to look for job or undergo training if made redundant
  - to attend antenatal clinics
  - to act as JP and certain public service duties

- Provisions relating to pregnancy and maternity (including pay)
- Sickness pay
- Health and safety rights
- Rights relating to TU membership and activities
- Bank holidays
- Guarantee payments
- Redundancy payment
- Medical suspension payment

Figure 17.3   Statutory rights (Employment Rights Act 1996)

Employment protection legislation required different lengths of continuous service as a condition of being eligible for these statutory rights, with part-timers having to serve for a longer period of time. However, this has been held to be discriminatory since more women are likely to be part-timers and an increasing number of statutory rights have no continuous service as a prerequisite (see below).

The minimum wage and the Working Time Directives

The National Minimum Wage Act 1998 aims to combat poverty pay. Subject to certain exceptions the national minimum wage will apply at the same rate to all workers, regardless of the sector in which they work. The Act creates a framework for the minimum wage to be implemented and enforced and the details are contained in regulations issued by the Secretary of State. The Act refers to workers, including agency workers and homeworkers, and created the Low Pay Commission (LPC), which works with the Secretary of State in creating the minimum wage and advising on policy matters. The LPC is an independent statutory non-departmental public body set up to advise the Government about the national minimum wage. Its permanent status was confirmed in 2001. Its most recent report in 2008[3] assessed the impact of the 2007 increase and recommended a minimum of £5.73 an hour from October 2008. Further information on the LPC can be found on its website.[4]

The Working Time Regulations,[5] which came into force from 1 October 1998 implement the Council Directive 93/104[6] (concerning certain aspects of the organisation of working time and provisions concerning working time) and Council Directive 94/33[7] on the protection of young people at work. The regulations were revised in 2002[8] to give enhanced rights to young workers. Obligations are imposed on employers concerning:

- a limit of an average weekly working time of workers of 48 hours;

- the average normal hours of night workers of 8 hours in any 24-hour period;
- the provision of health assessments for night workers;
- workers have a right to 11 hours rest in any 24-hour period;
- workers have a right to a day off each week;
- workers have a right to an in-work rest break if the working day is longer than 6 hours;
- workers have a right to 5.6 weeks paid leave a year (from 1 April 2009 – increased from 4.8 weeks);
- the keeping of records of workers' hours of work.

The right of employees to opt out of the regulations is being examined by the European Commission and is being negotiated throughout the EU. The rights to time limits and health assessments are enforced through the Health and Safety Executive and local authority environmental health departments. Entitlements to rest and leave are enforced by individuals through the employment tribunals. Further information is available from the Department for Business Enterprise and Regulatory Reform (which replaced the Department of Trade and Industry) on its website[9] and also from the Employments Tribunal Service. The NHS Employers also provide information on the working time regulations in their applicability to the NHS including the significance of on call times and the prevention of abuse of the ability to opt out.[10] The CSP has published a briefing paper on the Working Time Regulations.[11]

Performance of the contract

Both parties under the contract of employment have a duty to fulfil the express, implied and the statutory requirements in the contract of employment. Failure by the employee to fulfil his/her contractual requirements could result in him/her facing disciplinary proceedings. Failure by the employer to fulfil its contractual obligations could result in the employee claiming that he/she has been constructively dismissed (see Glossary) by the employer, i.e. the employer has shown an intention of no longer abiding by the contract of employment and this therefore gives the employee the right either to see the contract as ended by this breach of contract or of treating the contract as continuing but being able to claim damages or compensation for this breach of contract. Rights in connection with constructive dismissal are considered below.

It is a basic principle of contract law that one party to a contract cannot unilaterally change the terms of the contract without the consent of the other person. Thus an employer who required an employee to work in a different capacity or in a different location could be seen as being in breach of the contract of employment if the capacity and the location were express terms in that contract.

Termination of the contract

A contract of employment can come to an end in the following ways:

- performance
- expiry of a fixed term contract
- giving notice
- breach of contract by one or other party
- frustration.

Performance

A contract which specifies that a stated service is to be provided will come to an end when those services have been given. Thus a physiotherapist in private practice might agree that he/she will attend for 10 sessions. On the completion of those 10 sessions the contract, unless renewed, will come to an end.

Fixed-term contract

A fixed-term contract will come to an end at the passing of the specified time unless the contract is renewed.

Notice

Under the employment protection legislation the employee is entitled to a minimum length of notice terminating the job. The period depends upon the length of continuous service. However, there will usually be agreed in the contract of employments notice provisions which are in excess of the statutory requirements. Such terms will require the employer to give the employee notice of an intention to end the contract and vice versa. Where the employer dismisses an employee without regard to the length of notice this constitutes a wrongful dismissal and damages calculated at the rate of pay for the proper notice period are due. However, the employee might also have a case for unfair dismissal if there are not adequate grounds for ending the contract or if the employer has acted unreasonably in treating certain grounds as justifying dismissal and further compensation will be due (see below).

Breach of contract

By the employer If the employer is in fundamental breach of the contract of employment, the employee might see herself as being constructively dismissed and bring an application for unfair dismissal (see below).

By the employee Where an employee is in breach of contract the employer can, if the circumstances justify, see the contract of employment as at an end and dismiss the employee. The employee does however have the right to claim that the dismissal is unfair if the circumstances do not justify such action (see below).

Frustration

Where an event occurs that was not in the contemplation of the parties at the time the contract was agreed and this makes the performance of the contract impossible, then the contract will end by law without any requirement for the employer to terminate it. Each case depends on its own facts and the following events have been seen as frustrating and therefore bringing to an end a contract of employment – death, imprisonment and blindness (in a pilot). (The law of contract is further considered in Chapter 19 in relation to the private practitioner.)

Protection against unfair dismissal

One of the most important statutory rights has been the right not to be unfairly dismissed. This is given to those employees who have worked continuously for the same employer for 1 year (4 months in the case of an employee dismissed on medical grounds in consequence of certain health and safety requirements), and in many situations there is no continuous service requirement.

Exceptions to the continuous service requirement

The situations where there is no continuous service requirement include:

- dismissal in connection with TU activity and membership, lawful industrial action (of 12 weeks or less), TU recognition procedures;
- dismissal in connection with pregnancy, paternity leave, adoption leave, parental leave and taking time off for dependants;
- dismissal in connection with request for flexible working;
- dismissal in connection with discrimination;
- dismissal in connection with disciplinary and grievance hearings;
- dismissal in connection with health and safety;
- dismissal for asserting a statutory right, including right to a minimum wage, part-time workers rights, fixed term employees' rights;
- dismissal on grounds of jury service;
- dismissal in a protective disclosure situation;
- dismissal on grounds relating to the Information and Consultation of Employees Regulations (from 6 April 2007 organisations

with over 100 employees, from 6 April 2008 organisations with over 50 employees);
- from 1 October 2006 dismissal in connection with a meeting to discuss a request not to retire.

Grievance and dispute resolution

New disciplinary and grievous procedures regulations place new duties upon employers and employees. A statutory dispute resolution is set out in Schedule 2 to the Employment Act 2002. There are two forms: a standard three-step procedure and a modified two-step procedure. There are separate procedures for dealing with grievance issues and for disciplinary matters. Schedule 2 Part I sets out the dismissal and disciplinary procedures. In addition to the new procedures for disciplinary and grievance matters, Schedule 2 to the Employment Act 2002 sets out general requirements which must be followed by the parties. These include the following:

- Each step and action under the procedure must be taken without unreasonable delay.
- Timing and location of meetings must be reasonable.
- Meetings must be conducted in a manner that enables both employer and employee to explain their cases.
- In the case of an appeal meeting that is not the first meeting, the employer should, as far as is reasonably practicable, be represented by a more senior manager than attended the first meeting (unless the most senior manager attended that meeting).
- The employee has a right to be accompanied to these meetings (Section 10 of the Employment Relations Act 1999; Section 37 of the Employment Relations Act 2004 clarified the role of this person).

The ACAS (Advisory, Conciliation and Arbitration Service) Code of Practice on Disciplinary and Grievance Procedures is available from its website.[12]

These dispute resolution procedures were repealed by the Employment Act 2008, which gives powers to employment tribunals to amend awards if parties have failed to comply with a relevant statutory code (see below on Employment Act).

Application for unfair dismissal

If an allegation of unfair dismissal arises, and the employee has failed to win an internal appeal, an application to an employment tribunal can be made. The time limit for making such an application is 3 months from the date of dismissal (but can be extended with the discretion of the tribunal). If the setting up of the internal appeal is protracted the employee may need to protect his/her rights by applying to the employment tribunal within the time limit and then asking for an adjournment pending the hearing of the internal appeal.

New rules have been introduced relating to intervention by the ACAS, which receives a copy of the application to the employment tribunal and a conciliator is appointed. The conciliator from ACAS will contact the employee in an attempt to conciliate between the parties, so that a hearing of the case is unnecessary. ACAS has a general duty of promoting the improvement of industrial relations. It can provide advice on employment legislation and industrial relations and can also assist in the settling of disputes. It has also published a Code of Practice on disciplinary practice and procedures in employment. Failure by any employer to follow the ACAS guidelines will not make the employer liable to proceedings but this evidence could be used against the employer in evidence before an employment tribunal. ACAS is also able to offer an arbitration scheme for unfair dismissal disputes that is a voluntary alternative to the tribunal. Information is available on the ACAS website[12] and it also provides free advice on employment matters on a national helpline (08457 47 47 47). Information can also be obtained on the website for the Department of Business Enterprise and Regulatory Reform.[9]

Interim relief

In many of these situations where there is no continuous service requirement, an employee could make an application to a tribunal for interim relief within 7 days of the effective date of termination of the contract of employment. If the tribunal considers that it would be likely at the full hearing that it would uphold the complaint, then it can make an order for reinstatement or re-engagement or will make an order for the temporary continuation of the contract of employment.

Definition of dismissal

The employee must show that there has been a dismissal and not a resignation. A dismissal may be:

- an ending of the contract of employment by the employer, with or without notice;
- a constructive dismissal where the employee is able to regard the contract as ended by the employer's fundamental breach of contract;
- the failure to renew a fixed-term contract.

There is however the power for the employer to exclude from a fixed-term contract the employee's right to apply to an employment tribunal if the fixed term is not renewed.

Once the employee has established the dismissal then the employer has to show reasons why the dismissal was justified.

Defence to an unfair dismissal application

The employer must show the reason for the dismissal and the fact that the reason is recognised in law as capable of being a reason for dismissal. The tribunal will determine whether the employer also acted reasonably in treating this statutory reason as justifying the dismissal. The statutory reasons that can render a dismissal fair are:

- conduct;
- capability or qualification;
- redundancy;

- legal impossibility;
- other substantial reason;
- retirement (but employer must comply with the duty to consider the employee working beyond retirement).

The factors which are taken into account in determining the reasonableness of the dismissal and the employer's action are:

- consistency;
- following the ACAS Code of Practice;
- clarity;
- hearing the employee's case;
- allowing the employee to be represented;
- giving a series of warnings;
- making a fair investigation of the facts.

Sanctions of employment tribunal

If an employee wins the case for unfair dismissal, the tribunal has the following options:

- compensation: basic award, compensatory award, special award;
- reinstatement or re-engagement.

Further information on these remedies can be obtained from the Department of Business Enterprise and Regulatory Reform website.[9]

Case: *Watling v. Gloucestershire County Council*[13]

One of the conditions on which an occupational therapist was employed was that he would obtain permission to engage in any outside work and he would only see private clients in the evenings and at the weekend. In 1990 he was seen by an area manager seeing a private client during the normal working week. He was given a strong warning that when he saw his private clients for alternative therapy it was to be outside his normal working hours. In 1993 there was again evidence that he was seeing a patient in ordinary working hours and that he was calling up a private client during his working time.

A disciplinary hearing was held and he was found guilty of gross misconduct in two respects – first in seeing a private patient during working hours and second in ignoring the very clear and emphatic warning which he had been given. He was summarily dismissed for gross misconduct.

He failed in his application to the industrial tribunal (the former name of the employment tribunal), which found the dismissal to have been fair and he also failed in his appeal to the Employment Appeal Tribunal (EAT). His defence that he was doing no more than taking an early lunch was rejected on the grounds that lunch hours are for lunch and not for seeing private patients. It was also alleged on his behalf that the management were aware that he was seeing private clients during the day and that the flexibility which he was permitted in the ordering of his work and the taking of his lunch break enabled him to see private clients. However, the EAT was satisfied that the employers had conducted a reasonable and fair enquiry into what had happened and that the decision of the tribunal was beyond any sensible criticism.

Redundancy

Redundancy may be a reasonable cause to end an employment contract but the employer must ensure that it acts reasonably in the selection of employees and in giving them the requisite information. The CSP has provided guidance for members[14] and also for managers.[15]

Other statutory rights

Recent legislation has added to the statutory rights enjoyed by employees, including flexible working, rights for part-timers and adoption and paternity leave. The CSP has prepared guidance on the right to request flexible working[16] and adoption leave[17] and paternity leave[18] and introducing new working patters, including 7-day working.[19]

Employee protection and health and safety

The Trade Union Reform and Employment Rights Act 1993 (now consolidated in the Employment

[Dismissal in health and safety cases is unfair in cases where]

(a) having been designated by the employer to carry out activities in connection with preventing or reducing risks to health and safety at work, the employee carried out (or proposed to carry out) any such activities,

(b) being a representative . . . on matters of health and safety at work or member of a safety committee . . . [he] performed (or proposed to perform) any functions as such . . . ,

(c) being an employee [where there was no safety representative or committee or it was not reasonably practicable to use these means] he brought to his employer's attention, by reasonable means, circumstances connected with his work which he reasonably believed were harmful or potentially harmful to health or safety,

(d) in circumstances of danger which [he] reasonably believed to be serious and imminent and which he could not reasonably have been expected to avert, he left (or proposed to leave) or (while the danger persisted) refused to return to his place of work or any dangerous part of his place of work, or

(e) in circumstances of danger which he reasonably believed to be serious and imminent, he took (or proposed to take) appropriate steps to protect himself or other persons from the danger.

Figure 17.4   Employment Rights Act 1996 Section 100(1)

Rights Act 1996) has given to the employee considerable protection against dismissal where the employee is taking action on grounds of health and safety. There is no continuous service requirement placed upon the employee to obtain protection against dismissal or any other action short of dismissal. In Figure 17.4 is set out a summary of Section 100 of the Employment Rights Act 1996. The ambit of Section 100 was considered in a case brought against St George's Hospital[20] where it was held that Section 100 was not confined to the health and safety of the employees, but the employee's dismissal could relate to his or her fears about the health and safety of others.

The criteria for judging the appropriateness of the employee's actions are 'all the circumstances including, in particular, his knowledge and the facilities and advice available to him at the time.' (Section 100(2)).

A defence is available to the employer if the employee's actions were so negligent, that a reasonable employer might have dismissed him as the employer did (Section 100(3)).

Interim relief is available where an application is made to a tribunal in the case of a complaint of unfair dismissal (Section 128 of the Employment Rights Act 1996). The tribunal has the power to establish whether the employer is willing to reinstate the employee pending the determination of the complaint.

The provisions shown in Figure 17.4 give the employee much greater protection when bringing issues of health and safety hazards to the attention of the employer so that he/she should not be victimised (see also section on whistleblowing, below).

Local bargaining

Most physiotherapists are employed by NHS Trusts, some by social services departments and a minority are employed in the private sector. Within the NHS the framework of collective bargaining under the Whitley Councils was gradually being dismantled as local bargaining replaced centrally negotiated terms and conditions. However, the Agenda for Change (see below) has led to central terms and conditions prevailing. The physiotherapist needs to ensure that he/she understands the principles of contract law and employment law in order to make maximum use of the system of any local bargaining which still exists.

The introduction of NHS Trusts and the internal market with GP fundholding presented the healthcare-based physiotherapist with a very different environment from that which existed prior to the implementation of the NHS, Community Care Act 1990. Under the system of commissioning, physiotherapists were having to show the value of physiotherapy treatment to their patients in order to ensure the contracts for purchasing physiotherapy services are in place. The internal market has been abolished along with GP fundholding, but it is essential for the physiotherapist to convince those who arrange the commissioning of physiotherapist services that physiotherapy services provide added value for patients[21] (see below). The physiotherapist is still likely to face conflict over the number of recommended sessions for a patient. The commissioner may, for example, stipulate six sessions as a norm, when the physiotherapist may consider that a far greater number is justified.

Rights of the pregnant employee

Statutory rights given to the pregnant employee are:

- paid time off to attend for antenatal care for all pregnant employees;
- maternity leave: 52 weeks (26 weeks of ordinary and 26 additional maternity leave);
- maternity pay (if qualifying conditions are met, up to 39 weeks of Statutory Maternity Pay; if qualifying conditions are not met, Maternity Allowance may be payable);
- right to return after confinement;
- protection against dismissal on grounds of pregnancy or childbirth and sex discrimination.

The rights of the pregnant woman are contained in the Employment Rights Act 1996, the Employment Relations Act 1999, the Employment Act 2002 and the Work and Families Act 2006. Full details of all the entitlements are available on the Department of Business Enterprise and Regulatory Reform website.[9] All employed women whose babies were due on or after 1 April 2007 are now entitled to additional maternity leave: 39 weeks for statutory maternity pay and maternity allowance; 8 weeks (instead of 28 days) notice must be given if she wishes to change the date of her return from maternity leave. All women have the right to return to work after maternity leave regardless of the size of the employer.

The above rights are those given by statute. Many employers however give far more generous benefits than those given as a statutory right. The employee cannot, however, have both. The NHS conditions of service are in many ways superior to the statutory rights for those who have been in employment for more than 2 years. Any locally agreed conditions cannot, of course, be worse than those to which women are entitled by statutory right and these are subject to review under the Family Friendly Policies set out in the White Paper *Fairness at Work*.[22]

The CSP has prepared information on maternity leave and maternity pay.[23]

The Court of Justice of the European Communities held that the dismissal of a woman when her ova had been fertilised in an *in vitro* procedure, but had not been transferred to her uterus was not prohibited by the Community directive on the safety and health of pregnant workers but was prohibited by the equal treatment directive if it was established that the dismissal was based on the fact that she had undergone *in vitro* fertilisation.[24]

Work and Families Act 2006

The Work and Families Act 2006 followed a consultation on Work and Families: Choice and Consultation published in October 2005. As well as enhancing the rights of the pregnant employee, the Act:

- extended the right to request flexible working to carers of adults from April 2007;

- gave employed fathers a new right to up to 26 weeks Additional Paternity Leave;
- introduced measures to help employers manage the administration of leave and pay;
- introduced measures to improve communications during maternity leave.

Information on adoption leave and pay, flexible working and work life balance, paternity leave and pay, additional paternity leave and pay, parental leave, part-time work and time off for dependants can be obtained from the website of the Department for Business Enterprise and Regulatory Reform.[9]

Rights in relation to sickness

Employees are entitled to receive statutory sick pay from their employer when they are sick. Those who are not in work or are self-employed may be able to claim state incapacity benefits instead. These include sickness benefit, invalidity benefit, and severe disablement allowance.

Statutory sick pay is payable for up to 28 weeks of incapacity, with spells separated by a period of not more than 8 weeks counting as one. It is paid to all employees who are incapable of work and who satisfy the conditions for payment. Details of the conditions and actions to be taken by the employee and employer are set out on the website for the Department for Works and Pensions.[25]

Many employees receive superior sickness benefits under their contracts of employment. In the NHS most employees with the necessary continuous service have sickness cover of 6 months of full pay and 6 months of half pay.

Protection against discrimination

Race and sex discrimination

The main legislation protecting persons against discrimination over race and sex are the Race Relations Act 1976, the Sex Discrimination Act 1975 and subsequent amendments and regulations. Also the Equal Pay Act 1970 implies an equality clause into any employment contract, that a woman employed on like work to a man is entitled to have similar terms and conditions.

The basic principles under the race and sex discrimination laws, and these apply both within and outside the employment field, are shown in Figures 17.5 and 17.6.

A test case[26] on the Equal Pay Act 1970 was brought by speech therapists who claimed that they were employed on work of equal value with male principal-grade pharmacists and clinical psychologists employed in the NHS whose salaries exceeded theirs by about 60%. Part of the argument circulated around the nature of speech therapy and what was the relevant profession to it in comparative terms. The employers pointed out that speech therapists had been considered in the past to be a profession auxiliary to medicine, and were therefore grouped with almoners, chiropodists, dieticians, medical laboratory technicians, occupational therapists, physiotherapists and radiographers. In contrast, clinical psychologists had been treated as comparable to scientists such as physicists and biologists. The Court of Appeal referred the case to the European Court of Justice.[27] This decided that the fact that differences in pay were mainly arrived at through collective bargaining is not sufficient objective justification for the difference in pay between the two jobs. It is for the national court to determine whether and to what extent the shortage of candidates for a job and the need to attract them by higher pay constitutes an objectively justified economic ground for the difference in pay between the jobs in question.

A Code of Practice on Equal Pay came into force on 1 December 2003, replacing the 1997 edition.[28] The Equal Pay Directive 1975 and the Equal Pay Treatment Directive 1976 were brought together in the Consolidated Equal Treatment Directive 2006.[29] Member states must implement it by 15 August 2009.

The Sex Discrimination Act 1975 (Amendment) Regulations 2008[30] implements the 2002 Directive,[31] which applies the principle of equal

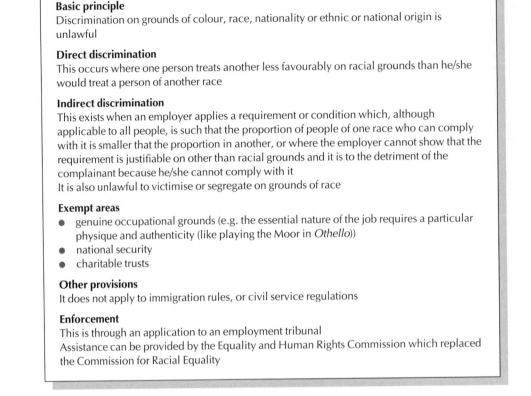

Basic principle
Discrimination on grounds of colour, race, nationality or ethnic or national origin is unlawful

Direct discrimination
This occurs where one person treats another less favourably on racial grounds than he/she would treat a person of another race

Indirect discrimination
This exists when an employer applies a requirement or condition which, although applicable to all people, is such that the proportion of people of one race who can comply with it is smaller that the proportion in another, or where the employer cannot show that the requirement is justifiable on other than racial grounds and it is to the detriment of the complainant because he/she cannot comply with it
It is also unlawful to victimise or segregate on grounds of race

Exempt areas
● genuine occupational grounds (e.g. the essential nature of the job requires a particular physique and authenticity (like playing the Moor in *Othello*))
● national security
● charitable trusts

Other provisions
It does not apply to immigration rules, or civil service regulations

Enforcement
This is through an application to an employment tribunal
Assistance can be provided by the Equality and Human Rights Commission which replaced the Commission for Racial Equality

Figure 17.5   Principles of protection against discrimination on grounds of race

treatment of men and women to access to employment, vocational training and promotion and working conditions. The Regulations amend the 1975 Act amending the definition of harassment and discrimination on grounds of pregnancy or maternity leave.

Discrimination on grounds of religion or belief or sexual orientation

New regulations came into force in December 2003 as a result of employment directives from the EC. The Employment Equality (Religion or Belief) Regulations[32] (guidance has been provided by the CSP[33]) and the Employment Equality (Sexual Orientation) Regulations[34] (guidance has been provided by the CSP[35]) protect employees and applicants and those in vocational

training against discrimination, victimisation or harassment on the grounds of religion or belief or sexual orientation. Exceptions to equality in respect of religion or belief are recognised for national security, positive action and the protection of Sikhs from discrimination in connection with requirements as to wearing of safety helmets. Exceptions to equality in respect of sexual orientation are recognised for national security and positive action and also for benefits that are dependent on marital status. Enforcement in respect of both sets of regulations is through the employment tribunal.

The first successful case under the sexual orientation regulations was the case of *Whitfield v. Cleanaway UK*,[36] where a manager won £35 000 for constructive dismissal as a result of suffering sustained abuse including references to 'queer', 'queen' and 'dear' from senior management.

Basic principle

To treat a person less favourably on the grounds of sex than a person of the other sex would be treated is unlawful. It is also unlawful for an employer to discriminate against a person on grounds of marital status, civil partnership, pregnancy, maternity or gender assignment.

Indirect discrimination

This occurs where an employer applies a requirement or condition which, even though it applies equally to all persons, is such that the proportion of people of one sex who can comply with it is considerably smaller that the proportion in the other and where the employer cannot show justification on other than sexual grounds and it is to the detriment of the complainant. It is also unlawful to victimise or segregate on grounds of sex.

Exempt areas
- Genuine occupational qualification

  - essential nature of the job requires a person of a different sex
  - authenticity, decency and privacy, personal services
  - work abroad which can only be done by a man
  - the job is one of two held by a married couple

- National security
- Work in private households
- Charitable trusts
- Ministers of religion
- Sports and sports facilities
- Police and police cadets (in respect of certain terms only)

Enforcement

This is through an application to the employment tribunal
Like the Commission for Racial Equality the Equal Opportunities Commission (EOC) (now replaced by the Equality and Human Rights Commission) had a duty to work towards the elimination of discrimination and in promoting the equality of opportunities. It kept the Sex Discrimination Act under review and could bring action itself in the event of advertising which indicates an intention to discriminate unlawfully. It could also bring an action for an injunction to prevent a person discriminating unlawfully

Figure 17.6   Principles of protection from discrimination on grounds of sex

Employment Equality Regulations[37] came into force on 1 October 2005 that brought sexual indirect discrimination in line with racial discrimination. Article 9 of the European Convention on Human Rights (ECHR) gives a qualified right in respect of freedom of thought, conscience and religion.

Disability discrimination

The Disability Discrimination Act 1995 gives the disabled person certain rights in relation to employment, pensions and insurance, the provision of goods and services, access to premises, education and public transport. The main provisions of the Act are set out below in Figure 17.7.

Implementation

The first rights under the Disability Discrimination Act 1995 Part III came into force on 2 December 1996. The remaining provisions of Part III were implemented in two stages. From October 1999, service providers had to take

Part I	Definitions of disability and disabled person
Part II	Employment: discrimination by employers, enforcement provisions, discrimination by other persons, occupational pension schemes and insurance services
Part III	Discrimination in other areas: goods, facilities and services, premises, enforcement.
Part IV	Education
Part V	Public transport: taxis, public services vehicles, rail vehicles
Part VI	National Disability Council (replaced by the Disability Rights Commission which has been incorporated into the Equality and Human Rights Commission)
Part VII	Supplemental: Codes of Practice, victimisation, help
Part VIII	Miscellaneous

Figure 17.7   The Disability Discrimination Act 1995

reasonable steps to change practices and pro-cedure that make it unreasonably difficult for disabled people to use a service. From 2004 service providers had to take reasonable steps to remove, alter or provide reasonable means of avoiding physical features that make it impos-sible for disabled people to use that service.

Definition of disability

The Disability Discrimination Act 1995 defines a person as having a disability if

> he has a physical or mental impairment which has a substantial and long-term adverse effect on his ability to carry out normal day-to day duties.

Schedule 1 supplements this definition of dis-ability. Further guidance is available in the statutory code of practice. This Code, which covers the duty to promote disability equality and clarifies the statutory duties, was published by the Disability Rights Commission in 2005.[38] It will be updated by the new Equality and Human Rights Commission (EHRC). A chief inspector of police claimed that he had been unfairly dis-criminated against on account of his dyslexia. The tribunal found that the dyslexia did not have a substantial adverse effect on his ability to carry out normal day-to-day activities and therefore

he was not disabled within the meaning of Section 1 of the Disability Discrimination Act 1995. The employee's appeal to the Employment Appeal Tribunal succeeded.[39] It held that once the tribunal had accepted that the employee was disadvantaged to the extent of requiring 25% extra time to do an assessment, it inevitably followed that there was a substantial adverse effect on normal day-to-day activities. He was therefore a disabled person within the meaning of the Act

Employment

In Part II, which covers discrimination in em-ployment, it is made unlawful for an employer to discriminate against a disabled person (i.e. unjustifiably treat the disabled person less favourably) in arrangements for recruitment, and also in the terms of employment which are offered, including opportunities for promotion and training and other benefits. The disabled employee is also protected against dismissal or other detriment on the grounds of disability. Regulations have been passed to cover these provisions and also to define further the duties of the employer in relation to physical arrange-ments. Small businesses are exempt from these provisions if the employer has fewer than 20 employees.

The disabled person has the right to apply to an employment tribunal over any discrimination. There are also provisions covering discrimination in respect of contract workers and discrimination by TU organisations. Discrimination on the part of occupational pension schemes and insurance services is also made illegal.

Goods, services, education and transport

Part III covers discrimination in the provision of goods, facilities and services. It is unlawful for a provider of services to discriminate against a disabled person by refusing to provide him with services, or in relation to the standard or terms of the service. There is a duty on service providers to take such steps as are reasonable to make alterations to buildings and the approach or access, and to provide auxiliary aids, such as audio tapes or sign language.

In the provisions relating to discrimination in education, it is a requirement for the annual report of each county, voluntary or grant-maintained school to include information on the arrangements for the admission of disabled pupils, the steps taken to prevent disabled pupils from being treated less favourably than other pupils and the facilities provided to assist access to the school by disabled pupils. Similar requirements are made in relation to further and higher education.

Taxi accessibility regulations have been passed to ensure that disabled persons and persons in wheelchairs can get into and out of taxis safely and also be carried in safety and in reasonable comfort. Taxi drivers also have a duty to carry the guide dogs and hearing dogs of passengers without making an additional charge. Regulations have also been made relating to public service vehicles and the access and carriage of disabled persons and wheelchairs.

The Disability Discrimination Act 2005

This Act puts into law some of the recommendations of the Disability Rights Task Force, which was set up by the Government in 1997. Section 18 of the Act extends the definition of disability in respect of those with a mental illness (it is no longer a requirement that mental illness must be clinically well recognised if it is to be the basis of 'mental impairment') and includes those diagnosed with cancer, multiple sclerosis and HIV infection from the point at which the disease was diagnosed rather than from the point at which their illness had an adverse effect on them. It also brings councillors and members of the Greater London Authority within the scope of the Disability Discrimination Act (DDA), places a new duty on public authorities to have due regard to the need to eliminate harassment of and unlawful discrimination against disabled person, to promote positive attitudes to disabled persons and encourage participation by disabled people in public life and promote equality of opportunity for them. New provisions are introduced in relation to rail vehicles.

The Court of Appeal has held that the rights recognised in the disability discrimination legislation applied to the services provided in prisons, police custody and detention centres for failed asylum seekers.[40] Whether an adverse effect on a person's ability to carry out normal day-to-day activities was likely to recur should be determined by an employment tribunal on the basis of evidence available at the time of the alleged disability discrimination.[41]

Age discrimination

Protection from discrimination on grounds of age came into force in October 2006 as a result of a European Directive[42] which was implemented by the Employment Equality (Age) Regulations 2006.[43] The Regulations only apply to employment and vocational training and only protect employees up to 65 years who can be dismissed after that age provided the employer satisfies the specified procedure set out in the regulations. If the employer agrees to keep the employee on after that age, the employee is protected against other forms of discrimination in relation to discipline, pay, harassment and job classification. Employees have the right to request working beyond 65 years, and in such a case employers have a duty to consider the request according to Schedule 6. In a case on 16 October 2007[44] involving a Spanish worker who challenged his forced retirement, the European Court of Justice said that the EU states can introduce and enforce mandatory retirement ages as long as they are justified. Heyday, an offshoot of the charity Age Concern, had awaited this ruling before pursuing its own case and is now unlikely to succeed. One possible distinction between the UK and the ruling in the Spanish case is that in the UK retirement ages are fixed by collective bargaining with individual employers and not by the Government.

The Age Discrimination Regulations do not only protect the older worker: in March 2008 a teenager won an age discrimination claim.[45] Leanne Wilkinson, who worked as an administrative assistant in Springwell Engineering, was sacked and told that she was too young for the job. She obtained £16 000 compensation, the tribunal concluding that she had been discriminated against on grounds of age. Provisions of a new Equality Bill 2009 would prohibit age discrimination beyond the work place (see below).

The Equality and Human Rights Commission

The EHRC was established on 1 October 2007 under the Equality Act 2006 replacing the Equal Opportunities, the Disabilities Rights Commission and the Commission for Racial Equality. It also assumes responsibility for promoting equality and combating unlawful discrimination in three new areas: sexual orientation, religion or belief and age. It also has responsibility for the promotion of human rights. The Commission has a general duty under Section 3 to exercise its functions with a view to encouraging and supporting the development of a society in which

(a) people's ability to achieve their potential is not limited by prejudice or discrimination;
(b) there is respect for and protection of each individual's human rights;
(c) there is respect for the dignity and worth of each individual;
(d) each individual has an equal opportunity to participate in society;
(e) there is mutual respect between groups based on understanding and valuing of diversity and on shared respect for equality and human rights.

More specific duties relate to equality and diversity (Section 8), human rights (Section 9), groups (Section 10), monitoring the law (Section 11) and monitoring progress (Section 12). It has powers to publish or disseminate ideas or information, undertake research, provide education or training, give advice or guidance, and issue codes of practice. It also has the power to carry out an investigation, to apply to court for an injunction against a person who it believes to be committing an unlawful act, to bring proceedings in its own name and to give legal assistance to an individual who alleges that he/she is a victim of behaviour contrary to the equality enactments. Further information can be obtained from the EHRC website.[46] The scope of the EC Directive on equal treatment in employment and occupation[47] was considered in a significant case. The EHRC supported Sharon Coleman, who had a disabled son, in claiming that she was discriminated against at work because of her child. She said that she was forced to resign from the law firm because it would not accommodate her responsibility to care for a disabled child. The case was heard by the European Court of Justice's (ECJ) advocate general who decided in her favour.[48] On 17 July 2008 the ECJ[49] ruled that the EU directive which outlawed discrimination or harassment at work on the ground of disability is not limited to disabled people themselves but extends to those caring for them. It is described as a landmark case, which could bring new rights for the 6 million carers in the UK.

Equality Bill 2009

In June 2008 the Government published, as part of its draft legislative programme for 2008/9, a new Equality Bill with the aim of simplifying and strengthening rights to equality by updating existing anti-discrimination laws. If the Bill is implemented, older people would no longer be refused medical treatment on grounds of age and should be offered a full range of insurance products. The Bill includes the following provisions:

- a single equality duty on public bodies;
- public bodies' performance will be monitored and evaluated in relation to the equality duty;
- employment tribunals to make recommendations to employers on equality issues;
- clarify and simplify the law by consolidating the legislation and regulations.

The Bill was welcomed by the EHRC, who saw its remit as assisting service providers (schools, hospitals, local authorities etc) to prepare for the changes which would extend the law against age discrimination to the provision of goods, facilities and services.[50]

Rehabilitation of Offenders Act 1974

The aim of this Act is to prevent discrimination against those who have had criminal convictions. It works by regarding certain offences as 'spent' after a certain length of time. This means that the person does not have to disclose the offence and to dismiss an employee on grounds that he or she failed to disclose a spent offence is automatically unfair. However, the Act does not apply to serious crimes and many occupations are excluded from its effects, including health service employment.[51] Under Schedule 1 to the Statutory Instrument detailing the exceptions all members of any profession coming under the aegis of the Professions Supplementary to Medicine Act 1960 (now the Health Professions Council) are excepted from the provisions of the 1974 Act and no convictions considered spent. All convictions will remain on the record and have to be disclosed to prospective employers.

Trade unions

Industrial action

The protection and immunities that trade unions (TUs) and their members enjoyed in the 1970s and 1980s have been eroded until they have very few rights in relation to protection as a result of industrial action. Industrial action itself is defined in narrow terms if it is to be construed as 'lawful'. Rules are laid down in relation to elections and the holding of secret ballots before a strike can commence. Secondary industrial action is prohibited, so that TUs are not immune from liability for the effects of any secondary action.

The individual citizen was given a right to prevent disruption to his/her supply of any goods or services because of unlawful industrial action. If he/she can show that he/she has been or will be deprived of goods or services and that the industrial action is unlawful then he/she can apply to the court for an order to restrain the action. The establishment of a Commissioner for protection against unlawful industrial action enabled legal advice and representation to be paid for, though the Commissioner could not itself bring proceedings on behalf of an individual. However, this Commission was abolished under Section 28 of the Employment Relations Act 1998.

Unlawful industrial action includes the following: that

- which constitutes a tort;
- which is not supported by ballot;
- of which proper notice is not given;
- which is not in furtherance of a trade dispute;
- which is secondary action;
- which promotes a closed shop;

- which is to support an employee dismissed whilst taking part in unofficial industrial action;
- which is unlawful picketing.

Members' rights

The law relating to the constitution, membership, elections, funds, accounts and other forms of control was consolidated in the Trade Union and Labour Relations (Consolidation) Act 1992. An employee's right to join an independent TU and to take part in its lawful activities is protected so that dismissal in relation to such activities is automatically unfair without any continuous service requirement.

The office of the Commissioner for the Rights of Trade Union Members was established following the Employment Act 1988. Its task was to assist TU members who have complaints against their TU. This Commission was however abolished on 29 October 1999 under the Employment Relations Act 1999. The Employment Relations Act 1999 established a statutory procedure for an employer to recognise a TU for the purpose of collective bargaining and also for derecognition.

The Employment Relations Act 2004 implemented the findings of the review of the Employment Relations Act 1999, which was carried out in 2002. Most of the provisions of the 2004 Act had come into force by April 2005. The 2004 Act introduced a statutory code of practice on access to workers during recognition and derecognition ballots. The Act also clarifies the powers of the Central Arbitration Committee (CAC) in relation to the holding of ballots on union recognition, strengthened the law in relation to industrial action and provided further protection for the rights of TU members, workers and employees.

In the European Court of Human Rights in the case of *Aslef* v. *UK* it was held that clearer rights of TUs to determine their membership were required. Provision to secure these changes is contained in the Employment Act 2008 (see below)

Whistle-blowing

This is the term that refers to a person (usually an employee) who draws attention to concerns which have health and safety implications. Because of a fear that such persons, many of whom have a professional duty to draw attention to dangers and hazards, would be victimised as a result of their actions, the Department of Health issued a circular recommending that each Trust and authority should set up a procedure whereby an individual employee could raise these concerns with the management internally without being victimised and thus not needing to bring in the media or other external bodies. Subsequently the Public Interest Disclosure Act was enacted.

The Public Interest Disclosure Act 1998

The Public Interest Disclosure Act received the royal assent on 2 July 1998. The basic provisions of this Act are shown in Figure 17.8.

The explanatory memorandum envisages that the Act will protect workers who disclose information about certain types of matters from being dismissed or penalised by their employers as a result. The Act applies to disclosures relating to:

- a criminal offence
- a breach of a legal obligation
- miscarriages of justice
- dangers to health and safety
- dangers to the environment
- deliberate covering up of information tending to show any of the above five matters.

To qualify for protection, the worker making the disclosure must be acting in good faith throughout and must have reasonable grounds for believing that the information disclosed indicates the existence of one of the above problems. Disclosures are protected if they are made to the employer or other person responsible for the matter; to a Minister of the Crown, in relation to certain public bodies, to a regulatory body

Section 1	Protected disclosures
Section 2	Right not to suffer detriment
Section 3	Complaints to employment (industrial) tribunal
Section 4	Limit on amount of compensation
Section 5	Unfair dismissal
Section 6	Redundancy
Section 7	Exclusion of restrictions on right not to be unfairly dismissed
Section 8	Compensation for unfair dismissal
Section 9	Interim relief
Section 10	Crown employment
Section 11	National security
Section 12	Work outside Great Britain
Section 13	Police officers
Section 14	Remedy for infringement of rights
Section 15	Interpretative provisions of 1996 Act
Section 16	Dismissal of those taking part in unofficial industrial action
Section 17	Corresponding provisions for Northern Ireland
Section 18	Short title, interpretation, commencement and extent

Figure 17.8   Basic provisions of the Public Interest Disclosure Act 1998

designated for the purpose by order and for the purpose of seeking legal advice. Further details of the legislation can be obtained from the website of the Department for Business Enterprise and Regulatory Reform.[9]

The Clothier, Bullock and Shipman reports

Following the offences by Beverly Allitt, the Clothier Inquiry made several recommendations to detect the possibility of personal disorder in applicants for nursing posts. It suggested that there should be procedures for management referrals to occupational health and the criteria to trigger such referrals should be clarified. There would therefore be a duty on any employee who suspects that a colleague is acting suspiciously to advise the appropriate manager. The Government accepted the recommendations of the Clothier Inquiry.[52]

The Clothier recommendations were reinforced by an inquiry chaired by Richard Bullock following the case of Amanda Jenkinson, a Nottinghamshire nurse who was jailed for harming a patient.

The Government have accepted the recommendations that all NHS staff will have a pre-employment health assessment. Information provided to occupational health staff will remain confidential unless disclosure is necessary because a member of staff is considered to be a danger to patients, other staff or themselves. In these circumstances there should be disclosure to the appropriate person or authority.

Six enquiries followed the conviction of Dr Harold Shipman[53] for the murder of 15 patients and significant changes were recommended to professional regulation, certification of death and the coronial system. These are considered in Chapters 4 and 25.

Protection of vulnerable adults and children

Employers now have duties under legislation relating to vulnerable adults and children including the Protection of Children Act 1999, the Protection of Vulnerable Adults scheme and the Sexual Offenders Act 1997 to establish if there are grounds for not employing prospective employees, and must carry out checks with the Criminal Records Bureau.

The Safeguarding Vulnerable Groups Act 2006 aimed at strengthening current safeguarding arrangements for individuals in the workplace and reducing the risk of individuals suffering harm at the hands of those employed in either paid or voluntary capacity to work with them. The Independent Barring Board (IBB) was set up on 2 January 2008 and people included in lists maintained under the Protection of Children Act 1999 or the Care Standards Act 2000 or who are subject to a direction under the Education Act 2002 Section 142 will be included or considered for inclusion by the IBB in the children's barred list of the adults' barred lists.

The IBB was renamed the Independent Safeguarding Authority (ISA), which was established to support the implementation of the Safeguarding Vulnerable Groups Act and bring together the existing barring schemes, Protection of Vulnerable Adults (POVA), Protection of Children Act and List 99. From the autumn of 2008 ISA will cover the following areas:

- coverage of all workforce areas where children or vulnerable adults may be exposed to abuse or exploited instead of just regulated social care settings;
- pre-employment vetting;
- independent and consistent decision-making by employers;
- continuous monitoring: ISA can review decision not to bar on receipt of new information;
- reduction in bureaucracy: on line and free of charge checking system, once people have joined the scheme;
- wide range of sources of information: duty of employers and service providers to give information to the scheme;
- coverage across the UK.

ISA issued a consultation paper on the barring process in June 2007 covering the time period for making representations, the minimum no-review period, the age boundary in relation to the minimum barred period and automatic barring offences. It is estimated that 11 million individuals will have to be passed through the ISA's checking process in the first 5 years of its

operations. Further details on the Vetting and Barring Scheme Programme can be found on the Home Office website.[54]

The Department for Children, Schools and Families (DCSF) has also developed a cross-government strategy for children and young people called 'Staying Safe', which can be accessed on the DCSF website and the police website.[55]

Agenda for Change

In 1999 the Government published *Agenda for Change: Modernising the NHS Pay System*. This included:

- a single job evaluation scheme to cover all posts in the NHS to support a review of pay and all other terms and conditions for health service employees;
- three pay spines for doctors and dentists; for other professional groups covered by the Pay Review Body and for remaining non-Pay Review Body staff;
- a wider remit for the Pay Review Body.

The Employment Relations and Union Services Department of the CSP published a briefing for the Agenda for Change relating to job descriptions in February 2004.[56] The Agenda for Change introduced a national modernised pay and grading framework into the NHS which required a specially designed NHS job evaluation scheme to be used as the basis for deciding the appropriate Agenda for Change grade for NHS posts.

A second edition of the *NHS Job Evaluation Handbook* was published in 2004.[57]

Graduate unemployment

Recent years have seen a growth in the number of physiotherapy graduates finding it difficult to obtain posts within the NHS. A survey in October 2005 by the CSP showed that 51% of the graduates of that year did not have a junior physiotherapist job. An action plan was launched to tackle graduate unemployment that included the CSP's participation in the Social Partnership Forum to promote graduate employment. The CSP has also issued an employment pack guide for physiotherapy students[58] to assist final year students in finding their first post. The CSP has also published guidance for managers and its members on the implications of the removal of physiotherapy from the shortage occupations list.[59]

Fairness at Work and the Employment Act 2008

The White Paper *Fairness at Work* was published in 1998.[60] Its principles are shown in Figure 17.9. The following 10 years since its publication were reviewed in a speech in May 2008 by the Secretary of State for Business, Enterprise and Regulatory Reform.[61] He envisaged that the UK had reached the end of any new regulations and believed that in future there would be a changing balance of rights and responsibilities; business success would be boosted by investing in employees; a need to ensure more effective enforcement of existing laws; recognising that consumers can drive up standards at work. Some of these ideas are contained in the Employment Act 2008. The Act aims to:

- improve the effectiveness of employment law to the benefit of employers, TUs, individuals and the public sector;
- bring together both elements of the government's employment relations strategy increasing protection for vulnerable workers and lightening the load for law-abiding businesses;
- promote compliance and help to ensure a level playing field for law-abiding businesses.

The Act's provisions are:

Rights for individuals:
- national minimum wage
- Public Interest Disclosure Act
- Employment Rights (Dispute Resolution) Act
- abolition of the cap on the compensation that employment tribunals can award in unfair dismissal cases
- a reduction from 2 years to 1 in the qualifying period for unfair dismissal claims
- consultation on removal of waiver of unfair dismissal rights in fixed term and zero hours contracts

Collective rights:
- implementation of European Works Council Directive
- changes in legislation on representation and recognition of TUs
- changes in law on industrial action ballots and notice
- abolition of Commissioner for the Rights of Trade Union Members (CRTUM) and Commissioner for Protection Against Unlawful Industrial Action (CPAUIA)

Family friendly policies:
- Working Time Directive
- Young Workers Directive
- Parental Leave Directive
- extension of maternity leave to 18 weeks
- reasonable time off for family emergencies
- protection against dismissal in exercising rights to parental leave and time off for urgent family reasons

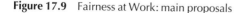

Figure 17.9   Fairness at Work: main proposals

- to repeal the Employment Act 2002 and the Dispute Resolution Regulations 2004 and thus abolish the existing statutory dispute resolution procedures and related provisions about procedural unfairness;
- to establish a new non-regulatory scheme for dispute resolution;
- to clarify and strengthen the enforcement framework for the National Minimum Wage;
- implement the changes required following the ECHR decision in *ASLEF* v. *UK*,[62] which ruled that clearer rights for TUs to determine their membership were required.
- employment tribunals are given discretionary powers to amend awards if parties have failed to comply with a relevant statutory code. Tribunals will be able to reach a determination without a hearing. Tribunals will also be able to award compensation for financial loss, in certain cases. The law relating to conciliation by ACAS is also to be amended.

Conclusions on employment law

Changes to employment rights and benefits are constant, partly as a result of European Directives, and the CSP has provided members with useful guidance on updates to employment legislation. The now pro-active role of ACAS in unfair dismissal cases has made it more likely that a dispute will be resolved internally and made it less likely that a case will go to the employment tribunal. The tighter laws on discrimination, and in particular the Equality Act 2006, have still to be embedded within the NHS, which still remains an organisation where racism and other blatant forms of discrimination abound. Considerable challenges thus remain for physiotherapists. The CSP is a member of NHS Together – an alliance of health service TUs and staff associations that is aiming for a more consultative, evidence-based and measured approach to reform of the NHS. More information on the NHS Together Campaign can be obtained from the CSP website.[63]

Statutory framework of the NHS

Following the NHS and Community Care Act 1990 NHS Trusts were established with the intention that they should become the principal providers of NHS secondary and community health care. Purchasers were either GPs, who were approved as fundholders to hold a budget to purchase secondary and community healthcare services for their patients, or health authorities.

In April 1996 health authorities were reorganised: the former district health authorities (DHAs) and family health services authorities (FHSAs) were abolished and in their place were established new health authorities which had the responsibility of commissioning and, in conjunction with GP fundholders, purchasing services from providers, as well as carrying out the responsibilities in relation to the primary healthcare services formerly undertaken by FHSAs. Subsequently GP fundholders were abolished and strategic health authorities (SHAs) established with primary care trusts (PCT) having a wider commissioning remit.

Other changes introduced by the 1990 Act relate to the functions of the local authorities in community care provision and these are considered in Chapter 18.

The White Paper on the new NHS

A White paper on the NHS,[64] published in 1997, envisaged that the internal market would be abolished, but proposed that long-term service level agreements covering at least 3 years for the provision of services should be in place. The CSP published guidance for physiotherapists on setting service specifications and negotiating service agreements in the light of the White Paper[65] and more recently a guide on commissioning.[21]

The main features of the White Paper on the NHS are shown in Figure 17.10.

Many of the recommendations contained in the White Paper were contained in the Health Act 1999 and re-enacted in the Health and Social

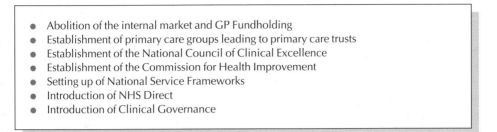

- Abolition of the internal market and GP Fundholding
- Establishment of primary care groups leading to primary care trusts
- Establishment of the National Council of Clinical Excellence
- Establishment of the Commission for Health Improvement
- Setting up of National Service Frameworks
- Introduction of NHS Direct
- Introduction of Clinical Governance

Figure 17.10   Main features of the White Paper *The New NHS: Modern Dependable* (1997)

Care (Community Health and Standards) Act 2003.

The basic duty placed on the Secretary of State to provide health care was contained in the NHS Act 1946 and re-enacted in the NHS Act 1977 and 2006. This is considered in Chapter 6 and shown in Figure 6.2. Chapter 6 looks at ways in which these duties can be enforced. In this chapter we consider the NHS organisations which have the responsibility of performing those duties on behalf of the Secretary of State.

The Secretary of State has the power (Section 7 of the 2006 Act) to direct a SHA, PCT or special health authority to exercise any of his functions relating to the heath service which are specified in the directions. The Secretary of State may also give directions to SHAs, PCTs, NHS trusts and special health authorities about their exercise of any functions.

An NHS contract is an arrangement under which one health service body (the commissioner) arranges for the provision to it by another health service body (the provider) of goods or services that it reasonably requires for the performance of its functions. Such a contract does not give rise to contractual rights and liabilities but any disputes over such arrangements may be referred to the Secretary of State for his determination.

The Secretary of State also has the power to make arrangements with other bodies or individuals or voluntary organisations to assist in the provision of any services under the Act.

Strategic health authorities

Health authorities were amalgamated to create SHAs with functions in relation to the planning and commissioning of health services. They are responsible for contracting for the provision of health services in a given area and ensuring that the health needs within their catchment area are met and work with the Secretary of State to an agreed plan and under his directions. Their constitution, powers, functions and duties are set out in the National Health Service Act 2006 Sections 13–17 and Schedule 2. Each SHA is a corporate body which consists of a chairman and members appointed by the Secretary of State. Each SHA is required to make arrangements to ensure that it receives advice from persons with professional expertise relating to the physical or mental health of individuals to enable it to exercise its functions effectively. (Section 17 of NHS Act 2006). Members of the SHA are required to comply with a Code of Accountability and a Code of Conduct, drawn up by the Department of Health.

NHS Trusts

Established under the NHS and Community Care Act 1990 (re-enacted in the NHS Act 2006 Sections 25–29 and Schedules 4 and 5), NHS trusts have a duty to exercise their functions in the provision of health services, effectively, efficiently and economically (S.26). Each NHS

Trust, which is a body corporate has a chairman appointed by the Secretary of State and non-executive and executive directors. The latter are employees of the NHS trust. Each trust is established under an NHS trust order. The Secretary of State has the power to dissolve any NHS trust if he/she considers it appropriate in the interest of the service. Consultation must be carried out unless the dissolution is a matter of urgency.

Foundation Trusts

Foundation hospital trusts were set up in April 2004. The statutory provisions have now been consolidated in the National Health Service Act 2006 Sections 30–65 and Schedules 7, 8, 9 and 10. The Act defines an NHS foundation trust as 'a public benefit corporation which is authorised to provide goods and services for the purposes of the health service in England'. A body corporate known as the Independent Regulator of NHS Foundation Trusts (called Monitor)[66] is set up under Section 31 of the 2006 Act with additional provisions relating to membership, tenure of office, general and specific powers, finance and reports set out in Schedule 8. Monitor has a duty to exercise its functions in a manner consistent with the performance by the Secretary of State of the duties under Sections 1, 3 and 258 of the NHS Act 2006 (duty as to health service and services generally and as to university clinical teaching and research). NHS trusts can apply to Monitor for authorisation to become an NHS foundation trust. The application must describe the goods and services it intends to provide together with a copy of the proposed constitution of the trust. Monitor must maintain a register of NHS foundation trusts together with a copy of its constitution, latest annual report and accounts and any notice relating to its being a failing NHS foundation trust. Once an NHS foundation trust is established, it ceases to be regarded as the servant or agent of the Crown or as enjoying any status, immunity or privilege of the Crown.

An NHS foundation trust is an independent public benefit corporation, not under the direct control of the Secretary of State. Ownership and accountability for the NHS foundation trust is in the hands of the local community rather than the Secretary of State.

If Monitor is satisfied that an NHS foundation trust is contravening or failing to comply with the terms of its authorisation then it may serve a notice on the trust that the board of governors is required to do a specified thing, or that all of the directors or the members of the board of governors are removed and replaced with interim directors or members or suspended. (S.52) The directors can be required to take steps to obtain a moratorium or propose a voluntary arrangement under insolvency legislation. Ultimately, Monitor can make an order (after following a specified procedure) providing for the dissolution of the trust and the transfer of its property or liabilities to another NHS foundation trust, a PCT, an NHS trust or the Secretary of State.

Primary Care Trusts (Local Health Boards in Wales)

Recent years have seen a devolution of funding and powers to primary care with more services being available from PCTs. Sections 18–24 and Schedule 3 of the NHS Act 2006 re-enacts the constitution, function and powers of the PCTs. They were established by the Secretary of State, who has the power to vary their areas, abolish them or establish a new PCT. A Strategic Health Authority may give directions to a PCT about the exercise of its functions. The PCT may provide services under an agreement for primary medical services and primary dental services and premises for pharmaceutical services and primary medical, dental and ophthalmic services. They can also manage health service hospitals. They have a duty, to enable them effectively to exercise their functions, to make arrangements to secure appropriate advice from persons with professional expertise about the physical and mental health of individuals. They are required to prepare and keep under review a plan which sets out the strategy for improving the health of the people for whom they are responsible and the provision of health services to them. Each local authority in the PCT catchment area must participate in the preparation or review of the plan. PCTs, SHAs and local authorities must have regard to these plans in the exercise of their functions. The National Audit Office reviewed the progress in implementing clinical governance in primary care and drew lessons for the new PCTs in January 2007.[67] It urged the NHS to ensure that a focus on quality and safety was at the top of the agenda in primary care. It noted that progress in implementing clinical governance was not uniform and the independence of primary care contractors, such as GPs, community pharmacists, dentists and practice nurses was a major challenge. The PCT did not have direct line management authority over individual contractors. PCTs needed to develop a strategy for engaging their independent contractors in improving quality and safety and create a professional culture within their organisations.

Care Trusts

The NHS Plan[68] envisaged that care trusts would be established to commission and provide social services as well as community health care. Further provisions to regulate care trusts are contained in the Health and Social Care Act 2001 Part 3. Care trusts enable social services as well as health services to be provided by the same trust. A PCT or NHS trust can apply to the Secretary of State for the recognition of their (proposed) delegation arrangements with a local authority as a care trust. The Secretary of State has the power to dissolve the PCT or NHS trust and designate a care trust (S.77 of the 2006 NHS Act).

Standards and guidelines

The concept of clinical governance was based on the statutory duty of quality under Section 18 of the Health Act 1999 which has now been replaced by Section 45 of the Health and Social Care (Community Health and Standards) Act 2003. It is shown in Box 17.1.

Box 17.1   Section 45 of Health and Social Care (Community Health and Standards) Act 2003.

(1) It is the duty of each NHS body to put and keep in place arrangements for the purpose of monitoring and improving the quality of healthcare provided by and for that body.

(2) Healthcare means the services provided to individuals for or in connection with the prevention, diagnosis or treatment of illness and the promotion and protection of public health.

Legal standards in the duty of care are discussed in Chapter 10 on the law of negligence and the extent to which clinical guidelines, protocols, procedures and practices are enforceable through the courts is considered in that chapter and also covered in a fascinating work by Brian Hurwitz.[69]

National Institute for Health and Clinical Excellence

This was set up on 1 April 1999 to promote clinical excellence and cost-effectiveness.[70] It is an independent organisation for providing national guidance on treatments and care for those using the NHS in England and Wales. It can be accessed on its website.[71] In discussing the legal status of guidance, the memorandum of the Department of Health[72] states that:

All guidance must be fully reasoned and written in terms which makes clear that it is guidance. Guidance for clinicians does not override their professional responsibility to make the appropriate decision in the circumstances of the individual patient, in consultation with the patient or guardian/carer and in the light of locally agreed policies. Similarly, guidance to NHS trusts and commissioners must make clear that it does not take away their discretion under administrative law to take account of individual circumstances.

However in more recent years NICE has been concerned at the failure by NHS trusts and PCTs to follow clinical guidance and has looked at ways of securing the implementation of its guidance. It has faced several legal challenges. For example, the drug manufacturers Eisai Ltd sought judicial review of the guidance issued by NICE on restricting the use of drugs for the treatment of Alzheimer's Disease.[73] The judge held that the processes of NICE were not flawed, but there were breaches of discrimination legislation As a consequence of the case, NICE was asked to revise its guidance within 28 days and the revised guidance can be seen on its website.[74] Subsequently Eisai Ltd won its appeal in the Court of Appeal.[75] The case is considered in Chapter 6.

Physiotherapists can access the NICE guidance across many of their specialties on its website.

Commission for Audit and Inspection

The Health Act 1999 led to the establishment of the Commission for Health Improvement (CHI), which was replaced by the Commission for Audit and Inspection (known as the Healthcare Commission) on 1 April 2004 as a consequence of the Health and Social Care (Community Health and Standards) Act 2003, which sets out its powers, functions and constitution. It has the overall function of encouraging improvement in the provision of health care by and for NHS bodies and undertakes inspections of NHS organisations, and is responsible for the registration of private hospitals and healthcare facilities under the Care Standards Act 2000. Further information on its functions, together with the copies of its reports and inspections can be obtained from its website.[76]

The Care Quality Commission

The Health and Social Care Act abolished the Health Care Commission, the Commission for Social Care Inspection and the Mental Health Act Commission and replaced them with a new Care Quality Commission with enhanced powers of inspection and enforcement. The Chairs of the Commissions which were to be replaced by the Care Quality Commission gave evidence to the scrutiny committee reviewing the Health and Social Care Act. The Chairs said that they had been presented with the changes as a fait accompli, that the £140 million it was estimated that it would cost would negate the savings already made, and it was not yet clear that a single regulator could effectively monitor a vast range of services from a 1000 bed hospital Trust to a six-bed unit for people with learning disability.[77] In spite of these objections the Government's plans to create a new superbody were implemented and the Care Quality Commission with additional powers came into being in April 2009.

National Service Frameworks

The White Paper on the NHS[78] set out a package of measures to raise standards within the NHS and these were further elaborated in the NHS Plan.[68] Included in this programme of action was the introduction of National Service Frameworks (NSFs). The intention was that the NSFs would set national standards and define service models for a defined service or care group; put in place strategies to support implementation; and establish performance measures against which progress within an agreed timescale would be measured. The CHI (now the Healthcare Commission) had the remit of ensuring through a programme of systematic service reviews that they are implemented. NSFs cover the following areas: cancer; children; coronary heart disease; diabetes; long-term health conditions; mental health; older people; paediatric intensive care; renal services and chronic obstructive pulmonary disease. Physiotherapists working in these fields would be expected to be aware of the contents of the relevant NSF and be involved in their implementation.

- What if an NHS trust ignores the implications of an NSF?

In such circumstances, the Care Quality Commission in its inspection would identify the failures by the NHS Trust and in serious situations, the NHS Trust could be put under special measures until compliance was achieved. Individual patients could refer to an NSF in an action for compensation for negligence if they were able to show that, as a result of a failure to implement the standards set in an NSF, they had suffered harm. An application for judicial review could also be brought but it is likely that the courts would insist that other internal methods of enforcement were used, before judicial review was considered appropriate

Selling physiotherapy

In 1995 the CSP issued an information pack for GPs on purchasing physiotherapy.[79] It covers the following areas:

- the aim of physiotherapy
- who should provide physiotherapy
- the development of Chartered Physiotherapists
- the contribution of physiotherapy to General Practice
- the effect on practice workload
- who may benefit from physiotherapy
- the range of clinical and other services offered by chartered physiotherapists
- physiotherapy service provision
- management and organisational issues
- quality issues.

There was also a pack provided by the Department of Health in 1996 on all the professions allied to medicine,[80] which includes examples of service level agreements.

Although the internal market has been abolished this guidance is still of value since it is still essential that physiotherapists can justify their work to health commissioners and to local health groups or primary care trusts and the managers of NHS Trusts. They will need to show the value added that physiotherapy can bring to a clinical situation, thereby justifying the investment in care and treatment by the physiotherapist. Even though the internal market might not exist in name there will still be value in developing managed care schemes for physiotherapy services. The CSP prepared guidance, *Patterns of Health Care Delivery: Managed Care,*[81] to assist its members to understand the economics of any given disease/disorder, to know the standards and guidelines governing delivery of health care and to understand care interventions and their interrelationships as part of the overall care process. It states:

> Physiotherapists need to carefully examine managed care and disease management schemes to ensure that they do not compromise their clinical autonomy in order to achieve short term cost benefits. Failure to preserve physiotherapists' clinical autonomy, perhaps swapping it for standardised, inflexible care packages in the name of cost control, may compromise patients' welfare.

Physiotherapy as part of primary health care

Situation: unmet need

> A GP practice arranges for services from the physiotherapy department for the rehabilitation of a patient. Six sessions are agreed. At the end of this time, the physiotherapy department recommends that the patient should have a further six sessions, but the GP is not prepared for them to be funded. What is the situation?
>
> The physiotherapist could appeal to the primary care trust (in Wales the local health board) to ascertain if it is prepared to ensure that funding remains available for the patient, since the PCT has the responsibility of commissioning services. Hopefully the dispute could be resolved, possibly through mediation with an expert.

The physiotherapist as manager

Managing a department

Many physiotherapists may be concerned at how the law impinges upon their role as a manager of a service and most of the general chapters in this book will provide specific information for many of the issues that confront a manager. They should of course also be able to look for assistance from solicitors to the Trust and personnel officers or health and safety and other specialists employed within the organisation.

Situation: liability of a manager

A senior physiotherapist who had charge of a department discovered that, during her annual leave, a basic grade physiotherapist had used a defective alarm clock and as a consequence a patient was injured. Is the manager liable?

The principle of vicarious liability, which means that the employer is liable for the negligence of an employee while acting in the course of employment (see Chapter 10) does not apply to the relationship of senior to junior members of staff. Provided that work has been appropriately delegated and supervised, a senior is not liable for the negligence of a junior. In this situation the manager is not personally liable because the basic grade has acted negligently. However, she may be liable on her own account. Was she aware that the alarm clock was defective? If so, she should have removed it from the work place for repair, so that it could not be used inadvertently. If there is evidence that she has failed to follow a reasonable standard of care in management issues such as these, then she would be personally and professionally liable.

It follows too that a failure in any field of management which is directly the responsibility of the physiotherapist could result in his/her liability. Thus failure in ensuring a safe system of work, failure to draw the attention of senior management to any inadequacies in resources (including staffing and equipment), or failure to establish an appropriate system for determining priorities, could all result in his/her personal liability, for which his/her employer will also be vicariously liable.

A manager will also have responsibilities for the health and safety of staff. The manager should be aware of any unreasonable stress being suffered by individual employees and should ensure that there is no bullying. It is also her responsibility that risk assessment is undertaken in the department (see Chapter 11 for health and safety laws).

Situation: manager's responsibilities

A physiotherapist complains to the manager that she is receiving unwelcome attention from a patient. The manager tells her that this is an expected part of her work with patients and that she should try to ignore the problem. Unfortunately, the physiotherapist is assaulted by the patient when she is alone with him in the gymnasium. She suffers significant injuries.

An inquiry should be undertaken into this incident. It is clear from the few facts given here that the manager acted entirely inappropriately and failed to take the situation seriously. The employee might well have grounds for suing the employer for compensation for the injuries which she suffered, because of the failure of the manager to take reasonable precautions to ensure her safety.

Some of the main topics of concern for the allied health professionals manager are considered in two books edited by Robert Jones and Fiona Jenkins, *Key topics in Healthcare Management*[82] and *Managing and Leading in the Allied Health Professions*.[83]

Managing a clinical interest or occupational group

Some physiotherapists may find that they are involved in running a clinical interest or occupational group. They may be unfamiliar with the administrative demands of such work and it is essential that they take advice on the responsibilities involved. It is hoped that such work is unlikely to lead to legal disputes, but clarity of role, responsibility and procedure is essential to prevent any possible arguments. The CSP issued guidance in 1997[84] for the 31 clinical interests and occupational groups that were then in existence. The number has since grown and revised criteria issued by the Professional Practice Committee in March 2001 are shown in Figure 1.3. At the time of writing no new groups are being recognised as a review is being undertaken of processes and resources. This work is expected to be finished by December 2008 and may result in a change of the recognition criteria.

Conclusions

Significant changes have taken place in both employment law and in the structure and roles within the NHS. This chapter has sought to identify the main developments, but following the NHS review by the Health Minister and surgeon Mr Darzi a further reorganisation is anticipated. The reforms to the NHS include the possibility of placing failing NHS hospitals in the hands of private healthcare managers – a suggestion which has led to an outcry claiming that it would amount to the privatisation of the NHS.[85] The Darzi reforms are considered in more detail in Chapter 28. Both developments within employment law and within the NHS place considerable burdens upon the physiotherapist individually and as manager.

Questions and exercises

1   Consider the implications of the Agenda for Change on the physiotherapist as manager.
2   Look at the letter setting out your contract conditions and identify the source of each term i.e. statutory, express as a result of personal agreement, express as a result of collective bargaining. What terms would be implied?
3   There are very few men who are employed as physiotherapists or physiotherapist assistants. What action do you consider your NHS Trust or social services employer could take to encourage the recruitment of more men, without breaking the law on sex discrimination?
4   Take any NSF relevant to your area of work and analyse the extent to which the service provided by your department meets with the standards set by the NSF. What steps would you initiate to implement any changes to meet the required standards?
5   You have just been appointed as a senior manager within the physiotherapy department. How does the law impact upon your new responsibilities?

References

1   Chartered Society of Physiotherapy (2002) *Emergency Respiratory on Call Working: Guidance for Physiotherapists.* Information Paper 53. CSP, London.
2   *Johnstone* v. *Bloomsbury Health Authority* [1991] ICR 269.
3   Secretary of State for Business, Enterprise and Regulatory Reform (2008) *National Minimum Wage Low Pay.* Commission Report Cm 7333. Stationery Office, London.
4   www.lowpay.gov.uk
5   The Working Time Regulations 1998 SI 1833.
6   Council Directive 1993/104; [1992] OJL 307/18.

7   Council Directive 1994/33; [1994] OJL 216/12.

8   Working Time (Amendment) Regulations 2002 SI 3128.

9   www.berr.gov.uk/employment

10   www.nhsemployers.org

11   Chartered Society of Physiotherapists (2002) *Working Time Regulations*. CSP, London.

12   www.acas.org.uk

13   *Watling* v. *Gloucestershire County Council* 1994 EAT/868/94, Lexis transcript.

14   Chartered Society of Physiotherapy (2007) *Redundancy – A Guide of Law and NHS Provision*. ERUS IP 05. CSP, London.

15   Chartered Society of Physiotherapy (2007) *Redundancy – A Guide for Managers*. ERUS IP 06. CSP, London.

16   Chartered Society of Physiotherapy (2003) *Right to Request Flexible Working*. ERUS Factsheet No 21. CSP, London.

17   Chartered Society of Physiotherapy (2003) *Adoption Leave*. ERUS Factsheet No 20. CSP, London.

18   Chartered Society of Physiotherapy (2004) *Paternity Leave*. ERUS Factsheet No 19. CSP, London.

19   Chartered Society of Physiotherapy (2007) *Introducing New Working Patterns Including 7 Day Working*. CSP, London.

20   *Von Goetz* v. *St George's Hospital Employment Appeal Tribunal* EAT/1395/97 18 October 2001.

21   Chartered Society of Physiotherapists (2007) *Making the Business Case: a Physiotherapist's Guide to Commissioning*. CSP, London.

22   Board of Trade (1998) White Paper *Fairness at Work* CM 3968. Stationery Office, London.

23   Chartered Society of Physiotherapy (2006) *Maternity Leave and Maternity Pay*. IP 08. CSP, London.

24   *Mayr* v. *Backerel und Konditorei Gerhard Flockner OHG*. The Times Law Report 12, March 2008 Case C-506/06.

25   www.dwp.gov.uk/lifeevent/benefits/statutory_sick_pay.asp

26   *Enderby* v. *Frenchay Health Authority and the Secretary of State for Health* [1991] IRLR 44.

27   *Enderby* v. *Frenchay Health Authority and Health Secretary* (C-127/92) October 1993 (ECJ) [1994] Current Law 4813, [1994] 1 All ER 495.

28   Code of Practice on Equal Pay Order 2003 SI 2003 No. 2865.

29   Directive 2006/54/EC.

30   The Sex Discrimination Act 1975 (Amendment) Regulations 2008 SI 656.

31   Directive 2002/73 (2002) OJ L269/16.

32   The Employment Equality (Religion or Belief) Regulations SI 2003 No. 1660.

33   Chartered Society of Physiotherapy (2004) *Employment Equality (Religion or Belief) Regulations 2003*. Information Paper ERUS 1P 22. CSP, London.

34   The Employment Equality (Sexual Orientation) Regulations SI 2003 No. 1661.

35   Chartered Society of Physiotherapy (2005) *Employment Equality (Sexual Orientation) Regulations 2003*. Information Paper. ERUS Factsheet No 33. CSP, London.

36   Wainwright, M. (2005) Landmark ruling on homophobic taunts. *The Guardian*, 29 January.

37   Employment Equality (Sex Discrimination) Regulations SI 2005 No 2467.

38   Disability Rights Commission (2005) *The Duty to Promote Disability Equality*. Stationery Office, London.

39   *Paterson* v. *Metropolitan Police Commissioner* [2007] All ER (D) 346 July.

40   *Gichura* v. *Home Office*. The Times Law Report, 4 June 2008.

41   *McDougall* v. *Richmond Adult Community College*. The Times Law Report 22 February 2008.

42   Council Directive 2000/78 ([2000] OJL303/16).

43   Employment Equality (Age) Regulations 2006 SI 2006 No 1031.

44   *Felix Palacios de la Villa* v. *Cortefiel Servicios SA ECJ* [2007] 16 October Case C-411/05; [2008] All ER (EC) 249; The Times Law Report, 23 October 2007.

45   Gibb, F. (2008) Teenager Wins Age Discrimination Claim. *The Times*, 4 March p. 27.

46   www.equalityhumanrights.com

47   OJ 2000 I 303 p. 16.

48   Coleman (Social Policy) [2008] EUECJ C-303/06 31 January 2008.

49   Coleman (Social Policy) [2008] EUECJ C-303/06 17 July 2008.

50   www.equalityhumanrights.com/en/newsandcomment

51   HMSO (1975) *Rehabilitation of Offenders Act 1974* (Exceptions) Order 1975 SI No. 1023.

52   DGM (95) 71 The Allitt Inquiry.

53   Shipman Inquiry First Report Death Disguised published 19 July 2002; www.the-shipman-inquiry.org.uk/reports.asp; Shipman Inquiry Second Report, The Police Investigation of March 1998, published 14 July 2003; Shipman Inquiry

Third Report, Death and Cremation Certification, published 14 July 2003; Shipman Inquiry Fourth Report, the Regulation of Controlled Drugs in the Community, published 15 July 2004 Cm 6249 Stationery Office; The Shipman Inquiry Fifth Report, Safeguarding Patients: Lessons from the Past – Proposals for the Future. Command Paper CM 6394, December 2004, Stationery Office. The Shipman Inquiry Sixth, Shipman: The Final Report, January 2005, Stationery Office. Available from www.the-shipman-inquiry.org.uk/reports.asp

54 http://police.homeoffice.gov.uk/about-us/police-policy-operations

55 http://police.homeoffice.gov.uk/operational-policing/bichard-implementation

56 Chartered Society of Physiotherapy Agenda for Change Briefing No 1 Job Descriptions and Supporting Information for Matching Panels ERUS. CSP London.

57 Department of Health (2004) *NHS Job Evaluation Handbook*. DH, London.

58 Chartered Society of Physiotherapy (2005) *Employment Pack Guide for Physiotherapy Students*. CSP, London.

59 Chartered Society of Physiotherapy (2007) *Removal of Physiotherapy from the Shortage Occupations List*. CSP, London.

60 Board of Trade (1998) White Paper. *Fairness at Work* CM 3968. Stationery Office, London.

61 www.berr.gov.uk/aboutus/pressroom

62 *Associated Society of Locomotive Engineers & Firemen (ASLEF)* v. *the United Kingdom* 11002/05 [2007] ECHR 184 (27 February 2007) http://www.bailii.org/eu/cases/ECHR/2007/184.html

63 www.csp.org.uk

64 DoH (1997) *The New NHS: Modern Dependable*. HMSO, London.

65 Chartered Society of Physiotherapy (2000) *The New NHS – Modern, Dependable: Making the Best of Physiotherapy Services*. CSP, London.

66 www.dh.gov.uk

67 National Audit Office (2007) *Improving Quality and Safety – Progress in Implementing Clinical Governance in Primary Care: Lessons for the new Primary Care Trusts*. HC 100 2006–7. Stationery Office, London.

68 Department of Health (2000) *The NHS Plan: a Plan for Investment, a Plan for Reform*. Cm 4818-1. The Stationery Office, London, July.

69 Hurwitz, B. (1998) *Clinical Guidelines and the Law*. Radcliffe Medical Press, Oxford.

70 National Institute for Clinical Excellence (Establishment and Constitution) Regulations SI 1999 No. 220; amendments SI 2002 No. 1759 and 1760.

71 www.nice.org.uk

72 Department of Health (1999) *Memorandum of Understanding on Appraisal of Health Interventions*. DH, London.

73 *Eisai Ltd* v. *National Institute for Health and Clinical Excellence (Alzheimer's Society and Shire Pharmaceuticals Ltd Interested parties)* [2007] EWHC 1941.

74 http://guidance.nice.org.uk/TA111

75 *R (on the application of Eisai)* v. *National Institute for Health and Clinical Excellence and Shire Pharmaceuticals Ltd and the Association of the British Pharmaceutical Industry* [2008] EWCA Civ 438.

76 www.healthcarecommission.org.uk

77 Rose, D. Bonfire of Quangos 'is unnecessary and puts patient safety at risk'. *The Times*, 9 January 2008 p. 2

78 Department of Health (1997) *The New NHS – Modern, Dependable*. HMSO, London.

79 CSP Professional Affairs Department (1995) *Purchasing Physiotherapy: Information for General Practitioners and Fundholding Practice Managers*. CSP, London. and *In Touch* 1995, **74**, Winter, 38–40.

80 *Department of Health Getting Involved and Making a Difference: Purchasing and the Professions Allied to Medicine*. 1996.

81 CSP Professional Affairs Department (1995) Information Paper No. 28 (August 1995) *Patterns of Health Care Delivery: Managed Care*. CSP, London.

82 Jones, R.J., Jenkins Fiona (eds.) (2007) *Key Topics in Healthcare Management*. Radcliffe Medical, Oxford.

83 Jones, R.J., Jenkins Fiona (eds.) (2006) *Managing and Leading in the Allied Health Professions*. Radcliffe Medical, Oxford.

84 CSP Professional Affairs Department (1997) *Clinical interests and Occupational Groups*. CSP, London.

85 Rose, D. Anger Over 'Backdoor Privatisation' of the NHS. *The Times*, 6 June 2008 p. 21.

18 Community Care

In the last chapter we looked at the legal issues which arise in relation to employment law and at the organisation of care within the NHS. In this chapter we look at the legal issues arising from physiotherapy practice in the community, whether the physiotherapist is working for healthcare trusts or (very infrequently) the social services. The community role of physiotherapists has increased enormously over the past decade and most trusts providing community services would now have physiotherapy services in the community. Since 1993 major changes have resulted from the community care legislation with which the community physiotherapist should be familiar. This chapter considers the effect of these developments upon the role of the physiotherapist and the legal issues which can arise in community care.

Topics considered are:

- The community physiotherapist
- Community care changes
- Assessments
- Long-term care and NHS/social services responsibilities
- Residential and nursing home provision
- Inspection
- Legal concerns of the community physiotherapist

Reference should be made to Chapter 15 for equipment issues, to Chapter 16 for transport issues, to Chapter 19 for private practice and to Chapters 20–24 covering individual client groups. (Clients may of course come under more than one of the chapters.)

The community physiotherapist

A community physiotherapist needs to have an in depth understanding of the sociological, environmental and economic factors that influence people's lives and be able to adapt their intervention accordingly. The physiotherapist should have good working relationships with primary health care, local authority, voluntary and private sector personnel in their area.

This is set out by the Association of Chartered Physiotherapists in the Community, which produced *Standards of Good Practice* (1995) covering the following topics:

- The role of the community physiotherapist
- Resource management (Standard 1)
- Referrals (Standard 2)
- Professional matters (Standard 3)
- Management issues (Standard 4)
- Human resources (Standards 5, 6 and 7)
- The junior physiotherapist (Standard 8)
- The physiotherapist helper (Standard 9)
- Administrative support (Standard 10)
- Health promotion (Standard 11)
- Communication and team work (CSP Standards 1 to 6)
- Documentation (CSP Standards 8 to 10)
- Assessment/patient management (CSP Standard 11)
- Informed consent (CSP Standards 12 to 14)
- Health and safety (CSP Standard 20)
- Quality assurance (CSP Standards 21 to 25)

In addition of course the community physiotherapist would be expected to follow the Health Professions Council (HPC) *Standards of Conduct, Performance and Ethics*,[1] the Chartered Society of Physiotherapy (CSP) *Rules of Professional Conduct*,[2] the CSP core standards[3] and the CSP service standards.[4]

Multidisciplinary work

The physiotherapist working in the community will probably find that he/she is working as part of a multidisciplinary team, though the extent of team working varies considerably across the country. In mental health care community mental health teams are in some districts extremely sophisticated. The impact of the White Paper in 1997[5] which aimed at enhancing primary health care and the development of local health groups encouraged more multidisciplinary working for those suffering from physical disabilities. A White Paper published in 2006 on community health and social care (discussed below) envisaged more partnership working including co-location of services, including health and care services.

The law does not recognise a concept of team liability.[6] If, therefore, a physiotherapist is given an instruction from the team that he/she finds unacceptable professionally, the physiotherapist would have a duty to inform the team of the reasons why the instruction clashed with his/her professional duties. To say in a civil action for compensation 'I was obeying the instructions of the team' would not constitute a valid defence.

If the physiotherapist is appointed a key worker it is essential that he/she stays within his/her sphere of competence, and that the physiotherapist obtains the appropriate training and supervision if he/she is asked to perform activities and take on responsibilities which would not normally be seen as those of a physiotherapist.

Under Section 82 of the NHS Act 2006 local authorities and NHS bodies have a statutory duty to cooperate with one another in order to secure and advance the health and welfare of the people of England and Wales.

Research and development

The White Paper on the NHS encourages an emphasis on research-based practice. The physiotherapist is expected to be aware of recent research findings on clinical effectiveness and is also expected to take part in research projects herself. Research is carried out on all aspects of physiotherapy, including work in the community. This topic is considered in Chapter 26.

Community care changes

The Griffiths report

The debate on the value of developing community care goes back to the late 1950s and 1960s with a Hospital Plan published in 1962 and a Community Care Plan being published in 1963 with the aim of reducing dependence on long-stay hospitals and gradually closing them. Progress was made to a limited extent in reducing the size of long-stay NHS institutions, both for the mentally disturbed and for older people. The greatest impetus to the community care changes however was the report prepared by Sir Roy Griffiths.

In December 1986 the then Secretary of State, Norman Fowler, asked Sir Roy Griffiths, who had undertaken the report into hospital management, to undertake a review of community care policy. His terms of reference were as follows:

> To review the way in which public funds are used to support community care policy and to advise . . . on the options for action that would improve the use of these funds as a contribution to more effective community care.

In addition he was instructed

> that the review should be brief and geared towards advice on action as was the review of management in the health service in 1983.

The report was presented in February 1988. In his letter of response to the Government Sir Roy Griffiths made some radical suggestions which were initially not enthusiastically received. His main recommendations are summarised in Figure 18.1.

Basically, the recommendations were for a radical change in the funding of accommodation in the community and greater emphasis on clear lines of managerial accountability. Provision in the future had to be on the basis of an assessment of need and the development of local plans, drawn up by the local authorities in conjunction with health authorities and the voluntary sector.

White Paper

In November 1989 a White Paper was published, *Caring for People: Community Care in the Next Decade and Beyond*.[7] Figure 18.2 sets out the key objectives of the White Paper's proposals.

The White Paper explained how these objectives would be met in practice and outlined the roles and responsibilities of the social services authorities and also those of the health services. Emphasis was placed upon quality control and achieving high standards of care, collaborative working and service for people with a mental illness. It also considered the issue of resources and the links with social security. Separate chapters cover Wales and Scotland.

The NHS and Community Care Act 1990

Many of the recommendations of the White Paper were incorporated in the NHS and Community Care Act 1990. The main provisions of this Act in relation to community are listed in Figure 18.3.

It should be noted that Section 7 of the Local Government Social Services Act 1970 requires a local authority to act under the guidance of the Secretary of State in exercising its social services functions.

- Strengthening and clarifying the role of central government
- Clarifying the role of local social services authorities in assessing needs, developing local priorities and determining priorities
- Transferring to local authorities the responsibility for funding residential and nursing home accommodation for those unable to pay
- Enhancing the role of health authorities in the provision of medically required community health services and their role in the assessment of needs

Figure 18.1 Summary of Griffiths recommendations

(1) To promote the development of domiciliary, day and respite services to enable people to live in their own homes wherever feasible and sensible
(2) To ensure that service providers make practical support for carers a high priority
(3) To make proper assessment of need and good care management the cornerstone of high quality care
(4) To promote the development of a flourishing independent sector alongside good quality public services
(5) To clarify the responsibilities of agencies and so make it easier to hold them to account for their performance
(6) To secure better value for taxpayers' money by introducing a new funding structure for social care

Figure 18.2   Objectives of White Paper *Caring for People*

Section 46(3): Statutory definition of community care
Sections 42 to 45: The provision of accommodation and welfare services, charges for accommodation and the recovery of charges provided by local authorities
Section 46: The provision of a community care plan by each local authority (disapplied in relation to England for 2002/3)
Section 47: Assessment of needs for community care services
Section 48: Inspection of premises used for provision of community care services
Section 49: Transfer of staff from health service to local authorities
Section 50: Power of Secretary of State to give directions and instruct local authorities to set up complaints procedures
Section 51 to 58: Provisions for Scotland

Figure 18.3   The community care provisions of the NHS and Community Care Act 1990

Community care services

Section 46(3) provides the first statutory definition of community care services and it is given in Figure 18.4.

Two main topics in the community care provisions will be considered in the first part of this chapter: the duty to assess and the care management approach.

Community care plans

Section 46 of the 1990 Act required each local authority to prepare and publish a plan for the provision of community care in their area. Section 46 also required the local authority to

keep the plan, and any further plans prepared by them under this section, under review and empowered the Secretary of State to direct the intervals at which the local authority must prepare and publish modifications to the current plan or a new plan. The local authority was required to consult health authorities and voluntary organisations in the preparation of the plans. However, this section was disapplied in relation to England from 9 July 2003.[8]

Assessments

Statutory provision

Section 47 of the NHS and Community Care Act 1990 places upon the local authority a duty to

'Community care services' means services which a local authority may provide or arrange to be provided under any of the following provisions:

(a) Part III of the National Assistance Act 1948 [provision of accommodation for those over 18 who need it because of age, illness disability or any other circumstances];

(b) Section 45 of the Health Services and Public Health Act 1968 [covers arrangements for promoting the welfare of 'old people'];

(c) Section 21 of and Schedule 8 to the National Health Service Act 1977 [the provision of services for the care of mothers and young children; prevention, care and after-care; home help and laundry facilities];

(d) Section 117 of the Mental Health Act 1983 [the duty of the health authority and local social services authority to provide, in cooperation with relevant voluntary agencies, after care services for any person who has been detained under specified sections of the Mental Health Act 1983].

Figure 18.4   The NHS and Community Care Act 1990: Section 46(3)

carry out an assessment for any individual who appears to be eligible to receive its services.

The assessment is of the 'needs' of the individual for these services and it is on the results of the assessment that the local authority decides whether those needs call for the provision of services. There are, however, emergency provisions in Section 47(5) and (6) enabling urgent needs to be met temporarily without the formality of a prior assessment.

Disabled persons

There is a statutory requirement (Section 47(2)) upon local authorities to proceed under the Disabled Persons (Services, Consultation and Representation) Act 1986 if, at any time during the assessment of needs, it appears that the client is a disabled person. They need not wait for a request from the client but must inform him/her that they will be doing so and inform him/her of his/her rights under the 1986 Act (see Chapter 20).

Section 47(7) states that the section is 'without prejudice' to Section 3 of the Disabled Persons (Services, Consultation and Representation) Act 1986. This means that it does not affect the provisions of the 1986 Act that exist in parallel with the provisions for giving information under the 1990

Act. 'Disabled person' has the same meaning as that used in the 1986 Act.

Involvement of health and housing authorities

Under Section 47(3)(a) the local authority must notify the relevant health authority if, at any time during the assessment, it appears that the person may need services provided under the National Health Service Act 1977.

Under Section 47(3)(b) a similar provision exists if there is seen to be a need for the provision of any services which fall within the functions of a local housing authority.

In such circumstances the local authority has a duty not only to notify the health authority and/or housing authority but also to invite them to assist, to such extent as is reasonable in the circumstances, in the making of the assessment. In making a decision as to the provision of the services needed for the person in question, the local authority shall take into account any services that are likely to be made available for him/her by the health authority or housing authority.

Central government directions and guidance

The Secretary of State has the power to make directions relating to assessments (Section 47(4)).

Subject to this the local authority shall carry out the assessment in such manner and take such form as it considers appropriate.

Guidance was issued to local and other authorities for use in carrying out the assessments, *Caring for People: Community Care in the Next Decade and Beyond. Policy and Guidance*.[9] In addition, the Social Services Inspectorate prepared several handbooks on guidance in care management and assessment for managers and practitioners. Directions were issued by the Department of Health (DH) in 2004[10] about the involvement of carers in the assessment (see below) and can be obtained from the DH website which required the local authority to consider whether the person being assessed has any carers and, where they think it appropriate, consult those carers. In addition, the local authority must take all reasonable steps to reach agreement with the person and, where they think it appropriate, any carers of that person, on the community care services which they are considering providing to him/her to meet his/her needs. The local authority must provide information to the person and, where they think it appropriate, any carers of that person, about the amount of the payment (if any) which the person will be liable to make in respect of the community care services which they are considering providing to him/her.

Entitlement to assessment

Entitlement is not defined in the section other than in terms of eligibility to service provision. This is determined by residence.

- Could it be argued that if the local authority does not provide specific services then the assessment for those services need not be carried out?

The term 'any person for whom they may provide or arrange for the provision of community services' (Section 47(11)) covers all those services under the Acts specified in Section 46(3) which defines what is meant by community care

services. The fact that the local authority does not supply all the services the client may require cannot be a justification for not carrying out the assessment. After all it could be argued that until the assessment has been carried out it cannot be certain which services the client will or will not require.

The duty to assess is owed to those who are ordinarily resident within the local authority area. Guidance on the possibility of making arrangements with other local authorities for the provision of services stresses the need to take into account the desirability of providing services in the locality.

Carrying out the assessment

Stages in the process

The summary of practice guidance included in both the *Managers' Guide*[11] and the *Practitioners' Guide*[12] sets out the stages that should be followed in implementing the care management and assessment process. These stages are shown in Figure 18.5.

Levels of assessment

The *Practitioners' Guide* suggests that stage one requires an initial identification of the need and the determination of the level of assessment required. For example, it sets out six possible levels of assessment:

- *level one* simple assessment
- *level two* limited assessment
- *level three* multiple assessment
- *level four* specialist assessment either simple or complex
- *level five* complex assessment
- *level six* comprehensive assessment.

An example of an outcome from a level one assessment is a bus pass or disabled car badge. An example of an outcome from a level six assessment could be family therapy, substitute care or intensive domiciliary support.

Stage 1: Information to carers and prospective clients on needs for which the agencies accept responsibilities and the range of services currently available
Stage 2: The level of the assessment required is decided
Stage 3: A practitioner is allocated to assess the needs of the individual and of any carers
Stage 4: The resources available from statutory, voluntary, private or community sources that best meet the individual's requirements are considered. The role of the practitioner is to assist the user in making choices from these resources and to put together an individual care plan
Stage 5: The implementation of the plan, i.e. securing the necessary financial or other identified resources
Stage 6: Monitoring of implementation of the care plan
Stage 7: Review of the care plan with the user, carers and service providers; firstly, to ensure that services remain relevant to needs and, secondly, to evaluate services as part of the continuing quest for improvement

Figure 18.5   Care management and assessment process

Differing perceptions of need

The assessment of need is described in the *Practitioners' Guide* as being undertaken to 'understand an individual's needs, to relate them to agency policies and priorities, and to agree the objectives for any intervention'.

The practitioner is required by the guidance 'to define, as precisely as possible, the cause of any difficulty'. It recognises that need is unlikely to be perceived and defined in the same way by users, their carers, and any other care agencies involved. It suggests that:

the practitioner must, therefore, aim for a degree of consensus but, so long as they are competent, the users' views should carry the most weight. Where it is impossible to reconcile different perceptions, these differences should be acknowledged and recorded ...

Who carries out the assessment?

There is an emphasis on a multidisciplinary approach to the task of assessment with local authorities bringing in relevant professionals where necessary. The White Paper, *Caring for People: Community Care in the Next Decade and Beyond* suggests:

3.25 All agencies and professions involved with the individual and his or her problems should be brought into the assessment procedure when necessary. These may include social workers, GPs, community nurses, hospital staff such as consultants in geriatric medicine, psychiatry, rehabilitation and other hospital specialties, nurses, physiotherapists, occupational therapists, speech therapists, continence advisers, community psychiatric nurses, staff involved with vision and hearing impairment, housing officers, the Employment Department's Settlement Officers and its Employment Rehabilitation Service, home helps, home care assistants and voluntary workers.

3.26 Assessments should take account of the wishes of the individual and his or her carer, and of the carer's ability to continue to provide care, and where possible should include their active participation. Effort should be made to offer flexible services which enable individuals and carers to make choices.

Where the client is in hospital then the lead agency for carrying out the assessment will be the health services; where the client is in the community or in residential accommodation then the lead agency for carrying out the assessment will be the local authority.

What if the client refuses to co-operate in the assessment?

It would seem that there is a duty under Section 47(1)(a) of the 1990 Act for the assessment to be made even if the client refuses. Clearly, however, this may lead to a less than satisfactory assessment and any later objection by the client to the assessment should take account of this lack of cooperation. Where the client is incapable of assisting in the assessment, e.g. as a result of mental incapacity, the provisions of the Mental Capacity Act 2005 apply (see Chapters 7, 22 and 24). Where accommodation is being provided or rearranged, the local authority would have a duty to ensure that an independent mental capacity advocate was appointed, in the absence of any family or friends who could be consulted in determining the best interests of the client.

Disputes over care plans

In a case discussed in Chapter 23[13] a single mother failed in her application for judicial review of the Council's care plan for her disabled daughter on the grounds that its rejection of an independent review was both unreasonable according to the Wednesbury principle and a breach of Article 8 of the European Court of Human Rights.

In the following case the claimant alleged that the Council was failing to provide services according to the existing care plan, had failed to complete a lawful assessment on the claimant's accommodation and care needs and was failing to make arrangements for the provision of suitable accommodation pending the completion of an assessment of her accommodation under S 47(5) of the 1990 Act.

R (on the application of Irenschild) v. London Borough of Lambeth 2006[14]

Mrs Irenschild suffered an accident which left her with serious back and neck injuries and she had lost the ability to stand and move about unsupported, in constant pain and suffering from urinary and faecal incontinence. The judge allowed the application holding that the LA's community care assessment was unlawful: it had failed to take into account significant matters contained in the occupational therapist's report; it had not followed the guidance issued by the Department of Health in its Fair Access to Services paper and it was procedurally unfair in that certain issues had not been raised with the claimant (e.g. that the claimant had not had a fall in 8 years – which was contested by the claimant).

The physiotherapist and the assessment

In hospital

The physiotherapist is more likely to be involved in a healthcare-led assessment, especially when the patient is being assessed prior to discharge from hospital. It is essential that the physiotherapist is able to take a full part in this multidisciplinary process. The physiotherapist should also ensure that he/she records his/her assessment and the outcome.

Situation: report ignored

Prior to the discharge of a stroke victim, a physiotherapist carries out an assessment on the patient, together with an analysis of the carer's ability to cope with the patient at home. She recommends further in-patient care for the patient. To her surprise the consultant ignores her report and states that the patient should be discharged that day.

This is becoming an increasingly common problem as the pressure on beds, especially during the winter months, leads to early discharges. All the physiotherapist can do in this situation is:

- ensure that her report has been seen by all relevant parties and in particular the consultant;
- take all reasonable steps to provide support for the patient and carer in the community through liaison with social services, occupational therapy and other relevant departments;

- make arrangements to visit the patient if appropriate; and
- ensure that her records reflect the action that she has taken.

In the community

From April 1990 GPs have had, as part of their terms of service, the duty to carry out an annual assessment of every patient on their list who is aged 75 years or more. This work is increasingly delegated to practice nurses but there is no reason why physiotherapists should not take a greater responsibility in the assessment of these groups. From 2004 significant changes have taken place in the role of the primary care trust (PCT) and its relationship with GPs. PCTs receive a cash-limited allocation for the provision of primary care. They commission six directed enhanced services and other enhanced services. GPs have new contractual terms with the PCTs. Under contracts to provide general medical services GPs must provide essential services, have the expectation and right to provide additional services and the right to provide certain of the directed enhanced services.[15] Contractors are subject to statutory requirements relating to quality, including a new duty of clinical governance.

Long-term care and NHS/social services responsibilities?

Review of continuing care decisions

Each health authority in conjunction with local authorities and other agencies is required to establish a procedure for reviewing decisions in relation to the provision of continuing care. Guidance, published in 1995,[16] set out a recommended review procedure to be established in the context of high-quality discharge policies based on proper assessment and the provision of all relevant information and sensitivity to the needs and concerns of patients and their fami-

lies. The working of the review procedures has been monitored as part of the overall evaluation of the community care provisions.

The use of local eligibility criteria for access to continuing care (and therefore non-means-tested services from the NHS) has led to considerable diversity between different PCTs and local authorities, and many disputes over a refusal to provide NHS care. In July 2001 the DH published a consultation document *Guidance on Fair Access to Care Services* to ensure greater consistency in the use of eligibility criteria for access to care services. However, this failed to meet the problem and in 2006 the following case was heard:

Case: *R (on the application of Grogan)* v. *Bexley NHS Care Trust* 2006[17]

G. applied for judicial review of a decision by an NHS trust that she did not qualify for continuing NHS health care. If the NHS provided care it would be free; if it were the social services, she would be means tested. The high court held that an NHS trust should apply a primary health need test to determine whether accommodation should be provided by the NHS or social services. The criteria of the NHS trust for determining whether the patient had continuing care needs were fatally flawed and it failed to give reasons why it considered that the patient's continuing care needs were neither complex nor intense. The court ordered the trust's decision to be set aside and remitted for fresh consideration

Following the decision in the Grogan case, the DH announced that a national framework for continuing care would be implemented in October 2007. Assessments for continuing NHS care were to be carried out by a multidisciplinary team using the concept of 'a primary health' need as the criteria for the receipt of continuing healthcare.[18] New eligibility criteria were introduced in 2007, which are considered below and in Chapter 24.

Community Care (Direct Payments) Act 1996

On 1 April 1997 the Community Care (Direct Payments) Act came into force, which enabled social services departments to make payments in cash instead of kind to certain groups in receipt of community care. This enables a person to purchase their own care. However, the local authority originally retained its discretion and could not be compelled to offer cash rather than services. The level of payment must be sufficient to enable the recipient to buy the services the payments are intended to cover. New regulations came into force in 2003[19] under which there is now a duty to make direct payments to eligible individuals who appear to be capable of managing a direct payment by themselves or with such assistance as may be available to them. (Persons listed in Regulation 2 are ineligible.) These include persons under a community rehabilitation order for mental health or drug or alcohol dependency and those on Section 17 leave of the Mental Health Act 1983). If a person meets the criteria for direct payments and has had a community care assessment then the services needed are identified and he or she then has the choice of using the local social services or using the money provided to buy services from an alternative provider. In the DH circular *Transforming Social Care* in January 2008[20] it was estimated that only 54 000 out of a potential million recipients were receiving direct payments. The circular aimed at increasing the numbers of persons receiving direct payments or individual budgets (see below). Further information on direct payments is available from the DH publication in March 2008,[21] which can be downloaded from its website.

In the following case the defendant in a road traffic accident argued unsuccessfully that the amount of direct payments should be taken into account in calculating the compensation for future care costs.

Case: *Morgan v. Phillips*[22]

The claimant was 19 years when she suffered very severe injuries in an road traffic accident when she was knocked down by a car driven by the defendant. She suffered severe brain damage, which led to spastic tetraparesis. Her father acted as her litigation friend and receiver. The defendant was held liable for 55% of the damages. Following a community care assessment, the local authority offered the claimant a weekly sum to fund a certain level of support. The defendant argued that the claimant's father on behalf of the claimant was bound to accept the offer of the direct payment and that the sum fell to be deducted from the multiplicand in respect of the claimant's future care costs. The court held that the actual consent of the person was required under Section 57(1) of the Health and Social Care Act 2001 and her father as receiver did not have the power to give consent on her behalf. The defendant had not shown that there would be any direct payments and therefore the amount of direct payments should not be taken into account in calculating the compensation for future care costs.

Situation: protecting the public purse

A physiotherapist helps parent/carers to apply to the Social Fund for a chair for their adult son, in order to aid maintenance of a good posture. The Social Fund agree and a cheque is sent to the parents. When the physiotherapist makes inquiries about the chair she discovers that, as it was Christmas time, the money has been used for other purposes. What action should she take? Does she have a duty to inform the social services?

The simple answer to the last question is 'No'. It is not her responsibility to ensure that Social Fund moneys are used for the purpose they have been allocated. She has no duty to inform the Department of Social Security. However, since the client is still without the chair, she could encourage the family to try and save up for it since, without it, the client's condition will deteriorate.

Direct payments and liability for support workers

The following situation is of concern to physiotherapists.

Situation: accountability for the support worker?

Hugh has received from social services a care package which enables him to select and pay for his own support workers. His mobility is severely compromised and he needs to be hoisted into and out of his wheelchair. He employed carers sent to him from an independent care agency. Unfortunately, they had not been trained in manual handling and in attempting to transfer Hugh from his bed to the wheelchair, he fell to the floor, fracturing his pelvis. Who if anyone is accountable for this accident?

On the few facts given here, it would appear that the care agency did not hold itself out as being the employer of the carers. However, if the agency was recommending persons who could be employed as carers by Hugh, it should have ensured that the carers were trained in manual handling. It could be said that the agency owed a duty of care to Hugh, by failing to provide the necessary training, it was in breach of that duty and as a consequence reasonable foreseeable harm to Hugh has occurred (see Chapter 10 and the principles of negligence). It would therefore be liable to Hugh. If on the other hand, Hugh had employed a support worker who did not come via an agency, and this was known to health and social care professionals visiting Hugh, then they might have a duty of care to Hugh to advise him that any support worker should have a minimum training in manual handling. Such advice should be put in writing. If Hugh ignores that advice, then he could not hold the health or social care professionals liable (see Chapter 11 for manual handling).

Care management

The status of a claimant's case manager was considered in a case in 2005.

Case: *Wright* v. *Sullivan*[23]

The claimant was born in 1984 and was 20 at the time of the hearing. She had problems in learning and had one-to-one tuition. She was badly beaten up when she was 14 years old. Eleven months later she was knocked down by a car when crossing the road. Liability was eventually accepted by the defendant as 70% with 30% contributory negligence. A dispute arose as to the amount of compensation. She had suffered a very severe concussive head injury resulting in brain damage with physical and mental symptoms. She developed post-traumatic epilepsy for which there was a 70% chance of bringing under control, poor concentration and memory reduction in her powers of literacy and a personality change. It was said that she was fully capable of all acts of daily living, but she required daily supervision of her behaviour by others and daily care in the absence of her mother. It was considered that she would be incapable of managing and administering her own financial affairs or of independent living. Her chances of finding work were severely jeopardised and her affairs were managed by the Court of Protection. The daughter got into trouble and was placed under the probation service. She was evicted from a hostel for rule-breaking. She became pregnant and the mother was providing care for her and the child. The mother had failed to obtain help from social services or other agencies. An application for an interim payment was made to enable a clinical case manager to be appointed. The defendants asserted that damages would be reduced because of the 30% contributory negligence and the fact that some of the symptoms were the result of the beating prior to the accident and not attributable to the road accident and there was a dispute about her earning capacity. The defendant's insurers proposed that a clinical case manager should be instructed jointly to consider the claimant's needs and to prepare a report. Until the report was available the interim payment should be deferred. The claimant objected to the joint instruction, stating that the clinical case manager is a person engaged on behalf of the claimant and whose relationship with the claimant is therapeutic. Although an expert in her field, she would not be called on behalf of the claimant to give evidence in her capacity as an expert witness, but as a witness of fact. The judge ordered the payment of the interim sum of £50 000 with no conditions on the order. The defendant appealed and the claimant cross-appealed submitting that the clinical case manager should be seen as a witness of fact. The Court of Appeal considered the role of the clinical case manager as set out in the British Association of Brain Injury Case Managers in 2005 (see Figure 18.6). The court was told that an occupational or physiotherapist often fulfilled the role of clinical case manager. The Court of Appeal rejected the submission of the defendant that the clinical case manager should be seen as an expert witness. It said that the clinical case manager may receive suggestions from other experts, but ultimately she

must make decisions in the best interests of the patient and not be beholden to two different masters. The Court rejected the defence submission that the instruction of the clinical case manager should be joint instruction and neither party should be permitted to have 'behind closed doors' access to her. It held that the role of the clinical case manager, if she is called to give evidence at the trial, will clearly be one of a witness of fact. She is there to give evidence of what she did and why she decided to do it. She will not be giving evidence of expert opinion. The Civil Procedure Rules on expert witnesses do not therefore apply to her.

Carers

It is estimated that there are about 5.2 million carers in England and Wales with nearly half of them providing more than 20 hours' care a week

---

(a) A clinical manager must have a relevant professional qualification
(b) The responsibilities of a clinical case manager include:
   (i) Advocating for and on behalf of a client
   (ii) Protecting a client from vulnerability and abuse
   (iii) Maintaining effective communication systems for, amongst others, the client
   (iv) Coordinating a package of rehabilitation and care/support relevant to his/her needs
   (v) Managing such package using evidence-based practice and in line with National standards
   (vi) Undertaking an appropriate full needs and risk assessment
   (vii) Designing a case management plan to meet the assessed needs
   (viii) Implementing the plan taking account of quality, safety, efficiency and cost-effectiveness
   (ix) Monitoring progress/deterioration and updating goals and related documentation
(c) The relationship between clinical case manager and his/her client (injured party) is therapeutic and professional
(d) The clinical case manager owes a duty of care to the injured party
(e) The instruction to the clinical case manager should be from the client or from a representative of his or her behalf (e.g. a receiver)
(f) Joint instructions can lead to conflict and are not recommended
(g) The clinical case manager should be responsible for providing factual evidence as to work completed and the underlying reason for this, if so required
(h) The clinical case manager should only act as a witness of fact as regards the service provided for a case management client

Figure 18.6 Principles and guidelines for case management best practice from the British Association of Brain Injury

[I]n any case where:

(a) a local authority carries out an assessment under Section 47(1)(a) of the [1990] Act of the needs of a person ('the relevant person') for community care services, and

(b) an individual ('the carer') provides or intends to provide a substantial amount of care on a regular basis for the relevant person,

the carer may request the local authority, before they make their decision as to whether the needs of the relevant person call for the provision of any services, to carry out an assessment of his ability to provide and to continue to provide care for the relevant person; and if he makes such a request, the local authority shall carry out such an assessment and shall take into account the results of that assessment in making that decision.

Figure 18.7 Carers (Recognition and Services) Act 1995: Section 1(1)

and over a million providing more than 50 hours' care per week. The Carers (Recognition and Services) Act 1995, which came into force on 1 April 1996, places a duty on local authorities to provide for the assessment of the ability of carers to provide care and for connected purposes. The basic provisions are shown in Figure 18.7. The Carers and Disabled Children Act 2000 strengthened the provisions of the 1995 Act by making provision for the informal (i.e. not paid or working for a voluntary organisation) carers to have a right to an assessment. The Carers (Equal Opportunities) Act 2004 amended the 1995 and 2000 Acts to ensure that an assessment under Section 1(2) must include consideration of whether the carer works or wishes to work, and whether the carer is undertaking, or wishes to undertake, education, training or any leisure activity. These provisions came into force on 1 April 2001.

Directions were issued by the DH in 2004[10] about the involvement of carers in the assessment, which required the local authority to consider whether the person being assessed has any carers and, where they think it appropriate consult those carers. In addition, the local authority must take all reasonable steps to reach agreement with the person and, where they think it appropriate, any carers of that person, on the community care services which they are

considering providing to him/her to meet his/her needs. The local authority must provide information to the person and, where they think it appropriate, to any carers of that person, about the amount of the payment (if any) which the person will be liable to make in respect of the community care services which they are considering providing to him/her.

The duty to assess the carer on request also applies where the local authority makes an assessment of the needs of a disabled child for the purposes of Part III of the Children Act 1989 or Section 2 of the Chronically Sick and Disabled Persons Act 1970 and a carer provides or intends to provide a substantial amount of care on a regular basis for the disabled child or person. The local authority may take into account an assessment made under Section 1 or 6 of the Carers and Disabled Children Act 2000 in carrying out its assessment (S.1(2)(A) of 1995 Act

Excluded from those carers entitled to be assessed are those providing care by virtue of a contract of employment or other contract with any person, or as a volunteer for a voluntary organisation. The cases of *R (on the application of B)* v. *London Borough of Newham* and of *R (on the application of LH)* v. *London Borough of Lambeth* illustrate the working of the 1995 and 2000 Acts.

Case: *R (on the application of B) v. London Borough of Newham*[24]

Mr B was 64 years of age and suffered from depression and high blood pressure, a shoulder problem and other more minor medical problems. He left work to become a full-time carer for his family. His wife, the claimant was 38 years old, registered blind and suffered from osteoarthritis and asthma. Their eldest child C is aged 18 and lived at home. He was partially sighted and described as being in danger of social isolation if not given support and encouragement. He attended college and the Chicken Shed Theatre Company. A daughter of 13 was partially sighted and suffered from urinary incontinence. A brother of 8 suffered from Attention Deficit Hyperactive Syndrome (ADHS) and his behaviour demanded constant attention and was very disruptive to the family and was described as the principal cause of the family's stress. The youngest child was 3 and with no substantial disability but beginning to copy the behaviour of her ADHS brother. The defendants carried out a number of assessments that the claimant alleged were incomplete and unsatisfactory. An interim consent order whereby the family had 6 hours a day and 2 days a week in nursery was agreed as a temporary measure. The issues between the claimant and defendant related mainly to the extent of services provided, i.e. the extent of home care support, the extent of nursery provision for H, the girl of 3, and the issue of respite care for H. The claimant alleged that there was criticism of the inadequacy of Mr B's contribution to the support of his wife and his role vis-à-vis the children and also criticism that the behaviour of the boy with ADHS should have been treated by medication, when he was in fact on medication. The judge held that the local authorities' approach on the issue of home care support and on nurse provision was fatally flawed. The local authority had a duty to exercise its discretion and the statutory provisions (e.g. Section 2 of the 2000 Act) rationally and in a way that takes important relevant matters into account. Because the family had been so recently assessed it was suggested between the counsel before the judge that a round table meeting should resolve the issues and if another assessment was necessary it should be undertaken by a different person from before.

Case: *R (on the application of LH) v. London Borough of Lambeth*[25]

The claimant MH was the mother of the claimant LH who had autism, moderate learning disabilities, chronic long-term constipation, severe epilepsy and asthma. LH lived at home with his mother and attended a school for children with moderate or severe learning difficulties. The local authority was informed that LH's behaviour was causing serious difficulties and could result in a breakdown in the situation at home. The claimants requested an assessment under the Children Act 1989 and the Carers and Disabled Children Act 2000. A month later they requested a completion of the Special Educational Needs (SEN) Annual Review process and urgent consideration to the amendment of the SEN statement to enable a residential placement for LH at a school. Several assessments were made resulting in a core assessment dated 31 March 2006. That assessment concluded that a residential placement would be a last resort and that LH and his family could be supported within the community using a package of support. That package of support would include attendance at a play centre, play schemes during holidays and other strategies which would be formulated to help MH to deal with LH's behavioural difficulties. The claimants appealed for judicial review of that assessment.

The judge allowed the application. It was held that to conclude that a package of support, much of which remained to be identified, was to be preferred to a residential placement was seriously flawed and irrational. A declaration was granted that the defendant was in breach of its assessment obligations (See also Chapter 23 and Special Educational Needs).

There is evidence to suggest that this statutory duty to assess the carer is not working. The Public Accounts Committee (PAC) in its report on dementia[26] noted that:

> Between a half and two thirds of all carers do not receive the carer's assessment to which they are entitled.

It recommended that the DH should emphasise to local health organisations and their social care partners that they need to develop an action plan which gives priority to assessing and meeting the needs of carers and develop a commissioning tool kit to demonstrate the cost benefits of the different options for providing support including respite and domiciliary care.

The full report of the PAC is considered in Chapter 24.

Strategy for carers

A new deal for carers strategy was launched in February 2007 by the Government with £35 million granted for funding projects with several departments being involved including the DH, the Department of Work and Pensions, the Department for Business Enterprise and Regulatory Reform, the Department for Children, Schools and Families, the Department for Communities and Local Government and the Treasury. Four separate taskforces are considering equalities, employment, health, and social care and income. A major consultation of carers took place in the summer of 2007 and the report a *New Deal for Carers* was published in October 2007. This identified the main concerns of carers as being:

- physical and emotional pressure;
- lack of availability of respite care;
- need for improved access to information about support services;
- long delays in receiving help and support;
- a postcode lottery for support services;
- inconsistencies in the care provided for carers;
- a considerable amount of bureaucracy;
- financial problems as carers become worse off;
- little opportunity to be able to work;
- a need for more recognition of the role that they play.

In June 2008 the DH announced that more resources for more respite places would be provided as part of the 10-year plan to assist carers. Further information is available on the DH website.

Inevitably, the value of a statutory duty to assess carers will to a considerable extent depend upon the resources provided to assist the carer. There are many concerns raised about the support which should be provided for carers, the lack of respite beds and the fact that where such respite provision is made by local authorities it is on a means-tested basis. Yet it is clear that unless respite is made available many carers will not be able to continue for so long caring for a person at home.

The legal situation of carers should benefit from the decision of the European Court of Justice (ECJ) in the Coleman case,[27] where the ECJ held that the EU Directive against discrimination on the grounds of disability applied to the carers of disabled persons as well as to the disabled themselves. The case is considered in Chapter 17.

The Princess Royal has established the Association for Carers, which provides advice and guidance.[28]

Chapter 10 is relevant to legal issues relating to the carer's liability in negligence.

Reference should also be made to a recent case accepting that the local authority owed a duty of care to a couple with learning disabilities who were being bullied, assaulted and abused by a gang of youths.[29] The facts are set out in Chapter 22.

Strategic planning and community services

Green Paper on the future of social care for adults

In 2005 the Department of Health published a Green Paper called *Independence, Well-being and Choice*.[30] This aimed to develop a new vision for social care underlain by the principles that everyone has a positive contribution to make to society and they should have the right to control their own lives. Key proposals to deliver this vision include:

- wider use of direct payments and the piloting of individual budgets to stimulate the development of modern services delivered in the way people want;
- greater focus on preventative services;
- a strong strategic and leadership role for local government, working in partnership with other agencies particularly the NHS;
- encouraging the development of new and exciting models of service delivery and harnessing technology to deliver the right outcomes for adult social care.

The Report[31] on the responses to the Government's Green Paper stated that the five top areas of interest were direct payments/individual budgets; shift to prevention; risk management; vision and assessment.

White Paper: *Our Health, Our Care, Our Say*: a new direction for community services

Following the Green Paper *Independence, Well-being and Choice*[30] in 2005, a White Paper on community health and social care was published in 2006[32] that set four main goals:

- better prevention services with earlier intervention;
- more choice and a louder voice for patients;
- improving access to community services and tackling inequalities;
- support for people with long-term conditions.

Achieving these goals would include an expansion of the Expert Patients Programme, support for carers, including emergency home-based respite care services, the provision of care closer to home, including moving services out of acute hospitals for out-patients, day case surgery, and intermediate care and greater partnership working including co-location of services, including health and care services. In addition different providers would be allowed to compete for services. The White Paper can be accessed on the DH website. It was welcomed in a policy statement by the CSP, which was pleased that

the White Paper specifically referred to more self-referral physiotherapy services that could improve access to treatment, a reduction of waiting times and achieve significant savings in GP time.

The 2006 White Paper was followed by the DH circular[33] *Transforming Social Care*, which set out the information to support the transformation of social care signified in the Green Paper of 2005 and the White Paper of 2006. It describes the vision for the development of a personalised approach to the delivery of adult social care. The circular anticipated a rise in the numbers of persons over 85 to rise from 1 million in 2006 to 2.9 million in 2036. Direct payments and individual budgets were seen as enabling people to take control of their care. Further information is available on the DH website.[34] The social care reform agenda also envisaged further development of the care services efficiency delivery programme[35] (which was established in 2004) to implement the recommendations of independent reviews of public sector efficiency) that works in partnership with local councils, the NHS and service providers to deliver efficiency improvements. Six major, interconnected and interdependent workstreams were developed to deliver end-to-end efficiency improvements to all councils with social services responsibilities. The six workstreams are:

- Effective monitoring and modernisation of home-based care
- Assessment and care management
- Demand forecasting and capacity planning
- Homecare re-enablement
- Improved procurement practices
- Transforming community equipment and wheelchair services (TCEWS) (see Chapter 15).

Personalisation of social services

In supporting this principle objective of personalising social services, a ministerial concordat was launched in December 2007 called Putting People First a Shared Vision and Commitment to the Transformation of Adult Social Care. The concordat set out the shared aims and values (of the central and local government, professional leaders, providers and the regulator) that would guide the transformation of adult social care. The concordat was followed by a toolkit published in June 2008 to assist councils and partners in implementing the necessary changes. These publications can be downloaded from the DH webite.[36] Additional information is also available on individual budgets and the documents related to the commitment to individual budgets.

The key role playable by allied health professionals in social care was discussed by Joanne Lyall with David Behan, the Director General of Social Care in the DH. The conversation published in *Frontline* on 5 December 2007 is available on the CSP website.[37] He emphasised the key role which physiotherapy has to play in enabling people to live independent lives.

The National Service Frameworks for long-term care and for older people are discussed in Chapter 24.

Long-term care: the ideal of the 'seamless service'

In the Parliamentary debates on the community care provisions of the 1990 Act much emphasis was placed upon the need to secure a seamless provision of services from one organisation to another. Considerable difficulties however arose in the implementation of a seamless service and in ensuring close cooperation and collaboration between the various providers.

One difficulty was that of defining where the NHS statutory duty to provide ends and the statutory duty of the local authority begins. While local arrangements could resolve many disputes, the fact that the NHS care must be provided free at the point of delivery (unless there is specific statutory provision, as with prescription charges) but that most social services can be means tested makes the distinction extremely important from the client' or patient's point of view.

There have been several cases brought before the Health Service Commissioner about the failures of health authorities to make provision for the continuing care needs of their patients. The DH and Welsh Office issued advice setting the principles on which continuing care should be provided by the different statutory authorities. Each local authority was asked to prepare, in conjunction with the health authority and voluntary groups, local eligibility policies for continuing care. The Grogan case discussed above is one example of a court case where the claimant was disputing the basis of the assessment by the local authority. Following the Grogan case the DH published a National Framework of NHS continuing care and NHS-funded nursing care, which is considered in Chapter 24.[18]

Uneven provision

Situation: the right to live at home?

Ben is paraplegic, being cared for in hospital, but wants to return home. His wife would be happy for him to be nursed at home. The health authority has said that the costs of caring for him at home would be four times the cost of his remaining in hospital and have refused. Residential accommodation has been offered to him. Ben learns that in a neighbouring health authority area, a patient with a similar condition has been allowed home. What is the law?

Unfortunately, although we have an NHS, there has been a lack of uniformity of provision across the country and resources dictate the services which are available to local residents. In theory, Ben could seek judicial review of the refusal of the health authority to provide the facilities for his home care. However, on the basis of previous judicial decisions[38] (see Chapter 6), he would be unlikely to succeed unless he can show that the health authority has failed to follow DoH guidance in providing the home facilities.[39] The National Institute of Health and Clinical Excellence (NICE) was established with the aim of abolishing the postcode lottery and in making recommendations on effective treatments to apply across the NHS, but almost 20 years after its establishment, this has not been achieved and considerable variations still exist in the provision of health care (see Chapters 6 and 17 on NICE).

The provision of long-term care and strategies for the future are considered in Chapter 24 on older people.

Residential and nursing home provision: registration and inspection

The Registered Homes Act 1984 was replaced by the Care Standards Act 2000, which followed a White Paper in 1998 on social services.[40] The White Paper envisaged a single independent system of regulation and inspection with commissions for care standards. The White Paper also recommended a statutory body known as the General Social Care Council, which would register those involved in social care work together with a national training organisation and improve standards in social care. National required standards for residential and nursing homes for older people were published in a consultation document by the Department of Health.[41]

Care Standards Act 2000

The main provisions of the Care Standards Act 2000 are given below.

Part 1 establishes a new independent regulatory body for social care and private and voluntary healthcare services in England known as the National Care Standards Commission [subsequently replaced by the Commission for Social Care Inspection (CSCI)]. In Wales, the National Assembly for Wales set up a department or agency to be the regulatory body in Wales. These regulatory bodies are also responsible for the regulation of nursing agencies.

Part II sets out provisions in relation to registration, right of appeals and provisions for the regulation of establishments and standards and creates offences in respect of the regulations. National minimum standards have been issued for all homes. Local authority homes have to comply with the same standards as those set for independent homes.

Part III provides for the inspection of local authority fostering and adoption by the National Care Standards Commission and the National Assembly for Wales.

Part IV of the Act makes provision for the registration of social care workers by a General Social Care Council for England and a Care Council for Wales. These councils regulate the training of social workers and attempt to raise standards in social care through codes of conduct and practice. The Central Council for Education and Training in Social Work (CCETSW) has been abolished. The use of the title 'social worker' is also protected.

Part V of the Act, in response to the recommendations of the report of inquiry chaired by Sir Ronald Waterhouse,[42] established a Children's Commissioner for Wales (see Chapter 13).

Part VI makes arrangements for the regulation of childminding and day care provision, including checks on the suitability of persons working with children.

Part VII of the Act makes provision for the protection of children and vulnerable adults, including the duty of the Secretary of State to keep a list of persons considered unsuitable to work with children and vulnerable adults. There is a statutory duty on persons providing care for such individuals to refer potential individuals to the list holder.

Subsequent changes

As a consequence of the Health and Social Care (Community Health and Standards) Act 2003, the National Care Standards Commission was abolished and its functions under the Care Standards Act 2000 transferred to the Commission for

Health Audit and Inspection (CHAI) (known as the Healthcare Commission) and the CSCI. Part 2 Chapter 7 of the 2003 Act covers the functions of CHAI and CSCI under the Care Standards Act 2000. Each organisation has a general statutory duty to keep the Secretary of State informed about the provision in England of independent health services (CHAI) or registered social care services (CSCI) and in particular the availability and quality of the services. They are both also required to encourage the improvement in the quality of the services under their aegis. They may give advice to the Secretary of State on any changes that should be made to secure improvement in the quality of those services and must have particular regard to the need to safeguard and promote the rights and welfare of children. Additional functions can be placed on both organisations by regulations drawn up by the Secretary of State. Under the Health and Social Care Act 2008 from April 2009 there is a single regulatory body for all hospitals, NHS and private and residential care replacing the Healthcare Commission, the Mental Health Act Commission and the Commission for Social Care Inspection. This new body is known as the Care Quality Commission and has increased powers of control.

Legal concerns of the community physiotherapist

No witnesses

One concern of physiotherapists working in the community, is that if they visit homes on their own and they are falsely accused of theft or assault or another offence, then they are unlikely to have any witnesses to support them. In this situation it must be remembered (see Chapter 2) that in any prosecution it must be proved beyond all reasonable doubt that the accused is guilty. This will be difficult if there is no evidence against the physiotherapist other than the word of the client against that of the physiotherapist.

If the physiotherapist is aware from the client's attitude that false accusations could be brought against him/her, then the physiotherapist should discuss with his/her manager being accompanied by another person or a colleague taking over that case.

Mileage and expenses

What if the employer accuses the physiotherapist of a fraudulent claim? The physiotherapist should be able to prove from his/her records and diary, the length and time of each journey to establish his/her innocence of the charge. The physiotherapist should keep a copy of each claim form submitted to the finance department for mileage and other expenses. Whether the physiotherapist is in independent practice or an employee he/she will need to keep such records for tax purposes.

Health and safety

The physiotherapist who visits in the community will be entering premises that are not under the control or occupation of his/her employer. If therefore the physiotherapist suffers harm because of the condition of the premises, he/she would not be able to obtain compensation from his/her employer. The physiotherapist would be dependent upon the occupier having the funds or insurance cover (see Chapter 11).

It is therefore advisable for physiotherapists who visit in the community to have private accident insurance or check with their professional association that they are covered for such accidents.

Concern over abuse of vulnerable people

There is growing awareness now of the extent of abuse of the vulnerable adult in the community. Unfortunately, at present there is no legislation similar to the Children Act 1989 under which an older person or other mentally incompetent adult could be taken to a place of safety. The National Assistance Act 1948 enables a person to be taken to a place of safety on public health grounds (see Chapter 24) but this would probably not cover the possibility of more subtle abuse. The Law Commission[43] in 1995 recommended that there should be a statutory structure to make decisions for mentally incompetent adults and to care for them and this has been provided under the Mental Capacity Act 2005. The physiotherapist who suspected that a patient was being abused, would wish to seek the advice of social services and also of the health visitor to ensure that all reasonable action was taken to protect that person. The issue of abuse of the older person is considered in Chapter 24 and the protection of vulnerable adults in the employment context is considered in Chapter 17.

Conclusions

Recent years have seen a major shift from institutional care to community care with PCTs becoming the main commissioners for health care. The decision by the DH to have national criteria for continuing care should ensure that some of the wide divergences between different areas over access to NHS continuing care should disappear. In addition, the focus on local provision of hospital care should enable physiotherapists to provide an integrated community and hospital service to the benefit of clients and health professionals. The white paper on the future direction of community services in 2006 should provide an impetus for a new direction in social care. The consultation on the future of care and support and the setting up of a care and support website[44] (this is considered in Chapter 24) suggests that the Government is at last tackling the consequences of the huge demographic changes and the funding implications. These are challenges that will not be easy to resolve.

Questions and exercises

1 What do you see as the main problems that can arise in the community care of patients with long-term conditions? What solutions are needed to meet these problems?

2 An NHS physiotherapist carried out an assessment for a ventilated patient being discharged to his home and prescribes certain equipment. She also considers that certain adaptations are necessary in the home. She then discovers that her recommendation has been changed by a disability officer employed by social services who is not a registered occupational therapist or registered physiotherapist. What action, if any, should she take?

3 Parents of a child with cystic fibrosis are anxious to have a regular community physiotherapy service. Unfortunately, resources only permit physiotherapy to be provided for in-patients. What action could the parents take to obtain the community service?

4 What do you consider to be the main challenges in the provision of community physiotherapy and how are you meeting these?

References

1 Health Professions Council (2003 revised 2008) *Standards of Conduct, Performance and Ethics*. HPC, London.

2 Chartered Society of Physiotherapy (2002) *Rules of Professional Conduct*. CSP, London.

3 Chartered Society of Physiotherapy (2005) *Core Standards of Physiotherapy Practice*. CSP, London.

4 CSP Professional Affairs Department (2005) *Service Standards of Physiotherapy Practice*. CSP, London.

5 DoH (1997) *The New NHS: Modern Dependable*. HMSO, London.

6 *Wilshire* v. *Essex Health Authority* (CA) [1986] 3 All ER 801.

7   DoH (1989) *Caring for People: Community Care in the Next Decade and Beyond*. Command Paper, 849. HMSO, London.

8   The Community Care Plans (Disapplication) (England) Order 2003 SI 1716.

9   DoH (1990) *Caring for People: Community Care in the Next Decade and Beyond. Policy and Guidance*. HMSO, London.

10   Department of Health. Community Care Assessment Directions 2004; LAC (2004) 24. Available from DH carers' website: www.carers.gov.uk

11   Department of Health (1991) *Care Management and Assessment: Managers' Guide*. HMSO, London.

12   Department of Health (1990) *Care Management and Assessment: Practitioners' Guide*. HMSO, London.

13   *R (on the application of W.)* v. *Lincolnshire County Council* [2006] EWHC Admin 2365.

14   *R (on the Application of Irenschild)* v. *London Borough of Lambeth* [2006] EWHC 2354.

15   Department of Health (2003) *Delivering Investment in General Practice: Implementing the New GMS Contract*. DH, 2003.

16   HSG(95)39; LAC(95)17.

17   *R (on the application of Grogan)* v. *Bexley NHS Care Trust* [2006] EWHC 44 (2006) 9 CCL 188.

18   Department of Health (2007) *The National Framework for NHS Continuing Healthcare and NHS-funded Nursing Care*. DH, London.

19   The Community Care Services to Carers and Children's Services (Direct Payments (England)) Regulations 2003 SI 762.

20   Department of Health (2008) LAC (DH) 2008/1 *Transforming Social Care*. DH, London.

21   Department of Health (2008) A Guide to Receiving Direct Payments from your Local Council. DH, London.

22   *Morgan* v. *Phillips* [2006] All ER (D) 189 March.

23   *Wright* v. *Sullivan* [2005] EWCA Civ 656.

24   *R (on the application of B)* v. *London Borough of Newham* [2004] EWHC 2503 (Admin).

25   *R (on the application of LH)* v. *London Borough of Lambeth* [2006] EWHC 1190 Admin; [2006] All ER (D) 83 June.

26   House of Commons Committee of Public Accounts (2008) Improving Services and Support for People with Dementia Sixth Report of Session 2007–8 HC 228 Stationery Office.

27   Coleman (Social Policy) [2008] EUECJ C-303/06 17 July 2008.

28   www.carers.org

29   *X and Y* v. *London Borough of Hounslow* [2008] EWHC 1168 (QB), 23 June 2008.

30   Department of Health (2005) Green Paper. *Independence, Well-being and Choice*. DH, London.

31   Department of Health responses to the Consultation on adult social care in England: analysis of feedback from the Green paper *Independence, Well-being and Choice*, DH 2005.

32   Department of Health (2006) *Our Health, Our Care, Our Say: A New Direction for Community Services*. DH, London.

33   Department of Health (2008) LAC (DH) 2008/1. *Transforming Social Care*. DH, London.

34   www.dh.gov.uk/en/SocialCare/Socialcarereform

35   www.csed.csip.org.uk

36   www.dh.gov.uk/en/SocialCare/Socialcarereform/Personalisation

37   www.csp.org.uk/director/newsandevents/frontline/archiveissue

38   *R* v. *Secretary of State for Social Services, ex parte Hincks and others*. reported in *Solicitors Journal*, 29 June 1979, 436.

39   *R* v. *North Derbyshire Health Authority, ex parte Fisher* [1997] 8 Med LR 327.

40   Modernising Social Services Cm 4169, The Stationery Office, London, 30 November 1998.

41   Department of Health (1999) *Fit for the Future? National Required Standards for Residential and Nursing Homes for Older People* (consultation document). DH, London.

42   Lost in care – the report of the tribunal of inquiry (chaired by Sir Ronald Waterhouse) into the abuse of children in care in the former county council areas of Gwynedd and Clwyd since 1974 February 2000, The Stationery Office, London, HC 201.

43   Law Commission (1995) No. 231. *Mentally Incapacitated Adults*. HMSO, London.

44   www.careandsupport.direct.gov.uk

19

The Physiotherapist as a Private Practitioner

An increasing number of physiotherapists are deciding to work as self-employed independent contractors and there is every likelihood that this number will grow as NHS Trusts, practitioners, other health service bodies, social services authorities and groups such as charitable organisations and private healthcare providers have the capacity to contract with self-employed individuals for services. The Chartered Society of Physiotherapy (CSP) estimated in 2007 that there may be as many as 5000 physiotherapists who treat some patients privately. The CSP has provided a simple guide for physiotherapists who are thinking of private practice.[1] It covers the UK healthcare market and potential purchasers of physiotherapy services; what private practice is; and starting in private practice. It also lists the differences between working in the NHS and in private practice noting the many benefits which are lost through no longer being an employee and therefore entitled to employment benefits. It also sets out details of Physio First (formerly the Organisation of Chartered Physiotherapists in Private Practice). Members of Physio First receive a member's manual, which includes information on the organisation and constitution, members benefits, Physio First Information Papers on a business plan, buying and selling a

practice, debt collection, insurance and negotiating with private medical insurers, sample documents, complaints procedures, Health Professions Council (HPC) standards, CSP Rules and Standards and Audit tools.

This chapter covers the following topics:

- Variety of contracting partners and CSP guidance
- Legal issues for the self-employed
- Running a business
- Accountability and the private practitioner
- Essential contract law
- The practitioner and health and safety
- Professional issues
- Private practice and the NHS
- Areas of concern

Variety of contracting partners and Chartered Society of Physiotherapy guidance

Figure 19.1 shows some of the different contracting partners for the physiotherapist who works as an independent contractor.

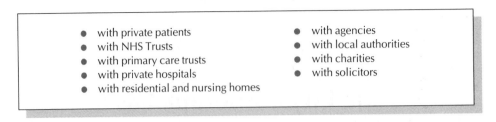

- with private patients
- with NHS Trusts
- with primary care trusts
- with private hospitals
- with residential and nursing homes
- with agencies
- with local authorities
- with charities
- with solicitors

Figure 19.1   Contracts and the private practitioner

Physio First (originally the Organisation of Chartered Physiotherapists in Private Practice (OCPPP)) also actively supports the work of those in private practice by providing a forum for concerns to be explored and to develop standards of practice and by publishing its journal In Touch. Private practitioners still have a duty to ensure that their own professional development is maintained and this is considered by Sally Roberts.[2] *Thinking of Private Practice?*[3] produced by Physio First examines the implications of going private and gives practical guidance on a range of topics such as money matters, insurance and tax. Physio First has also published a professional profile pack which assists in reflecting on and providing evidence of continuous professional development.

Legal issues for the self-employed

There are significant legal implications in becoming a self-employed practitioner and the CSP guidance warns practitioners very clearly about

the implications of leaving the NHS or the independent sector and going it alone.[4] The most obvious one is that as self-employed professionals they do not have an employer who will be vicariously liable for their actions and therefore pay out compensation arising from their negligence. Instead as self-employed, independent practitioners who offer a contract for services with others, they are personally responsible for their own negligence and also vicariously liable for any harm resulting from the negligence or other wrongful acts of their employees which are committed in the course of employment. Some of the differences are shown in Figure 19.2.

The relationship between the independent contractor and the contracting party is not a contract of employment but a contract for services. All the benefits which the employment legislation gives to employees (see Chapter 17) such as sick pay, time off work for specific purposes, protection against unfair dismissal and redundancy and guaranteed payments are not there for the self-employed. Serious considertion should therefore be given to taking out insurance to

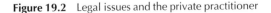

Contract for services **not** contract of employment

- No vicarious liability (except in respect of their own employees)
- No employee rights (except for those they employ)
- No indemnity *by* another (liability *for* others)
- Personal liability for health and safety of self and others
- Liability for breach of contract

If the private practitioner is an employer he/she will have the responsibility of complying with the statutory duties placed upon an employer and in accepting vicarious liability for the negligence of his/her employees.

Figure 19.2   Legal issues and the private practitioner

provide all or some of the benefits that they would have received had they been employees. In addition they cannot look to an employer for protection in relation to health and safety and should take out their own personal accident cover.

Since private practitioners have to pay personally any compensation arising out of their negligence, it is crucial that they are insured in respect of public liability and that the cover is adequate for what might be a very high claim (see Chapter 10 for typical quantum figures)

As employers themselves they must ensure that they recognise the employment rights of their employees, have relevant insurance cover and also provide all reasonable care to protect their employees' health and safety. Carmel Richard[5] sets out very clearly the health and safety responsibilities of the private practitioner as an employer, and the Health and Safety Executive's guide for small businesses should be of assistance.[6] Guidance is provided by Vince Owen[7] on recruiting staff and by Neil Andrews[8] on contracts of employment by the private practitioner.

Physio First provides its members with guidance on safeguarding self-employed status when sharing premises and a pro forma for a licence agreement for the use of the premises. Physiotherapists in private practice should also ensure that they and any persons whom they employ do not infringe the laws relating to the protection of children and vulnerable adults and ensure that the necessary checks take place with the Independent Safeguarding Authority (ISA) (which replaced the independent barring board). Further details on the Vetting and Barring Scheme Programme can be found on the Home Office website[9] (see Chapter 17).

Running a business

Practical business issues

CSP guidance assists any practitioner who is contemplating starting in private practice.[1] It sets out what should be the initial considerations and provides advice in determining the location, finding a position in the market, setting up trading arrangements, advertising and other considerations such as tax and insurance.

It is essential to plan the business. In the first of a series of management articles in *In Touch* Lesley McCann[10] describes how a business plan can be put together, including carrying out a SWOT (strengths, weaknesses, opportunities and threats) analysis and preparing a budget. Grahame Connor[11] discusses the advantages of setting up a limited liability company for private practitioners and the practical implications of such a step are considered by Elaine Atkins and Barbara Johnson.[12] The CSP has given guidance to its members who are intending to become independent practitioners on business planning.[13] As well as covering issues such as deciding on the location of premises, and the marketing of the service and choice of business name, it also gives advice on developing a business plan and writing it up. In its guidance on entering into private practice the CSP has a section on marketing,[1] which states the following:

A vital part of establishing a private practice is ensuring that those who can use your services – your potential market – know you exist. The Society's Rules of Professional Conduct deal with advertising, canvassing and publicity and what is and is not allowed. A document setting out the Rules and interpretations is available from the Society and is on the Society's website www.csp.org.uk.

The best way of making a practice known is to call upon general practitioners, consultants, district or superintendent physiotherapists in NHS and private hospitals, nursing or rest homes, secretaries of sports clubs, etc. You will have to decide whether to specialise in a client group – elderly people or sportsmen and women, for example – or be a generalist. Specialising means that your marketing effort can be more easily targeted. Many private practitioners work very hard at developing good relationships with local GPs and this is always going to be an important aspect of your marketing effort.

Before beginning any form of practice promotion it is advisable to produce a business plan to ensure that your effort and money is not wasted. Members of Physio First can obtain templates and advice on these.

Physio First encourages its members to participate in block advertisements in their local Yellow Pages telephone directory and members details on the Physio First website are searched by all the major health insurance companies.

David Grant,[14] who is a management consultant and business manager of his wife's physiotherapy practice, suggests using the SMART analysis for planning the objectives in the business plan. The characteristics of the chosen objectives should be:

- specific
- measurable
- attainable
- realistic
- trackable.

Ethical/professional issues

The CSP provided guidance on the *Standards of Business* Conduct[15] in 1995 covering such issues as:

- conflict of interests
- conflict of stance/position
- changes in employment status
- restrictive clauses
- incentives
- favouritism
- gifts and hospitality.

These apply both in employed and self-employed practice, so that the physiotherapist is beyond reproach in his/her professional work. Guidance on practice is also contained in the CSP Core Standards and Service Standards. Many ethical issues arise in relation to the financial relationship between therapist and patient. It is essential that any physiotherapist embarking on private practice clarifies from the start such issues as payment and services available from the NHS without payment, and is scrupulous to avoid any temptation to exploit her professional relationship for financial reward other than the receipt of appropriate fees. The CSP has provided guidance on patients who seek concurrent treatment from physiotherapists or other regulated or non-regulated practitioners[16] (see below).

Situation: increasing private practice

Della, a registered physiotherapist with a private practice, received a referral from the mother of a child with severe neurological problems following a road accident. Della knew that the parents were extremely wealthy and she planned a course of treatment of several sessions a week. She was aware that there was little research evidence to suggest that her treatments would be effective.

Della should discuss with the parents frankly the lack of any evidence that her proposed treatment would be clinically effective. They may be prepared to commence it on an experimental basis but provision should be made for the progress to be evaluated at reasonable intervals and the interventions reassessed.

Financial rewards should not lead to physiotherapists recommending treatments that cannot be professionally justified. The CSP guidance on private practice[1] includes information about fees and suggests that:

It is good business practice to give an indication of fees and the likely number and frequency of treatments before a treatment programme is begun. Patients with private health insurance e.g. BUPA, PPP etc – may claim reimbursement for treatment from physiotherapists/Chartered physiotherapists or you may choose to be paid directly by the health insurance company.

Cash flow can be enhanced by taking payment from every patient at the time of treatment. Acceptance of credit and debit cards can help make this easy for the patient.

John Spencer provides guidance to independent physiotherapy practitioners on breaking into the personal injury market.[17] He dispels the myth that this work inevitably means frequent appearances in court and emphasises that since claimants have a duty in law to mitigate their loss, this means that they must follow guidance on recommended treatment for their injuries, which could include physiotherapy. A claimant could utilise private physiotherapy treatment and this would be paid for from the compensation eventually received. There is no obligation on a claimant to obtain treatment from the NHS.

Tax issues

It is also essential that at the very beginning of commencing business, the physiotherapist should have an accountant to guide her in setting up a practice and the tax laws which apply. Alan Pink describes tax tips for private practitioners,[18] which includes a discussion on whether physiotherapy practices should be incorporated as limited companies and how to deal with a tax investigation.

Partnership issues

It is essential that the practitioner takes legal advice before deciding upon the type of arrangement he/she should have if working with another person or persons. For example, it may seem preferable to set up a partnership so that the profits and overheads can be shared. However, each partner would be responsible for the debts of the partnership even if he/she has not personally incurred them. Advice is provided by the CSP on trading status, copyright and patents,[19] but it emphasises that a practitioner should always take legal advice in determining the legal form that the business should take.

Summary

It is essential that all the legal responsibilities of becoming an independent practitioner are taken on board. Those intending to start a business on their own should seek professional help on the areas shown in Figure 19.3.

Accountability and the private practitioner

Figure 19.4 illustrates the arenas of accountability for private practitioners. For the most part they are similar to those of the professional who works as an employee. However, instead of being accountable to an employer the private practitioner has a contract of services with a purchaser (see Figure 19.1). If there is a breach of contract then the referral is not to the employment tribunal but to the civil courts.

Essential contract law

The private practitioner must have a good understanding of the law of contract. Some of the essential features of contract law are shown in Figure 19.5 and are also discussed in Chapter 17.

Formation of contract

There may often be a lengthy period of negotiation before a contract is formed. There may for example be an opening 'invitation to treat' by the one party which is on different terms to those eventually arrived at. The contract is eventually reached where one party can be said to have made an offer (either in response to the invitation to treat or as a 'counter offer') and the other party accepts that offer. If an offer is made and the other party responds by offering alternative conditions, this is a counter offer which, if accepted by the other party constitutes the agreement and therefore the contract. The contract

- Income tax/VAT
- National Insurance:
  - self
  - others
- Insurance and indemnity:
  - Personal accident cover
  - Public liability insurance
- Health and Safety regulations

Formation of business
- Type of business
  - Sole trader
  - Partnership
  - Limited company
  - Cooperative
- Name
- Protection:
  - patents
  - registered designs

- Contracts for supplies/services
- Training and development
- Employment law (for own employees)
- Data Protection
- Pensions and sickness:
  - for self
  - for employees

- Premises:
  - Planning permission
  - Building regulations
  - The lease
- Trading laws:
  - Sale of goods and services
  - Trade Descriptions Act
  - Unfair Contract Terms Act
- Taxation and starting up:
  - Capital allowances
  - Deciding on tax year

Figure 19.3   The private practitioner and business law

To the public:	criminal law, including Trade Descriptions legislation
To the patient:	civil law of negligence and contract law; and Sales of Goods and Services legislation
To the purchaser:	civil law; contract for services
To the profession:	Fitness to Practice Committee of the Health Professions Council

Figure 19.4   Accountability and the private practitioner

Formulation:	invitation to treat offer and acceptance	**Breach:**	remedies for breach right of election
Contents:	fundamental terms implied terms express terms	**Termination:**	by performance by breach by agreement by notice by frustration
Performance			

Figure 19.5   Elements of contract law

may not be entirely in writing. It may be partly in writing and partly by word of mouth. If, following a dispute, one party argues that additional terms discussed during negotiations became part of the contract and are therefore binding, it is a question of interpretation of what was said and any other evidence to establish what are the agreed terms of the contract.

The three essential elements to make a contract binding are:

1. an agreement
2. consideration
3. an intention to create legal relations.

Consideration need not necessarily be payment of money in return for the performance of the agreement by the other side. It could be a benefit in kind or it could be an agreement releasing the other from something that they had a duty to do.

It need not necessarily equate with what the other is prepared to do. For example, a physiotherapist who has a private practice may agree that, because a client is extremely short of funds but runs an aromatherapy clinic, she will forgo any payment on the understanding that she will be given two sessions of aromatherapy. On that basis the agreement is made and she provides the physiotherapy. If the aromatherapist client then goes back on that agreement she is in breach of contract. The physiotherapist has the right to seek damages for breach of contract in the civil courts. In practice, she may prefer not to attract the publicity which such an action would bring.

It is important that agreement upon fees payable should be reached before treatment commences and that this agreement is put into writing.

In commercial contracts the intention to create legal relations would normally be presumed. In domestic matters, there is a presumption that there is no such intention. Where a practitioner is carrying out private work it is essential for him/her to make it absolutely clear that it is the intention to create a binding agreement in order to be able to enforce the contract through the courts.

Where possible the private practitioner should ensure that all the terms of the contract are put in writing to protect him/herself in the event of a dispute. The CSP has provided guidance on an associate agreement for self-employed staff[20] that could also be used as the basis for private practice. It sets out clearly the essential terms on which agreement must be reached before a contract can be considered to exist.

Breach of contract

If it is claimed that one party is in fundamental breach of the contract then the innocent party has the right of election. He/she can either elect to see the contract as at an end and seek damages, i.e. compensation for the breach of contract, or he/she can elect to treat the contract as continuing but seek compensation for the loss to him/her (financial or otherwise) of it being less than he/she had bargained for. It is important that the innocent party makes it clear how he/she chooses since, if he/she delays and carries on regarding the contract as subsisting, it could be said that by his/her conduct he/she has treated the contract as continuing and has therefore lost the right of election.

Termination of contract

By performance/agreement/notice

It is advisable to consider at the beginning of the contract how it should end.

- Is it for a specific number of treatments?
- Is it for a certain length of time?
- Is it for a specified number of weeks after hospital discharge?
- Can it be ended on notice by one party to the other?
- How long should that notice be?

In the absence of notice provisions in an employment contract the courts will imply a reasonable notice provision into the contract and there are statutory minimum periods for contracts of employment. However, these statutory minimum periods do not exist for contracts for services and it would be more difficult to determine what is reasonable notice.

Frustration

Frustration of contract arises when an event takes place that is right outside the contemplation of the parties when the contract was made.

Situation: a cancelled match

A physiotherapist had a contract to provide assistance at a football match. Unfortunately, the match was cancelled because of very heavy snow falls. The physiotherapist claimed that she was still available to provide services and was therefore entitled to a minimum payment. The club argued that the snow frustrated the contract and therefore brought it to an end.

In this situation it would be surprising if the contractual agreement did not cover the possibility of matches being cancelled or postponed because of weather conditions and, if there are provisions covering this, then the doctrine of frustration would not apply. If however the contract is silent on such a possibility, then the law of frustration would apply and the contract, because of the existence of an event which makes the performance of the contract very different from that contemplated, would come to an end by operation of law. If the physiotherapist had actually spent some time or money, e.g. had travelled to the venue for the match, then she would be able to obtain reimbursement for the work she had already undertaken. As a result of the Law Reform (Frustrated Contracts) Act 1943, generally all sums paid before the contract was frustrated are repayable and any money due to be paid but not paid before frustration ceases to be payable. However, the court will look to the justice of the situation and work done will be paid for. This Act does not apply where the contract itself makes provision for any frustrating

event and it would therefore be possible for the private practitioner to include in the agreement provision defining what rights would exist were a frustrating event to occur.

What if the client refuses to pay?

Payment is the passing of consideration from the one party to the contract in return for the provision of some service. Time of payment is not normally a fundamental term unless the contract clearly makes it so. It is therefore advisable for the professional to include in the contract a term in relation to when the fee should be paid – in advance, in instalments at each session, after each session, monthly, etc. When the physiotherapist is negotiating with a health service body or NHS Trust there might not be much choice for him/her, but it is essential that this should be agreed, so it is clear when there has been a breach of contract and he/she is entitled to commence action for recovery.

Situation: failure to pay promptly

A physiotherapist contracted with a NHS Trust for physiotherapy services to be provided for four sessions a week on the basis that payment would be made every month in arrears on completion and submission of a return certified by the unit manager. The physiotherapist duly performed the services and submitted the return but several months later was still without payment. Should she cease to work?

Failure to pay could be regarded as breach of a fundamental clause of the contract and, looking back at the section on breach of contract, it will be recalled that the innocent party therefore has the right of election, i.e. to decide whether to continue to recognise the contract as continuing or see it ended by the breach of contract. The physiotherapist could therefore see the contract as at an end and sue for the outstanding payment and damages for the breach of contract. Alternatively, if there is every likelihood that she would eventually be paid, she might well prefer to elect to see the contract as continuing and continue to perform her sessions meanwhile chasing them for the outstanding payments. Should she eventually be forced into taking legal action she could, depending upon the amount outstanding, take the case to the small claims court, to the County Court or (in theory if the sums were large enough) to the High Court. With the contract in writing and evidence of the sessions she has carried out she should obtain her payments with no valid defence being available against her.

However, if she were suing an individual rather than an organisation, the practicalities of getting the money from someone who may have no assets and no job is another matter.

Case: physiotherapy debts

In a case[21] concerning judicial separation there were many debts which the husband had not paid. These included a debt of £2050 to the physiotherapist. The husband explained that he had not paid in accordance with the undertakings because he had not got the money.

It is essential that the physiotherapist does not allow debts owed by a private individual to build up, since the dangers of non-payment increase and, as seen from the above case, could become tied up in matrimonial settlements.

A physiotherapist who provides services for a private hospital will probably do so on the basis that he/she has a personal contract with the patient. It is important therefore that she keeps an account of the debt and ensures early payment.

Contract law and the tort of negligence contrasted

It may be bewildering to non-lawyers that there are two overlapping duties – the duty owed to a client under the law of negligence and the duty owed to a client under the law of contract.

However, this is the legal situation and an aggrieved client who had suffered harm as a result of the activities of the private practitioner could sue both for breach of contract and also for breach of the duty to care at common law.

The duties are not identical, since the former derives from the contract that has been agreed between client and practitioner, including the implied terms, and the latter is set by law. It has been stated by the Court of Appeal that, where a duty of care in tort arose between the parties to a contract, wider obligations could be imposed by the duty of care in tort than those arising under the contract.[22]

The practitioner and health and safety

Responsibility for others

Although there exists no employer who is responsible for the self-employed practitioner, he/she may be an employer him/herself and therefore have responsibilities to his/her employees. The duty to take reasonable care of the health and safety of the employee exists whether the employee is full or part time. He/she also has a duty under the health and safety legislation to take care of the safety of others who may be affected by her work and if he/she operates from premises which clients attend he/she could be liable as 'occupier' if harm befalls them as a result of a foreseeable hazard (see Chapter 11). The health and safety laws considered in Chapter 11 apply to the private practitioner. The Core Standards of the CSP state that:

Medical Devices Regulations (2002)

These require a practitioner to ensure that medical devices are properly maintained and comply with current standards. Healthcare Trusts should have appropriate protocols in place to comply with these regulations. Private practitioners need to be aware of, and ensure compliance with, these standards themselves.

> **(2)**   Every self-employed person shall make a suitable and sufficient assessment of:
>
>   (a)   the risks to his own health and safety to which he is exposed whilst he is at work; and
>   (b)   the risks to the health and safety of persons not in his employment arising out of or in connection with the conduct by him of his undertaking,
>
>   for the purpose of identifying the measures he needs to take to comply with the requirements and prohibitions imposed upon him by or under the relevant statutory provisions.
>
> **(3)**   Any assessment such as is referred to in paragraph (1) [employers] or (2) shall be reviewed by the employer or the self-employed person who made it if:
>
>   (a)   there is reason to suspect that it is no longer valid; or
>   (b)   there has been a significant change in the matters to which it relates;
>
>   and where as a result of any such review changes to an assessment are required, the employer or self-employed person concerned shall make them.

Figure 19.6   Regulation 3(2) and (3): the self-employed

Regulation requirements

The Management of Health and Safety at Work Regulations 1999[23] refer specifically to the self-employed as shown in Figure 19.6.

Threatened violence and self-defence

Situation: violence in private practice

A private practitioner, who has her own premises which clients attend, was carrying out a session when a client became extremely violent and threatening. The professional was working on her own and there was no-one who could come to her aid.

In such a situation she is entitled to use reasonable force in self-defence. What is reasonable depends upon the circumstances:

- the danger she is in and the amount of violence which she faces;
- the nature of the training she has received;
- her own size and that of her assailant;
- the type of weapons to hand.

Where grievous bodily harm is feared, more force might be justified. Her actions should however always be defensive not aggressive.

Professional issues

Client-led practice

Situation: unjustified demands

A physiotherapist works as a self-employed practitioner and has a caseload of clients for whom she provides services. One client is extremely demanding and is very anxious to obtain a chair lift from the social services. The physiotherapist forms the view that a lift is neither appropriate nor practicable and in fact given the client's particular circumstances could be dangerous. The physiotherapist is told by the client that unless she is prepared to support her claim their contract for services will be ended. What should the physiotherapist do?

The answer should be clear: she must abide by her professional standards and not be demand-led by the client into recommending equipment that is entirely unsuitable. The difference between the employee status and the self-employed status however is apparent. If NHS employees refuse to agree with patients on professional grounds, their employment should not be endangered. If it is the employer who is putting pressure on them to act unprofessionally then, provided they have the continuous service requirement, they could claim constructive dismissal in the employment tribunal (see Chapter 17). However, the self-employed professionals have no such protection. If they keep to their professional standards then they might lose that client and suffer economically. However, there is no alternative if they wish to remain as registered professionals.

NHS refusal to purchase services

Not everyone is content with healthcare developments outside the NHS. There may for example be some practitioners who refuse to contract with private practitioners. What action can the private practitioners take? Even under the NHS following the White Paper,[24] primary healthcare groups have the freedom to buy services from those providers that they consider would be best for their patients. They cannot be forced to go outside the NHS nor can they be forced to stay within it. If a GP practice refuses to use the services of the private sector there is no action which can be taken other than to hope that in terms of quality and price the private service will eventually succeed in providing services to those within the NHS. The DH[25] has provided guidance for doctors in private practice that would apply to physiotherapists and this is quoted by the CSP in its 2008 publication on patients seeking concurrent treatment from physiotherapists or other regulated or non-regulated practitioners which is considered below.

Compensation claims: expert witness

An increasing part of the practitioner's work is the provision of expert reports for those who have been involved in litigation and are seeking compensation. The practitioner might be asked by the claimant's (formerly plaintiff) solicitor or the defendant's solicitor for an expert report on the situation and the prognosis in order to assess the amount of compensation (known as quantum). This and the need to give the true picture even if it does not 'help' the client's case is considered on Chapter 13 on giving evidence in court.

Complaints and unprofessional conduct by others

Because the private practitioner often works on his/her own, he/she is more vulnerable in pointing out low standards of care provided by other professionals. The private practitioner lacks a management hierarchy and does not belong to a large organisation (other than his/her own professional association) to be able to take action effectively and without becoming a scapegoat or losing out financially.

Situation: unacceptable standards in residential care

> A physiotherapist provides private services at a residential care home. She is horrified to discover that the residents have a very low standard of care. Some seem to be in pain and there is evidence of low standards of cleanliness both of the residents and the premises. She tries to point this out discreetly to the manager, but unfortunately the manager reacts badly at the implied criticism, and says the funds do not exist for more carers and cleaners to be appointed.

There are several options open to the physiotherapist but all are likely to end her association with the home.

- She could report the situation to the owners or senior management.
- She could complain to the Commission for Social Care Inspection (CSCI) under the Care

Standards Act 2000 which would have to investigate her complaint. [CSCI has been replaced by the Care Quality Commission from April 2009 (see Chapter 17)].

- She could report the situation to the contract department of the local authority that purchases places in the home for clients.
- In extremely serious cases where it would appear that criminal activities are taking place, she could report the situation to the police.

Unfortunately, none of these courses of action are likely to ensure that her work with the home will continue.

- What if the unsound or unsafe practice she witnesses is the conduct of another professional?

Situation: unacceptable practice by colleagues

A physiotherapist visits an older person who lives alone and is always profusely grateful for the help and attention she receives. She notices that on the dresser the client keeps a few notes of money. She questions her about the advisability of keeping money in the house and on the dresser. The client explains that she always gives the ambulance driver £5 after each visit to the day hospital. The physiotherapist fears that the ambulance man might be exploiting the old lady. What action, if any, should she take?

One course would be to explain to the client that the service provided by the ambulance is free and no payment need be made. If the client says that the ambulance men expect it, what does the physiotherapist do then? One possibility is for her to take up the complaint to the director of the ambulance service. This would be preferable to writing an anonymous letter or complaining indirectly. However, she may find that she becomes ostracised as a result.

It is essential, however, that she takes appropriate action and does not ignore the dangers to the client. She has a duty of care to the client and

if harm were eventually to befall the client and it were ascertained that the professional had been aware of the situation but had taken no action, she could face professional conduct proceedings (see section on whistle-blowing in Chapter 17).

Private practice and the NHS

The internal market and its abolition

An internal market was established in the NHS following the NHS and Community Care Act 1990 and GP fundholders were able to purchase physiotherapy services. With the abolition of fundholding, primary care trusts (in Wales local health boards) are able to purchase services which include physiotherapy services. There are signs at the time of writing that fewer physiotherapists are being employed within the NHS and therefore dependence on private physiotherapy services might develop. Many graduates from the 2007 graduates are still unemployed and many may have to look to the private sector.

Shared facilities

Private practitioners such as independent midwives and physiotherapists in private practice might make use of NHS facilities. The CSP has provided guidance on the use of NHS facilities for private practice,[26] emphasising that members should avoid a conflict of interest. NHS facilities may be used by private practitioners outside of NHS hours, e.g. for sports injuries, but the basis on which they are so used must be made absolutely clear and a proper contract should be drawn up setting out the responsibilities of both parties. Fees charged should reflect the value of the services provided.

Shared clients

Difficulties can arise for both physiotherapists within the NHS and in private practice where their clients are receiving help from both sectors. In such a situation it is essential that the therapists are communicating with each other and not being derogatory about each other to the patient. If it becomes apparent that the two practitioners are using different and possibly conflicting methods of treatment, then it is essential that this is discussed with the patient and the patient invited to choose. Sometimes arbitrary rules are followed, such as always leave 2 weeks between the treatment provided by an NHS physiotherapist and treating that patient privately. The thinking behind such a rule is that, if harm befalls the patient, the 2-week gap may identify which therapist caused the harm. However, this is not a rule of law and it is preferable if there can be communication between the NHS and private physiotherapist as to the continuing treatment of the patient. Clearly, documentation on the activities of each physiotherapist is essential.

The same problem can arise when an NHS patient or patient being treated by an independent physiotherapist seeks treatment from a person practising in an alternative or complementary therapy, e.g. osteopathy or reflexology. Issues in connection with complementary medicine are considered in Chapter 27.

The problems which can arise when a patient receives both private treatment and NHS treatment are considered by the CSP in its paper published in 2008.[27] It quotes from the Department of Health guidance given to the CSP in 2007 which refers to advice of the DH for doctors published in 2003.[25] The CSP in its key points emphasises that

- any referral for NHS treatment and the priority to be given must be based on clinical need;
- that patients seeking a private physiotherapist or an alternative practitioner via an NHS physiotherapy service can be given guidance on information to acquire about a potential practitioner in terms of regulation, registration, rules of professional conduct and standards of proficiency;
- an NHS physiotherapist must declare any potential conflicts of interest such as

providing a private service outwith their NHS contract;
- it is good practice for each NHS service to hold a list of local private practitioners. This list must be held in a central administrative area, a waiting room or reception. The treating clinician must not directly give out the list;
- NHS practitioners don't have an automatic right to refuse to take on the management of a patient, however if the clinician has evidence to suggest that two clinical interventions will be detrimental to the patient they may suggest to the patient that they need to choose, without prejudice, which service to attend in the first instance;
- the reasoning behind rationing and resource management decisions should be explained openly and objectively to a patient where the rationing or resource management decisions may have a negative impact on the implementation of an appropriate treatment management plan.

Concerns have been raised recently at a policy decision taken by NHS trusts that any patient who opts to purchase medicines for cancer treatment which are not available from the NHS must either forgo all their NHS care for cancer (and fund it privately, if at all) or stop using the private medicines.[28] The argument in favour of this policy is that this leads to a two tier NHS with those who can afford paying privately for medicines which the NHS cannot supply. However, this is a rule that does not apply in other specialties. For example, a person may go to a private doctor for diagnosis and then seek NHS treatment, including surgery, for the condition. There are legal actions being contemplated, and signs that the NHS is rethinking this policy.

Accreditation of private practice

The accreditation process endeavours to identify standards of practice for physiotherapists and also provides a form of reassurance for members of the public and was undertaken by the Organisation of Chartered Physiotherapists in Private Practice (OCPPP). It published an accreditation manual, which was revised in 1996 following a review of the accreditation process and it set up an Accreditation Management Panel, which offered advice and help to those participating in the scheme.[29] This work has not been continued by Physio First in view of the many other bodies which review standards in private practice including insurance companies. Physio First does offer advice and support for those in private practice. Information on the work of Physio First can also be obtained from the CSP website.

Part-time private practice

Some physiotherapists might try to develop a private practice as well as being employed part-time. In such a situation they must ensure that they do not exploit their employed situation to increase their private practice by taking clients away from their employer. This would be regarded as a breach of the implied term of loyalty to their employer in their contract of employment (see Chapter 17). Similarly, they should keep their private practice entirely separate from their employment and not attempt to see private clients in working hours without the express consent of their employer nor use any of the employer's facilities for their private work (e.g. telephones, equipment, secretarial services or stationery). In the case of *Watling* v. *Gloucestershire County Council*[30] (see Chapter 17 for the full facts), Mr Watling, an occupational therapist employed by the County Council, was fairly dismissed since he continued to see private clients during his working hours, despite the specific prohibition of his employers.

If the physiotherapist has the agreement of his/her employer to him/her undertaking private practice in her own area, there should be no difficulty in doing private work. However, it is essential that the physiotherapist makes sure that patients are aware of their entitlements to have NHS treatment without paying. There are dangers in the physiotherapist or a colleague treating the same patient as part of NHS at the same time as the patient is receiving private treatment from the physiotherapist. However, it depends upon the circumstances.

Situation: private and NHS?

The mother of a child with cystic fibrosis was concerned that, because she was working full time, the child was not receiving sufficient physiotherapy. She mentioned this to a physiotherapist at the hospital who said that she did private work and would come in her off-duty hours to give physiotherapy to the child. The mother was not told that there was a community physiotherapy paediatric service.

In this situation the mother may well have grounds for complaint if she was not told that the child could be given physiotherapy in the community under the NHS. If, however, the kind of service the mother wanted would not have been available, then the offer of private help would be acceptable. The physiotherapist should ensure that her employer knows of the arrangements and that the mother has been offered full information of what is available within the NHS. The CSP paper published in 2008 patients seeking concurrent treatment from physiotherapists or other regulated or non-regulated practitioners (which is discussed above) emphasises the duty of fidelity that the physiotherapist owes to her employer.[27] For a physiotherapist to encourage NHS patients to see her privately may constitute a conflict of interest and a breach of the implied duty of fidelity to the employer and lead to disciplinary action. See also the CSP paper on patients seeking treatment in the public and private sector.[31] It considers the problem of when an in-patient seeks to have treatment from a private practitioner and states that NHS trusts should have a policy covering this possibility since the issue arises with other professional groups. The CSP states that if this occurs, everybody involved should be aware that issues, such as ongoing management of the patient and liability have been agreed and documented.

Areas of concern

Insurance

Membership of the CSP provides insurance cover for physiotherapists in private practice and the CSP has negotiated additional business cover to protect businesses against exposure to be being sued as a business. Physio First also provides guidance on insurance cover for those in private practice. The CSP has also issued guidance on insurance cover on its website (Ins and outs of insurance) and published guidance for physiotherapy students and individualised insurance cover for practice-based learning.[32] Details of the members' professional and public liability insurance scheme published in 2007 is available from the CSP and would clarify concerns over cover for private practice.[33]

Lasers and licensing

The DH announced in 2001 that independent healthcare practitioners registered with the HPC would not need to register with the National Care Standards Commission (now the Care Quality Commission) to use class 3B lasers. The CSP had been campaigning for many years to have physiotherapists exempt from the licensing requirements, since the high registration fees demanded meant that many physiotherapists in the private sector were not using Class 3B lasers.

Documentation

It should be obvious from the many conflicts which can arise in private practice that the documentation that the private practitioner

keeps is extremely important – not only in establishing the care that is given to each patient and the terms on which it is to be given in the event of any referral or dispute, but also in relation to the management of a small business. The private practitioner needs to ensure that he/she is able to respond to the many statutory requests for information about his/her practice from HM Revenue and Customs as well as answering any queries from statutory health and social services providers. (Record keeping is discussed in Chapter 12.)

A private practitioner is responsible for registering personal records with the Information Commissioner (IC). The IC provides a helpline for any queries.

Situation: registration under the Data Protection Act

A physiotherapist has records from a previous clinic. She is registered with the Information Commissioner under the Data Protection Act for her new records. What about registration for the records from her former clinic?

She must be registered for all personal records in her keeping and should seek further advice from the Information Commissioner.

Going abroad

Some physiotherapists may wish to consider working abroad. With a shortage of physiotherapists worldwide and freedom of work within the EU the opportunities are considerable. Often they will be taking employment overseas but, where they consider offering services privately, then the topics covered in this chapter are essential, bearing in mind the fact that they will be working in a different legal context and therefore local advice will be necessary on the legal implications of offering services privately. The CSP has prepared guidance on going abroad.[34] It strongly advises its members to have at least 2 years' good rotational experience before going overseas and gives advice on tax, insurance and pensions. Information is also provided by the CSP on insurance and working overseas.[35]

Consumer protection regulations

New consumer protection regulations implementing an EU Directive on unfair commercial practices require businesses to act fairly towards consumers and will outlaw disreputable trading activities. Fortune-tellers, tarot readers, faith healers, spiritualists and other personal services may have to advise the customer that their services are not research based. In the future, prosecutions by trading standards officers will be based on 'is it an unfair commercial trade practice?' rather than 'is there a false or misleading trade description?' Anyone offering a service must not engage in unfair commercial practice, misleading statements or omission or aggressive sales practice. Convictions can be followed by fines up to £5000 or 2 years' imprisonment. Physiotherapists in private practice should be aware of these regulations.

Conclusion

The increase in the numbers of physiotherapists who are self-employed offering their services in the community and to hospital trusts is continuing. To move outside employed status is often a courageous step and the physiotherapist who is considering taking such step should seek professional advice and take note of the topics briefly discussed in this chapter. Reference should be made to general law books (see bibliography) and to the publications recommended by the CSP[36] and Physio First.

Questions and exercises

1   Identify the differences in law between the situation of the physiotherapist in private practice and the employed physiotherapist.
2   A colleague has suggested that there may be considerable advantages in the physiotherapists withdrawing from employed status within the NHS and setting up a group of private practitioners to sell their services to the NHS Trusts and PCTs. Draw up a list of benefits and weaknesses of this suggestion.
3   A physiotherapist in private practice has two sessions at a private nursing home. She is concerned at the low standards of patient care. What action could she take?

References

1   Chartered Society of Physiotherapy (2007) *Thinking of Private Practice*. PA 7 CSP, London.
2   Roberts, S. (2003) Continuing Professional Development: The Implications for Private Practitioners. *In Touch* **103**, 26–30.
3   Physio First (2004) *Thinking of Private Practice? A Practical Guide for Chartered Physiotherapists*. OCPP, Towcester.
4   CSP Professional Affairs Department (no date) *Self-employed Status*. PA No. 44. CSP, London.
5   Richards, C. (2006) Health and Safety Issues as Employers. *In Touch* **116**, 24–29.
6   Health and Safety Executive (2004) *An Introduction to Health and Safety; Health and Safety in Small Businesses*. HSC, London. www.hse.gov.uk
7   Owen, V. (2006) Recruiting Staff. *In Touch* **114**, 26–29.
8   Andrews, N. (2006) Contracts of Employment and Service Contracts – Getting it Right. *In Touch* 114, 29–31.
9   http://police.homeoffice.gov.uk/about-us/police-policy-operations
10   McCann, L. (1998) The Practice Management Series – Putting Together a Business Plan. *In Touch* **82**, 16–17.

11 Connor, G. (2006) Going Limited. *In Touch* **115**, 47–48.

12 Atkins, E. Johnson, B. (2003) Becoming a Limited Company – an Inside Story. *In Touch* **103**, 32–37.

13 CSP Professional Affairs Department (1996) *Business Planning*. No. 42. CSP, London.

14 Grant, D. (1995) Thriving on Chaos? *In Touch* **76**, 22–24.

15 CSP Professional Affairs Department (1995) *Standards of Business Conduct*. No. PA 26. CSP, London.

16 Chartered Society of Physiotherapy (2008) *Patients Seeking Concurrent Treatment*. CSP London.

17 Spencer, J. (2002) Personal Injury Law – How to win referrals. *In Touch* **99**, 29–32.

18 Pink, A. (2004) Tax Tips for Private Practitioners. *In Touch* **108**, 29–31.

19 CSP Professional Affairs Department (no date) *Trading Status, Copyright and Patents*. No. PA 45. CSP, London.

20 CSP Professional Affairs Department (1998) *Associate Agreement (Self-employed staff)*. No. PA 46. CSP, London.

21 *W* v. *W (Judicial separation ancillary relief)* [1995] 2 FLR 259.

22 *Holt and Another* v. *Payne Skillington (a firm) and Another* (1995) *The Times*, 22 December 1995.

23 Management of Health and Safety at Work Regulations 1999 SI No 3242.

24 Department of Health (1997) *The New NHS: Modern Dependable*. HMSO, London.

25 Department of Health (2003) *A Code of Conduct for Private Practice: Guidance for NHS Medical Staff*. London, DH. http://www.dh.gov.uk/en/Publicationsandstatistics/Publications/PublicationsPolicyAndGuidance/DH_4100689

26 CSP Professional Affairs Department (1995) *Use of NHS Facilities for Private Practice*. No. PA 3. CSP, London.

27 Chartered Society of Physiotherapy (2008) *Patients Seeking Concurrent Treatment From Physiotherapists or other Regulated or Non-regulated Practitioners. Guidance for Chartered Physiotherapists*. PD002. CSP London.

28 Templeton, S.-K. (2008) Cancer Patients 'Betrayed' by the NHS. *Sunday Times*, 1 June.

29 England, S. (1996) Accreditation – Take a New Look – We Have It. *In Touch* **82**, 26.

30 *Watling* v. *Gloucestershire County Council* EAT/868/94, 17 March 1995, 23 November 1994, Lexis transcript.

31 Chartered Society of Physiotherapy (2004) *Patients Seeking Treatment in the Public and Private Sector*. PA 05. CSP, London.

32 Chartered Society of Physiotherapy/Graybrook Ltd (2008) *Students and Insurance Cover*. CSP London.

33 Chartered Society of Physiotherapy (2007) *Members' Professional and Public Liability Insurance Scheme*. CSP, London.

34 Chartered Society of Physiotherapy (2003) *Guidance for CSP working Abroad*. ERUS IP44. CSP, London.

35 Chartered Society of Physiotherapy (2004) *Insurance and Working Overseas*. No. PA 320. CSP, London.

36 Chartered Society of Physiotherapists (2007) *Thinking of Private Practice*. PA 7. CSP, London.

Section E

Specialist Client Groups

20 Care of Those with Physical Disabilities, Sports and Road Traffic Injuries and Neurological Disorders

This chapter considers legal issues which mainly arise in the course of caring for those with physical disabilities, with sports and orthopaedic injuries and suffering from neurological disorders, but there are, of course, many clients with multi-handicaps and who therefore come under other client groupings covered in Chapters 21–24. Reference should also be made to the general chapters in Sections B and C that discuss legal issues arising across all client groups. Possible situations of negligence in relation to this group and in relation to equipment and adaptations are considered in Chapters 10 and 15, and complaints from this client group are discussed in Chapter 14. Legal issues arising in relation to children are considered in Chapter 23. The National Service Framework (NSF) on long-term conditions is considered in Chapter 24.

This chapter will look at the following issues:

- The Chronically Sick and Disabled Persons Act and related legislation
- Inter-agency and inter-professional cooperation
- Limitations on resources and priority setting
- Legal issues arising from sports injuries
- Legal issues arising in musculoskeletal conditions
- Road traffic victims and legal issues
- Legal aspects of respiratory care
- Legal issues arising in patients with neurological conditions
- Pain management
- Smoking and the physically disabled

Chronically Sick and Disabled Persons Act 1970 and related legislation

The general duties placed upon local authorities in respect of the needs of the disabled are set out in the Chronically Sick and Disabled Persons Act 1970. The principal duties are shown in Figure 20.1. It should be noted that the provisions apply to those suffering from mental disabilities as well as those with physical disabilities, but for

(1)   It shall be the duty of every local authority having functions under Section 29 of the National Assistance Act 1948 to inform themselves of the number of persons to whom that section applies within their area and of the need for the making by the authority of arrangements under that section for such persons.

(2)   Every such local authority:

(a)   shall cause to be published from time to time at such times and in such manner as they consider appropriate general information as to the services provided under arrangements made by the authority under the said Section 29 which are for the time being available in their area; and

(b)   shall ensure that any such person as aforesaid who needs any of those services is informed of any other *service provided by the authority (whether under any such arrangements or not)* which in the opinion of the authority is relevant to his needs *and of any service provided by any other authority or organisation which in the opinion of the authority is so relevant and of which particulars are in the authority's possession*

[words in italics introduced by the Disabled Persons (Service, Consultation and Representation) Act]

Figure 20.1   Duties under the Chronically Sick and Disabled Persons Act 1970: Section 1

convenience these are dealt with here and not repeated in Chapters 21 or 22.

Section 2 of the 1970 Act lists the provisions that the local authority has a duty to make in the following circumstances:

● The local authority has the functions under section 29 of the National Assistance Act (NAA) 1948.

● It is satisfied that the section applies to an individual.

● The person is ordinarily resident in their area.

● It is necessary, in order to meet the needs of that person,

● To make arrangements for all or any of the matters set out in Figure 20.2.

(The duties referred to in section 29 of the NAA 1948 are that the local authority may make arrangements for promoting the welfare of persons over 18 who are blind, deaf, dumb or who suffer from mental disorder, and other persons who are substantially and permanently handicapped by illness, injury or congenital deformity or such other disabilities.)

The right to enforce provision under Section 2 was considered by the High Court, Court of Appeal and House of Lords in a case[1] where disabled persons applied for judicial review of the decision by Gloucester County Council to cut social services for the disabled (see the section on resources and priority setting below). It is inevitable, given the range of services required and the limited resources of local and health authorities that services for individual patient groups will vary. In a case involving the closure of a day centre, J a person with learning disabilities applied for permission to seek judicial review of the action taken by the local authority alleging that he was ordinarily resident within the catchment area of the local authority and entitled to receive services under Section 2 of the Chronic Sick and Disabled Persons Act 1970. It was also alleged that the closure was an infringement of Article 8(2) of the European Convention on Human Rights. Permission to seek judicial review was granted on the grounds that J came within Section 2 of the 1970 Act and the local authority's approach to those for whom the service was a central part of their life was unnecessary or disproportionate or both.[2]

A novel way to avoid paying the accumulated fees in respect of a person's residential care after their death was attempted in vain in the following case.

(a) The provision of practical assistance for that person in his home;

(b) the provision for that person of, or assistance to that person in obtaining, wireless, television, library or similar recreational facilities;

(c) the provision for that person of lectures, games, outings or other recreational facilities outside his home or assistance to that person in taking advantage of educational facilities available to him;

(d) the provision for that person of facilities for, or assistance in, travelling to and from his home for the purpose of participating in any services provided under arrangements made by the authority . . . or in any services provided otherwise than as aforesaid which are similar to services which could be provided under such arrangements;

(e) the provision of assistance for that person in arranging for the carrying out of any works of adaptation in his home of the provision of any additional facilities designed to secure his greater safety, comfort or convenience;

(f) facilitating the taking of holidays by that person, whether at holiday homes or otherwise and whether provided under arrangements made by the authority or otherwise;

(g) the provision of meals for that person in his home or elsewhere;

(h) the provision for that person of, or assistance to that person in obtaining, a telephone and any special equipment necessary to enable him to use a telephone.

Figure 20.2   Arrangements which the local authority has a duty to make: Section 2 Chronically Sick and Disabled Persons Act 1970

Case: *Sandford and another v. London Borough of Waltham Forest*[3]

The claimants were executors of the deceased's estate. In an assessment of the deceased's home-based needs, an occupational therapist recommended the provision of cot-sides for her bed. In April 2003 the deceased fell while getting out of bed and fractured her right femur. Following her recovery she was admitted to a nursing home where she died in October 2006. She was required to contribute to the fees for her accommodation. The claimants brought proceedings, claiming that the failure to fit cot-sides was a breach of the defendants' statutory duty for which they could recover damages in respect of the costs of her accommodation in the nursing home and damages in respect of the pain, suffering and loss of amenity caused to the deceased by the injuries she had suffered as a result of her fall.

The claim failed. The authority had not owed the deceased a common law duty of care arising out of the statutory duty. The duty was not actionable at the suit of a private individual, and, in any event, in performing its duties, the authority had not voluntarily assumed any responsibility but was doing that which was required of it by statute. Further, on the evidence the claimants had failed to make out that, on the balance of probabilities, if the cot-sides had been fitted then the deceased would not have suffered her injury.

Disabled Persons (Independent Living) Bill

At the time of writing a Disabled Persons (Independent Living) Bill is being debated in Parliament. If enacted the following provisions would be introduced:

- each disabled person to make decisions about their own independent living arrangements by choosing whether allocated resources are provided in cash, services or a combination of both;

- advocacy to be provided where there are disputes between careers and disabled persons;

- new rights to ensure a disabled person is not placed in care against their wishes;

- amend the Mental Health Act 1983 to ensure independent living options are investigated before authorities decide to section or provide compulsory treatment;
- care homes will come within the definition of public authority for the purposes of the Human Rights Act 1998 (see Chapter 6 for the significance of this);
- the Care Standards Act 2000 is to be amended to ensure that disabled people in residential care have an individual living agreement;
- a duty would be placed on local housing authorities to provide disabled people with accessible and affordable homes.

Social security provisions for the disabled

It is impossible to cover in detail the benefits which are available to those suffering from mental and physical disabilities and reference must be made to the publications of the Royal Association for Disability and Rehabilitation (RADAR) and others that are updated on an annual basis. An excellent guide to the rights and benefits which are available is provided by the Disability Rights Handbook. This provides far more detail that can be given in this chapter. Information is also available from the direct government website.[4]

The main benefits include:

- Taxable benefits:
  - Bereavement allowance
  - Incapacity benefit for the first 28 weeks
  - Some income support benefits
  - Pensions payable under the Industrial death benefit scheme
  - Carer's allowance
  - Jobseeker's allowance
  - Retirement pension
  - Statutory sick pay
  - Statutory maternity pay
  - Widowed parent's allowance
- Non-taxable benefits
  - Attendance allowance
  - Back to work bonus

- Bereavement payment
- Child benefit
- Child's special allowance
- Child tax credits
- Cold weather payments
- Council tax benefit
- Constant attendance allowance
- Disability Living Allowance
- Exceptionally Severe Disablement Allowance
- Guardian's allowance
- Housing Benefit
- Incapacity benefit for first 28 week of entitlement
- Income Support
- Industrial injuries benefit
- Invalidity benefits
- Maternity allowance
- Pensioner's Christmas Bonus
- Reduced earnings allowance
- Retirement allowance
- Severe Disablement Allowance
- Social Fund payments (and interest free loans) to help with maternity expenses, funeral costs, financial hardship and community care grants
- War widow's pension
- Winter fuel payment
- Working tax credit

Physiotherapists should be careful to ensure that they know the limitations of their knowledge in this very complex area which is constantly changing. They could be liable for giving negligent advice if clients relied on advice to their financial loss. It is preferable for physiotherapists to ensure that they know how to guide clients to the best sources of advice available.

Accommodation

Local authorities have a duty to provide accommodation for those suffering from physical and mental disabilities under the provisions of Section 21 (as amended) of the National Assistance Act 1948 and other legislation.

The duties under the amended Section 21 cover:

- Residential accommodation for persons aged 18 or over who by reason of age, illness, disability or any other circumstances are in need of care and attention not otherwise available to them.
- Temporary accommodation for persons who are in urgent need where the need for that accommodation could not reasonably have been foreseen.
- Accommodation
  - for persons who are or have been suffering from mental disorder; or
  - (to prevent mental disorder) for persons who are ordinarily resident in the area or have no settled residence.
- Accommodation in order to:
  - prevent illness;
  - care for those suffering from illness; and
  - provide after care of those so suffering.
- Arrangements specifically for persons who are alcoholic or drug dependent.
- Residential accommodation for expectant and nursing mothers (of any age) who are in need of care and attention which is not otherwise available to them.

Services for residents

Further arrangements (in relation to persons provided with accommodation) cover all or any of the following purposes:

- The welfare of all such persons.
- Supervising the hygiene of the accommodation so provided.
- Enabling such persons to obtain:
  - medical attention
  - nursing attention
  - services provided by the National Health Service.

The local authority is also required to review the accommodation and the arrangements. However it is not required to provide any accommodation which it is the duty of the NHS to provide.

Local authorities may also, in such cases as the authority considers appropriate, provide for the conveyance of persons to and from the accommodation that is provided.

Developments after the 1990 Act

The result of changes introduced by the NHS and Community Act 1990 was that, although the basic duties of the local authority to provide accommodation to specific categories of people have been slightly modified, the range of organisations with whom they can contract has increased. In addition the purchasing of the accommodation for persons since 1 April 1993 is the responsibility of the local social services authorities, who can recover fees from residents on a means-tested basis, rather than the Department of Social Security. A National Framework for NHS Continuing Healthcare was published in October 2007, which was designed to resolve the disputes over whether it was an NHS or social services duty to provide care. (This is considered in Chapter 18.)

Factors in the placement decision

Psychological needs as well as physical ones have to be taken into account.

Case: *R v. Avon County Council, ex parte M*[5]

The applicant was 22 and suffered from Down's syndrome. In 1989 the local authority began an assessment of the applicant's needs. In 1991 he was offered a place at Milton Heights where he spent 3 weeks. He and his family were set on his going there, but the local authority proposed various alternatives that were not acceptable. In January 1992 a review panel recommended that he should be placed at Milton Heights. The social services committee rejected the recommendation. After the threat of judicial review proceedings and further delay for a joint assessment of the applicant's needs the review panel in January 1993 found that the applicant had formed an entrenched wish to go to

Milton Heights and recommended that he should be placed there. The social services committee declined to accept this recommendation and decided to place the applicant elsewhere. As a result the applicant revived his application for judicial review to challenge the local authority's decision.

The High Court held (quashing the local authority's decision)

1. Residential accommodation should be appropriate to the needs of the individual applicant, which properly included his psychological needs. In the present case the applicant's entrenched wish to go to Milton Heights was not mere personal preference, but part of his psychological needs.
2. The social services committee could not overrule the recommendation of the review panel without a substantial reason. The review panel had properly arrived at its decision on the evidence before it and the strength, coherence and apparent persuasiveness of that decision had to be addressed head on if it were to be set aside and not followed. Anybody required, at law, to give reasons for reconsidering and changing such a decision must have and show a good reason for doing so. The local social services committee had failed to do so and its decision must be quashed.

A dispute be provided over the accommodation to for the disabled person arose in the following case.

Case: *R (on the application of A) v. London Borough of Bromley*[6]

A, a young man of 19 years, profoundly autistic with severe learning disabilities and petit mal epilepsy had been in a boarding school run by the Hesley group in Purbeck in Dorset. His time there had come to an end and all agreed that he needed a placement on a 52-week basis. His parents wished him to go to Hesley Village and College in Yorkshire but the local authority disagreed and

wished him to go to Robinia Care in Horndean. The local authority also had suggested a home in Lee on Solent. Judge Crane found the decision making of the local authority to be flawed: Hesley was ruled out as too expensive before any alternatives had been considered. He stated his role was not to substitute his decision for that of the local authority, but to determine the lawfulness of the local authority's actions and if he made a positive order to send the claimant to Hesley Village in Yorkshire the court would be substituting its decision for that of the local authority. He therefore quashed the local authority's decision and left his judgment to speak rather than grant declarations. Discussions then took place between the barristers and the judge in order to reach agreement over the immediate care of A, whose condition would deteriorate unless he was immediately placed in the appropriate accommodation.

Disabled facilities grants

Under section 114 of the Local Government and Housing Act 1989 the local housing authority had a duty to approve applications for grants for facilities for the disabled. These are known as disabled facilities grants (DFGs). The Housing, Grants, Construction and Regeneration Act 1996 replaced many of the mandatory grants under previous legislation by discretionary grants, except for DFGs that remain mandatory for specified purposes. Section 23(1) of the 1996 Act now details the provision of DFGs for the purposes shown in Figure 20.3. Further information on DFGs is available on the website for communities and local government[7] and a booklet has been published.[8]

A comment by the judge in the case[9] brought against Birmingham (see below) was:

In enacting the 1996 Act Parliament chose to downgrade statutory duties to discretions in relation to the approval of other types of grant, save for the disabled facilities grants for section 23(1) purposes. In making the decision to treat section 23(1) disabled facilities grants differently, it recognised the importance of obliging local housing authorities to approve

(1) The purposes for which an application for a disabled facilities grant must be approved . . . are the following:

(a) facilitating access by the disabled occupant to and from the dwelling or qualifying house boat or caravan or the building in which the dwelling or, as the case may be, flat is situated;

(b) making the dwelling or qualifying house boat or caravan or building safe for the disabled occupant and other persons residing with him;

(c) facilitating access by the disabled occupant to a room used or usable as the principal family room;

(d) facilitating access by the disabled occupant to, or providing for the disabled occupant, a room used or usable for sleeping;

(e) facilitating access by the disabled occupant to, or providing for the disabled occupant, a room in which there is a lavatory, or facilitating the use by the disabled occupant of such a facility;

(f) facilitating access by the disabled occupant to, or providing for the disabled occupant, a room in which there is a bath or shower (or both), or facilitating the use by the disabled occupant of such a facility;

(g) facilitating access by the disabled occupant to, or providing for the disabled occupant, a room in which there is a wash hand basin, or facilitating the use by the disabled person of such a facility;

(h) facilitating the preparation and cooking of food by the disabled occupant;

(i) improving any heating system in the dwelling or qualifying house boat or caravan to meet the needs of the disabled occupant or, if there is no existing heating system there or any such system is unsuitable for use by the disabled occupant, providing a heating system suitable to meet his needs;

(j) facilitating the use by the disabled occupant of a source of power, light or heat by altering the position of one of more means of access to or control of that source or by providing additional means of control;

(k) facilitating access and movement by the disabled occupant around the dwelling or qualifying house boat or caravan in order to enable him to care for a person who is normally resident there and is in need of such care;

(l) such other purposes as may be specified by order of the Secretary of State.

Figure 20.3   The Housing, Grants, Construction and Regeneration Act 1996: Section 23

grants to disabled occupants whose applications fulfilled the purposes enumerated in section 23(1).

There is also provision for a disabled facilities grant to be available for making the dwelling or building suitable for the accommodation, welfare or employment of the disabled occupant in any other respect (Section 23(2)).

Disabled occupant is defined as 'the disabled person for whose benefit it is proposed to carry out any of the relevant works' (Section 20).

Disabled person is a person, over 18 years, registered under Section 29(1) of the National Assistance Act 1948, or is a person for whom welfare arrangements have been made under Section 29 or, in the opinion of the social services authority, might be made under it (Section 100(2) of the 1996 Act).

The social services authority, means the council that is the local authority for the purposes of the Local Authority Social Services Act 1970 for the area in which the dwelling is situated (Section 100(4) of the 1996 Act).

A grant is not automatic. By Section 24(3), (4) and (5) the local authority in making a decision can consider whether:

- the relevant works are necessary and appropriate to meet the needs of the disabled occupant;
- it is reasonable and practicable to carry out the relevant works, having regard to the age and condition of the dwelling or building;
- the dwelling is fit for human habitation;
- (in the case of an application that requires works to the common parts of a shared building) that building meets the requirements of Section 604(2) of the Housing Act 1985;
- (in respect of works to the common parts of a building containing one or more flats) the applicant has a power or is under a duty to carry out the relevant works.

These statutory provisions can give rise to many difficulties for physiotherapists. Although the local housing authority should ensure that the social services authority is consulted over the decision to give a grant this is not always implemented. It may happen that applications go straight to the housing authority which places them upon a waiting list without first obtaining the advice and assessment of a registered physiotherapist or registered occupational therapist.

It is inevitable that priorities have to be established to meet the demand for DFGs and physiotherapists may be encouraged to make an assessment in the light of the available resources rather than in the light of the needs of the disabled person.

Nevertheless, it was held by the High Court in the case of *R* v. *Birmingham City Council*[9] that financial resources are not relevant when a local authority is deciding whether to provide someone with a disabled facilities grant under Section 23(1) of the Housing, Grants, Construction and Regeneration Act 1996. The judge allowed an application for judicial review of a decision of Birmingham City Council that took account of financial resources when deciding whether to offer the applicant a disabled facilities grant.

However, entitlement to receive a disabled facilities grant is means tested, and this fact may dampen demand. The decision in the Birmingham case was considered together with the nature and ambit of Section 23 of the 1996 Act in the following case:

Case: *B* v. *Calderdale Metropolitan Council*[10]

The claimant was the father of four children, the eldest of whom, D, was autistic and thought to suffer from Asperger's syndrome. The family lived in a rented three-bedroom house, in which D shared a bedroom with his brothers. D was uncontrollably aggressive towards S, frightening him while he slept and attacking him when they were in the bedroom together. The family wanted a grant to build an additional bedroom in which D can sleep on his own. The Council refused a grant and B's application was rejected in the High Court. The Court of Appeal allowed the appeal, quashing the decision to refuse a DFG and ordering the Council to reconsider the application in the light of the judgment of the Court. Lord Justice Sedley stated that while the additional bedroom would not completely remove the risk of harm to the brother, it would obviate the risk caused by their sharing a bedroom. He considered the facts fell within Section 23(1)(b) of the 1996 Act (see Figure 20.3).

It should also be remembered that, in addition to its powers under Section 23(1), the local housing authority has the power to make grants in respect of improvements and repairs depending upon the age of the property, its condition and the nature of the applicant's interest in the property. The maximum grant for disabled facilities grant is £25 000 per application in England and £30 000 in Wales. However, where the cost of the eligible work is more than the grant limit, the council may use its discretionary powers under the Regulatory Reform (Housing Assistance) (England and Wales) Order 2002 to bridge the part or all of the gap between what they are required to pay and the full cost of the works. Social services can also provide community care equipment and minor adaptations which a person has been assessed to need and for which he is eligible, free of charge, provided the cost, including fittings, is less than £1000.

It is possible that where parents are separated a dispute could arise between them over which house should be adapted to meet the disability needs of a child. This situation is considered in Chapter 23 on children.

Education and training and employment facilities

Duties are placed upon local authorities under the National Assistance Act 1948, the Chronically Sick and Disabled Persons Act 1970 and the Disabled Persons (Employment) Acts 1944 and 1958 (as amended by subsequent legislation) to provide education and training and employment facilities for those with physical and mental disabilities.

Sheltered employment facilities for the seriously physically or mentally disabled have therefore been established by local authorities. The local authority's duty extends to those disabled people who are resident within its catchment area.

The National Network of Assessment Centres[11] is a UK wide network of specialist services that work together to facilitate access for disabled people to education, training, employment and personal development. Assessment centre services include quality assessment and support in the use of assistive technology and/or specialised learning strategies. Students in higher education in the UK claiming the Disabled Students Allowance are often referred to an Assessment Centre for DSA-funded Study Aids and Strategies Assessment on behalf of higher education students.

Physiotherapists may have a role in the management and planning of such facilities and in bringing to the attention of the social services authority deficiencies and shortcomings in the arrangements and facilities, as well as being involved in the assessment of clients for the use of such facilities.

Duty of Care owed by local authority

In Chapter 22 a case is discussed where it was held that the local authority owed a duty of care towards a husband and wife with learning disabilities who were being victimised and assaulted by a gang of youths.[12] The case, which was heard in June 2008, is likely to go to appeal, so the full implications of the decision are not yet clear. Although the case concerned persons with learning disabilities the principles could be extended to those persons who are physically disabled.

Inter-agency and inter-professional cooperation

Local authorities have a statutory duty to cooperate with other statutory authorities and the voluntary sector in the provision of services. In practical terms the cooperation between health staff and local authority staff is vital to the interests of the client and can cause the physiotherapist considerable problems.

Integrated care pathways

The Chartered Society of Physiotherapy (CSP) published a paper on integrated care pathways to help members understand what integrated care pathways are, what their background is and how a pathway can be developed.[13]

The CSP describes the integrated care pathways (ICPs) as one means for improving the delivery of care to patients. It cites the definition provided by the National Pathways Association:

An Integrated Care Pathway determines locally agreed multidisciplinary practice, based on guidelines and evidence where available for a specific patient/client group. It forms all or part of the clinical record, documents the care given and facilitates the evaluation of outcomes for continuous quality improvement.

Physiotherapist involvement might be:

- developing a pathway for a specific client group, e.g. total hip replacement;
- reviewing a pathway that has been developed;
- using one in practice;
- assessing the results of an audit of a pathway;
- implementing changes as a result of an audit;
- instructing other staff members in the use of the pathway.

Legal issues can arise in their use such as:

- What if the pathway is followed to the detriment of the patient? Can the pathway be held responsible?

If any reasonable physiotherapist would have realised that the specific circumstances of an individual patient meant that the ICP was inappropriate, then the physiotherapist slavishly following the ICP would be negligent. Professional discretion cannot be abandoned because an ICP exists. This same principle applies to National Institute for Health and Clinical Excellence (NICE) guidelines and NSFs and other protocols and procedures (See Chapter 10).

- What if the physiotherapist disagrees with the view of the multidisciplinary team on the ICP?

The CSP in its ICP document points out that professional autonomy and discretion should be preserved if members collaborate with their colleagues from the beginning in the development of the pathway. The law does not recognise a concept of team liability (see Chapter 10) and if an ICP is developed which is not in accordance with the reasonable standard of care of the physiotherapist, this should be brought to the attention of the team. The physiotherapist could not in his/her defence, if he/she has been negligent in providing care to the patient, argue that he/she was only following the ICP.

Use of volunteer agencies and other non-statutory bodies

Local authorities are increasingly using non-direct labour for the provision of services and entering into contracts with other organisations, usually of a non-profit making kind, for them to provide the services that the local authority has a statutory duty to ensure exist. Such arrangements can create complex issues relating to responsibility and accountability. It is advisable for the physiotherapist who may have to deal with complaints about the services provided by these non-statutory organisations to have sight of the agreements drawn up with the local authority in order to be certain of the terms on which their services are given and to be aware of which duties are enforceable.

The use of such organisations and agencies does not, however, remove the primary responsibility from the local authority to ensure that the services are available.

Limitations on resources and priority setting

In 1995 certain disabled people in Gloucester challenged, by judicial review, the decision by Gloucestershire County Council to reduce or withdraw certain welfare assistance provided to them under Section 2 of the Chronically Sick and Disabled Persons Act 1970.

The court had to decide the issue of resources and statutory duties.

Case: *R v. Gloucester County Council, ex parte Mahfood and others*[14]

> Disabled persons complained when services had been curtailed following withdrawal of a government grant upon which the County Council's plans had been based and the Council gave greater priority to the more seriously disabled. The Council had not reassessed in the light of the cutbacks but had simply sent out a standard letter withdrawing services.

The High Court at first instance refused to grant a declaration that in carrying out the reassessment the local authority was not entitled to take into account the resources available to it. A local authority was right to take account of resources both when assessing needs and when deciding whether it was necessary to make arrangements to meet those needs.

One applicant, Mr Barry, appealed to the Court of Appeal.

The Court of Appeal[15] allowed the appeal, granting a declaration that in assessing or reassessing whether it was necessary to make arrangements in order to meet the needs of a disabled person, a local authority was *not* entitled to take into account the resources available to it. The local authority appealed to the House of Lords.

The House of Lords[16] held that, for the purposes of Section 2 of the 1970 Act, the needs of a chronically sick or disabled person were to be assessed in the context of, and by reference to, the provision of certain types of assistance for promoting the welfare of disabled persons using eligibility criteria (decided upon by the local authority) as to whether the disability of that particular person dictated a need for assistance, and if so at what level. Those criteria were to be set by taking into account:

- current acceptable standards of living,
- the nature and extent of the disability, and
- the relative cost balanced against the relative benefit and the relative need for that benefit.

In deciding how much weight was to be attached to the cost of providing the benefit, the authority had to make an evaluation about the impact which the cost would have on its resources, which in turn would depend on the authority's financial position. It followed that a chronically sick and disabled person's need for services could not sensibly be assessed without having some regard to the cost of providing such services, since his need for a particular type or level of service could not be decided in a vacuum from which all considerations of cost were expelled.

The House of Lords therefore allowed the appeal.

The House of Lords ruling in the Gloucester case was applied in *R v. E. Sussex CC ex parte Tandy*,[17] which is considered in Chapter 23. In the following case the High Court held that it was lawful for the local authority to charge for services provided under the Chronically Sick and Disabled Persons Act 1970.

Case: *R v. Powys County Council ex parte Hambridge*[18]

The applicant who was disabled received care services provided by the local authority for which she paid £10 per week. She applied for judicial review arguing that the local authority had not power to demand payment for services provided under the 1990 Act. Her application was dismissed. Section 17 of the Health and Social Services and Social Security Adjudications Act 1983 enabled a local auhtority to charge for services provided under Section 29 of the National Assistance Act 1948. The local authority was not providing services under Section 2 of the 1970 Act; they were making arrangements under the 1948 National Assistance Act for the provision of their services. The charge for welfare services was lawful.

At the same time as the Gloucester case, the court heard an application by Mr McMillan[16] for judicial review of the decision of Islington Borough Council not to provide him with home help cover when his carers were ill or away. This application failed on the grounds that the Council had conducted a proper balancing exercise taking into account resources and the comparative needs of the disabled in its area. The court held that the Council was not in breach of the duty that it owed to the applicant.

The Gloucester case was followed in a case[19] involving adaptions and aids for two severely disabled children aged 17 and 13 years. The local authority asked for details of the parents' means. The parents said they could not afford to pay for the alterations but refused to provide information about their means and sought judicial review of the authority's action. The High Court held that the authority was entitled to take into account the parents' financial resources when deciding whether or not to provide and pay for alterations. The claimants appealed, arguing that Section 2 of the 1970 Act created a free-standing duty on the authority to provide services without any right to charge. The Court of Appeal dismissed the appeal holding that the local authority could charge for the provision of services provided under Section 2 of the 1970 Act and Section 17 of the Children Act 1989 and could reasonably expect that parents who could afford the expense would make any alterations to their home that were necessary for the care of their disabled children. The local authority was entitled to decline to provide services to meet the needs of disabled children until it was demonstrated that having regard to their means, it was not reasonable to expect their parents to provide them.

In the case of *R (on the application of Hefferman)* v. *Sheffield City Council*,[20] the claimant who suffered from Still's disease and was almost totally blind and had both hips and knees replaced argued that the amount he was paid to enable him to obtain care was insufficient and that he required 27–30 hours per week as opposed to the $24^1/_2$ provided. The court held that it could not be said that the allocation of care was perverse. It was not at all generous but it did not have to be: it had to be adequate to meet the proper needs. The claimant's condition was deteriorating and there had to be regular reviews of his care, but such a reconsideration would not inevitably result in more hours of care.

In 2005 the Department of Health published a Green paper called *Independence, Well-being and Choice*,[21] which placed considerable emphasis on users of social care and local authority services having individual budgets to buy in the care services they require. This is considered in Chapter 18. Reference should also be made to Chapter 24 and the care of older people.

Legal issues arising from sports injuries

The Association of Chartered Physiotherapists in Sports Medicine

The Association of Chartered Physiotherapists in Sports Medicine (ACPSM) was founded in 1971 to provide quality sports physiotherapy, rehabilitation and counselling to athletes and recreational participants before, during and after injury. Its objectives are shown in Figure 20.4. The ACPSM works closely with the International Federation of Sports Physiotherapists and World Federation of Athletic Training and Therapy and with many British and national sports and exercise organisations. It has developed a programme of three-tier continuing professional development awards.

Numerous legal issues arise in this field of physiotherapy practice including:

- The liability of those who volunteer help and take on the duty of care (this is considered in Chapter 10).
- The liability of the physiotherapist who provides help at sports events (see below on initiatives to ensure that only chartered physiotherapists provide services on the football field).
- The physiotherapist in private practice specialising in sports injuries (the problems

---

- To improve the techniques and facilities for the prevention and treatment of sports injuries
- To inform all interested individuals and bodies of the existence and availability of Chartered and State Registered Physiotherapists
- To provide a specialised service to meet the demands of sports people
- To encourage education, and to develop and publish research in the field of sports physiotherapy in the UK

Figure 20.4   Objectives of the Association of Chartered Physiotherapists in Sports Medicine

relating to private practice are considered in Chapter 19).

- Keeping within one's competence (this is discussed in Chapter 4 on the scope of professional practice).
- Giving advice as to whether the patient should continue on the field (liability arising from negligent advice is considered in Chapter 10 but a situation relating to a sports injury is discussed below).
- Administration of pain killers on the field (see below).
- Acting as an expert witness in a case brought by an international sports person against another player on the field (the role of the expert witness is considered in Chapter 13).

Negligent advice on the sports field

A physiotherapist specialising in sports physical therapy could be liable in several different circumstances:

- providing treatment designed to enable continued play with an injury before it is fully healed;
- informing athletes of the potential health risks on continued athletic activity in their physical condition; and
- treating, evaluating and advising athletes on their ability to resume athletic activity.

In an emergency situation where time is of the essence and there is an absence of diagnostic aids and specialist advice, the physiotherapist would still be expected to comply with the Bolam test of the standard of the reasonable physiotherapist in those circumstances (see Chapter 10). A recent discussion has taken place over whether physiotherapists have sufficient skills to treat athletes effectively. A sports physiotherapist, Sean Fyfe, stated that a knowledge of strength and conditioning training was essential for physiotherapists to plan long-term rehabilitation and maintenance programmes for acute and chronic injuries. However, this element was missing from basic physiotherapy education. This claim

was refuted by the CSP and the education chair of the ACPSM since the association had developed continuing professional development pathways for physiotherapists working in sport.[22] In April 2008 it was reported that a private physiotherapy practice in Scotland had set up the first specialist training academy for newly qualified graduates.[23] The nature and sufficiency of the training of a physiotherapist would be essential evidence in any case brought on the grounds of alleged negligence in the situations listed above.

Situation: tension stress fracture

Alan, a registered physiotherapist, assists a local football team. He is not paid a fee for his work, but is allowed free entrance for all matches including away games. He is called onto the pitch following an injury to one of the players, Billy. He gives Billy a speedy examination. Billy is clearly in a lot of pain in the groin region and Alan sprays an analgesic over the affected area and when asked by Billy if he should come off, he says that Billy could carry on playing. Subsequently, Billy is diagnosed as having a tension stress fracture and his continuing to play has exacerbated his injury. Billy who is likely to be off work for many months is claiming compensation from Alan for the extra work time he has lost because of Alan's negligent advice. Is he likely to succeed?

In the above situation, whether the footballer's case will succeed will depend upon whether he can prove that he was given advice that no reasonable physiotherapist would have offered. In addition, he will have to prove that he relied on the advice he received and would have come off the field if that advice had been given instead. It is possible that, with the adrenalin of the match, he was anxious to continue and would have ignored advice to come off if the physiotherapist had so advised him.

Liability of the unregistered physiotherapist

- What would be the legal situation if, in the above situation, the physiotherapist assisting at the game was not registered?

Because of the protection of title introduced under the Health Professions Council (HPC) any physiotherapist who acted as a sports physiotherapist without being registered would be acting illegally and could be prosecuted (see Chapter 3). However, persons who claim to act as sports therapists, athletic trainers, masseurs and sports scientists do not have registered status under the HPC and as long as they do not use the title of physiotherapist or profess themselves to be acting as a physiotherapist or use any other registered title would not be committing a criminal offence. Such persons may still have their place in the multidisciplinary sports medicine team, provided a registered physiotherapist was also a member of the team. The Football Association and other national organisations for sports would require a registered physiotherapist to be in attendance. Any person giving advice on sports injuries could be liable for breach of a duty of care if further harm occurred as a result of negligent advice. If he or she also falsely held themselves out to be a physiotherapist then he or she would be committing a criminal offence.

The club's liability

What of the local team? Does it have a duty to confirm that it is insured for Billy's injuries and that it only employs a registered physiotherapist?

Much would depend upon Billy's status – whether he is an amateur or an employee of the club. The club itself would not necessarily be defined as a legal entity and capable of being sued (it depends upon how it has been formed and its constitution), but individuals who had specific responsibilities may be liable.

The fact that players are amateurs rather than professionals would not automatically change any principles in relation to insurance cover. However, much will depend upon what the players are told. If they are told to obtain their own insurance cover then they could not look to the club for that protection.

The fact that they have not used a chartered physiotherapist may be significant if club members consider that they are entitled to have a reasonable standard of professional care. Under the new protection of title rules under the HPC, a physiotherapist must be registered to practise. The club would therefore be required to ensure that any person calling themselves a physiotherapist was registered.

Vicarious liability of the club

In a recent case the Court of Appeal held that a rugby club was vicariously liable for a player punching a member of the opposing team on the field and causing a fracture which required reconstructive orbital surgery.[24] The player had a contract with Redruth Rugby Football Club by which it employed him to play rugby for it. The Court of Appeal held that the employer was vicariously liable for the acts of its employees committed while in the course of employment. There was a close connection between the punch and his employment. He was employed to play rugby and that was what he was doing at the time. There was a melee going on of the kind that frequently took place during rugby matches. The melee was part of the game. It was just the kind of thing that both clubs would have expected to occur. Unfortunately, the throwing of punches was not uncommon in such situations. The player was acting in the course of employment when he punched the claimant and the club was therefore vicariously liable for his actions.

Children

Clearly, no player should be compelled to return to a game and care should be taken with children. In a school situation Corinne Williams,[25] 16 years old, obtained damages of £1500 when she was forced to join in a PE class despite having an injured ankle. The girl's mother, an orthopaedic nurse, had written to the school notifying them that the girl had a sprained ankle but, believing the letter to be forged by the girl, the school teacher forced her to take part (see also Chapter 23).

Sports preparation

A physiotherapist may be involved in the preparation for sports activities as well as dealing with the aftermath. (See Chapters 10 and 26 on liability for negligent advice and instruction.)

Dance specialists

There are other areas of specialism that could involve physiotherapists. For example, Dance UK[26] has established a national list of health professionals who are used to working with dancers and so will understand their needs and problems. Any physiotherapist wishing to be on the register has to complete a form of application and provide a recommendation from a dancer or dance company.

Representing the multidisciplinary team

The physiotherapist should be aware of any limits on her own competence in rehabilitation and recognise the contribution that other professionals could make.

Situation: physiotherapy advice ignored

A footballer player for an amateur team who had hopes of becoming a professional was injured during a match and was attended by the physiotherapist on duty. She examined his injury and advised him not to continue. Because he was so ambitious to become professional and therefore to be seen in the match, he ignored her advice and carried on playing and was selected for later matches. Subsequently his injury exacerbated and he had to give up work. He blamed the physiotherapist for not being clear enough about the dangers of continuing to play and the club for selecting him for later matches and took legal action against them. What are the likely legal repercussions?

Inevitably, cases are won in the main on what facts can be established in court. If the physiotherapist can provide evidence of her clear advice for him not to play and has witnesses to establish what she said to the player, it is likely that he will fail in his claim against her. She has not been in breach of the duty of care owed to him. He ignored her instructions and therefore is entirely responsible for the worsening of his injuries. There is no evidence that he lacked the mental capacity to make his own decisions and he takes the consequences of so doing.

What is the club's position? It has a duty of care towards its members. Was it in breach of this duty? Much depends upon the evidence of his injuries and unfitness to play. If the club ignored evidence about his unfitness to play, then it could be seen to be in breach of its duty of care by selecting him to play. However, there would be a large element of contributory negligence by the player who knew from what the physiotherapist had told him that he was not fit. If the club did not know about his unfitness, then was it failing to ensure that there was in place a safe system for checking the fitness of players before selection? If so, the club could be seen to be partly to blame, but there would still be an element of contributory negligence by the player himself. (See Chapter 10 on contributory negligence.)

Further reading

Medicine, Sport and the Law edited by Simon D.W. Payne[27] provides more detailed information relating to specific conditions such as patients with organ transplants and the transplant games, rowing, golf, water sports and most other sports, including the Firearms Act and mental health. See also *Sports Medicine: Ethics and Law* by E. Grayson and C. Bond.[28]

Legal issues arising in musculoskeletal conditions

This is one of the most difficult areas of physiotherapy practice including back pain, rheumatology and other conditions. Of frequent concern are such issues as:

- deception by patient;
- limits of competence;
- the use of other specialists in this field, e.g. osteopaths, chiropractors, neurologists and neurosurgeons;
- giving advice;
- prognosis decisions and advice;
- sickness and disability laws;
- management of chronic pain and legal aspects which arise;
- the scope of professional practice, e.g. TENS (transcutaneous electrical nerve stimulation) being applied by the physiotherapist;
- acupuncture and electro-acupuncture (see Chapter 27 on complementary therapies).

The CSP published in 2005 advice for physiotherapists on preventive strategies for work-related musculoskeletal disorders that affect physiotherapists, which is considered in Chapter 11.

The Manipulation Association of Chartered Physiotherapists

This Association was formed in 1967 to provide a specialist approach in the treatment of musculoskeletal disorder and is a member of the International Federation of Manipulative Therapy (IFOMT).[29]

The aims of the Association are shown in Figure 20.5.

Membership of the Association is gained via either a postgraduate diploma or MSc in manual therapy, or a membership examination. A minimum of 2 weeks' clinical supervision under someone with an Manipulation Association of Chartered Physiotherapists (MACP) education is strongly recommended. The Association has adopted a continuing education policy for members. It also encourages research into manipulative therapy and to this end has appointed a research officer and allocated funds to assist individual members with their projects.

In 1992 the MACP together with related organisations formed an umbrella organisation known as the British Association of Chartered Physiotherapists in Manipulation (BACPIM). It aims to maintain connections with all the manipulative groups, to promote manipulative skills among its members and to make the public, the government and medical practitioners aware that there are several thousand highly trained chartered physiotherapists capable and willing to treat patients with neuromusculoskeletal problems by manipulation and associated therapies. Among its achievements has been the development of an integrated course on the management of low back pain for physiotherapists and the production of an information pack aimed at promoting physiotherapy in the management of low back pain. The CSP has published guidance for the safe teaching of manipulation to undergraduates.[30]

Advice the physiotherapist specialising in this field might give would include:

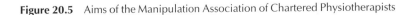

- To promote the concept of a broad based approach to the overall management of musculoskeletal disorders
- To develop highly skilled clinicians who are able to draw upon a vast bank of knowledge, and analyse, evaluate and treat often extremely complex problems of neuromusculoskeletal origin
- To provide an opportunity for those actively engaged in the practice of manipulative therapy to exchange knowledge and improve their professional skills

Figure 20.5   Aims of the Manipulation Association of Chartered Physiotherapists

- advice on posture
- advice on dynamic lifting
- instruction on ergonomics
- muscle strengthening exercises e.g. abdominal exercises
- flexibility exercises
- advice on overall fitness.[31]

Communication problems

The patient's knowledge of anatomy may be poor, and he is likely to use colloquial expressions. When pain is felt 'in the hip', it usually means the buttock or greater trochanteric region. Patients rarely volunteer 'the buttock'. When pain is felt 'in the shoulder' it often means the supraspinous region of the scapula.[32]

The way in which a patient might refer to symptoms may be extremely important in ensuring good communication between professional and patient. Liability can arise for negligence on the part of the professional in the duty to inform and communicate (see Chapters 7 and 10).

Hutson[31] gives a list of headings in history taking for back pain. They include:

longevity of symptoms	terminology
onset of symptoms	relationship to activity
intensity of symptoms	general health enquiry
change in symptoms	past health
site of pain	effect on lifestyle
accompanying symptoms	

Lower limb amputation and risk management

J. Kulkarni and others describe[33] a study of patients attending the Manchester Disablement Service Centre. Fifty-eight per cent of patients with unilateral amputations and 27% of patients with bilateral amputations reported at least one fall in the last 12 months. Of the unilateral patients, 12% of these falls related to prosthesis alone. The authors recommend a multidisciplinary intervention for all such patients and education for both patients and professionals.

Only a quarter of patients recall being instructed in how to get up from a fall and the authors have prepared a small booklet with diagrammatical illustrations showing patients how to do this with the physiotherapist providing supporting demonstration and instruction. Risk management is considered in Chapter 24 on the care of older people and in Chapter 11 on health and safety law.

Road traffic victim and the legal issues

The following situation is an example of a case (taken from Lynch and Grisogono[34]) giving rise to multiple legal issues. The text in italics emphasises the legal problems that arise and where they are considered in this book.

Situation: Dawn, a road traffic accident victim

Dawn was a 26-year-old victim of a road traffic accident in which her friend, who was driving a sports car in which she was a passenger, died. She was resuscitated at the accident site and placed on life support. She needed a transfer to a nearby hospital so that she could be given a CAT scan. *Dawn's parents had to give their written permission for the transfer, which added to their anxieties about the situation (Chapter 7 on the law of consent). This chapter shows that where a patient is unable to give consent, then carers and the clinical team must act in her best interests under the Mental Capacity Act 2005. Written consent from the relatives to the transfer was not necessary and the relatives did not have the power to withhold consent on behalf of a mentally incapacitated adult contrary to the patient's best interests. The professionals should have acted in the best interests of the patient and not sought the written consent of the relatives. In determining the best interests of Dawn they are required in law to consult with the relatives and close friends over what Dawn's wishes, views and beliefs would have been had she been able to express her wishes. The clinicians would also have to ascertain if Dawn had drawn up a living will or appointed a person under a lasting power of attorney.*

The parents were initially told that she would be unlikely to survive. CAT scan showed no brain damage. When she came round from the coma, she was found to be suffering from a left hemiplegia. The parents never understood at what stage she suffered brain damage. They found this confusing, and, to a certain extent, it became a cause of resentment. *Reference should be made to the law relating to giving information to relatives, the duty of care and liability for negligent information (see Chapters 7 and 10).*

She suffered from bouts of severe depression and at one stage was referred to a clinical psychologist for counselling. *The standard of care to which the patient is entitled requires the involvement of other health professionals and a physiotherapist would be failing in her duty of care if she failed to bring in the appropriate person at the correct time (see Chapter 10).*

The psychologist worked on the basis that Dawn would always be dependent and referred her to a neurosurgeon who promised that he could operate to cure the spasticity that kept causing her muscles to tense up involuntarily. The parents only discovered that the operation would leave her paralysed and wheel bound for the rest of her life when they questioned the neurosurgeon about the operation. *There is a duty to inform according to the reasonable standard of care; the duty includes not simply information about serious risks but also inevitable consequences of any operation (see Chapters 7 and 10).*

Most of her treatment was done privately, because she could not obtain adequate long-term treatment through the National Health Service. *The right to have continuing care is considered in Chapter 6 and responsibilities for the provision of rehabilitation and continuing care is considered in Chapters 18 and 24 and private care in Chapter 19.*

She had to make a claim against the insurers because her friend had not had full cover for his sports car. *See Chapter 16 for mention of the Motor Insurer's Bureau, which covers liability where the driver is not insured or in a hit-and-run case, but only provides compensation for personal injuries and death, not property.*

The case dragged on and the insurers made an offer of settlement. *It is important to consider the effect of court proceedings on patients; the role of the physiotherapist who may have to give evidence in court about the patient's condition is considered in Chapter 13. The dangers that patients are unwilling to do exercises, because any improvements might reduce the amount of compensation, are considered in Chapter 7 and in this chapter. Legal significance of a settlement is considered in Chapters 2 and 10.*

Dawn was advised that she might obtain more money if she went to court, but she felt that this would be too hard for her emotionally, even though she had no memory of the accident or indeed of the friend who had died. She accepted the offer. *See Chapter 13 on giving evidence in court.*

She was able to buy a specially adapted car. *See Chapter 16 about transport and disabled drivers, Road Traffic Act rules and insurance issues. The physiotherapist may be involved in providing confirmation that a disabled person is fit to drive.*

She took up sports, javelin, shot and discus, but her coach misunderstood the nature of her spasticity and believed that controlling spasticity was a matter of trying harder. As a result of his persuasion to run into a throw, she fell over and suffered a broken ankle. *See Chapter 10 for liability of people who do not understand the condition and who give advice and instructions that cause harm. See also Chapter 26 for liability of the instructor. The possibility that a patient might assume the risks of harm (volenti non fit injuria) is discussed in Chapter 10.*

She married. *In order to be able to give consent to marriage she must be mentally capable, otherwise the marriage would be void. There are social security provisions for a married person with disabilities.*

Non-compliance in road traffic accident cases

Physiotherapists often come across situations where patients are awaiting compensation following road accidents to be settled and there is a reluctance on the patient's part to make rapid progress which would reduce the amount of compensation they receive.

Situation: non-compliance following a road traffic accident

Jim had severe leg injuries following an accident on his motorbike for which he was not to blame. He was hesitant to take part in mobility exercises since he was anxious to obtain maximum compensation for his injuries. What is the legal situation of the physiotherapist?

The physiotherapist should do all she can to encourage Jim to make as full a recovery as possible as quickly as possible. She should advise Jim:

- that the law requires an injured person to mitigate their loss, i.e. to do as much as is reasonable to reduce the effects of the harm which has been suffered;
- that the courts will take into account the pain and suffering that the patient has borne during the recovery process; and
- that ultimately money is a poor substitute for the loss of amenities.

The courts could find that there has been contributory negligence by Jim in failing to follow a recommended treatment and exercise plan thus reducing the compensation. (This is discussed in Chapter 10.) Ultimately, however, the physiotherapist cannot force Jim to undertake the exercises if persuasion and reasoning fail (see Chapter 7 on the law of consent).

Assessing for compensation (quantum)

Even where liability is admitted, there may still be disputes over the amount of compensation due in road traffic accident cases. The physiotherapist who is caring for a road traffic accident victim may have a responsibility in drawing up figures on the likely costs of future rehabilitation which may be used in a subsequent court case. The figure may include the costs of adaptations and equipment and services required by the patient. Other physiotherapists may be called as expert witnesses and would have to assess the accuracy of such an estimate (see Chapter 13).

Care of young adults

The care of young adults following road traffic injuries can present special problems for the physiotherapist as the following situation shows.

Situation: joking around

Tom, a lad of 19 years of age, had severely fractured his leg in a road accident and hated being confined in hospital for traction. He was full of high spirits and encouraged other patients to play jokes on the nursing and therapy staff. What action can be taken?

Legally an occupier of premises is entitled to ask any person whose presence has become intolerable to leave the premises. Even a patient can be asked to leave if their conduct is unacceptable, unless the cause is mental disorder or the patient lacks the requisite mental capacity to understand the situation. There will therefore be certain limits beyond which Tom's behaviour need not be accepted and he could be warned of this possibility. Even though it is clinically inadvisable for him to leave hospital, if his conduct becomes dangerous to others then in an extreme situation it may be necessary to discharge him.

Legal aspects of respiratory care

The Association of Chartered Physiotherapists in Respiratory Care (ACPRC) have prepared clinical guidelines on physiotherapy management of the spontaneously breathing, acutely breathless, adult patient.[35] Topics covered include: assisted ventilation, entonox, humidification, bronchodilation, NFR (which in this context means neurophysiological facilitation of respiration – and not 'Not for resuscitation') and TENS. If it were alleged that a physiotherapist providing respiratory care was negligent reference could be made to these guidelines in determining the reasonable standard of care which should have been followed, on the understanding that the guidelines were kept up to date and reflected the reasonable standard of care at the time.

Situation: a tetraplegic

Mavis, a tetraplegic, is extremely abusive to staff, especially the physiotherapy staff and this has led to several physiotherapists applying for posts in other hospitals. What action can be taken?

Unlike the Situation: joking around described above, it would be impossible to tell Mavis that if she continued such abuse she would have to leave hospital. However, it is possible that her aggression arises from underlying factors of depression and the non-acceptance of her condition. It may be that a psychologist or other counsellors could provide assistance. It is essential that senior management provide support to staff, ensuring that the care of Mavis is shared around the department, since employers can be liable for mental illness arising from stress at work (see Chapter 11).

Legal issues arising in patients with neurological conditions

This covers a vast group of patients, including those who have had strokes, cerebral palsy, Parkinson's disease and many forms of brain damage. Each of these fields gives rise to many different legal issues. Thus in Parkinson's disease[36] the legal issues which arise include:

- consent from a patient who may not be able to communicate but is able to understand the clinical situation (see in Chapter 7);
- the rights of the patient to receive appropriate care, including the right to receive drugs or surgery as appropriate (see in Chapter 6);
- the standards of care to be provided (see Chapter 10).

Treatment of undressed patients

One well-known method for treating patients with muscle weakness and neurological disorders is the Bobath method of treatment. Its philosophy is for a hands-on approach to patient treatment. Many legal concerns can arise for the Bobath physiotherapist.

Situation: accused of assault

The mother of a child with severe cerebral palsy made a complaint about the actions of a physiotherapist when she discovered that the physiotherapist took off her son's clothes in order to carry out the treatment. She had assumed that the exercises would be carried out with the boy fully clothed.

There has been a clear failure of communication in this situation between physiotherapist and mother. Had the mother been properly informed about the nature of the treatment, she could have refused on behalf of her son, or she could have made sure that she was present during the treatment and saw that no assault was taking place. The physiotherapist must be highly sensitive to any discomfort felt by a patient during such treatments and examinations that involve intimate procedures, and clarify the patients' or parents' consent or cease to provide that personal treatment (see Chapter 7).

Clinical effectiveness

Situation: slow progress

A Bobath physiotherapist considers that she has made considerable progress with realigning muscles in a patient and she is supported by the mother. However, she has now learnt that resources for the work she is doing are to be discontinued on the grounds that there is no identifiable clinical progress.

Many treatments in physiotherapy show only gradual progress and there is a danger that, with the emphasis on clinical effectiveness, minute stages of progress in patient comfort and care may be ignored and resources refused because identifiable results are not apparent. Moreover, often treatments may prevent further damage or distortion rather than leading to a complete cure. Record keeping is essential so that the physiotherapist can point to a clear record of benefit to such patients, as expressed by the patients themselves or by the relatives.

Litigation fears

Situation: fears of litigation

A physiotherapist trained in the Bobath method was so concerned at the possibility of litigation for assault or for negligence that she decided to give up practice.

It would be unfortunate if the increase in litigation and complaints led to practitioners withdrawing their services or turning to other careers. It is impossible to prevent a person deciding to sue (although in extreme cases, an order of the court can be sought to ban a vexatious litigant from pursuing a hopeless claim). However the physiotherapist should be able to defeat any such claim by pointing to her records, and to the fact that she has followed a reasonable standard of care and has obtained the consent of the patient (or parent) to any touching of the person.

Pain management

Physiotherapists are involved in all aspects of pain management with all client groups, so this topic has been placed in this chapter for convenience. This is a field where major developments are taking place and the management of pain relief is becoming less of an ad hoc process of trial and error and more systematically managed. Hospices have developed considerable expertise in pain control among the terminally ill. Physiotherapists will be expected to be aware of developments in understanding which treatments are clinically effective. The Bolam test (see Chapter 10) requires that the individual physiotherapist will be providing the reasonable standard of care in the circumstances of the case and will keep up with developments in the field. Thus, it is essential that treatments that are no longer seen to be effective are only provided where there are clear clinical indications for them, although things such as infra red treatments and shortwave diathermy may still have their place, but are in very restricted use. Similarly, wax treatments may have only limited application. The physiotherapist has to keep up to date with research developments. The legal issues arising from pain management are considered in the author's work.[37]

Back pain and contributory negligence

The patient's cooperation is essential in the implementation of any treatment plan devised by a physiotherapist. What are the legal implications if a patient fails to follow the advice of the physiotherapist and carry out recommended exercises as in the following example?

Situation: failure to follow advice

Bob Evans was provided with a personalised exercise programme for the restoration and maintenance of adequate lumbar function by his physiotherapist to treat his low back pain. However, he failed to carry out the exercises and blamed the physiotherapist for providing inadequate treatment and care. What is the legal situation of the physiotherapist?

In this situation the physiotherapist would have to show that her advice and guidance was in accordance with the reasonable practice of a physiotherapist. Any legal action could also be defended on the grounds that Bob was contributorily negligent in failing to follow the treatment plan and failing to carry out the programme of exercises. Where there has been some failure on the part of the physiotherapist, the lack of compliance by the patient could be an important factor in determining the amount of compensation payable in a case of litigation. (This issue of patient non-compliance because compensation has not been settled is considered above.)

Smoking and the physically disabled

Situation: assisted smoking

> A patient who is tetraplegic insists on being assisted in smoking. Does the physiotherapist have to help? What if she disagrees with smoking?

Often the physiotherapist might find that her personal views conflict with those of her patients/clients. She does not have any right to impose her beliefs on others (although the law does recognise a statutory right for health professionals to object to involvement in the termination of pregnancy or fertilisation and embryology). On the other hand there is no statutory right for the patient to smoke. Smoking in public places was prohibited under Section 1 of the Health Act 2006 from 1 July 2007. Some exemptions were granted temporarily under the Smoke-free (Exemptions and Vehicles) Regulations 2007.[38] All NHS trusts have had to introduce a no-smoking policy. It would have seemed reasonable for long-term patients to have a private area where smoking could be permitted and this would include tetraplegic patients but there is no right recognised in law as the following case shows.

Case: *R (G)* v. *Nottingham Healthcare NHS Trust* 2008

> A challenge by detained patients in Rampton special hospital that the ban on smoking breached their human rights under Article 8 and 14 failed.[39] The High Court dismissed an application for judicial review. Lord Justice Pill was not prepared to exempt detained mental health patients from the effect of the statute.

If smoking is permitted in an area to which the public have no access any dangers to safety and compatibility with anti-smoking legislation must be taken into account.

Situation: smoking dangers in the community

> A severely disabled person at home wishes to smoke but because of his condition drops the cigarette and causes fires. He has been burnt on several occasions, but still continues to smoke. Fire alarms and smoke detectors have been fitted to his premises and they keep going off. Even if social services try to prevent him having access to matches, he obtains them from neighbours. What is the law? Can he be allowed to remain a menace to public safety?

Unlike the preceding situation where the patient is in hospital, here the person is in the community, presumably living on his own and there are no laws banning smoking in private premises. There are provisions to take a person to a place of safety under the National Assistance Act 1948 and the Mental Health Act 1983 if the statutory conditions are present (see Chapters 21 and 24). However, it is likely that these conditions would not be present in these circumstances and it may be necessary to prepare a care package which takes account of the dangers from his smoking and the need for persons to be in attendance. Neighbours could be warned of the dangers of giving him matches and then leaving him on his own.

Situation: enveloped in smoke

> A physiotherapist visits a patient with multiple sclerosis. Both he and his wife smoke and the room reeks of tobacco. The physiotherapist is concerned about her own health as a passive smoker in this environment. Does she have any rights?

The physiotherapist cannot be compelled to enter a situation that damages her health. It would be uncertain how damaging spending half an hour in this environment three times a week is likely to be. Certainly, it would be reasonable for the physiotherapist to ask the couple not to smoke while she is visiting. However, it is unlikely that the circumstances here are sufficient to justify any refusal to attend. The anti-smoking legislation would not apply to a person's private home. It may be that the physiotherapist could agree with a colleague for the visits to be shared or transferred.

Conclusions

It is not possible in a work of this kind to consider every possible type of physical disability and physical injury or condition which physiotherapists might treat and consider the legal implications of each. Emphasis has to be placed on the general principles. However, it is apparent that considerable criticisms can be made about the facilities which are available for those suffering from physical disabilities. The implementation of the Disability Discrimination Act 1995 (see Chapter 17) and its extension in further legislation should ensure that the situation will improve.

The National Audit Office reported on health services for physically disabled people aged 16 to 64 years[40] in 1992 and concluded that more action needed to be taken to provide more rehabilitation services generally and in particular the treatment of incontinence and prevention of pressure sores. Specific recommendations were made for health authorities to ensure that rehabilitation services were provided to meet identified need including services for brain-damaged people. Gaps in the provision of respite care should be identified and action taken to fill them. In addition, there should be improvements in the timeliness, quality and availability of information on services available for physically disabled people. The picture however does not seem to have improved greatly. A Commission for Social Care Inspection report on the state of social care in England 2006–7[41] describes a gloomy picture of the social care for older and disabled people. This is discussed in Chapter 24. Physiotherapists have a key role to play in identifying the gaps in service provision and in ensuring that the appropriate services are monitored.

✏️ **Questions and exercises**

1 A client suffering from multiple sclerosis who lives on her own complains to you that her home help visits have been reduced to three a week. What advice do you give her and what action do you take?

2 Your assessment of the physical needs of a person suffering from arthritis and your treatment plan for physiotherapy is rejected by your departmental manager who considers that only six sessions rather than the 12 you have recommended should be provided and reminds you of the pressure placed on the physiotherapy services. What is the legal situation and what action would you take? (See also Chapters 6 and 10.)

3 Draw up a protocol that identifies the role and function of the physiotherapy assistant in the care of those suffering from physical disabilities.

4 You have been asked by your local rugby club to provide a service on the field. What considerations would you take into account before accepting the offer?

5 You are involved in the care of a patient suffering from back pain, but are not convinced that her symptoms are real. You see her shopping in a supermarket with no apparent discomfort. What action, if any, would you take?

6 The parents of a 25-year-old boy are asked to give consent to his having brain surgery that the surgeon considers essential as a consequence of a stroke which he has suffered. They refuse to give consent. What is the legal situation? (Refer to Chapter 7 and the Mental Capacity Act 2005.)

References

1 *R* v. *Gloucester County Council, ex parte Mahfood (et al).* [1997] AC 584; [1997] 2 All ER 1 HL; [1996] 4 All ER 421 CA; Times Law Report, 21 June 1995.

2   *R (on the application of Jones)* v. *Southend-on-Sea BC* [2005] EWHC 1439 (admin), (2007) 10 C.C.L. Rep 428.

3   *Sandford and another* v. *London Borough of Waltham Forest* [2008] EWHC 1106 (QB).

4   www.direct.gov.uk/en/DisabledPeople/FinancialSupport/index.htm

5   *R* v. *Avon County Council, ex parte M* [1994] 2 FLR 1006.

6   *R (on the application of A)* v. *London Borough of Bromley* [2004] EWHC 2108 (Admin).

7   www.communities.gov.uk/publications/housing/disabledfacilitiesgrant

8   Department for Communities and Local Government and Welsh Assembly Government (2007) *Disabled Facilities Grants*. Stationery Office, London.

9   *R* v. *Birmingham City Council, ex parte Mohammed* [1998] 3 All ER 788; The Times Law Report, 14 July 1998.

10   *R* v *Calderdale Metropolitan Council* [2004] EWCA Civ 134.

11   www.nnac.org

12   *X and Y* v. *London Borough of Hounslow* [2008] EWHC 1168 (QB) 23 June 2008.

13   Chartered Society of Physiotherapy (2002) *Integrated Care Pathways*. CSP, London.

14   *R* v. *Gloucester County Council, ex parte Mahfood, et al. R* v. *Islington London Borough Council, ex parte McMillan* (QBD) The Times Law Report, June 21 1995.

15   *R* v. *Gloucester County Council and another, ex parte Barry* [1996] 4 All ER 421.

16   *R* v. *Gloucestershire County Council* [1997] AC 584 HL [1997] 2 All ER 1.

17   *R* v *E. Sussex CC ex parte Tandy* (1995) 95 LGR 745.

18   *R* v. *Powys County Council ex parte Hambridge* [1998] 1 F.L.R. 643; 7 October 1997.

19   *R (on the application of Spink and another)* v. *Wandsworth London Borough Council* [2005] EWCA Civ 302.

20   *R* (on the application of Hefferman) v. *Sheffield City Council* [2004] All ER (D) 158 June.

21   Department of Health (2005) Green Paper. *Independence, Well-being and Choice*. DH, London.

22   www.csp.org.uk. Frontline News Issue 20 June 2007 available on the CSP website.

23   www.csp.org.uk. Frontline News Issue 18 April 2008 available on the CSP website.

24   *Gravil* v. *Carroll and Another* Times Law Report, 22 July 2008.

25   Fletcher, V. (1998) Damages for Injured Girl Made to do PE. *The Times*, 6 August.

26   www.danceuk.org.metadot/index.pl

27   Payne, S.D.W. (ed.) (1990) *Medicine, Sport and the Law*. Blackwell Scientific Publications, Oxford.

28   Grayson, E., Bond, C. (1996) *Sports Medicine: Ethics and Law*. Butterworth-Heinemann, Oxford.

29   Exelby, L. (1994) The Manipulation Association of Chartered Physiotherapists. *In Touch* **73**, 17.

30   Chartered Society of Physiotherapy (2003) *Guidance for the Safe Keeping of Manipulation to Undergraduates*. CSP, London.

31   Hutson, M.A. (1993) *Back Pain Recognition and Management*, p. 51. Butterworth-Heinemann, Oxford.

32   Hutson, M.A. (1993) *Back Pain Recognition and Management*, p. 39. Butterworth-Heinemann, Oxford.

33   Kulkarni, J. *et al.* (1996) Falls in Patients with Lower Limb Amputations: Prevalence and Contributing factors. *Physiotherapy* **82**, 2, 130–5.

34   Lynch, M., Grisogono, V. (1991) *Strokes and Head Injuries*. John Murray, London.

35   The Association of Chartered Physiotherapists in Respiratory Care (1996) *Clinical Guidelines: Physiotherapy Management of the Spontaneously Breathing, Acutely Breathless, Adult Patient*. ACPRC, Solihull.

36   Sagar, H. (1991) *Parkinson's Disease*. Macdonald Optima, London.

37   Dimond, B. (2002) *Legal Aspects of Pain Management*. Quay Books, Dinton.

38   Smoke-free (Exemptions and Vehicles) Regulations 2007 SI no 765.

39   *R (G)* v. *Nottingham Healthcare NHS Trust; R (N)* v. *Secretary of State for Health* and *R (B)* v. *Nottingham Healthcare* NHS Trust The Times Law Report, 28 May 2008 QBD.

40   National Audit Office (1992) *Report on Health Services for Physically Disabled People aged 16 to 64*. HMSO, London, *see also* NAHAT Briefing Summary, September 1992.

41   Commission for Social Care Inspection (2008) *The State of Social Care in ENGLAND 2006–7*. CSCI, London.

21 Care of the Mentally Ill

This chapter aims to give the physiotherapist an understanding of the law in relation to the care of those suffering from a mental illness (both the detained and the informal patient). Legal issues arising from the care of those with neurological conditions are considered in Chapter 20. Reference should also be made to textbooks on physiotherapy and mental health.[1] A concise summary of mental disorders and the potential value of physiotherapy in their care and treatment is given by Jean Picton-Bentley.[2] Useful sources of law relating to the care of the mentally ill are given in the bibliography.

The following topics are covered in this chapter:

- Physiotherapists practising in the field of mental health
- The Mental Health Act 1983 (as amended by the Mental Health Act 2007)
- Care in the community
- Informal patients
- General issues involving physiotherapists
- The future

Physiotherapists practising in the field of mental health

Physiotherapy has been seen in the past as essentially dealing with the physical and therefore its role in mental illness has been doubted. Thus in 1992, in reporting the results of research into the recruitment of physiotherapists into psychiatry, Helen Ainsworth[3] stated that psychiatry had not been part of physiotherapy training and even then was covered patchily, that senior physiotherapists therefore had little or no experience in the field and were reluctant to take on the unknown.

The situation is changing however. Inevitably the main contribution of physiotherapists in the field of mental health has been a traditional one with the emphasis on physical problems, but physiotherapists realise that they can make a significant contribution in the treatment of psychiatric and psychological problems. The physiotherapist working in the field of mental health needs to be multi-skilled with a knowledge of mental illness as well as physical problems.

Some physiotherapists who specialise in the care of the mentally ill will be working in secure psychiatric units where most patients will be detained under the Mental Health Act 1983 (as amended by the Mental Health Act 2007). Other physiotherapists specialising in mental health care may be involved in community care and / or with long-stay chronic mentally disordered patients who are not detained under the Act and others who suffer from depression, anxiety states and behavioural problems.

National Service Framework for Mental Health

The National Service Framework (NSF) was published in 1999 and set standards for mental health in the following areas:

- Standard One: Mental Health Promotion
- Standards Two and Three Primary Care and access to services
- Standards Four and Five Effective services for people with severe mental illness
- Standard Six Caring about carers
- Standard Seven Preventing suicide.

As well as setting national standards and defining service models, the NSF put in place underpinning programmes to support local delivery and established milestones and performance indicators against which progress would be measured.

In response to the NSF the CSP research and clinical effectiveness unit published an evidence briefing paper in the form of a report on the clinical effectiveness of physiotherapy in mental health.[4] The report stated that the evidence suggests that exercise training and increased physical activity produces definite improvements in reduction in depression and anxiety, improved physical status, improved cognitive function and can facilitate behavioural lifestyle change. It outlines the ways in which physiotherapists working in mental health can provide an extensive range of physical treatments aimed at relieving symptoms and improving quality of life. The treatments include:

- physical activity, exercise and sport
- balance, postural and movement re-education
- management of chronic and acute pain
- relaxation techniques
- hydrotherapy
- manual therapy and complementary therapies
- the core skills in treating musculoskeletal and orthopaedic problems and neurological deficits.

The Chartered Physiotherapists in Mental Health Care

The Chartered Physiotherapists in Mental Health Care (CPMH) (formerly the Association of Chartered Physiotherapists in Psychiatry formed in 1982) publishes a biannual journal and facilitates the exchange of information and the development of the understanding of physiotherapists practising in this field. Its aims are shown in Figure 21.1. The CPMH has prepared

- To provide a representative body of physiotherapists in psychiatry
- To establish standards of good practice through education and research
- To facilitate the exchange of ideas and information
- To improve multidisciplinary communication and understanding
- Formation of regional groups
- To encourage communication and interaction with physiotherapists in other spheres
- To encourage the involvement of community physiotherapists with psychiatric patients

Figure 21.1   Aims of the Chartered Physiotherapists in Mental Health Care

guidelines for good practice for physiotherapists working in this area. This covers the role of the physiotherapist in mental health care, standard setting and quality, key points of competence, quality measures, developing a physiotherapy service in mental health and examples of physiotherapy input.[5] The CPMH published a physiotherapy effectiveness bulletin on mental health in October 1999. The CSP contributed a response to the White Paper *Our Health, Our Care, Our Say* for the Mental Health Allied Health Professionals Advisory Project as part of the New Ways of Working for AHPs.[6] Further information is available through the Chartered Society of Physiotherapy (CSP) (see list of websites). In 2007 the CPMH published a strategy for physiotherapists in mental health.[7] This aimed to support and promote the unique role of physiotherapy in the holistic approach to physical and mental health care for people with mental health needs and to provide a framework for physiotherapy practice in all healthcare settings based on an up-to-date evidence base and client-centred practice in mental health care. An action plan in the four countries of the UK is being developed with four main project groups:

- Education
- New roles and team working
- Policy and national guidelines
- Networking, promoting physiotherapy profession.

The Healthcare Commission in July 2008 raised concerns that about 5000 patients abscond from mental health wards each year causing more than 200 violent incidents and harm to themselves and the public. It was also concerned about the level of violence in mental health in-patient wards partly caused by overcrowding. It stated that guidelines recommended 85% occupancy, where more than one in ten trusts has a rate of more than 100% occupancy.

The Mental Health Act 1983 (as amended by the Mental Health Act 2007)

The philosophy of the Mental Health Act 1983 is that admission to a psychiatric hospital should be avoided if there is alternative treatment and care available outside and compulsory admission should not be used if the patient will agree to be admitted as an informal patient or if alternative services outside the hospital are possible. Since only about 5–10% of psychiatric patients are detained under the statutory provisions, the physiotherapist working with the mentally disordered is more likely to be caring for informal rather than detained patients unless she works in a regional secure unit or special hospital. However, they should all have an understanding of the basic provisions of the Act.

Fundamental principles

The 2007 Act required the Secretary of State to include in the Code of Practice (prepared under Section 118 of the 1983 Act) a statement of principles. Each of the following matters must be addressed in this statement:

(a) respect for patients' past and present wishes and feelings
(b) respect for diversity generally including, in particular, diversity of religion, culture and sexual orientation (within the meaning of Section 35 of the Equality Act 2006)
(c) minimising restrictions on liberty
(d) involvement of patients in planning, developing and delivering care and treatment appropriate to them
(e) avoidance of unlawful discrimination
(f) effectiveness of treatment
(g) views of carers and other interested parties
(h) patient well-being and safety and
(i) public safety.

The Secretary of State is also required to have regard to the desirability of ensuring the efficient

Section 4   emergency admission for assessment for up to 72 hours
Section 2   admission for assessment for up to 28 days
Section 3   admission for treatment for up to 6 months: this section can be renewed,
            initially for 6 months, and thereafter for 12 months at a time

Figure 21.2   Compulsory admission for mental disorder

use of resources and the equitable distribution of services.

In addition of course, all patients have the protection of the European Convention on Human Rights as set out in Schedule 1 of the Human Rights Act 1998 (see Appendix 1 of this book and Chapter 6).

Definition of mental disorder

Nobody can be compulsorily detained under the Mental Health Act 1983 (as amended) unless they are suffering from mental disorder as defined in the Act. The definition has been revised by the 2007 Act and is now 'any disorder or disability of the mind'. (The distinctions in the earlier Act are no longer retained.) Dependence on alcohol or drugs is not considered to be a disorder or disability of the mind for the purposes of the definition of mental disorder.

Compulsory admission

There are three main Sections for the compulsory admission of the mentally disordered person (other than through the courts). These are shown in Figure 21.2.

Admission for assessment: Sections 4 and 2

The requirements for the medical recommendation for admission under Sections 2 and 4 are shown in Figure 21.3.

The applicant is usually an approved mental health professional (which replaces the approved social worker (ASW) under the 1983 Act) though, as with the other two Sections, it could be the 'nearest relative' (a term defined by the Act – see below). Mental Health Professionals are 'approved' because they have had to undergo a special training in mental health.

Section 4 is an emergency admission section and enables a person to be detained for up to 72 hours on the basis of one medical recommendation. In applying for a Section 4 emergency admission the approved mental health professional (AMHP) has to explain why a second medical recommendation for admission could not be obtained. The application is made to the managers (see below) of the appropriate hospital and the application gives authority to the ambulance men or police to transfer the patient

(a)   [The patient] is suffering from mental disorder of a nature or degree which warrants the detention of the patient in a hospital for assessment (or for assessment followed by medical treatment) for at least a limited period; and
(b)   he/she ought to be so detained in the interests of his/her own health or safety or with a view to the protection of other persons.

Figure 21.3   Medical requirements for Sections 2 or 4 admission

(a)   The patient is suffering from mental disorder and his/her mental disorder is of a nature or degree which makes it appropriate for him/her to receive medical treatment in hospital, and

(b)   it is necessary for the health or safety of the patient or for the protection of others that it cannot be provided unless he/she is detained under this section, and

(c)   appropriate medical treatment is available

Figure 21.4   Medical requirements for Section 3 admission

to the hospital. When a second doctor can be contacted the admission under Section 2 with the longer period for assessment can be made.

Section 2 is an application for assessment and under this the person can be detained for up to 28 days. There must be two medical recommendations, one of them from a doctor who is recognised as having the required expertise in psychiatric medicine, i.e. he is approved under Section 12 of the Act – colloquially called 'a Section 12 approved' doctor. (Regulations have been passed permitting mutual recognition of approved doctor status between England and Wales.[8]) One of the two doctors should have had previous acquaintance with the patient and, if this is not possible, the approved mental health professional must explain the reasons why on the application form. The medical requirements shown in Figure 21.3 must be present.

Admissions for treatment: Section 3

This is an admission for treatment (sometimes following an initial assessment under Section 2) and can last up to 6 months, and it can be renewed. Two medical recommendations are required and following the amendments from the 2007 Act no specific form of mental disorder need be stated (see Figure 21.4). The other requirements shown in Figure 21.4 must also be present. Under the 2007 Act, appropriate medical treatment must be available for compulsory admission to be justified. One of the medical recommendations must be by a Section 12 approved doctor and preferably at least one of the doctors should have had previous acquaintance with the patient. The nearest relative should be consulted over the application by the AMHP and has the right to object to the application being made.

Definition and powers of the nearest relative

The nearest relative has a significant role to play in the statutory provisions for compulsory admission of the mentally disordered. The relative who is 'nearest' is defined by statute (Section 26 of the Mental Health Act 1983). The order of priority in determining the nearest relative is shown in Figure 21.5.

(a)   Husband or wife or civil partner or cohabitee (after 6 months)
(b)   Son or daughter
(c)   Father or mother
(d)   Brother or sister
(e)   Grandparent
(f)   Grandchild
(g)   Uncle or aunt
(h)   Nephew or niece

Figure 21.5   Definition and order of priority of nearest relative

A cohabitee would count as the nearest relative where the couple had been living together for a period of not less than 6 months. A person other than a relative could be classified as a relative if he or she had been ordinarily living with the patient for at least 5 years. A relative who ordinarily lives with or cares for the patient would take precedence over the others.

The functions and powers of the nearest relative include the following:

- Application for admission of the patient: under Section 2 for assessment, or Section 3 for treatment, or Section 4 emergency admission for assessment – in practice the approved mental health professional usually makes the application.
- Application for the patient to be placed under guardianship (Section 7).
- Must be consulted by the approved mental health professional and can object to an application by an approved mental health professional for admission for treatment or for a guardianship order.
- Must be notified of application for admission for assessment and in an emergency (Sections 2 and 4).
- Has the power to discharge the patient from compulsory admission under Section 2 or 3 but must give 72 hours notice to the managers of such an intention.

Treatment for mental disorder

Compulsory treatment for mental disorder can be given under the Act to the patient detained under either Section 2 or Section 3 but not to the patient who is detained under Section 4. This is so even though Section 2 is described as admission for assessment. Figure 21.6 shows the treatments that can be given and the conditions required.

The second-opinion appointed doctor

It should be noted that if medication is required after 3 months and the patient is either unable or unwilling to give consent, a second opinion appointed doctor (SOAD) must be called in to decide if the treatment should be given. Regulations have been passed to ensure the independence of the SOAD[9] and prevent a conflict of interest for financial, business, professional or personal relationship reasons. The SOAD has a duty:

- to examine the patient;
- to determine whether the patient is incapable of giving consent or is refusing consent;
- to talk to the responsible clinician or the approved clinician in charge of the treatment in question) about the proposed treatment; and
- to decide whether the treatment should be given against the patient's will.

Before the SOAD decides he or she must consult with two people – one a nurse who is professionally concerned with the treatment of the patient and the other who is neither the responsible clinician or the approved clinician in charge of the treatment in question nor nurse but who is professionally concerned with the patient.

Involvement of the physiotherapist

The second person whom the SOAD is obliged to consult before agreeing to treatment under Section 58 could be a physiotherapist if he/she is professionally concerned with the treatment of the patient. The SOAD merely has to record on the statutory form (form 39) the names of the nurse and the other professional whom he/she has consulted. Their advice does not have to be recorded. If the physiotherapist were to be the second professional to be consulted it would be advisable for him/her to ensure that he/she records in the patient records the content of his/her advice to the SOAD.

A physiotherapist may also be consulted in a treatment decision involving brain surgery for mental disorder or hormonal implants to reduce sexual drive in the male. Before the physiotherapist consents to be formally consulted he/she must have a good knowledge of the patient and

Section 57	Surgery destroying brain tissue, hormonal implants to control sexual urge. The patient must consent and the understanding of the patient to consent should be certified by three persons appointed by the Mental Health Act Commission, one of whom must be a registered medical practitioner. The latter must certify that the treatment should be given
Section 58	Medication after 3 months and electroconvulsive therapy (subject to qualifications – see below). The patient must either consent or a second opinion must be obtained from an independent doctor appointed by the Mental Health Act Commission (replaced by the Care Quality Commission in April 2009)
Section 63	Any treatment not covered by Sections 57 and 58 which is given for mental disorder under the direction of the approved clinician in charge of the treatment
Section 62	The provisions of the above Sections to be dispensed with in an emergency situation
Section 62A	A new Section 62A has been added to the Mental Health Act 1983 to enable treatment to be given to those community patients who have been recalled. The patient is to be treated as if he/she had remained liable to be detained since the making of the community order

ECT and other specified treatments

A person shall not be given such treatments unless he or she falls within certain specified conditions.

These conditions include:

(1) where the patient is at least 18 years, has consented to the treatment and his capacity to consent has been certified by the approved clinician in charge of it or by the appointed registered medical practitioner

(2) the patient is below 18 years, has consented to the treatment and an appointed registered medical practitioner (not being the approved clinician in charge of the treatment) has certified in writing the patient's capacity to consent and that it is appropriate for the treatment to be given or

(3) an appointed registered medical practitioner (not being the responsible clinician/approved clinician in charge of the treatment) has certified in writing:

    (a) that the patient is not capable of understanding the nature, purpose and likely effects of the treatment; but that it is appropriate for the treatment to be given but

    (b) that it is appropriate for the treatment to be given and

    (c) that giving him/her the treatment would not conflict with:

        (i) an advance decision which the registered medical practitioner concerned is satisfied is valid and applicable or

        (ii) a decision made by a donee or deputy or by the Court of Protection.

Before a certificate is given in circumstance 3, the appointed registered medical practitioner must consult two persons who have been professionally concerned with the patient's medical treatment, one must be a nurse and the other neither nurse nor a registered medical practitioner. In addition neither shall be the responsible clinical or the approved clinician in charge of the treatment in question

Figure 21.6 Treatment for mental disorder

the earlier treatments and be able to give his/her views on the use of Section 57 treatments.

Definition of treatment

Treatment is defined in the Act as amended by the 2007 Act: 'Medical treatment' includes 'nursing, psychological intervention and specialist mental heath habilitation, rehabilitation and care (Section 145(1)). Any reference to medical treatment, in relation to mental disorder shall be construed as a reference to medical treatment the purpose of which is to alleviate, or prevent a worsening of, the disorder or one or more of the symptoms or manifestations. (S.145(3)).

It has been held[10] that preliminary care given to enable the treatment for mental disorder to be given was within the original definition and so covered by Section 63. Thus, a detained patient who was anorexic could be tube-fed, even though that was not the treatment that justified admission under Section 3. The Court of Appeal held that compulsory feeding by tube came under Section 63.

This definition would, of course, cover most of the therapy provided by physiotherapists, which in theory could therefore be given compulsorily under Section 63. However, there are very few treatments offered by physiotherapists that in practice can be given compulsorily against the will of the patient. For the most part treatments rely for their success upon the active involvement and participation of the patient.

There are considerable difficulties in persuading acutely ill or chronically sick patients to accept attendance at therapy sessions. However, the patient's involvement can be obtained through a quasi-contract in the form of an agreement whereby the treatment plan includes attendance at various sessions and rewards are then forthcoming. Turning up at the treatment venue does not necessarily imply consent by the patient to the treatment and the physiotherapist should be aware of the legal status of the patient and any rights to give treatment under a section. In Chapter 7 the nature and form of consent to treatment is considered in detail.

Individual treatment plans

The physiotherapist may be involved in the multidisciplinary preparation of a patient's treatment plan. Where this involves medication or electroconvulsive therapy, and the detained patient has originally agreed to the plan but then changes his/her mind, treatment can be continued under Section 62 if discontinuance of the treatment would in the view of the approved clinician in charge of the treatment cause serious suffering to the patient (Section 62(2)). Arrangements should be made for the SOAD to attend as soon as possible.

Treatment and common law powers

Common law powers (recognised by the House of Lords in the case of *Re F*[11]) to act in the best interests of a mentally incapacitated person were replaced by the statutory powers under the Mental Capacity Act 2005. (For further discussion on this see Chapters 7, 22 and 24.)

The informal in-patient and the Mental Health Act 1983

Many patients enter psychiatric hospital voluntarily and Section 131(1) of the Mental Health Act 1983 emphasises that there is nothing in the Act to prevent patients being admitted without any formality or remaining in hospital after being discharged from their detention. However, in the Bournewood case[12] the Court of Appeal interpreted this section as requiring the consent of the patient. The House of Lords[13] upheld the Department of Health's appeal against the Court of Appeal decision and confirmed that mentally incapable adults can be admitted to and cared for in hospital under the common law powers to act out of necessity recognised by the House of Lords in *Re F*. The European Court of Human Rights[14] declared that the detention of a patient under common law powers was contrary to his/her Article 5 rights. As a consequence of this decision the government, introduced amendments to the Mental Capacity Act 2005 to enable restrictions of patients to be lawfully made. These amendments are known as the Bournewood safeguards.

Bournewood safeguards

The Mental Health Act 2007 amended the Mental Capacity Act 2005 (MCA) to introduce the safeguards necessary to justify loss of liberty of residents in hospitals and care homes. They are set out in the new Schedule A1 to the MCA as introduced by the Mental Health Act 2007 and can be found in a briefing paper available from the Department of Health.[15.]

Who are covered by the Bournewood provisions?

Those over 18 years:

- who suffer from a disorder or disability of mind;
- who lack the capacity to give consent to the arrangements made for their care; and
- for whom such care (in circumstances that amount to a deprivation of liberty within the meaning of Article 5 of the European Convention on Human Rights) is considered after an independent assessment to be a necessary and proportionate response in their best interests to protect them from harm.

What procedures are required?

1. Application for authorisation:
   - The care home, i.e. the managing authority, must identify a client/patient as lacking capacity and who risks being deprived of his/her liberty. It must apply to the supervisory body i.e. the local authority in which the client/patient was ordinarily resident, for the authorisation of deprivation of liberty.
2. Assessments required:
   - Age assessment: client/patient must be over 18 years

- Mental Health Assessment: client/patient must be suffering a mental disorder
- Mental Capacity Assessment: client/patient must lack the capacity to decide whether to be admitted to or remain in the hospital or care home
- Eligibility assessment: the client/patient must:
- Not be detained under the Mental Health Act
- Not be subject to a conflicting requirement under the Mental Health Act
- Not be subject to powers of recall under the Mental Health Act nor
- A treatment order in hospital to which the client/patient objects
- Best interests assessment – the authorisation would be in the client/patient's best interests and is a proportionate response to the likelihood of suffering harm and the seriousness of that harm
- There is no conflict between the authorisation sought and a valid decision by a donee of a lasting power of attorney or a deputy and does not conflict with a valid and applicable advance decision made by the client/patient.

3. Appointment of Representative for the client/patient:
   - If the best interests assessor concludes that the client/patient has the capacity to appoint his/her own representative, then he/she can do this. Otherwise the best interests assessor can appoint a representative. If the assessor notifies the supervisory body that a representative has not been appointed for him/her, then it can appoint a representative who can be paid to act as the client/patient's representative. Regulations came into force in November 2008 on the appointment of the representatives.[16]
4. Authorisation granted:
   - If all the assessments are satisfactory then authorisation by the supervisory body can be granted for the deprivation of the client/patient's liberty for up to 12 months.

5. Review and Monitoring:
    - The supervisory authority should keep under review the client/patient's deprivation of liberty and the whole process of the assessments and authorisation will be monitored to ensure that all the required procedures were followed.

Detention under the Mental Health Act 1983 of an informal patient already in hospital

If the patient is already in hospital as an informal patient and wishes to take his/her own discharge and it would be dangerous to his/her health or safety or to the safety of other people for him/her to do so, the patient could be detained under the following provisions.

Holding power of the nurse: Section 5(4)

This enables an appropriately qualified nurse (i.e. one whose field of practice is registered with the Nursing and Midwifery Council as mental health nursing or learning disability nursing[17]) to prevent an informal patient who is being treated for mental disorder from leaving the hospital. The detention can continue for up to 6 hours but it will end as soon as the patient's own doctor (or the doctor's nominee) arrives to see the patient. The doctor may then, following an examination of the patient, decide to detain the patient further.

Power of doctor to detain an in-patient Section 5(2)

This enables the patient's doctor or approved clinician or the doctor's nominee to detain the patient for up to 72 hours to enable an application to be considered for admission under the Mental Health Act 1983. It may be that after the doctor has examined the patient it is decided that compulsory admission is not necessary. The effect of the section will then end and the patient will revert to informal status. Alternatively,

following examination by the patient's own doctor, by another doctor and an approved mental health professional an application may be made under Section 2 or Section 3.

Limitations on these powers

It must be emphasised that the provisions set out in Section 5(2) and Section 5(4) apply only to in-patients – the doctor's power applying to any in-patient, the nurse's only to in-patients being treated for mental disorder. This means that if a physiotherapist is working in an out-patient day hospital, or other such facility, and an informal patient becomes dangerous to him/herself or others, the patient can only be detained under Section 5(2) or 5(4) if the patient is an in-patient and, in the case of Section 5(4), already being treated for mental disorder.

The physiotherapist must be very clear about which category the patient comes under. If an out-patient becomes very disturbed and it appears that statutory powers of detention need to be investigated, then an approved mental health professional would have to be summoned together with one registered medical practitioner for detention under Section 4 (in an emergency) or two registered medical practitioners for detention under Section 2 or 3 to be considered.

Renewal

Section 4, Section 2, Section 5(4) or Section 5(2) are not renewable. A patient on Section 2 who needs to be detained for longer can only be further detained on Section 3. Section 3 can be renewed for a further 6 months and then for 1 year at a time. The procedure for the renewal is that the responsible clinician in charge of the patient's care examines the patient, within the period of 2 months ending with the date the section is due to end and, if it appears to him/her that the specific condition of mental disorder is present and the other conditions required by

Section 20 (similar to those set out in Figure 21.4) are present, he/she must furnish to the managers (a defined term – see below) a report to that effect and the patient's detention is then renewed. The managers in their review can later decide that the patient should be discharged.

Appeals against detention

The patient can appeal to a Mental Health Review Tribunal (MHRT) for discharge or to the managers of the hospital under Section 23 of the Mental Health Act 1983. There are set times for applying to the MHRT but not to the managers. The Mental Health Act 2007 amended Section 23 to include the right of a patient under a community order to apply to the managers for an order to discharge him from the liability to be recalled to hospital. The nearest relative also has the right to apply to an MHRT if his or her attempt to discharge the patient under Section 23 (the power to apply for a detailed patient's discharge) has been barred by the responsible clinician under Section 25 (the option to veto that application if certain specified circumstances seem to justify doing so).

Where a patient has not applied him/herself for an MHRT hearing during the first 6 months (and after that at least once every 3 years) the managers of the hospital have a duty to refer the patient to the MHRT. (In the case of patients under 16 years, the time limit is every year.)

It may be that the physiotherapist is asked to provide a report and/or oral evidence at the hearing, whether MHRT or managers' hearing, to give his/her views upon the discharge. Reference should be made to Chapter 12 on record keeping and to Chapter 13 on report writing and giving evidence in court for the professional principles to be followed. The Court of Appeal has held that the statutory scheme dealing with the referral of a recalled mental patient to a mental health review tribunal was not incompatible with the patient's rights under Article 5.4 of the European Convention on Human Rights (see Appendix 1).[18]

Information

To the patient

One of the duties on the managers introduced by the 1983 Act is to ensure that patients receive, both in writing and orally, information relating to the section under which they are detained, the right to apply to the managers and the MHRT, and the rules relating to consent to treatment. This duty is usually delegated by the managers to the nursing staff or the medical records staff. Leaflets are available giving the information for each of the different sections and are available in a wide variety of languages.

A physiotherapist who is concerned that a detained patient does not appear to understand the provisions of the Act or the section he/she is under, should ask to see the leaflet so that the physiotherapist him/herself understands the implications of the section the patient is under and can explain it to him/her.

To the nearest relative

The information that is given to the patient must also be given in writing to the nearest relative. However, the patient has a statutory right to object to this information being given to the nearest relative.

Independent mental health advocates

The Mental Health Act 2007 amends the Mental Health Act 1983 to make provision for independent mental health advocates (IMHAs) to be available to help qualifying patients. Regulations are to be drawn up to specify the circumstances in which the IMHAs should be appointed and the conditions for their approval. New Sections 130A, B, C and D are inserted into the 1983 Act to cover the details of these appointments, the qualifying patients and the information to be given to the IMHA.

The managers

The managers are the NHS Trust, primary care trust (PCT) or special health authority responsible for the administration of the hospital (S.140). In respect of a NHS trust the managers are the non-executive board members and only they, with their co-opted members, can carry out the function of hearing appeals to the managers by the patient against detention or renewing the patient's detention following a report from the responsible clinician. These functions of hearing appeals from patients or approving a renewal cannot be delegated to officers. Other functions in respect of the Mental Health Act can however be so delegated.

The Mental Health Act Commission

In 1983 a watchdog for detained patients was established known as the Mental Health Act Commission (MHAC). It consists of about 90 different professionals and lay people whose jurisdiction is to visit detained patients and to take up any complaints from them where they are not satisfied by the response from the managers, or any other complaint relating to the exercise of powers and duties under the Mental Health Act.

It also has statutory duties in relation to the withholding of mail in the special hospitals (i.e. Broadmoor, Rampton and Ashworth). The managers at special hospitals can withhold any postal package sent by the detained person if they consider it likely that it will cause distress to the addressee or to any other person (except hospital staff and other specific public persons such as MPs) or if it is likely to cause danger. Equally, packages sent to a detained patient in a special hospital may be withheld if, in the opinion of the managers, it is necessary do so in the interests of the safety of the patient or for the protection of other persons. These decisions are subject to review by the MHAC.

It also has a duty every other year to provide a report to the Secretary of State that must be placed before each House of Parliament. The Health and Social Care Act 2008, made provision for the MHAC, together with the Healthcare Commission and the Commission for Social Care Inspection, to be combined into a single Inspection Body known as the Care Quality Commission. This came into force in April 2009.

Role of the physiotherapist in assessment

Even though the physiotherapist is not among those professionals who have the responsibility of admitting the patient for treatment or assessment, the physiotherapist may have a role to play in taking part in the multidisciplinary work of assessment of the patient's mental health and treatment. In addition, the physiotherapist will have his/her own assessment procedures with regard to:

- health and fitness
- mobility
- physical assessment of musculoskeletal injuries.

The Code of Practice

The Secretary of State has a duty to prepare a Code of Practice[19] on the Mental Health Act which physiotherapists, who care for those suffering from mental disorder, would find a useful tool of reference. Some of its comments and recommendations apply also to the care of the informal patient.

Care in the community

Mental Health Act patients

The Mental Health Act 2007 introduced a new supervised community treatment order (SCT) which is considered below. Even physiotherapists working in the community may find that they are caring for patients who are under the provisions of the Mental Health Act 1983 (as amended by the 2007 Act). Some patients may also be placed under a guardianship order or be on Section 17 leave from the hospital.

Guardianship

Section 7 of the Mental Health Act enables a patient to be placed under a guardianship order where a guardian (which may be a social services authority) can be appointed to provide some supervision. Under the order the patient may be required to reside at a specified place, attend specified places at specified times for treatment, occupation, education and training and may also be required to permit access to the patient by any responsible clinician, approved mental health professional or other specified person. As a result, of the new supervised community treatment order, it may be that less use is made of guardianship orders.

Section 17 leave

Some patients who have been detained under the Mental Health Act 1983 may be on Section 17 leave. This is leave of absence granted by the responsible clinician (RC) (replacing the responsible medical officer by Mental Health Act 2007). Although there is no statutory requirement for the leave to be granted in writing, there are strong reasons in practice why this should be so.[20] The RC decides the conditions on which the patient can have leave of absence – escorted or unescorted, overnight or any other terms. An amendment by the Mental Health Act 2007 states the longer term leave may not be granted to a patient unless the responsible clinician first considers whether the patient should be dealt with under Section 17A instead. Longer term leave means that the leave of absence is granted either indefinitely or for a specified period or more than 7 consecutive days or a specified period of extended leave is granted so that the total period for which leave of absence will have been granted exceeds 7 consecutive days. The RC has the right to withdraw the leave of absence at any time but this revocation has to be put in writing. The patient must then return to the hospital. If the patient fails to do so, then he/she is unlawfully at large and could be returned under Section 18 or under the Police and Criminal Evidence Act.[21] Sections 17A, 17B, 17C 17 D, 17E, 17F and 17G were added to the Mental Health Act 1983 by the Mental Health Act 2007 and relate to supervised community treatment order (see below).

If a physiotherapist is attending a patient who is under Section 17 leave and is concerned about a deteriorating mental condition, the physiotherapist should ensure that he/she takes the appropriate action for the patient's return to hospital to be considered.

An absconding patient who is liable to detention under the Act or refuses to return to hospital when leave of absence under Section 17 expires or is revoked can be brought back to hospital under the provisions of Section 18. This does not apply to an informal patient who can only be returned to the hospital if he/she satisfies the compulsory admission provisions of the Act and the correct procedures are carried out.

Section 117 after care

Certain detained patients have a specific right under the Mental Health Act 1983 to receive after care. The right is given by Section 117, which is shown in Figure 21.7.

This statutory right exists alongside the provisions of the NHS and Community Care Act 1990, which are discussed in Chapter 18. The statutory right is enforceable by the patient against the health authority and/or the local authority.[22] Patients who had been detained under Section 3 and were then discharged and provided with residential accommodation under Section 117 argued that there was no right to charge for the accommodation. The Court of Appeal held that Section 117 imposed a free-standing duty to provide after-care services and charges could not be levied for the accommodation under Section 21 of the National Assistance Act 1948.[23]

(1) This section applies to persons
- who are detained under Section 3 [admission for treatment],
- or are admitted to a hospital in pursuance of a hospital order made under Section 37 [a court order]
- or who are transferred to a hospital [from prison] under Sections 45A, 47 or 48 and then cease to be detained and leave the hospital

(2) It shall be the duty of the primary care trust (or local health board) and of the local social services authority to provide, in cooperation with relevant voluntary agencies, after-care services for any person to whom this section applies until such time as the primary care trust (or local health board) and the local social services authority are satisfied that the person concerned is no longer in need of such services; but they shall not be so satisfied in the case of *community patient while he/she remains such a patient* (words in italics to be brought into force under Mental Health Act 2007 replacing patients subject to after-care under supervision)

(3) In this section 'the primary care trust' (or local health board) means the primary care trust (or local health board) and 'the local social services authority' means the local social services authority for the area in which the person concerned is resident or to which he/she is sent on discharge by the hospital in which he/she was detained.

Figure 21.7   The Mental Health Act 1983: Section 117

In the case of *R (on the application of B)* v. *Camden LBC*,[24] the court held that the duty to provide accommodation under Section 117 of the Mental Health Act 1983 does not arise until the patient ceased to be detained and left hospital. It also held that the duty to carry out an assessment under Section 47 of the NHS and Community Care Act 1990 (see Chapter 18) did not impose an obligation on a local authority to monitor a detained patient in hospital in case he/she should at some later time be in need.

The physiotherapist and after care planning

Ideally care planning for post-discharge should be considered before the admission of the patient, so that the treatment aims of the in-patient stay can be decided and the long-term care planned. The physiotherapist will have a role to play in this multidisciplinary planning and care and should ensure that his/her involvement is weighty and meaningful. The physiotherapist should also make certain that his/her input and

the outcome in terms of the team's decision is recorded. The physiotherapist has a further important role in ensuring the involvement of patients in after care planning and should discuss with them long-term plans for rehabilitation, employment and accommodation.

Supervised Community Treatment Order

The provisions on after-care under supervision, or supervised discharge introduced by the Mental Health (Patients in the Community) Act 1995 were replaced by the supervised community treatment order introduced by Section 32 of the Mental Health Act 2007 which added new Sections 17A, 17B, 17C 17 D, 17E , 17F and 17G into the Mental Health Act 1983.

Under the Section 17A the responsible clinician may by order in writing discharge a detained patient from hospital subject to his being liable to recall in accordance with Section 17E. The details of the provisions are shown in Figure 21.8.

Under 17A(4) the responsible clinician may not make a community treatment order unless:

    (a)   in his opinion, the relevant criteria are met; and

    (b)   an approved mental health professional states in writing:

        (i)   that he agrees with that opinion; and

        (ii)   that it is appropriate to make the order.

(5)   The relevant criteria are:

    (a)   the patient is suffering from mental disorder of a nature or degree which makes it appropriate for him to receive medical treatment;

    (b)   it is necessary for his health or safety or for the protection of other persons that he should receive such treatment;

    (c)   subject to his being liable to be recalled as mentioned in paragraph (d) below, such treatment can be provided without his continuing to be detained in a hospital;

    (d)   it is necessary that the responsible clinician should be able to exercise the power under Section 17E(1) below to recall the patient to hospital; and

    (e)   appropriate medical treatment is available for him.

(6)   In determining whether the criterion in sub-section (5)(d) above is met, the responsible clinician shall, in particular, consider, having regard to the patient's history of mental disorder and any other relevant factors, what risk there would be of a deterioration of the patient's condition if he were not detained in a hospital (as a result, for example, of his refusing or neglecting to receive the medical treatment he requires for his mental disorder).

17B Conditions for a community treatment order

(1)   A community treatment order shall specify conditions to which the patient is to be subject while the order remains in force.

(2)   But, subject to sub-section (3) below, the order may specify conditions only if the responsible clinician, with the agreement of the approved mental health professional mentioned in Section 17A(4)(b) above, thinks them necessary or appropriate for one or more of the following purposes:

    (a)   ensuring that the patient receives medical treatment;

    (b)   preventing risk of harm to the patient's health or safety;

    (c)   protecting other persons.

(3)   The order shall specify:

    (a)   a condition that the patient make himself available for examination under Section 20A below; and

    (b)   a condition that, if it is proposed to give a certificate under Part 4A of this Act in his case, he make himself available for examination so as to enable the certificate to be given.

(4)   The responsible clinician may from time to time by order in writing vary the conditions specified in a community treatment order.

(5)   He may also suspend any conditions specified in a community treatment order.

(6)   If a community patient fails to comply with a condition specified in the community treatment order by virtue of sub-section (2) above, that fact may be taken into account for the purposes of exercising the power of recall under Section 17E(1) below.

(7)   But nothing in this Section restricts the exercise of that power to cases where there is such a failure.

Figure 21.8   Community Treatment Order under Supervision

17C Duration of community treatment order

A community treatment order shall remain in force until:

(a)   the period mentioned in Section 20A(1) below (as extended under any provision of this Act) expires, but this is subject to Sections 21 and 22 below;

(b)   the patient is discharged in pursuance of an order under Section 23 below or a direction under Section 72 below;

(c)   the application for admission for treatment in respect of the patient otherwise ceases to have effect; or

(d)   the order is revoked under Section 17F below, whichever occurs first.

17D Effect of community treatment order

(1)   The application for admission for treatment in respect of a patient shall not cease to have effect by virtue of his becoming a community patient.

(2)   But while he remains a community patient—

(a)   the authority of the managers to detain him under Section 6(2) above in pursuance of that application shall be suspended; and

(b)   reference (however expressed) in this or any other Act, or in any subordinate legislation (within the meaning of the Interpretation Act 1978), to patients liable to be detained, or detained, under this Act shall not include him.

(3)   And Section 20 below shall not apply to him while he remains a community patient.

(4)   Accordingly, authority for his detention shall not expire during any period in which that authority is suspended by virtue of sub-section (2)(a) above.

17E Power to recall to hospital

(1)   The responsible clinician may recall a community patient to hospital if in his opinion—

(a)   the patient requires medical treatment in hospital for his mental disorder; and

(b)   there would be a risk of harm to the health or safety of the patient or to other persons if the patient were not recalled to hospital for that purpose.

(2)   The responsible clinician may also recall a community patient to hospital if the patient fails to comply with a condition specified under Section 17B(3) above.

(3)   The hospital to which a patient is recalled need not be the responsible hospital.

(4)   Nothing in this Section prevents a patient from being recalled to a hospital even though he is already in the hospital at the time when the power of recall is exercised; references to recalling him shall be construed accordingly.

(5)   The power of recall under sub-sections (1) and (2) above shall be exercisable by notice in writing to the patient.

(6)   A notice under this Section recalling a patient to hospital shall be sufficient authority for the managers of that hospital to detain the patient there in accordance with the provisions of this Act.

17F Powers in respect of recalled patients

(1)   This Section applies to a community patient who is detained in a hospital by virtue of a notice recalling him there under Section 17E above.

(2)   The patient may be transferred to another hospital in such circumstances and subject to such conditions as may be prescribed in regulations made by the Secretary of State (if the hospital in which the patient is detained is in England) or the Welsh Ministers (if that hospital is in Wales).

Figure 21.8   (cont'd)

(3) If he is so transferred to another hospital, he shall be treated for the purposes of this Section (and Section 17E above) as if the notice under that Section were a notice recalling him to that other hospital and as if he had been detained there from the time when his detention in hospital by virtue of the notice first began.

(4) The responsible clinician may by order in writing revoke the community treatment order if:

  (a) in his opinion, the conditions mentioned in Section 3(2) above are satisfied in respect of the patient; and

  (b) an approved mental health professional states in writing:

    (i) that he agrees with that opinion; and

    (ii) that it is appropriate to revoke the order.

(5) The responsible clinician may at any time release the patient under this Section, but not after the community treatment order has been revoked.

(6) If the patient has not been released, nor the community treatment order revoked, by the end of the period of 72 hours, he shall then be released.

(7) But a patient who is released under this Section remains subject to the community treatment order.

(8) In this Section:

  (a) 'the period of 72 hours' means the period of 72 hours beginning with the time when the patient's detention in hospital by virtue of the notice under Section 17E above begins; and

  (b) references to being released shall be construed as references to being released from that detention (and accordingly from being recalled to hospital).

Section 20A Community treatment period

A community treatment order shall cease to be in force on expiry of the period of six months beginning with the day on which it was made and this period is referred to in this Act as "the community treatment period". The community treatment period may be extended for a period of six months and then on for further periods of up to one year at a time. Section 20A sub-sections 4–10 set out the conditions for renewal and the procedure to be followed.

20B Effect of expiry of community treatment order

When the community treatment order expires, the community patient shall be deemed to be discharged absolutely from liability to recall under this Part of this Act, and the application for admission for treatment ceases to have effect.

Treatment provisions for those on a community treatment order

The Mental Health Act 2007 inserts into the Mental Health Act 1983 a new Part 4A which sets out the provisions for the treatment of community patients who are not recalled to hospital.

Figure 21.8   *(cont'd)*

Multidisciplinary team and key worker

In certain cases the physiotherapist may be the identified key worker for the care of the patient in the community. If the physiotherapist takes on this role he/she should ensure that he/she works within his/her professional competence. The physiotherapist must have an understanding of the role and competence of other health professionals and also those in other spheres in order to make appropriate referrals for further interventions. There should be clear operational policies on the terms of referral.

The physiotherapist working in the field of mental health may also find that he/she is relied upon by nurses who are not dual-trained, but only trained in mental health nursing and look to the physiotherapist for expert advice on the physical care of the patient. Again it is essential that the physiotherapist does not work outside his/her professional competence.

Informal patients

If a patient is not formally detained under the provisions discussed earlier in this chapter or subject to the Bournewood safeguards or prevented from leaving under Section 5(2) or 5(4), then the patient can leave hospital or care home at any time. Many patients however remain in hospital without their active consent simply because they do not have the capacity to make a decision for themselves. There are concerns about the large number of persons who are not detained, and who are outside the provisions of the Mental Health Act 1983 but remain in hospital as passive patients. These patients now come under the provisions of the Mental Capacity Act 2005, which is explained in Chapter 7. Actions and decisions must be taken in their best interests according to the statutory provisions. They may also come under the Bournewood safeguards, which are explained above.

The physiotherapist would have a duty to ensure that he/she takes action if he/she is aware that a patient who lacks the mental capacity to make his or her own decisions would benefit from the protection provided by the Mental Health Act 1983 or the provisions of the Mental Capacity Act 2005. There are several advantages to the patient if he/she is formally detained under the Mental Health Act including:

- visits from the Care Quality Commission;
- provision for the CQC to investigate complaints made by him/her or on his/her behalf;
- automatic regular review of his/her detention by the CQC;

- the appointment of a SOAD before any treatment is given compulsorily or without his/her consent (after the first 3 months of medication);
- being formally notified of these and other rights under the Mental Health Act.

The physiotherapist should also ensure that he/she is aware of the provisions of the Code of Practice prepared and monitored by the CQC on behalf of the Department of Health, which has useful guidance for the care of informal patients. For example, there may be informal patients who are cared for behind locked doors. This could constitute a false imprisonment of these patients unless the Bournewood safeguards (considered above) are in place.

The seclusion of patients must be closely monitored and there should be in existence a clear policy that sets out the maximum intervals within which a patient should be examined by a registered medical practitioner. Managers should review both the policy and its implementation and physiotherapists should ensure that they have copies of the policy and are involved in both its implementation and monitoring.

General issues involving physiotherapists

Danger to the physiotherapist from aggressive patients

The tragic death of the occupational therapist who worked at the Edith Morgan Unit is a sad reminder of the fact that working with the mentally disordered can be dangerous. Those physiotherapists working in acute and specialist units should be aware of the recommendations of the Blom-Cooper report.[20] Employers have a duty to ensure that reasonable care is taken of the health and safety of each employee and also of the general public, and this is further discussed in Chapter 11. Physiotherapists should be involved in the risk assessment of any unit for the care of the mentally ill and take active steps to ensure that recommendations for improving health and safety and preventing accidents are implemented. A risk assessment should also be carried out of dangers resulting from home visits. Where the risk assessment indicates it, physiotherapists should also have training in control and restraint procedures and receive regular training in the management of aggression and potential violence.

It is essential that careful records should be kept of any incident, including near misses, since these are vital in carrying out a useful and productive risk assessment.

Danger to patient from equipment

The physiotherapist who works with the mentally disordered should also be aware of the dangers of any equipment he/she is using, not only from the point of view of the patient accidentally or intentionally harming him/herself, but also from the dangers of the patient harming another person.

The physiotherapist needs to have full information regarding the patient's clinical condition and the risks of any harm which could arise. The physiotherapist must be prepared to carry out this risk assessment and management. Should harm befall a person in a department under his/her control, the physiotherapist may have to answer for that, both professionally and in relation to his/her employer and the civil courts. The physiotherapist therefore needs to know the differences that exist in law in relation to his/her powers and duties towards detained patients compared with informal patients.

Clinical risks may be different from health and safety risks and the physiotherapist must assess for both.

Death of a patient: suicide fears

In the event of an untoward death of an informal patient or the death of a detained patient, the coroner would be informed. In the case of a detained patient, the Care Quality Commission would also be informed. The physiotherapist may be required to give a statement on his/her knowledge of the patient and the events leading to the death (see Chapters 13 and 25).

Monitoring and evaluation

It is essential that the physiotherapist takes part in the monitoring process and assesses the quality and output of his/her work. Where possible the physiotherapist should try to obtain patient feedback on the services since this could lead directly to improvements.

Relationship with patients

Any improper relationship with a patient would be regarded as misconduct and could therefore be subject to disciplinary proceedings by the Health Professions Council. This would cover not only sexual impropriety but also the exploitation of vulnerable and mentally incapable adults. There should be a clear procedure relating to the acceptance of gifts (see Chapter 4) so that no suspicions could arise.

Older mentally infirm patients

One of the biggest difficulties in caring for the mentally ill is that fact that many patients lack the competence to give consent, or suffer from intermittent mental capacity. Where there are doubts about the mental competence of a patient, it is advisable to obtain a determination of competence by a person not directly involved in the care of the patient. There is now a statutory definition of competence under Sections 2 and 3 of the Mental Capacity Act 2005 (see Chapters 7 and 24). Reference should be made to Chapter 24 on older people and consent issues and to Chapter 25 on living wills and to the provisions of the Mental Capacity Act 2005 considered in Chapter 7.

Conclusions

The implementation of the amendments introduced into the Mental Health Act 1983 by
the Mental Health Act 2007 and in particular
the supervised community treatment order,
together with the provisions of the Mental
Capacity Act 2005 and the Bournewood safeguards, should have a major impact in the protection of the rights of those who are mentally
disordered or who lack the mental capacity
to make their own decisions. In addition, the
advocacy provisions that exist under both sets
of legislation should ensure that there is independent representation of the most vulnerable.
Unfortunately the right to advocacy (for those
detained for more than 72 hours) contained in
the Mental Health Act 1983 as amended will not
be brought in before April 2009. In addition,
resources are likely to affect the extent to which
independent advocacy and the rights of those
who are mentally disturbed are implemented
and protected. The Mental Health Act Commission in its biennial report[25] in January 2008
reported that practitioners are being told to
delay sectioning people with urgent mental
health needs until primary care trusts ascertain who should pay for their treatment.
Those physiotherapists who work in the field
of mental health will continue to be presented
with considerable challenges. They should be
assisted by the strategy drawn up by the CPMH
for mental health care,[7] which provides an action
plan following the New Ways of Working
Initiative.

References

1 Everett, T., Donaghy, M., Feaver, S. (eds) (2003)
   Interventions for Mental Health. Elsevier, London.
2 Picton-Bentley, J. (2007) Mental Health Disorders:
   Cause and Effect. A Discussion Paper for Physiotherapists *In Touch* **120**, 23–27.
3 Ainsworth, H. (1992) Recruiting physiotherapists
   into psychiatry. *Journal of the Association of Chartered Physiotherapists in Psychiatry* **IX**, 31–34.

Questions and exercises

1 An out patient, who has a history of mental
   health problems, comes to the physiotherapy department and is clearly highly
   disturbed and may need to be detained.
   What is the legal situation?
2 A physiotherapist is asked by the SOAD
   for her views on the giving of electroconvulsive therapy to an older patient who is
   extremely depressed and has been starv-
   ing herself. What information should she
   obtain and what principles should she
   follow in providing her recommendation
   and what are the implications of the
   changes introduced by the Mental Health
   Act 2007?
3 A detained patient asks a physiotherapist
   to accompany her to a Managers' hearing
   on her application for discharge. What
   action should the physiotherapist take?
4 The physiotherapist is a member of a
   community mental health team which
   is caring for a former detained patient
   who has been placed under a supervised
   community treatment order. What are the
   implications of this for the work of the
   physiotherapist?

4 Donaghy, M., Durward, B. (2000) *A Report on
   the Clinical Effectiveness of Physiotherapy in Mental
   Health*. CSP, London.
5 ACPMH (1995) *Physiotherapy in Mental Health
   Care*. CSP, London.
6 Chartered Society of Physiotherapy (2007) *Project
   Group 3 New Ways of Working in Psychiatry*. CSP,
   London.
7 Chartered Physiotherapists in Mental Healthcare (2007) *Strategy for Physiotherapists in Mental
   Healthcare*. CSP, London.
8 The Mental Health (Mutual Recognition) Regulations 2008 SI 1204.
9 Mental Health (Conflicts of Interest) (England)
   (Regulations) 2008 SI No 1205.

10 *B* v. *Croydon Health Authority* [1994] The Times Law Report, 1 December 1994, [1995] 1 All ER 683.

11 *F (re)* v. *West Berkshire HA* [1990] 2 AC 1; [1989] 2 WLR 1025; [1989] 2 All ER 545.

12 *L* v. *Bournewood and Community and Mental Health NHS Trust* in *The Times*, 3 December 1997; [1998] 2 WLR 764.

13 *R* v. *Bournewood Community and Mental Health NHS Trust, ex parte L* (HL) *The Times*, 30 June 1998, (also available on the internet).

14 *HL* v. *United Kingdom* [2004] ECHR 720 Application No 45508/99 5 October 2004; The Times Law Report, 19 October 2004.

15 Department of Health Briefing Sheet Bournewood November 2006 Gateway Reference 6794.

16 The Mental Capacity (Deprivation of Liberty: Appointment of Relevant Person's Representative) Regulations 2008 SI No 1315.

17 The Mental Health (Nurses) (England) Order 2008 SI No 1207.

18 *R (Rayner)* v. *Secretary of State for Justice*. The Times Law Report, 26 March 2008.

19 Department of Health (1999) *Code of Practice on the Mental Health Act*. Stationery Office, London.

20 Blom-Cooper, L., Hally, H., Murphy, E. (1995) *The Falling Shadow – One patient's Mental Health Care 1978–1993*. Duckworth, London (Report of an Inquiry into the death of an Occupational therapist at Edith Morgan Unit, Torbay 1995).

21 *D'Souza* v. *DPP, sub nom. R* v. *D'Souza* (HL) [1992] 4 All ER 545.

22 *R* v. *Ealing District Health Authority, ex parte Fox* [1993] 3 All ER 170.

23 R. v. Richmond Borough Council ex parte Watson [2000] 58 BMLR 219.

24 *R (on the application of B)* v. *Camden London Borough Council and other* [2005] EWHC 1366; [2006] LGR 19.

25 Mental Health Act Commission Risks, Rights and Recovery Biennial report January 2008.

Care of Those with Learning Disabilities

The topics to be covered in this chapter include:

- Philosophy behind the care of those with learning disabilities
- Physiotherapy and learning disabilities
- Living and working in the community
- Risk assessment and risk taking
- Horse riding for the disabled
- Decision making and incapacity
- Non-compliance or refusal by client or carer
- Sexual relations and related issues
- Property and exploitation

Introduction: statutory and common law duties

It should be pointed out, that while for convenience the different client groups (those with physical disabilities, mental illness, learning disabilities, children and older people) are considered in separate chapters, many clients may come into more than one category and reference should be made to the other relevant chapters. It should also be noted that the statutory duties

that are placed on local and health authorities in respect of those with disabilities apply to both physical and learning disabilities. To avoid repetition, an account of these duties and the financial benefits that are available is included in Chapter 20 on physical disabilities.

Reference should also be made to Chapter 23 on children for a discussion on the assessment and statementing of children with special educational needs. Chapter 11 covers the law relating to health and safety, including manual handling.

The High Court[1] has recently held that a duty of care is owed by a local authority.

Case: *X(1) and Y(2) v. London Borough of Hounslow*

The claimants had learning disabilities and lived in a council house with their two children, one of whom had learning difficulties. They were assaulted and abused by a group of youths who virtually imprisoned them in their home. The claimants brought an action against the Council on the grounds that the Council was negligent and in breach of the claimants rights under Articles 3 and 8 of the European Convention for the Protection of Human Rights (see Appendix 1). The Council defended on the grounds that no duty of care was owed to the claimants. The judge held that the injury and loss suffered was reasonably foreseeable and the relationship between defendants and claimants was sufficiently proximate to warrant the imposition of the duty of care. The Council, which was well aware of the circumstances (two independent reports had been commissioned on the situation), should have invoked the emergency transfer scheme to move the claimants to alternative accommodation. The judge found it unnecessary and too complex because of the timings to determine whether in fact there was a breach under the Human Rights Act 1998.

The implications of this decision are considerable for local social services authorities who may in future have to give evidence of the steps which they have taken to fulfil the duty of care they owe, and also the steps which they have taken to fulfil any statutory duties they may have.

Learning disabilities, mental capacity and mental disorder

Mental capacity

Mental capacity is now statutorily defined in the Mental Capacity Act 2005. This is explained in Chapter 7 as the two stages of defining capacity: (a) is there an impairment in the functioning of brain or mind and (b) if so, does this cause an inability to make decisions?

A person is unable to make decisions if he or she is unable:

(a)   to understand the information relevant to the decision,
(b)   to retain that information,
(c)   to use or weigh that information as part of the process of making the decision, or
(d)   to communicate his/her decision (whether by talking, using sign language or any other means) (S.3(1))

It should be noted however that under Section 3(2) a person is not to be regarded as unable to understand the information relevant to a decision if he/she is able to understand an explanation of it given to him/her in a way that is appropriate to his/her circumstances (using simple language, visual aids or any other means). This means that when attempting to assess the capacity of someone with learning disabilities and assisting them in communicating their wishes, every practicable means must be used to assist. This might include using the services of a speech therapist, obtaining specialist equipment, speaking to those who can communicate with that person and generally using any available means of communicating with the client.

Mental disorder

The provisions of the Mental Health Act 1983 (as amended by the Mental Health Act 2007) may become relevant in the situation where compulsory powers are being considered. The amended definition of mental disorder is 'any disorder or disability of the mind' and would therefore include those who suffer from mental impairment with associated specified conditions. Learning disability (which is defined as 'a state of arrested or incomplete development of the mind which includes significant impairment of intelligence and social functioning') is not considered to come under the definition of mental disorder unless the disability is associated with abnormally aggressive or seriously irresponsible conduct on the person's part. (Section 2 of 2007 Mental Health Act) (see Chapter 21 on mental illness).

The Association of Chartered Physiotherapists for People with Learning Disabilities

The Association of Chartered Physiotherapists for People with Learning Disabilities (ACPPLD) (up to 1991 the Association of Chartered Physiotherapists in Mental Handicap) provides a forum for the interchange of information and research developments between members and also publishes a newsletter/journal. Following the death in 1991 of Ann Russell, founder member of the ACPMH, which preceded the ACPPLD, a memorial trust was established and there are annual prizes for members who make a contribution to the advancement of the practice of physiotherapy in services for people with learning disabilities. It follows a holistic approach to the care of those with learning disabilities and in multidisciplinary working uses rebound therapy, hydrotherapy, pedal power, jabadao/ dance and movement, horse riding, sports/leisure, outward bound/challenging pursuits, seating and positioning, orthotics and footwear, and manual handling advice. The ACPPLD has a website, regional networks and a quarterly newsletter. It provides guidance on long-term management of physical disabilities, hydrotherapy, rebound therapy, orthotics and health promotion.

An example of the role of the physiotherapist in learning disabilities was given in an article reprinted in a ACPPLD newsletter.[2] A person discharged from a long-stay hospital wanted to be able to fasten the buttons on her coat and this instruction task was assigned to the physiotherapist who treated the patient holistically, a treatment which involved dieting and exercise.

The work which physiotherapists can do for those with learning disabilities includes:

- help with movement problems
- help prevent deformity
- encourage maintenance of good posture
- promote good health
- support and advise carers.

White Paper: *Valuing People*

The White Paper *Valuing People – a new Strategy for Learning Disability for the 21st Century,*[3] (which held that long-term hospitals were not an appropriate home environment for people with learning disabilities) recognised four key principles: rights, independence, choice and inclusion as lying at the heart of the Government's proposals. The White Paper is described by the government as taking a life-long approach, beginning with an integrated approach to services for disabled children and their families and then providing new opportunities for a full

and purposeful adult life. The proposals should result in improvements in education, social services, health, employment, housing and support for people with learning disabilities and their families and carers. The White Paper estimates that there are about 210 000 people with several learning disabilities and about 1.2 million with a mild or moderate disability. It sets out the following proposals:

- new national objectives for services for those with learning disabilities;
- a new Learning Disability Development fund;
- a new central implementation support fund;
- disabled children and their families to be an integral part of the Quality Protects Programme, the Special Educational Needs Programme of Action and the Connexions Service;
- development of advocacy services to assist them in having as much choice and control over their lives as possible;
- supporting carers by implementing the Carers and Disabled Children Act 2000 (see Chapter 18) and by funding the development of a national learning disability information centre and helpline in partnership with Mencap;
- improving health of those with learning disabilities by providing the same rights of access to mainstream health services as the rest of the population by appointing health facilitators, ensuring registration with a GP and a health action plan for each client;
- giving greater choice over where they live with more appropriate accommodation;
- more local day services to assist them in leading a full and purposeful life;
- new targets for increasing numbers of people with learning disabilities in work;
- raising of standards and quality of services provided for those with learning disabilities including training and qualifications for care staff through a learning disability awards framework;
- effective partnership working through Learning Disability Partnership Boards.

To implement these changes a Learning Disability Task Force was set up to advise the government, supported by an Implementation Support Team to promote change at regional and local level.

In December 2007 the Department of Health (DH) published a consultation document *Valuing People Now*,[4] which set out the next steps on the Valuing People policy and its delivery. It saw the main priorities for 2008–2011 to be personalisation; what people do during the day; better health; access to housing and making sure that change happened. The wider agenda would include an emphasis on advocacy and human rights; partnership with families; ensuring all those with learning disabilities were included; working with the criminal justice system and the Department of Transport and local groups to ensure those with learning disabilities can become full members of their local communities; providing the same opportunities as others in the transition from childhood to adulthood and supporting those who work with those with learning disabilities. The consultation ended in March 2008 and the outcome is awaited.

The Chartered Society of Physiotherapy (CSP) set priorities for physiotherapy research for those with mental health and learning disabilities in 2002. Mencap also provides a significant resource base for those involved in caring for persons with learning disabilities. It has published advice on areas of good practice including standards of care, person-centred approaches, health, employment and personalisation, the use of individual budgets and guidance for those who care for those who have profound and multiple learning disabilities (PMLD).[5]

Philosophy behind the care of those with learning disabilities

The White Paper recognised four key principles: rights, independence, choice and inclusion, as being central to government in the provision of services for those with learning disabilities. These implicitly include: autonomy, normalisation and maximum potential of each individual.

Autonomy

A basic principle that has been accepted by most twentieth-century Western philosophers is that the autonomy of the adult person should be respected and enhanced. Autonomy or self-rule or self-determination is based on the principle of respect for the person. It does not follow that because a person has learning disabilities that he or she is unable to act autonomously. There may be some decisions that are within the person's competence and the aim of any carer – informal or professional – should be to maximise the person's ability to enjoy his or her autonomy. It therefore follows that the rights of the person with learning disabilities should be protected. The Mental Capacity Act 2005 sets out a general principle that a person must be assumed to have capacity unless it is established that he/she lacks capacity (see Chapter 7). Any rebuttal of the presumption of capacity is on a balance of probabilities.

The rights shown in Figure 22.1 were identified by Knapp and Slade[6] in relation to the socio-sexual developmentally disabled person.

Normalisation

It follows from the principle that the autonomy of an individual should be respected that, as far as is possible, those with learning disabilities should be supported in enjoying as 'normal' a life as possible.

Figure 22.2 shows the rights that these same authors considered essential to implement the principle of normalisation.

Normalisation has as its aim to ensure the full potential of such clients and to attempt to prevent any restriction on their life and opportunities that is not an inevitable consequence of their condition. In this work the physiotherapist has an important role to play. It is clear that in the setting of priorities considerable sums should be available for staffing and equipment.

However, carers always have a duty to act in the best interests of their clients and these are not

- The right to equal educational opportunity
- The right to education and habilitation, which includes the right to receive information about sex and contraception
- The right to be free unless proven dangerous
- The right to privacy, especially concerning one's intimate bodily functions, including the right to sexual expression
- The right to equal access to medical services
- The right to have relationships with one's peers, including the members of the opposite sex – this right includes the right to sexual expression
- The right to equal opportunities for housing
- The right to equal and fair treatment by public agencies and officials

Figure 22.1   Rights of the socio-sexual developmentally disabled person.

- The right to a normal rhythm to the day (regular mealtimes, work and leisure time)
- The right to experience the normal life cycle
- The right to grow up, to leave parents and to move into the community
- The right to live in and experience male/female relationships
- The right to the same economic standards
- The right to make choices
- The right to fail – if developmentally disabled persons are offered as much autonomy as they are capable of, this necessarily will include the possibility of failing, just as everyone experiences this possibility

Figure 22.2   Rights to implement the normalisation principle

necessarily achieved by forcing a concept of 'normality' on clients who may be distressed by pressure to make decisions for themselves. Also it is often the case that learning disabilities are accompanied by physical problems and so a 'normal' lifestyle might not be that which is most comfortable for clients or, indeed, best for their physical health.

Situation: being normal

The physiotherapist assessed a patient as requiring a shoe raise. However, the staff in the community home considered that it was not normal to have a raise on one's shoes so, in the interests of the normalisation principle, these shoes were withdrawn. What is the legal situation?

This would appear to be an extremely odd implementation of the normalisation principle – comparable to denying spectacles to a person with extreme shortsightedness because people do not usually wear glasses. The physiotherapist has a responsibility to show the staff the importance to the physical health and safety of the patient that she should wear shoe raises, that long-term damage could occur if they were not worn and advise on how shoes could be obtained which took into account aesthetic or fashion considerations.

Maximum development of potential

The principles that govern the care of those with learning disabilities include not only that of normalisation but also the aim of ensuring the maximum development of the potential of each individual. This requires individual assessment and the preparation of an individual care plan covering all aspects of life – education, health, and social and economic development. The physiotherapist must play her part in this strategic planning for each individual as part of a multi-disciplinary team.

Physiotherapy and learning disabilities

Direct patient contact

Physiotherapy treatments often require more intimate contact with patients than those of other health professionals. Clients may be asked to remove their clothes. Often those with learning disabilities are unable to give a valid consent to such treatments and the removal of clothing.

Situation: massage for constipation

A physiotherapist advises that massage might assist an extremely constipated client, who suffers from severe learning disabilities. She is concerned that her treatment could be misinterpreted both by the client and others.

Every effort should be made to explain to the patient what the physiotherapist is intending to do. There would be strong reasons to ensure that the physiotherapist is chaperoned, both for her own protection and for that of the client. Clearly, if the client refused this treatment, then its value would have to be reassessed. The Mental Capacity Act 2005 enables action to be taken in the best interests of those who lack the requisite capacity to give consent and in certain circumstances restraint can be used. These circumstances are considered in Chapters 7 and 24.

Equipment for those with physical learning disabilities

Chapter 15 considers legal issues arising from the use of equipment. In this chapter further situations relating to those with learning disabilities will be considered.

Situation: a bad case of housemaid's knee

A 24-year-old patient with severe cerebral palsy, no verbal communication, extremely poor sitting balance and very strong extensor thrusting on excitement was fitted with a Gill II seating system. However, due to his fluctuating tone when excited or anxious his extensor thrusting was so strong he broke the hinge between the back and the base. This was repaired with reinforcing struts. A knee brace was used to limit his extensor thrust but the carers were unable to strap his feet to the footplates. His athetoid movements resulted in his shins pistoning up and down against the knee brace resulting in a bad case of double housemaid's knee. He was treated with ultrasound and resting from the knee brace for 10 days. (Taken from Maureen Grimmer[7].)

The lesson learnt from the above case was that an athetoid patient should not be fitted into a Gill II seating system with a knee brace unless one can strap the feet securely to the footplate. One would expect this lesson to be incorporated into the standard of care as measured by the Bolam test (see Chapter 10). One concern raised by this situation is whether the strapping of the feet would be classified as restraint. If the only safe way of transporting such a patient in a wheelchair was by using this strapping, then it would be seen as restraint, but justifiable in the best interests of the patient, like a seat belt in a car, in accordance with the Mental Capacity Act 2007. If the patient refuses to agree to the strapping then it should be made clear that he could not go in the wheel chair. If the patient lacked the mental competence to appreciate this reasoning, then the temporary restraint might be justified on the basis that the physiotherapist was acting in the best interests of the patient according to the principles set out in the Mental Capacity Act 2005 which replaces the common law principles set down by the House of Lords in the case of *Re F*.[8]

Situation: tied to the toilet

> In order to preserve the privacy and dignity of the client, a physiotherapist used a belt to tie the client to the toilet. This was so that she would not fall off and could be left alone. Is this lawful?

This would appear to be a degrading practice even if the intention was laudable. It would seem preferable to stay with the client, providing personal support than to use such a dangerous and unlawful method of restraint.

Situation: splints to prevent harm to the face

> Rachel, a woman of 32 with severe disabilities, scratches her face and eyes and arm splints are used to protect her.

There would appear to be justification in the short term to prevent Rachel from harming herself, but long-term methods of behavioural therapy and other treatments should be used to obtain a fundamental change in the patient's behaviour. An assessment is required under the Mental Capacity Act 2005 (as amended by the Mental Health Act 2007) to determine the lawfulness of the restraint used. The restraint must be in the best interests of the patient who lacks the mental capacity to make his/her own decision and the conditions laid down in the Act must exist, i.e. the person using the restraint must reasonably believe that it is necessary to use restraint in order to prevent harm to the patient and second the act of restraint must be a proportionate response to (a) the likelihood of the patient's suffering harm, and (b) the seriousness of that harm.

Records should be kept of the use of the splints and regular monitoring should take place to ensure that alternative ways of preventing her harming herself, e.g. by staff being in attendance on her, are used as often as possible.

Manual handling

Care for those with learning disabilities may often involve manual handling. Chapter 11 looks at this subject in more detail and also considers the physiotherapist's liability in instructing staff and providing guidance on manual handling in residential homes. Negligent instructions could give rise to liability if in reliance upon those instructions a person was harmed or caused harm to others.

Situation: lifting a patient with cerebral palsy

> Social services staff sought guidance from a physiotherapist in lifting a client who has cerebral palsy. He is well able to walk, but insists upon sitting down on the pavement and even in the road. What legal aspects arise?

Unless the behaviour of this client can be changed, it may be that a risk assessment would result in a recommendation that he should only be permitted outside the grounds of his home if he is in a wheelchair. He could possibly be taken to a safe area such as a park and assisted in walking. Much depends upon the practicality of staff lifting him off the road and to his feet. If he were of any significant weight this may not be safe practice unless there were at least three staff able to carry out the manoeuvre.

Any physiotherapist who is involved in instructing others in manual handling or in giving guidance on specific situations, should ensure that records are kept of this instruction or guidance, including the details of those present and what was said.

Restraint

A restriction on the liberty of a person may be a false imprisonment unless there is a lawful justification. Such justification could include a lawful arrest by a police constable or citizen exercising the right to arrest under the Police and Criminal Evidence Act 1984. Acting temporarily in the best interests of an adult who lacked mental capacity could also be lawful if it is in accordance with the principles of the Mental Capacity Act 2005 (see Chapter 7) or comes within the Bournewood safeguards as explained in Chapter 21. Thus to hold back a person with learning disabilities from running across the road would be defensible under the principle of acting in the best interest of an adult lacking mental capacity under the Mental Capacity Act 2005 and a justifiable restraint under Section 6 of the Act.

Situation: restraint

John Turner has severe learning disabilities and is always trying to leave the home. Staff tie him to the chair to keep him from wandering off. What is the law?

To tie a person into a chair would be an unlawful act, a false imprisonment, and also a breach of the Human Rights Act 1998 as degrading treatment under Article 3. In exceptional circumstances restraint may be justified as a temporary measure, but:

- it must be in the best interests of the mentally incapacitated adult;
- the person using the restraint must reasonably believe that it is necessary to use restraint in order to prevent harm to the patient;
- the act of restraint must be a proportionate response to
  - the likelihood of the patient's suffering harm;
  - the seriousness of that harm.

Records should be kept and any restraint should be regularly monitored. In certain situations restraint may be required by law such as the wearing of seat belts. The use of the Bournewood safeguards may be justified here.

GP contacts

A physiotherapist working with people with learning disabilities is part of a multidisciplinary team providing care. An important member of this team, though unfortunately not always playing a full part, is the GP. The following situation may be familiar to many.

Situation: no response

A patient with learning disabilities is referred to a physiotherapist by social services. She informs the GP of her involvement, and her planned treatment and asks if there is any reason why the patient should not receive the proposed treatment or participate in a certain activity. She receives no reply and wonders if she can assume that the absence of a reply implies that there is agreement to the treatment plan.

Silence does not imply agreement. In this situation to ensure that no harm occurs to the patient the physiotherapist needs to have access to the patient's medical records. The referral form should also include on it any information relating to the patient's condition of which the physiotherapist should be aware but this cannot be relied on.

In this situation of getting no reply to a request for information the physiotherapist would have to act as a reasonable physiotherapist would do in the circumstances (i.e. in accordance with the Bolam test), which might well be not to commence treatment but consult with her managers for them to take the issue further. If the patient's condition would seriously deteriorate if the treatment did not start immediately, the physiotherapist would have to weigh the risk of delay against the risk of proceeding without possibly relevant information. The patient's inability to consent to the treatment would require the provisions of the Mental Capacity Act 2005 to be followed. Where serious treatment is required an independent mental capacity advocate should be appointed in the absence of relations or friends who could be consulted.

Gender issues

A female physiotherapist caring for an adult client with learning disabilities can be confronted with practical difficulties arising from different genders.

Situation: swimming pool problems

A female physiotherapist uses a standard public swimming pool with a male client who needs help to undress. What should she do?

There are various choices in this situation:

- she could go with him into the male changing room, which would probably embarrass her more than the men in the room;
- she could take the patient into the female changing room which would disturb any other females changing there;
- she could ask the manager if there are any available rooms where she could take the client to change him (the possibility is extremely unlikely).

The answer would appear to be that only a male physiotherapist takes this particular client to the swimming pool or the female physiotherapist ensures that, if she goes, she is accompanied by a male care assistant.

Situation: undressing in an adult training centre

A physiotherapist attends an adult training centre and considers that treatment is best provided for a patient with learning disabilities if she is undressed. What is the law?

If the treatment is clearly indicated according to the Bolam test (see Chapter 10) and any

reasonable physiotherapist would require the patient to be undressed, then this would be justified. However, it is essential that the patient's dignity and privacy are respected and a chaperon is recommended. In January 2008 the Council for Healthcare Regulatory Excellence (CHRE) issued three sets of guidance (for the registration bodies to pass onto registrants; to those in education and training; and to advise fitness to practise panels) on the maintenance of clear sexual boundaries between healthcare professionals and patients. The guidance can be obtained from the CHRE website.[9]

Situation: suspected abuse

A physiotherapist visits a patient who lives with her parents and brother and suspects that she may be the victim of sexual abuse. What action should she take?

She has a duty of care to the client and this would include taking appropriate action if she suspected physical or mental abuse. The Mental Capacity Act 2005 makes it a criminal offence to ill treat or wilfully neglect a person who lacks capacity. Local authorities now have procedures for dealing with the abuse of the older and vulnerable adults. The physiotherapist should discuss her concerns with the multidisciplinary team and ensure that social services are brought in (if not already represented on the team). In some circumstances, it may become a police matter and lead to prosecution (see also Chapter 24).

The appropriate adult

It is a requirement that where a person with learning disabilities is involved in any police investigations or court proceedings an appropriate adult should be appointed to protect their interests. Under the Mental Capacity Act 2005 an Independent Mental Capacity Advocate (IMCA) must be appointed in specified circumstances. Where a NHS body or local authority are proposing or have taken protection measures in relation to a person P who lacks capacity to agree to one or more of the measures then the NHS or local authority may instruct an IMCA to represent P if it is satisfied that it would be of particular benefit to P to be so represented. An advocate can be appointed even it the person in an adult protection situation has friends or family who could be consulted.

Situation: an appropriate adult

> A physiotherapist was asked to attend the police station with a client with severe learning disabilities whom she had known for many years. He was suspected of committing the offence of indecency. What action should she take?

Such a request could be very unnerving for the physiotherapist. It may well be that in the actual situation here described she would need to ensure that a solicitor attended to represent the client legally. She could, however, as a person known to the client, ensure that the client was not harassed or bullied and ensure that practical arrangements were made for his care. She should keep records of her involvement. Under the regulations under the Mental Capacity Act 2005 an Independent Mental Capacity Advocate should be appointed in an adult protection case.[10]

Living and working in the community

Community homes for those with learning disabilities

The effect of the community care initiative has meant that fewer clients with learning disabilities are cared for in institutions administered under health service organisations and more are cared for either within the family setting or in community homes especially built or adapted for the needs of those with learning disabilities. Some of this accommodation has been provided by Housing Associations, which may work in conjunction with care organisations which undertake the day-to-day management of the home. These organisations often provide a code of practice covering the rights that the client/tenant/resident should enjoy and setting quality standards.

Many clients with learning disabilities are therefore under the care of professionals employed by the social services departments rather than NHS trusts.

The physiotherapist, within the context of the multidisciplinary team, should have a role to play in these community homes, not only in the selection of clients for each home but also in providing support and guidance on the health and mobility of those clients.

Sheltered workshops

Clients, whether living in their family homes or in community homes should have the facility of attending sheltered workshops and other forms of industrial therapy. However, provision is patchy across the country. Physiotherapists can work with the multidisciplinary team and provide expert advice on the most appropriate activities, taking into account any physical handicaps of the client group.

Record keeping

Health professionals visiting on an occasional basis need to be aware of changes in the client's condition.

Situation: 'I was not informed'

> Each time a physiotherapist visited a client in a residential home, she said to the staff, please notify me of any changes to the patient's condition and provided an information sheet for any changes to be recorded. On her next visit, she noted that nothing had been recorded and commenced her treatment with the client, who screamed loudly when she touched his shoulder. She was then told that he had had a bad fall 2 days before.

The physiotherapist clearly understood the importance of knowing the client's recent history and tried to meet this by providing the information sheet and asking the question. Unfortunately, the staff asked might not have been on duty at the time and might themselves have had no cause to consult the records where the fall should have been noted. The physiotherapist's own information sheet left at the home for noting such changes, although a laudable attempt to get relevant information, might have confused the issue. It would amount to a second and separate place where the incident should be noted – always difficult when staff are working under pressure (see Chapter 12 on the problems of more than one set of records).

The above situation is an example of the importance of record keeping. At each visit to the home the physiotherapist should see the client's records and should therefore have read of this incident. She should herself be noting her own treatments and care in these records so that other professionals are aware of her interventions. If records are not being kept, then, through the multidisciplinary team, she should be urging higher standards of patient care and record keeping.

Conflict with carers

Refusal to grant accommodation

The rights of relatives to refuse to take back an adult client who has been in respite care also need to be considered. In the case of an adult person suffering from mental impairment, if the relatives refuse to take the person back home this is their right and they cannot be compelled to look after him or her. Health and social services professionals would have to look for other accommodation for the client.

Reference should be made to the discussion in Chapter 18 on the guidelines for the division between health services and social services responsibilities on continuing care.

Protection of the autonomy of the client

It may happen that an extremely diligent parent/carer is unwilling to allow a son or daughter with learning disabilities to leave home and enter sheltered accommodation. In an extreme case a mother had been placed under an injunction not to visit her son who had been moved to alternative accommodation. The Court of Appeal ruled that the injunction should be lifted as it was not appropriate to threaten her with imprisonment but the case illustrates the difficulties of 'letting go'. The situation is now covered by the Mental Capacity Act 2005, which requires decisions to be taken in the best interests of an adult who lacks the capacity to make his or her own decisions. Where accommodation decisions are to be made an Independent Mental Capacity Advocate must be appointed, unless there is a relative or friend whom it would be appropriate to consult. It is hoped that where it is known that the parents are acting contrary to the client's best interests, then they would not be seen as appropriate and an IMCA could be appointed.

The role of the physiotherapist

If physiotherapists are aware of a conflict between the rights (as shown in Figure 22.2) of the person with learning disabilities and the wishes of the carer, they should (within the context of the multidisciplinary team) ensure that action is taken to protect the client and endeavour to secure a harmonious outcome, bearing in mind the rights of the client. The Mental Capacity Act 2005 and the Code of Practice drawn up under it recognises the rights of the mentally incapacitated adult and provides a statutory framework for decision making on their behalf.

Risk assessment and risk taking

The philosophy of normalisation requires that health and social services professionals working with those with learning disabilities should be acquainted with and implement a risk assessment strategy in relation to each individual client. It would be possible to prevent any harm arising by keeping the client indoors under close supervision and denying him or her opportunities to go shopping, to go to work and to undertake everyday activities. However, the quality of life would be severely reduced if the opportunities were not taken for holidays, trips and other activities.

The law requires that reasonable precautions are taken to prevent reasonably foreseeable risks of harm. Thus a risk assessment in respect of each individual client would be required to identify the risks of possible harm to the client or other people arising and to determine what action would be reasonable to prevent such risks occurring.

It is essential that records are kept of this risk assessment so that should the client's condition deteriorate or improve, it is possible to identify the significance of these changes to the proposed participation in the activities and so that other healthcare workers can identify through the treatment plan what a client should or should not be encouraged to do. Records are also of extreme importance if harm arises to the client or another person and the professional is required to justify her action before the civil courts, criminal courts, disciplinary proceedings, or professional conduct proceedings. If it can be established that the actions of the professional were reasonable in relation to reasonably foreseeable risks, then civil liability should not exist.

In Chapter 11 the use of a risk assessment strategy is considered in the context of health and safety and this strategy could also be used in relation to individual care planning.

In Chapter 24 the Green Paper *Independence, Well-being and Choice*[11] and the White Paper on *Our Health, Our Care, Our Say*,[12] published in 2006, are discussed in relation to risk management, together with the subsequent guidance published by the DH on independence, choice and risk[13] which provides a risk management framework for use by everyone involved in supporting adults using social care within any setting, including NHS staff working in multidisciplinary or joint teams.

Risk assessment and client compliance

Situation: cycle helmet – a necessity

> The physiotherapist has carried out a risk assessment of cycling and recommended that cycle helmets should be worn. One particular client refuses to wear a cycle helmet. What is the legal situation? Can he be allowed to cycle without a helmet at his own risk or should he be refused the chance of cycling?

If the client's learning disabilities make it impossible for him to appreciate the risks of cycling without a helmet, he cannot, in law, voluntarily accept the risk of being harmed. The defence of *volenti non fit injuria* (see Chapter 10) would therefore not apply. Those caring for this person must ensure that all reasonable care is taken during any activities. Reasonable care would include wearing a helmet. Failure to wear a helmet would therefore preclude cycling. It may be that skilful teaching, showing the client other persons wearing helmets, letting him choose the colour and other ways of involvement may lead to his cooperation in accepting that cycling requires that helmets have to be worn. Under the Mental Capacity Act 2005, limited restraint can be justified provided that that the decision maker must reasonably believe that it is necessary to do the act in order to prevent harm to the client/patient and that the action is a proportionate response. Proportionate means that the act of restraint is

> proportionate to both the likelihood of harm to the client/patient and the seriousness of the harm.

Restraint is defined as:

> including both the decision maker using or threatening to use force to secure the doing of an act which the client/patient resists and also restricts P's liberty of movement, whether or not P resists.

Situation: water sports

A physiotherapist arranges with a local yacht club that the club facilities can be used by clients with learning disabilities. She is concerned about the safety of one client who often fails to obey instructions. Would it be too risky to permit this client to take part in activities?

At the heart of the answer to this situation should be a risk assessment. The physiotherapist has a duty to take reasonable care of the safety of the client. She can reasonably foresee that this client might refuse to obey extremely important instructions and jeopardise his own safety and that of others. She needs therefore to balance the risks with the benefits and also consider how any risks could be reduced. If on balance the risks of harm cannot be avoided or reduced, then it would be reasonable to refuse to permit the client to take part. Much of course depends upon the mental capacity of the client and it could be that behavioural therapy methods could lead to compliance by the client, so that the risks were reduced.

Risk management and rebound therapy

Rebound therapy has been found useful in work with clients with learning disabilities. A clear risk assessment should be carried out before the therapy commences. *Safe Practice in Rebound Therapy* was published in 2007 by the ACPPLD[14] and covers a definition of rebound therapy, the scope of professional practice, consent, monitoring performance delegation to assistants, safety procedures, care factors and safety in relation to the environment, the trampoline and the physiotherapist

Situation: rebound therapy and pregnancy

A physiotherapist assessed a client for rebound therapy following the guidance issued by the ACPPLD. She failed to ascertain whether the client was pregnant. During the therapy, the client complained of severe stomach cramps and subsequently miscarried. The client's parents are now threatening to sue the physiotherapist for negligence.

It was ascertained that the physiotherapist had asked the client if she had had any recent medical attention, but did not ask her specifically if she was pregnant. Her failure to ask this specific question would be judged against the reasonable practice of a competent physiotherapist practising in the field of rebound therapy, whether or not a specific question on pregnancy was on the guidelines set by the ACPPLD.

If a client is incapable of understanding the question or the importance of it, enquiries should be made of the parents or carers as to the client's situation and whether pregnancy is a possibility.

Horse riding for the disabled

Horse riding can be a useful activity in the care and treatment for both the physically and mentally handicapped, but for convenience the topic is included in this chapter on learning disabilities. The Association published standards of practice in 1999.[15] There are three classifications recognised by the Association of Chartered Physiotherapists in Therapeutic Riding:

- therapeutic riding – where the client is taught to ride by an instructor and the physiotherapist assesses the rider;
- hippotherapy – treatment using the movement of the horse;
- recreational riding.

Such activities inevitably involve some element of risk and, particularly in working with those with learning disabilities, there is a duty on the health professionals to be vigilant on behalf of clients who might lack the capacity to appreciate and accept risks for themselves. The defence of *volenti non fit injuria*, or the voluntary assumption of risk on the part of the claimant (formerly plaintiff), would not be available (see Chapter 10). The benefits are to be weighed against the risks in accordance with the Bolam test and changing circumstances kept under review.

Situation: biting the horse[2]

> Cathy, recently discharged from a long-stay hospital, joined a Riding for the Disabled Group. People were nervous about how she would cope. She stroked the horse and was placed upon it and then suddenly leant forward and bit the horse.

In this situation it was explained that this was Cathy's way of indicating that she liked someone. However, if as a result the horse had bolted with Cathy upon it would those responsible have been liable? There is no doubt that they would have a duty of care for Cathy. However, liability would depend upon the extent to which they could have foreseen the specific risk of Cathy biting the horse and the horse therefore bolting. Once, of course, the event has occurred, the risk is foreseeable and should be taken into account. Thus, in Cathy's case the author noted that Cathy was banned from riding, but proved to be a great water baby.

Situation: assessing for competition categories in riding for the disabled

> A physiotherapist, who assisted in riding for the disabled, was asked to provide an assessment profile of a disabled person for the correct category for a competition. Subsequently the disabled person challenged the physiotherapist for a negligent assessment, disagreeing with the category within which she had been placed. Would the disabled person win any case?

The fact that the physiotherapist has volunteered her services does not imply that she has no duty of care to the client. Once she voluntarily accepts that task then she would be obliged to use all reasonable care, relevant to the circumstance, in fulfilling the duty of care. It would have to be shown that no reasonable physiotherapist would have assessed in the way in which she did. If the volunteer has carried out her duties reasonably according to the Bolam test (see Chapter 10) she should not be liable. Moreover, the disabled person would also have to show that harm has been suffered as the result of the negligent assessment. Harm could include financial loss, and this may mean proving that had the disabled person been in a different category then prizes could have been won. This might be difficult to establish.

However, this scenario shows the advisability of the physiotherapist keeping clear, comprehensive records even in situations where she is volunteering help.

Situation: recommending an activity

> A physiotherapist suggested that a particular client would benefit from horse riding. When the appointment came, the horse riding exacerbated a pre-existing shoulder injury. Whose responsibility is it to ensure that the client is fit to undertake the activity?

A physiotherapist would not be following the Bolam test in providing a reasonable standard of care for a client, if she recommended a particular activity without ensuring that the client was fit to undertake it. However, once her assessment has been made, any subsequent changes in the client's condition should be assessed by the carer, or the individual supervising the activity, to ensure that the client is still safe in undertaking it.

Decision making and incapacity

Many clients with learning disabilities may still have the capacity to make decisions on their own account. Clearly, the client's capacity must be related to the nature of the decision to be made. The client may be able to choose what clothes to wear or to buy but may not have the capacity to decide whether or not to undergo an operation to be sterilised. The basic principle of law is that a mentally competent adult has the right to give or refuse consent and cannot be compelled to have treatment even if it is life saving (see Chapter 7). The Mental Capacity Act 2005 fills the vacuum in decision making on behalf of those lacking capacity that had been temporarily filled by the common law. The House of Lords[8] had held that where an adult lacked the appropriate capacity, decisions could be made on his or her behalf in their best interests. This was known as 'The *Re F* principle' It derives from a case where it was considered to be in the best interest of a woman with learning disabilities to be sterilised.

The House of Lords stated that a professional had the duty to act in the best interests of any adult person who lacked the necessary mental capacity and should follow the Bolam test (see glossary) in providing a reasonable standard of care.

The Mental Capacity Act 2005

The Law Commission, following an extended period of consultation on the issue of decision making and mental incapacity, prepared draft legislation[16] in 1995. The Lord Chancellor issued a consultation document in December 1997,[17] *Who Decides*. Following this consultation a bill was introduced into Parliament to enact the Law Commission's recommendations. The Mental Capacity Act 2005 received royal assent in 2005 and was brought into force in October 2007. The Act is discussed in full in Chapter 7. The Act sets out statutory principles that should apply and can be found in Box 7.1. The Act defines mental capacity and also sets out the steps to be taken to determine the best interests of those lacking the requisite mental capacity. Independent mental capacity advocates are to be appointed in specific circumstances to provide information on the best interests of the patient. The Act recognises the power to appoint a lasting power of attorney (discussed in Chapter 24) and sets up a new Court of Protection with jurisdiction over personal welfare decisions as well as matters relating to property and affairs. The Court of Protection can appoint deputies, who come under the supervision of a new Office of Public Guardian, to make decisions. Further information can be found in the author's work.[18]

Case: the Bournewood case

A House of Lords decision in 1998[19] held that the power of acting out of necessity in the best interests of a person who lacks mental capacity can also apply to the admission of such patients to psychiatric care. The House of Lords had overruled a Court of Appeal decision which had held that any adult who lacked the mental capacity to give consent to voluntary admission to psychiatric care had to be examined with a view to detention under the provisions of the Mental Health Act 1983 (see Chapter 21). The carers applied to the European Court of Human Rights holding that its decision was contrary to Article 5 in the European Convention. The European Court of Human Rights held that there had been a breach of Article 5 of the European Convention on Human Rights.[20] The Bournewood case and the Bournewood safeguards are considered in more detail in Chapter 21.

The issue of capacity arose in the following case.

Case: *Local Authority X* v. *MM* 2007[21]

The local authority brought the case seeking orders that M lacked capacity to conduct litigation, make decisions where she should reside, determine with whom she should have contact, manage her own affairs or enter into marriage. It also wanted a declaration that it was in M's best interests to reside in supported accommodation and have limited contact with K, her partner. M was a vulnerable adult who suffered paranoid schizophrenia and learning disabilities. She had been with K for 15 years. The local authority received information that K was intending to move M from her supported accommodation and disengage from psychiatric services. They therefore applied for an interim injunction to prevent M being moved from her supported accommodation or have unsupervised contact with K.

The judge held that the test of mental capacity to consent to medical treatment was also applicable to decisions over residency and with whom the person was to have contact. There was no relevant distinction between the test in *Re MB*[22] and the statutory definition in the Mental Capacity Act 2005 (see Chapter 7). The capacity to consent to sexual intercourse depended on a person having sufficient knowledge and understanding of the sexual nature and character of the act of sexual intercourse and of the reasonably foreseeable consequences of sexual intercourse, to have the capacity to choose whether or not to engage in it. It was issue specific not partner specific. M had the capacity to consent to sexual intercourse, but lacked the capacity to litigate; to manage her finances; to decide where and with whom she should live, to marry and to decide with whom she should have contact. M's human rights had to be taken into account and her wishes and feelings should be considered and the court had to pay regard to M's wishes to have an ongoing sexual relationship with K. The judge made the order required by the local authority subject to the qualification that her contact with K did not have to be supervised. The local authority was directed to file a care plan setting out its final proposals.

Non-compliance or refusal by client or carer

The client

The care of those with learning disabilities should be aimed at ensuring the maximum autonomy and decision making by the clients (see above). However, difficulties can arise if the client refuses to undertake exercises which are necessary as part of a treatment plan designed by a physiotherapist. There is no statutory power to compel clients to cooperate in treatment unless the patient is formally detained under the Mental Health Act 1983 (see Chapter 21) and the treatment is seen as part of the treatment for mental disorder. Physiotherapy cannot usually be undertaken without the client's cooperation. It may be possible as part of a treatment plan to build in incentives for the client to be involved and thus encourage participation.

Situation: compulsory treatment?

A client, with severe learning disabilities, has a fractured femur and was attended by a physiotherapist after surgery. The client refused to come out of bed to commence mobilisation. Can he be compelled to do so?

If the client were mentally competent the answer would be 'No' (see Chapter 7). However, here the client lacks the mental capacity to make an appropriate decision. The Mental Capacity Act 2005 now provides a statutory framework for making decisions on behalf of a mentally incapacitated adult. The Act enables limited restraint to be used (see above). However, it is essential that all non-forceful means of compulsion should first be employed to persuade the client to cooperate in attempting to walk. A risk assessment would be necessary to ensure that the risks of harm were avoided or reduced and to identify the number of staff needed to walk the patient safely.

Non compliance by carer

Situation: non-cooperation by carer

The physiotherapist, following an assessment on a patient with learning disabilities, makes several recommendations as to what she thinks is best for the client, including daily passive movements to be carried out by the carer. She fears however that the care workers who look after the client may not carry out these exercises. What is the legal situation?

In this situation a distinction has to be made between the carer as an employee and the carer as a relative/friend in a non-employment situation.

Carer as an employee

If the physiotherapist has recommended a treatment plan that is to be implemented by the care worker, this should be discussed with the multidisciplinary team as part of the treatment plan for that patient, taking into account the resources available. The home manager would then have the responsibility of ensuring that staff implemented the agreed care plan. Care assistants should be supervised to ensure that treatment plans were carried out. Failures by the care assistant should be followed by disciplinary measures, initially counselling and subsequently oral or written warnings.

Carer as a relative/friend

Where the carer is a relative or volunteer, then there is no contract which is enforceable against them to ensure that a treatment plan was implemented. Clearly, explanations would be given of the importance of following any recommendations by the physiotherapist (see Chapter 7). If they fail to comply and this lack of compliance affects the health and safety of the patient, then action could be taken with social services cooperation to remove the adult patient to other accommodation where the necessary care and treatment could be provided. Clearly, this would only take place in an extreme situation. If the patient is a child, then the Children Act 1989 provides the mechanism for such action (see Chapter 23). The Mental Capacity Act 2005 has provided a framework for decision making on behalf of the mentally incompetent adult and procedures for such decision making should be available in every department. Relatives are not able to prevent action being taken in the best interests of the client. In the event of a dispute over what were in the best interests an application could be made to the new Court of Protection, which might in an ongoing situation consider the appointment of a deputy to make decisions on behalf of a mentally incapacitated adult. In extreme situations a carer may commit an offence in wilfully neglecting the care of a mentally incapacitated adult. Section 44 of the Mental Capacity Act 2005 has created an offence where a person has the care of a mentally incapacitated person and ill treats or wilfully neglects him or her.

Situation: deliberate obstruction by a relative

David was 35 years old with severe learning disabilities and epileptic fits. He lived in a community home but was regularly visited by his mother, who insisted on playing a major decision-making role in all aspects of his life. She stated that he was not safe to walk and objected when staff helped him to walk unaided. She also refused to let him attend at the day centre for assessments and treatment by the physiotherapist. It was suggested that David should wear a helmet because of the frequency of his epileptic fits, but his mother objected to that. What is the legal position?

David is over 18 years. He appears to lack the mental capacity to make decisions for himself. Carers and professionals looking after him have a duty under the Mental Capacity Act 2005 to make decisions and act in his best interests. It is clear that the mother is not, according to professional opinion, acting in his best interests. In theory, it would be possible to obtain a declaration of the court about his best interests and the action which health professionals should take. The Court of Protection would determine what are the best interests in the event of a dispute. The difficulty in this case is that David is probably gaining considerable benefit from the continuing relationship with his mother and any attempt to overrule her, albeit in David's best interests, might lead to difficulties between them. This is essentially a balancing act: would David benefit more by action being taken to enforce the mother to accept the treatment recommended by the physiotherapists for David, with a possible loss of contact or at least strained relations between them, or would David benefit more from the continued contact with his mother, unchanged without the treatment? Clearly all should be done to persuade the mother of the value to David of having the assessments, treatment and helmet. The Court of Protection has the power to appoint a deputy to take decisions on behalf of a mentally incapacitated adult and who could act on a day-to-day basis on behalf of David.

Appointment of deputy

The Court of Protection can make a single order or appoint a deputy in relation to a matter within its jurisdiction, which includes personal welfare as well as finance and property. Section 16 makes provisions for the Court of Protection to make decisions and for the appointment of deputies. The deputy must act on behalf of the patient in accordance with the principles set out in the Mental Capacity Act 2005, in the best interests of the patient (see Chapter 7) and within the powers granted him by the Court of Protection. The deputies can be given powers (with specified limitations) over matters of personal welfare which extend in particular to:

- deciding where P (the person lacking mental capacity) is to live, (where a deputy makes a decision on this, it is subject to the restrictions on deputies);
- deciding what contact, if any, P is to have with any specified persons; (the deputy has no power to make an order prohibiting a named person from having contact with P);
- giving or refusing consent to the carrying out or continuation of a treatment by a person providing health care for P.

A deputy cannot give a direction that a person responsible for P's health care allows a different person to take over that responsibility: only the Court of Protection has that power.

Where the deputy is given powers over a person's property and affairs, they could include the following:

- the control and management of P's property;
- the sale, exchange, charging gift or other disposition of P's property;

- the acquisition of property in P's name or on P's behalf;
- the carrying on, on P's behalf, of any profession, trade or business;
- the taking of a decision which will have the effect of dissolving a partnership of which P is a member;
- the carrying out of any contract entered into by P;
- the discharge of P's debts and of any of P's obligations, whether legally enforceable or not;
- the settlement of any of P's property, whether for P's benefit or for the benefit of others;
- the execution for P of a will (unless P is under 18 years old) (subject to restriction on deputies);
- the exercise of any power (including a power to consent) vested in P whether beneficially or as trustee or otherwise;
- the conduct of legal proceedings in P's name or on P's behalf.

The Code of Practice identifies the following list as duties to be followed by the court-appointed deputy.[23] It notes that when agreeing to act as deputy, whether in relation to welfare or financial affairs, the deputy is taking on a role that carries power that he/she must use carefully and responsibly. The standard of conduct expected of deputies involves compliance with the following duties as an agent and with the statutory requirements:

- to comply with the principles of the Act;
- to act in the best interests of the client;
- to follow the Code of Practice;
- to act within the scope of their authority given by the Court of Protection;
- to act with due care and skill (duty of care);
- not to take advantage of their situation (fiduciary duty);
- to indemnify the person against liability to third parties caused by the deputy's negligence;
- not to delegate duties unless authorised to do so;
- to act in good faith;
- to respect the person's confidentiality;

● to comply with the directions of the Court of Protection.

To be appointed as a deputy an individual must be 18 years or over. An individual of at least 18 years or a trust corporation can be appointed as a deputy in respect of powers relating to property and affairs. The deputy must give consent to the appointment. The holder of a specified office or position may be appointed as deputy. Two or more deputies could be appointed to act jointly or jointly and severally. (Jointly means that they act together in making decisions and exercising the powers; severally means that they act as individuals separately.)

The deputy is entitled to be reimbursed out of P's property for his/her reasonable expenses in discharging his/her functions. In addition, if the court so directs when appointing the deputy, the deputy can receive remuneration out of P's property for discharging his/her functions. The court can give the deputy powers to take possession or control of all or any specified part of P's property and to exercise all or any specified powers in respect or it, including such powers of investment as the court decides.

The Office of Public Guardian acts as supervisor of the deputy and any complaints about the conduct of a deputy can be made to that Office. Further information on the role of the deputy, the Office of Public Guardian and the Court of Protection can be obtained from the Ministry of Justice website.[24] See also the author's work.[18]

Sexual relations and related issues

Implicit in the concept of normalisation is the view that those suffering from learning disabilities should be able to participate in sexual activity according to their mental understanding.

Protection by the criminal code

The law protects those who do not have the capacity to give consent to sexual intercourse.

It is an offence for a man to have unlawful sexual intercourse with a woman who is a defective (Sexual Offences Act 1956, Section 7). However, it is a defence if a man is able to prove that he did not know and had no reason to suspect that the woman was defective. In the case of *R* v. *Hudson*[25] the Court of Criminal Appeal allowed the appeal of the defendant against conviction on the grounds that a subjective test should have been applied to determine whether he had reason to suspect this.

The Sexual Offences Act 2003 repealed the provisions of Section 128 of the Mental Health Act 1959, which made it an offence for a man on the staff of or employed by a hospital or mental nursing home to have extra-marital sexual intercourse with a woman who is receiving treatment for mental disorder in that hospital or home either as an out-patient or an in-patient.

Under the Sexual Offences Act 2003 the following offences are created in relation to carers:

● Section 38 care worker: sexual activity with a person with mental disorder;
● Section 39 care worker: causing or inciting sexual activity;
● Section 40 care worker: sexual activity in the presence of a person with mental disorder;
● Section 41 care worker: causing a person with a mental disorder to watch a sexual act;
● Section 42 includes in the definition of care worker a person who has functions in a home in the course of employment which have brought him/her or likely to bring him/her into regular face-to-face contact with the person with mental disorder. The definition also covers the situation where the patient is receiving NHS-independent hospital or clinic services and the person functions to perform in the course of employment. Those who have regularly face-to-face contact with B as a result of providing care, assistance or services to him/her in connection with his/her mental disorder, whether or not in the course of employment also come within the definition.

Protecting the vulnerable

The practical problem for carers is on the one hand protecting a person with learning disabilities from abuse and exploitation and on the other hand ensuring that where the capabilities exist the client should enjoy the rights set out in Figure 22.1.

Physiotherapists, working within the multidisciplinary team, should be aware of the importance of protecting vulnerable people who may not have the capacity to consent and who may be exploited in sexual relationships. It is also important to ensure that they are protected against the risk of AIDS/HIV or other infections. Preventing pregnancy is only one aspect of safe sex.[26]

The right to procreate

The rights set out in Figures 22.1 and 22.2 relate only to the client, no other person's rights are affected. However, the right to procreate involves the rights of the future child. There is considerable debate whether a person with severe learning disabilities has a right to procreate.[27]

Sterilisation

As the result of the case of *Re D* in 1976[28] (where a mother sought a declaration that her daughter, a sufferer of Sotos syndrome, could be sterilised) it became a requirement that those seeking non-therapeutic sterilisations (i.e. one which was not required for the physical ill health of the patient) should first obtain a declaration of the court. In this case, the judge refused to permit the sterilisation of a girl of 11 years, since it was not established that the child would not have the ability to make a decision for herself at a later date. On the other hand, in Jeanette's case[29] the House of Lords gave its approval to the sterilisation of a girl of 17 years who suffered from learning disabilities and in the case of *Re F*[8] (see above) the House of Lords declared that it would be lawful to sterilise a mentally incompetent adult woman if it were in her best interests and the doctors acted according to the Bolam test.

The situation is now covered by either the Children Act 1989 or the Mental Capacity Act 2005. Where the person is under 16 years an application for sterilisation would be made to the Family Division of the High Court. Where the person is over 18 years an application could be made to the Court of Protection. A young person or 16 or 17 could be referred to either court as appropriate. If there is a request from a relative that the client be sterilised then the professional should raise this issue with the multidisciplinary team and ensure that, if necessary, an application is made to the appropriate court. The decision to sterilise an individual is one of the most significant that can be taken and it is essential that any health professional who is involved in the court proceedings and the evidence which is required should follow the principles considered in Chapter 13. The Code of Practice on the Mental Capacity Act (issued by the Department of Constitutional Affairs (DCA) and now available from the website of the DCA's successor, the Ministry of Justice[24]) notes in paragraph 8.22:

> that cases involving non-therapeutic sterilisation will require a careful assessment of whether such sterilisation would be in the best interests of the person who lacks capacity and such cases should continue to be referred to the court.

In the case of *Re A* a mother applied for a declaration that a vasectomy was in the best interests of A, her son, (who had Down's syndrome and was borderline between significant and severe impairment of intelligence), in the absence of his consent. After balancing the burdens and benefits of the proposed vasectomy to A, the Court of Appeal held that the vasectomy would not be in A's best interests.[30]

Abortion

A person with learning disabilities who has the capacity to give a valid consent could sign the form for an abortion to be carried out provided that the requirements of the Abortion Act 1967 (as amended by the Human Fertilisation and Embryology Act 1990) are met, unless an emergency situation exists. Where the adult with learning disabilities lacks competence, then the Mental Capacity Act 2005 would now apply. Paragraphs 6.18–6.19 of the Code of Practice point out that some treatment decisions are so serious that they must be made by the Court and it includes within this category termination of pregnancy in certain circumstances. The court has also given guidance on when certain termination of pregnancy cases should be brought before the court.[31]

Property and exploitation

The duty of care owed by the health professional to care for a client would also include a duty of care in relation to any property of the client. Where the client has the capacity to look after his or her own property, then the health professional does not become responsible for that property unless it has been specifically entrusted to his/her care or unless the client has become incapacitated and cannot care for the property him- or herself. The new Court of Protection set up in October 2007 has a remit to make decisions on behalf of mentally incapacitated adults in respect of personal welfare and property and financial decisions. A deputy could be appointed to make decisions in relation to any property or financial interests of an adult lacking mental capacity. The jurisdiction of the Court of Protection is normally restricted to those over 16 years but where it is anticipated that the lack of the requisite mental capacity could continue beyond 16 years then it can hear cases involving persons who are younger than 16 years. For example, if a child was severely injured in a road accident that led to serious brain damage and received a payment for several million pounds as a consequence, the Court of Protection could hear an application relating to his/her case since the disability will persist beyond 16 years.

Situation: care of property

A physiotherapist visits a community home for five people with learning disabilities. Her client has wealthy parents who have provided him with expensive electrical goods. She sees him in his room and suggests that they go outside to carry out some exercises. When they return, a compact disc player, stereo system and cassette player have been stolen. Does the physiotherapist have any liability for these missing goods?

Normally such goods would be the responsibility of the resident but where the mental competence of the resident was such that he could not be expected to take care of the property the home would be expected to arrange safe custody. The physiotherapist, before leaving the room, should have checked if it were normal practice for the room to be locked and who had custody of the key. If, on the other hand, the resident had the mental capacity to secure his own room and had been provided with a key but failed to do so, then neither the physiotherapist nor the home manager would be liable.

Special precautions have to be taken in the care of those with learning disabilities who may be vulnerable to exploitation and who may not have the capacity to care for their own property. Any moneys belonging to the client and handled by staff must be strictly accounted for and records kept. Facilities should be provided for cash or other valuables to be safely stored and care should also be taken to prevent one client misappropriating property belonging to another. The Court of Protection and the Office of Public Guardian provide for the security of property of those who, by reason of mental incapacity, are unable to care for it themselves. (See Chapter 10 for further discussion on liability for property.)

For a discussion of the Community Care (Direct Payments) Act 1996 see Chapter 18.

Future strategy

The White Paper, *Valuing People*,[32] in 2001 set out the aim of investing at least £1.3 million a year for the next 3 years to develop advocacy services for people with learning disabilities in partnership with the voluntary sector in order to enable people with learning disabilities to have as much choice and control as possible over their lives and the services and support they receive. The eligibility for direct payments was to be extended through legislation. In addition, a national forum for people with learning disabilities was to be set up to enable them to benefit from the improvement and expansion of community equipment services now under way. New guidance on person-centred planning was to be issued with resources for implementation through the Learning Disability Development Fund.

In spite of the White Paper, it was reported on 15 June 2005 in *Frontline* (available from the CSP website)[33] by Caroline Hodges that the future of learning disabilities as a specialty within physiotherapy was uncertain, partly because so few undergraduates are aware of this area of work or of the opportunities it offers. Following a scandal in Cornwall, where significant failings were found at Buddock Hospital (a unit for 14 patients with severe disabilities) the Healthcare Commission carried out a national audit of learning disability services and then consulted on a 3-year plan.[34] The 3-year plan envisaged:

- audit of all in-patient care being provided for learning disability service users across the NHS and independent sector, including commissioning arrangements;
- investigation into long-stay hospitals to ensure that they are providing a safe and acceptable service;
- review of the care of people with learning disabilities who are placed outside their local area away from family and friends;
- increase the accessibility of the Commission's services so that people with a learning disability can better raise complaints and concerns about their care;
- establish champions at the regional offices of the Healthcare Commission responsible for monitoring services for people with a disability.

The response from the CSP to the 3-year strategy consultation can be found on its website.

In December 2006 as a result of the Equality Act, public bodies were placed under a new disability equality duty to ensure that their organisations had a policy to identify and eradicate discrimination against disabled people. Public authorities are required to carry out six duties:

- to promote equality of opportunity between disabled and other persons
- to eliminate discrimination that is unlawful under the Disability Discrimination Act 1995;
- to eliminate harassment related to their disabilities;
- to promote positive attitudes;
- to encourage participation in public life;
- to take account of their disabilities, even where that involves them more favourably than other persons.

It remains to be seen how effective this duty is in relation to those with learning disabilities.

Conclusion

It is apparent that this topic could form a book in its own right and it has only been possible to touch the surface of the many legal issues that arise for the physiotherapist who cares for those with learning disabilities. The strategy set out in the White Paper *Valuing People* should in theory lead to the appropriate resources being made available for this client group. The follow up consultation document, *Valuing People Now*, should ensure that the implementation of the policy remains a high priority for the DH. The consultation recognised that strong local and national leadership would be required over the next 3 years to ensure the vision became a reality. In addition, the establishment of a new multi-inspection agency in the form of the Care Quality Commission (see Chapter 17) should reinforce appropriate standards of care in health and social care settings. Mencap[35] is a useful source for further information on good practice, standards of care and many other aspects in the care of those with learning disabilities. The regulation of children's services moved from CSCI to the Office for Standards in Education, Childrens Services and Skills (Ofsted in 2007. Reference should be made to the other general chapters covering areas such as professional accountability, health and safety and the different rights of the client, and to the more specialist works included in the bibliography.

✍️ Questions and exercises

1 It is suggested that one of your clients with learning disabilities should go for a week's holiday by the seaside. In carrying out a risk assessment for this client, what aspects would you take into account?

2 The mother of a girl with severe learning disabilities who is now 13 years has asked you to assist in ensuring that she will be sterilised as soon as possible. What action would you take and what advice would you give the mother?

3 You are aware that one of your clients with learning disabilities, who lives in a community home and who has a private income from a family trust fund, is extremely generous with his money and is being exploited by the other residents. What action would you take and what is the law?

4 You have been asked to assist a charity that organises outdoor activities for those with learning disabilities. You would like to help but are uncertain of the legal situation. What are the legal implications of accepting the invitation?

5 What are the implications of the Mental Capacity Act 2005 for the making of decisions on behalf of those who have severe learning disabilities? (See Chapter 7)

References

1 *X and Y* v. *London Borough of Hounslow* [2008] EWHC 1168 (QB) 23 June 2008.
2 Fraser, R. (1994) Physiotherapy in Learning Disability. *ACPPLD Journal*, October, 10–14.
3 Department of Health (2001) White Paper. *Valuing People: A New Strategy for Learning Disability for the 21st Century.* CM 5086. The Stationery Office, London.
4 Department of Health (2007) White Paper. *Valuing People Now – From Progress to Transformation* – a consultation on the next three years of learning disability policy. DH, London.
5 www.mencap.org.uk
6 Knapp, M.B., Strade, C.L. (1984) Sexuality and the Developmentally Delayed Teenager. In: *Human Sexuality* (ed. N. Fulgate-Woods). Mosby, London.
7 Grimmer, M. (1993) A bad case of housemaid's knee. *ACPPLD Journal*, January, 2.
8 *F* v. *West Berkshire Health Authority and Another* [1989] 2 All ER 545.
9 www.chre.org.uk
10 The Mental Capacity Act 2005 (Independent Mental Capacity Advocates) (Expansion of Role) Regulations 2006 SI 2006 No 2883.
11 Department of Health (2005) Green Paper. *Independence, Well-being and Choice.* DH, London.
12 Department of Health (2006) *Our health, Our Care, Our Say: A New Direction for Community Services.* DH, London.
13 Department of Health (2007) *Independence, Choice and Risk: a Guide to Best Practice in Supported Decision Making.* DH, London.
14 Chartered Society of Physiotherapy (2007) *Safe Practice in Rebound Therapy.* PA 89 CSP, London.
15 Chartered Society of Physiotherapy with ACPTR (1999) *Standards of Physiotherapy Practice in Therapeutic Riding.* CSP, London.
16 Law Commission (1995) Report No. 231. *Mental Incapacity.* HMSO, London.
17 Lord Chancellor's Office (1997) *Who Decides?* HMSO, London.
18 Dimond, B. (2008) *Legal Aspects of Mental Capacity.* Blackwell Publishing, Oxford
19 *R* v. *Bournewood Community and Mental Health NHS Trust, ex parte L.* (HL) reported in *The Times*, 30 June 1998, [1998] 3 All ER 289.
20 *HL* v. *United Kingdom* [2004] ECHR 720 Application No 45508/99 5 October 2004; Times Law Report, 19 October 2004

21 *Local Authority X* v. *MM* [2007] EWHC 2003 Fam.

22 *Re M B (Caesarian Section)* [1997] 2 FLR 426; [1997] 2 F.C.R. 541; The Times Law Report, 18 April 1997.

23 Code of Practice Mental Capacity Act 2005 Department of Constitutional Affairs February 2007 Paragraph 8.56.

24 www.justice.gov.uk

25 *R* v. *Hudson Court of Criminal Appeal* [1965] 1 All ER 721.

26 Royal College of Nursing/Society of Mental Handicap (1991) *Nursing AIDS – a Proactive Approach to Mental Handicap.* Scutari Press, Harrow.

27 Dimond, B.C. (1988) *Ethical and Legal Issues Raised by the Sterilisation of the Mentally Handicapped.* MA thesis, University College Swansea.

28 *In Re D (a minor) (wardship: sterilisation)* [1976] 1 All ER 326.

29 *In Re B (a minor) (wardship: sterilisation)* [1987] 2 WLR 1213.

30 *Re A (medical treatment: male sterilisation)* (1999) 53 BMLR 66

31 *D* v. *An NHS Trust (Medical Treatment: Consent: Termination)* [2004] 1 FLR 1110

32 White Paper *Valuing People A New Strategy for Learning Disability for the 21st Century.* CM 5086. March 2001, The Stationery Office

33 www.csp.org.uk

34 Healthcare Commission (2005) *Three Year Plan for Adults with Learning Disabilities.* Stationery Office, London.

35 www.mencap.org.uk

23 Care of Babies, Children and Young Persons

The physiotherapist can make a considerable contribution to the care of children, from the special care baby unit to the child with special needs and working with the adolescent. Each division within a childcare and young person's specialty requires its own procedures and protocols.

It is not possible in a work of this kind to cover all the many laws that relate to the care of the child and the physiotherapist may need to refer to some of the more specialist works on child law. The aim in this chapter is to give to the physiotherapist who works with these groups an overview of the main principles of law applying to the care and rights of the child and young person.[1] Some of the textbooks on physiotherapy in paediatrics cover the legal dimensions. For example, in Chapter 1 in *Physiotherapy for Children*,[2] edited by Teresa Pountney, Julia Graham provides an ethical and legal framework of paediatric physiotherapy practice and in Chapter 2 Sarah Crombie sets out the legislation and government guidance covering special needs and education. Physiotherapists would also find *Disabled Children and the Law* by Read et al.[3] a useful resource. The Chartered Society of Physiotherapy (CSP) has published information to guide good practice for physiotherapists working with children.[4] It covers the legal and ethical framework, key factors that support the delivery of paediatric physiotherapy services, and provides useful general information on sports and leisure, specialist holidays and voluntary agencies and support groups. Information is also available from the website of the Department for Children, Schools and Families[5] and from the specific website set up by the Department of Health for child protection.[6]

The following topics will be covered in this chapter:

- The Rights of the Child
- The Children Act 1989
- Child protection
- The Children Act 2004
- Education and training requirements
- Special educational needs
- Consent by children
- Confidentiality of child information
- Access of the child to health records
- Standards in the care of children: the National Service Framework

Reference should also be made to Chapters 20, 21 and 22, which cover the law relating to the physically disabled, mentally ill and those with learning disabilities. Chapter 13 on giving evidence in court will also be useful for those who are involved in child protection issues. For the law in relation to the dying child reference should be made to Chapter 25.

The Rights of the child

The United Nations Convention on the Rights of the Child was ratified by the UK government in 1991 but it has not been incorporated into the laws of the UK. The opportunity to include its recognition in the Children Act 2004 was not taken. There is, however, a biennial review that reports on the extent of compliance by the UK with the convention requirements. In contrast, the European Convention on Human Rights (ECHR) was incorporated into the law of the UK under the Human Rights Act 1998. Schedule 1 of the Human Rights Act 1998 (which can be seen in Appendix 1 of this book) sets out those rights that are binding on public authorities or organisations exercising functions of a public

nature. Article 14 states that these rights must be recognised without any discrimination. Although age is not listed as a type of discrimination in that Article, it is implicitly included. This means that any child or young person is entitled to bring (or be represented in bringing) an action against a public authority that has ignored his or her rights. Other rights are recognised in specific legislation such as the Children Act of 1989 and 2004, and the Family Law Reform Act 1969.

The Children Act 1989

This Act set up a new framework for the protection and care of children and established clear principles to guide decision making in relation to their care. The principles that the court should take into account are shown in Figure 23.1. The overriding principle is that 'the child's welfare shall be the court's paramount consideration'.

The involvement of the child in the decision making is also a major principle and Figure 23.2 sets out the considerations which the court

---

(1) The welfare of the child is the paramount consideration in court proceedings
(2) Wherever possible children should be brought up and cared for in their own families
(3) Courts should ensure that delay is avoided, and may only make an order if to do so is better than making no order at all
(4) Children should be kept informed about what happens to them, and should participate when decisions are made about their future
(5) Parents continue to have parental responsibility for their children, even when their children are no longer living with them. They should be kept informed about their children and participate when decisions are made about their children's future
(6) Parents with children in need should be helped to bring up their children themselves
(7) This help should be provided as a service to the child and his family, and should:
    (a) be provided in partnership with parents
    (b) meet each child's identified needs
    (c) be appropriate to the child's race, culture, religion, and language
    (d) be open to effective independent representations and complaints procedures and
    (e) draw upon effective partnership between the local authority and other agencies including voluntary agencies

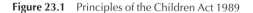

Figure 23.1 Principles of the Children Act 1989

(a)   The ascertainable wishes and feelings of the child concerned (considered in the light of his/her age and understanding)

(b)   his/her physical, emotional and educational needs

(c)   the likely effect on him/her of any change in his/her circumstances

(d)   his/her age, sex, background and any characteristics of his/her which the court considers relevant

(e)   any harm that he/she has suffered or is at risk of suffering

(f)   how capable each of his/her parents, and any other person in relation to whom the court considers the question to be relevant, is of meeting his/her needs

(g)   the range of powers available to the court under this Act in the proceedings in question

Finally, in deciding whether or not to make an order, the court shall not make the order or any of the orders unless it considers that doing so would be better for the child than making no order at all. (Section 1(5) [i.e. whoever started the proceedings, there has to be a positive advantage to the child in moving away from the status quo]

Figure 23.2   Circumstances to be taken into account by the court under the Children Act 1989: Section 1(3)

should take into account in making certain orders.

Although the considerations set out in Figure 23.2 apply to specific decisions to be made under the Children Act 1989, there is good reason for the physiotherapist to follow these same considerations in his/her care of the child.

It is not possible to cover the full contents of the Children Act 1989 but Figure 23.3 sets out the parts of the Act and the main areas which the Act covers. The House of Lords held that where care proceedings under the Children Act 1989 were being held, the test to be used was the civil test of the balance of probabilities. Care proceedings were there to protect the child from harm. The consequences for the child of getting it wrong were equally serious either way.[7] The duties and powers of the local authority under

Part I	Introductory (general principles relating to the welfare of the child, 'parental responsibility' and the appointment of guardians)
Part II	Orders With respect to Children in Family Proceedings
Part III	Local Authority Support for Children and Families
Part IV	Care and Supervision
Part V	Protection of Children
Part VI	Community Homes
Part VII	Voluntary Homes and Voluntary Organisations
Part VIII	Registered Children's Homes
Part IX	Private Arrangements for Fostering Children
Part X	Child Minding and Day Care for Young Children
Part XI	Secretary of State's Supervisory Functions and Responsibilities
Part XII	Miscellaneous and General (including the duty to notify the local authority of children accommodated in different establishments, tests to establish paternity, criminal offences, search warrants, and the jurisdiction of the courts)

Figure 23.3   Summary of main areas of the Children Act 1989

the Chronically Sick and Disabled Persons Act 1970 (see Chapter 20) can be combined with those under the Children Act 1989. For example in the case of *R (on the application of BG)* v. *Medway Council*[8] the Court held that the funding by the local authority to provide adaptations to the family home to provide for a disabled child was acceptable. The boy was 3 years old with severe mental and physical disabilities, including four-limb cerebral palsy, epilepsy, asthma and sleep problems. He needed assistance with all aspects of daily living and mobility. The family was suffering from sleep deprivation because there was insufficient space to cater for his needs. Adaptations were required to create more space, so that he could have his own room, and for more storage space for his equipment and to provide room for his treatment such as daily physiotherapy. The adaptations would cost £65 000. The local authority planned to meet the shortfall in the costs of the works remaining after the maximum available disability facility grant (DFG) by a loan secured on the home, which would be discharged after 20 years without any requirement for repayment. The loan was subject to conditions, so that the authority would not seek repayment unless the claimant ceased to live at the home during these 20 years. The father sought judicial review of the conditions on the loan. The court held that the relevant conditions were not unreasonable.

Children in need

Section 17 of the Children Act 1989 places a general duty on the local authority in relation to children in need.

It shall be the duty of every local authority (in addition to the other duties imposed on them by this Part):

- to safeguard and promote the welfare of children within their area who are in need;
- so far as is consistent with that duty, to promote the upbringing of such children by

their families, by providing a range and level of services appropriate to those children's needs.

This section was considered by the House of Lords in three appeals[9] over the responsibilities of local authorities for the accommodation of children who were in need.

R (on the application of A) v. Lambeth London Borough Council; R (on the application of G) v. Barnet London Borough Council and R (on the application of W) v. Lambeth Borough Council 2003

The claimants' case was that Section 17(1) required a local social services authority to assess the needs of a child who was in need, and to meet his needs when they had been assessed. They also considered whether a local authority might insist on providing accommodation for a child alone, as distinct from a child and his mother, when a child was in need of accommodation and it would cost no more to provide accommodation for both of them. The first appeal concerned two children who were in need because they were disabled, in the other two appeals, the children were in need because their mothers, with whom they were living were homeless. The House of Lords held in a majority judgment that Section 17(1) did not impose on local social services a duty to meet the assessed needs of a child. The section set out duties of a general character that were intended to be for the benefit of children in need in the local social services authority's area in general. Although the services under Section 17 could include the provision of accommodation, the provision of residential accommodation to re-house a child in need so that he could live with his family was not the principal or primary purpose of the legislation. Housing was the function of the local housing authority, for the acquisition and management of whose housing stock detailed provisions were contained in the Housing Acts. The local authority could insist on providing accommodation for a child alone. A local authority is entitled to adopt a general policy under which it is made clear that it will make accommodation available to the children of the family in order to prevent the children becoming homeless, but will not permit parents to use the children as stepping stones by means of which to obtain a greater priority to be re-housed than that to which they would otherwise be entitled.

In another dispute over Section 17 of the Children Act 1989 and Section 2 of the Chronically Sick and Disabled Persons Act 1970 and the provision of services to a child in need, the claimant argued that the local authority had failed to act reasonably and infringed the Article 8 rights of the child Z.[10] Z suffered from Sanfilippo syndrome, a disease like juvenile dementia, which was degenerative and life limiting. Her mother was her sole carer and an independent review recommended a care plan that suggested that the mother should no longer remain the primary carer and that there should be two carers around the clock. The plan was rejected by the council and the mother on behalf of the child claimed that this action amounted to Wednesbury unreasonableness (the Wednesbury[11] case laid down the principle that court will intervene to prevent or remedy abuses of power by public authorities if there is evidence of unreasonableness or perversity). The High Court judge analysed the independent review and concluded that the council had not acted unreasonably in deciding that the current care plan was adequate nor did he find any breach of Article 8 in that there was no evidence that the disabled person was not so circumscribed and so isolated as to be deprived of the possibility of developing his personality.

Child protection

Where a physiotherapist is concerned that a child in his/her care, or the sibling or child of one of his/her patients, is being abused, whether physically, sexually or mentally, the physiotherapist should take immediate action to ensure

that this is drawn to the attention of the appropriate persons. This means that he/she must be familiar with the provisions for child protection and who are the persons to be contacted. It is not always easy to decide if action is necessary and the physiotherapist should see as his/her main priority the safety of the child. As the guidelines on inter-agency cooperation state:[12]

> The difficulties of assessing the risk of harm to a child should not be under-estimated. It is imperative that everyone who deals with allegations and suspicions of abuse maintains an open and inquiring mind. (Paragraph 1.13)

Should the physiotherapist be wrong in her fears, and it appears that there is no abuse, his/her name could not be divulged to the parents.[13] Nor if his/her actions were reasonably taken in the best interests of the child would a parent have a right of action against the physiothrapist[14] (see below). Abuse may include an over-zealous dietary or religious regime. For example, a 12-year-old girl was brought up on a strict vegan diet and was admitted to hospital with a degenerative bone condition said to have left her with the spine of an 80-year-old woman.[15]

Procedure for the management of child abuse

There should be in existence an agreed procedure for the management of child abuse cases and the physiotherapist should be acquainted with this. The procedure should specifically refer to the role of the physiotherapy department if child abuse is suspected. This would require any professional staff working in the department who suspect that there is a possibility of ill treatment, serious neglect, or sexual or emotional abuse of a child to inform the senior physiotherapist in charge of the department who should contact a consultant paediatrician. If the consultant confirms the possibility of abuse, then the social services department should be informed immediately.

Children Act 2004

The death of Victoria Climbié led to an inquiry conducted by Lord Laming. His report is available from the internet.[16] The Department of Health published a detailed response, *Keeping Children Safe*,[17] and this was followed by a single source document for safeguarding children.[18] This document aims to provide a single set of advice for all those involved in the care of children, which replaces local guidance. It was followed by a Green Paper, *Every Child Matters*,[19] published in September 2003. The Green Paper focuses on four main areas:

(1)   supporting parents and carers
(2)   early intervention and effective protection
(3)   accountability and integration – locally, regionally and nationally
(4)   workforce reform.

The Children Act 2004 provides the legal underpinning for *Every Child Matters* and its provisions are shown in Figure 23.4 and was followed by the publication *Working Together to Safeguard Children*.[20] Significant features of the Children Act 2004 include the new Local Safeguarding Children's Boards (LSCBs) (which each local authority is required to set up under Section 13), and the duty on local authorities to appoint a director of children's services and a lead member for children's services. The LSCBs, which came into being on 1 April 2006, are designed to ensure that the agencies work effectively together to protect children. The old area child protection committees which they replace are in effect placed on a statutory footing. The core membership includes local authorities, health boards, the police and others. Guidance on the functioning of the LSCBs is obtainable on the Every Child Matters website.[6] The guidance is incorporated as Chapter 3 of *Working Together to Safeguard Children*, which was published in 2006. The guidance describes the LSCBs as 'the key statutory mechanism for agreeing how the relevant organisations in each local area agree to co-operate to safeguard and promote the welfare of children in the locality and for ensuring the effectiveness of what they do'.

Advice for LSCBs on safeguards for protecting disabled children was published in February 2006.[21] Disabled children are more vulnerable to abuse or neglect than non-disabled children. The resource is intended to help those with a strategic or planning responsibility for children to understand their particular needs and consider how best to safeguard and promote their welfare. Supplementary guidance has also been published for LSCBs on safeguarding children in whom illness is fabricated or induced.[22]

Part 1 Children's Commissioner
Part 2 Children's services in England: Co-operation to improve wellbeing
Arrangements to safeguard and promote welfare
Information databases
Local Safeguarding Children Boards:
establishment, functions, procedure and funding;
Children and young people's plans
Director of children's services
Lead member for children's services
Inspections of children's services
Part 3 Children's Services in Wales
Part 4 Advisory and support services for family proceedings

Figure 23.4   Main Provisions of Children Act 2004

Following the Lord Laming inquiry into the death of Victoria Climbié the Joint Chief Inspectors reported on safeguarding arrangements for children and young people in England. The Healthcare Commission is contributing to the third joint Chief Inspector's Report on Safeguarding children which was published in July 2008. The regulation of children's services moved from the Commission for Social Care Inspection to the Office for Standards in Education, Children's Services and Skills (Ofsted) in 2007. This Office reviews the work of local safeguarding children boards.

In spite of the changes following the Children Act 2004, serious failings in protecting children still arise. A baby girl died at 54 days old after she was abused and then murdered by her father. She might have been saved had 30 health and social services staff not missed vital signs that she was being ill treated.[23] In May 2008 Khyra Ishaq, 7 years old, apparently starved to death, despite an initial welfare check on the family in January 2008. Her mother and her mother's partner were accused of causing or allowing her death contrary to Section 5 of the Domestic Violence, Crime and Victims Act 2004. The House of Lords criticised the fact that the Housing Services and the Children's services did not communicate with each other in a case brought by a girl of 18 who was held not to be entitled to further council support in her own right. She had been provided with accommodation by the local authority's housing department but had not come to the attention of the children's services department and so was not entitled to further support.[24] The Housing Department should have referred her to the children's services so that she would have become a relevant child for the purposes of the duties of the children's department. The Court of Appeal held that there was no breach of the mother's right to a fair hearing under Article 6 of the European Convention on Human Rights when she was represented by the Official Solicitor in a case concerning a care order for her child. The Court of Appeal held that the Official Solicitor was right to concede that the threshold criteria under Section 31 of the Children Act 1989 were satisfied and that a care order was in the child's best interests.[25] The employment checks required for those who work with children and vulnerable persons are considered in Chapter 17.

The role of the physiotherapist

What if the doctor disagrees with the physiotherapist?

The physiotherapist should ensure that his/her concerns are made known to a senior member of the physiotherapy department who should decide whether it is appropriate to bring the consultant in to see the child. It is important to ensure that the physiotherapist records in writing all the facts that have given rise to his/her suspicions and fears and keeps a copy of this document. If the consultant subsequently takes the view that there is no abuse, then the physiotherapist has to accept this, but he/she should remain vigilant about the safety of the child and continue to report any concerns. The Department for Children, Schools and Families has published a statement on the duties of doctors and other health professionals in investigations of child abuse which is available on line.[26]

Errors in suspecting child abuse

The House of Lords has held that there is no right of action by parents, where children have been taken into care as a result of suspected child abuse, which has subsequently been shown not to exist.[14] In this case in East Berkshire, a mother was suspected of Munchausen's syndrome by proxy when her son suffered from allergic reactions following birth and he was placed on the 'at risk' register. However, it was subsequently discovered that he did have allergy problems. The mother claimed compensation on the grounds that the original diagnosis was made negligently. The House of Lords held that it would not be fair, just or reasonable to impose a duty of care on a doctor in respect of a negligent clinical diagnosis where there was a concurrent and potentially conflicting duty of care towards a child patient. No duty of care was owed to the parents. The East Berkshire case was followed in a case where a father of a child, who had been suspected of sexual abuse, brought a claim against the local authority. It was held that a duty of care was not owed by the social workers to the parents where the children were the subject of an investigation, whether the social workers were carrying out operational functions such as interviewing or relaying the results of the interview, or evaluating evidence and deciding whether intervention was necessary.[27]

What about the physiotherapist's duty of confidentiality?

Reference to Rule 3 of the *Rules of Professional Conduct*[28] on confidentiality will show that the Rule recognises that certain apparent breaches of confidentiality are justified:

> 3.3 Evidence of abuse
> Physical, sexual or psychological – either of the patient or another involved party. Immediate discussions with a senior colleague and referral to an appropriate professional, such as a doctor, a health visitor or an agency such as Social Services is essential. The Children Act (1989) provides clear guidance to professionals when abuse of children is discovered.

If the physiotherapist is in doubt, then he/she should seek advice. Any reasonable suspicion of child abuse should be notified to the appropriate agencies without fear of a successful action for breach of confidentiality by the parents (see Chapter 8).

If a suspected case is reported to the police, social services, or NSPCC and it turns out that the suspicions are unfounded, the parents have no right to be given the name of the person reporting them. The House of Lords has held that it is not in the public interest for such information to be disclosed to the parents.[13] The following is a situation encountered in private practice.

Situation: don't tell any one

A physiotherapist practising privately was treating the elbow of a girl of 14 years. At the second visit, the daughter did not want her mother in the room. The physiotherapist saw evidence of self-harm on the girl's arm. She asked the physiotherapist not to tell her mother. The physiotherapist promised the girl that she would not disclose this. Subsequently she changed her mind when the mother phoned to inquire as to why the daughter had wanted to be seen alone. They did not come for a further appointment. What action should the physiotherapist have taken?

A girl under 16 years old is able to give consent to treatment if she is mentally capable of understanding the issues and is considered to be 'Gillick competent' (see below). She can also request that her confidentiality is respected. However, a refusal to give consent to treatment which is considered to be necessary in her best interests can be overruled and an exception to the duty of confidentiality is where disclosure is justified in her best interests. In view of these principles, it is extremely unwise for a physiotherapist to offer confidentiality in a situation where there are exceptions to it. The physiotherapist should not have promised the girl that she would not tell her mother. Perhaps it would have been advisable, if reasonably practicable, for the mother to have been brought into the consulting room to talk together with physiotherapist and daughter over future action. A breach of confidentiality is only justified in these circumstances if serious harm is feared for the life of the patient or another person. The physiotherapist should document carefully the factors that led her to make her decision.

The Integrated Children's System (replacing child protection registers)

In *Working Together to Safeguard Children* the Government stated that child protection registers would be phased out by 1 April 2008 and replaced by the Integrated Children's System

(ICS). Each local authority is required to ensure that its local ICS is able to use data from the ICS child protection plans. The ICS has been developed to improve outcomes for children defined as being in need, under the Children Act 1989. It provides a conceptual framework, a method of practice and a business process to support practitioners and managers in undertaking the key tasks of assessment, planning, intervention and review. It is based on an understanding of children's developmental needs in the context of parental capacity and wider family and environmental factors. It is supported by an electronic case record system. A key aim of ICS is to provide frontline staff and their managers with the necessary help, through information communication technology, to record, collate, analyse and output the information required. Further information on the ICS and the technical details are available from the Every Child Matters website.[29] The aims of ICS are set out in Figure 23.5. All authorities were required to have the ICT support for all new referrals in place by 1 January 2006 and to be fully operational by 1 January 2007.

- What if the child is not known to social services and abuse is not certain?

If the consultant was not able to confirm that this was a case of suspected child abuse and there were no medical grounds for requiring the child to be detained in hospital, then the parent could not be stopped from taking the child home.

However, there should be arrangements in place for all such concerns to be notified to the appropriate health visitor or school nurse, and also to the appropriate GP.

When suspected child abuse is confirmed

If the consultant paediatrician confirms the suspected child abuse the agreed procedures and the inter-agency arrangements should be followed immediately. The provisions of the Children Act 1989 enable the following orders to be made. For further details of these orders and the other provisions of the Children Acts of 1989 and 2004 reference should be made to the Department of Health guides to the Children Acts 1989 and 2004.[30]

Child assessment order: Section 43

This is available where:

- the court is satisfied that the applicant has reasonable cause to suspect that the child is suffering or likely to suffer significant harm;
- an assessment is required to determine whether or not the child is suffering or is likely to suffer significant harm; and
- it is unlikely that an assessment can be carried out without an order being made.

Notice must be given of an application for a child assessment order to:

- All practitioners and managers, responsible for children in need, should work in accordance with the ICS conceptual framework, from case referral to case closure
- Assessments of children in need should be completed with the necessary detail and within the required timescales
- Case-based information should be aggregated through computer systems into management information, required for day-to-day service planning
- All practitioners should feel they are supported in their work by working directly with Information Communication Technology (ICT) systems that support ICS

Figure 23.5   Aims of the Integrated Children's System (ICS)

- the child's parents;
- any person, not the parent, but who has parental responsibility for the child;
- any other person caring for the child; and
- others who have a contact order.

The child assessment order cannot not be made if the court is satisfied that there are grounds for making an emergency protection order (see below) and that it ought to make that order rather than an assessment order.

The order must specify the date by which the assessment is to begin and have effect for a specified period not exceeding 7 days beginning with that date. The effect of the order is to authorise any person carrying out the assessment, or any part of the assessment, to do so in accordance with the terms of the order (Section 43(7)). The child has the right, if he/she is of sufficient understanding to make an informed decision, to refuse to submit to a medical or psychiatric examination or other assessment (Section 43(8)).

Emergency protection order: Section 44

If the court is satisfied that there is reasonable cause to believe (in the case of a personal application) that the child is likely to suffer significant harm if

- he/she is not removed to accommodation provided by or on behalf of the applicant, or
- he/she does not remain in the place in which he/she is then being accommodated, then the court can order that an emergency protection order be made.

Where the applicant is a local authority it must show that:

- enquiries are being made under Section 47(1)(b) (the local authority's duty to investigate);
- these enquiries are being frustrated by access to the child being unreasonably refused;
- and the applicant has reasonable cause to believe that access to the child is required as a matter of urgency (Section 44(1)(b)).

An application may also be made by the NSPCC as an authorised person.

Removal and accommodation of children by police in cases of emergency: Section 46

This section enables the child to be taken in to police protection. Where a constable believes that a child would be likely to suffer significant harm he/she may remove the child to suitable accommodation and keep the child there. The constable may also take reasonable steps to ensure that the child's removal from hospital, or any other place in which he/she is being accommodated, is prevented. The section, once invoked, lasts a maximum of 72 hours.

A new scheme is being piloted by Community Service Volunteers in Bromley and Sunderland with volunteers who do not have a social work background working with the families of children on the at-risk register.[31]

Education and training requirements

The physiotherapist who works with children should ensure that as far as possible arrangements are made for the child to receive education. She should therefore liaise with the local authority in whatever arrangements have been made and are appropriate for a specific child. Arrangements for the education of the sick child might include the following:

- the establishment of hospital special schools.
- hospital teaching units/hospital classes which are not formally classified as hospital schools;
- home tuition.

The following section considers the effect of the statutory duties upon home tuition and the next one looks at the law on assessing and meeting special educational needs. Further information is available from the website of the Department for Children, Schools and Families.[5] A debate has been commenced on the CSP interactive site on the role of physiotherapists in schools in order to develop guidelines.[32]

Home tuition

The statutory duty

The Education Act 1993 (Section 298(1) now consolidated in Section 19(1) of the Education Act 1996) placed a duty on local education authorities (LEAs) to provide suitable education for children out of school for reasons of illness or otherwise. The full subsection is set out in Figure 23.6.

The duty set out in Figure 23.6 applies to children of compulsory school age and the duty is mandatory, i.e. the LEA *shall make arrangements*. In contrast, the duty in relation to those above compulsory school age is permissive. This is set out in Section 19(4) of the Education Act 1996 and is shown in Figure 23.7.

Suitable provision is defined in relation to a child or young person in Section 19(6) as 'efficient education suitable to his age, ability and aptitude and to any special educational needs he may have'.

Government guidance

Home tuition is not expected to be provided for very short absences from school. Four weeks or more away from school is considered to be the point at which home tuition can be provided. Below that length of time it would normally be expected that the school would itself provide home work to be done outside school. However, it is a question of discretion, and some LEAs provide home tuition for 3 weeks away from school if the need exists. Calculation would obviously take into account the length of time that the child has already been in hospital with or without tuition.

LEAs should have a written policy on home tuition that covers the organisation and staffing of the service, the timing of provision and giving a named contact for parents, hospital teachers and others. Parents who brought an application to review a reduction in the hours of home tuition from 5 hours to 3 hours per week won in the High Court but the local authority's appeal succeeded. The Court of Appeal applied the ruling in the Gloucester case[33] (see Chapter 20), where the House of Lords accepted that resources were relevant in fulfilling a statutory duty. The Court of Appeal held that the authority was justified in balancing the individual's requirements against the cost of making arrangements.[34]

Each local education authority shall make arrangements for the provision of suitable full-time or part-time education at school or otherwise than at school for those children of compulsory school age who, by reason of illness, exclusion from school or otherwise, may not for any period receive suitable education unless such arrangements are made for them.

Figure 23.6　Section 19(1) Education Act 1996

The local education authority may make arrangements for the provision of suitable full time or part time education otherwise than at school for those young persons who, by reason of illness, exclusion from school of otherwise, may not for any period receive suitable education unless such arrangements are made for them.

Figure 23.7　Section 19(4) Education Act 1996

The contribution of the physiotherapist

With fewer children staying in hospital for long periods, and more caring and treatment taking place in the community, those children suffering from a chronic condition are more likely to benefit from home tuition. The physiotherapist should ensure that he/she works closely with the tutor and the school in caring for the child.

The National Association for the Education of Sick Children (NAESC) was set up to relieve the educational disadvantages suffered by sick children. It published the results of a survey on the provision by LEAs, the teaching available, home tuition and the falling number of hospital schools.[35] The NAESC has a government grant to monitor the effects of implementing the new duty.

Special educational needs

Part IV of the Education Act 1996 (replacing Part III of the Education Act 1993) covers provision for children with special educational needs. A summary of its main provisions is shown in Figure 23.8. A Green Paper, *Excellence for All Children: Meeting Special Educational Needs*, was published by the Government in 1997 and led to revised regulations. A report, *Special Education Needs: a Mainstream Issue*, was published in 2002, which identified continuing challenges in the provision of special educational needs (SEN)

services. The Green Paper *Every Child Matters* (2003) envisaged early intervention, inclusion and the raising of expectations and achievement and the development of partnership networks. In 2004 the Department for Education and Skills published a strategy for SEN[36] which identified weaknesses in the services offered at that time and set out objectives for improvement and makes specific commitments for future action. Under this strategy children trusts were required to review the policies on SEN and the support available to ensure:

- effective delegation of resources to support early intervention and inclusion;
- reduced reliance on SEN statements;
- appropriate provision;
- better specialist advice and support to schools and information to parents;
- a reduction in bureaucracy.

A Good Practice Guidance on commissioning placements and services for looked after children and children with special educational needs and disabilities in residential placements was published by the DfES in June 2005 and is available from its website.

Definition of disability and special educational needs

Under the Children Act 1989 Section 17(11) a child is disabled

---

- Meaning of 'special educational needs' and 'special educational provision' etc. – Section 312 Education Act 1996
- Code of Practice – Sections 313 to 314
- Special educational provision – Sections 315 to 320
- Identification and Assessment of children with special educational needs – Sections 321 to 332
- Special Educational Needs Tribunal (SENT) – Sections 333 to 336 (now SENDIST)
- Special Schools and Independent Schools – Sections 337 to 348
- Variation of deeds (changing a school's constitution) – Section 349

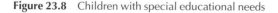

Figure 23.8 Children with special educational needs

> (1) For the purposes of the Education Acts, a child has 'special educational needs' if he has a learning difficulty which calls for special educational provision to be made for him.
> (2) For the purposes of this Act, subject to subsection (3) below, a child has a 'learning difficulty' if:
>   (a) he has a significantly greater difficulty in learning than the majority of children of his age;
>   (b) he has a disability which either prevents or hinders him from making use of educational facilities of a kind generally provided for children of his age in schools within the area of the local education authority; or
>   (c) he is under compulsory school age and is, or would be if special educational provision were not made for him, likely to fall within paragraph (a) or (b) when over that age.
>
> [The definition of child includes any person who has not attained the age of 19 years and is a registered pupil at a school]

Figure 23.9   Definition of special educational needs: Section 312 Education Act 1996

if he is blind, deaf or dumb or suffers from a mental disorder of any kind or is substantially and permanently handicapped by illness, injury, or congenital deformity or such other disability as may be prescribed.

Under the Disability Discrimination Act 1995 Section 1(1) a person has a disability for the purposes of the Act if:

He has a physical or mental impairment which has a substantial and long-term adverse effect on his ability to carry out normal day-to-day activities.

The definition of special education needs given in Section 312 of the Education Act 1996 is shown in Figure 23.9.

It has been decided by the courts that dyslexia can constitute a 'disability' for the purposes of Section 312 (2)(b).

Case: *R v. Hampshire County Council, ex parte J*[37]

The judge found that dyslexia which affected the capacity of a boy aged 13½ for continuous reading, spelling, and essay writing, whilst not preventing him from making use of educational facilities, clearly hindered him.

The definition (under a previous Act) can extend to what might otherwise be regarded as medical treatment.

Case: *R v. Lancashire County Council, ex parte Moore*[38]

A child born in 1979 had hearing and speech problems and required speech therapy on an intensive basis. The dispute arose as to the definition of special educational needs and as to whether speech therapy could be regarded as educational provision rather than medical treatment. It was noted that in the Government's White Paper on Special Needs in Education[39] it was recognised that:

for many children with special educational needs, a wide range of services needs to be made available by social services departments and health authorities ... Health authorities may have to provide a wide range of medical and nursing skills, including those of health visitors, district and school nurses, physiotherapists, and speech and occupational therapists, as well as providing personal aids and equipment. (paragraph 69)

The Court of Appeal held that speech therapy could be regarded as special educational needs provision and the authority's appeal was dismissed.

Case: *R (M)* v. *Suffolk County Council*[40]

M was nearly 17 years old and had severe learning, behavioural and health problems. The local authority assessed her as having needs falling within Section 17 of the Children Act 1989. A dispute arose as to whether the local authority was precluded by regulation 7 of the Community Care, Services for Carers and Children's Services (Direct Payments) (England) Regulations 2003 from making any payments in respect of the fees of the residential school she attended. The father argued that the direct payments were used to pay for the social and practical care elements of the school fees, but not the education or basic residence components of the fees. The judge made a declaration that the local authority was not precluded by regulation 7 from making direct payments in connection with the social and practical care of a child during term time by reason of the fact that she was at a boarding school.

The Education (Special Educational Needs) (England) (Consolidated) Regulations 2001

These regulations,[41] which came into force on 1 January 2002, amend and revoke for England the regulations issued in 1994 and cover the following topics:

Part 1 General
- Delegation of functions from head teacher to other qualified teachers.

Notices and Service of Documents.

Part II Assessments
- Notices relating to assessments, advice to be sought, matters to be taken into account, in making assessment, time limits, prescribed information and children without statements in special schools.

Part III Statements
- Notices, form of the statement, time limits, review of the statement, transfer of statements, restriction on disclosure of statements (see below).

In Schedule 1 to the Regulations, forms are provided for giving notice to a parent accompanying a statement of special educational needs (Part A) and a form for a notice of amendment to a parent (Part B). Schedule 2 sets out the format for a statement of special educational needs and has the following sections:

- Part 1 Introduction (name and address of child and parent or person responsible)
- Part 2 Special Educational Needs: in terms of the child's learning difficulties that call for special educational provision
- Part 3 Special Educational Provision: objectives, educational provision to meet needs and objectives, monitoring
- Part 4 Placement
- Part 5 Non-Educational Needs
- Part 6 Non-Educational Provision

The appendices cover written representations and other statutory requirements for advice as follows:

- parental advice
- educational advice
- medical advice
- psychological advice
- advice from the social services authority
- other advice obtained by the authority.

These regulations can be downloaded from the Every Child Matters website or the Office of Public Sector Information (OPSI) website.

The Code of Practice

The Secretary of State has a statutory duty, following consultation, to issue and from time to time to revise and publish, a Code of Practice giving practical guidance on the carrying out of the duties by the local education authorities under Part IV of the 1996 Act. They and the relevant governing bodies must have regard to the Code and, on any appeal, the Tribunal must have regard to any provision of the code which appears to it to be relevant. Any draft code must be placed before both Houses of Parliament for

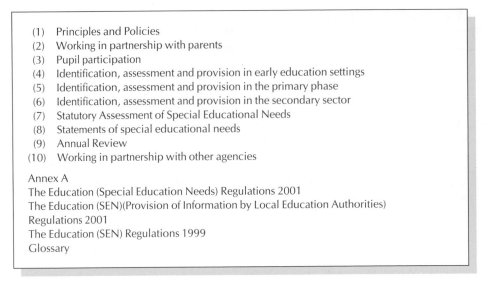

(1)   Principles and Policies
(2)   Working in partnership with parents
(3)   Pupil participation
(4)   Identification, assessment and provision in early education settings
(5)   Identification, assessment and provision in the primary phase
(6)   Identification, assessment and provision in the secondary sector
(7)   Statutory Assessment of Special Educational Needs
(8)   Statements of special educational needs
(9)   Annual Review
(10) Working in partnership with other agencies

Annex A
The Education (Special Education Needs) Regulations 2001
The Education (SEN)(Provision of Information by Local Education Authorities)
Regulations 2001
The Education (SEN) Regulations 1999
Glossary

Figure 23.10   Code of Practice on special educational needs and assessment

approval before it is issued. The Code of Practice was revised in 2002.

The Code of Practice[42] issued in 1994 was revised in 2002 covers the areas shown in Figure 23.10.

The Association of Paediatric Chartered Physiotherapists has provided guidelines for paediatric physiotherapists on the Code of Practice for Special Education needs.[43]

The fundamental principles identified in the Code are shown in Figure 23.11. and the critical success factors in Figure 23.12.

Any physiotherapist who is involved in the assessment of special educational needs and the preparation of a statement on a child should ensure that he/she obtains a copy of the Code of Practice. There is also guidance from the Association of Paediatric Chartered Physiotherapists, which has published a document entitled *Statutory Assessment of Children with Special Educational Needs.*[44]

Duty to secure the education of children with special educational needs in ordinary schools

Section 316 requires those responsible under the Act to ensure that a child with special educational needs is educated in an ordinary school if certain conditions are satisfied, unless this is incompatible with the wishes of his/her parent. The conditions are:

●   A child with special educational needs should have their needs met
●   The special educational needs of children will normally be met in mainstream schools or settings
●   The views of the child should be sought and taken into account
●   Parents have a vital role to play in supporting their child's education
●   Children with special educational needs should be offered full access to à broad, balanced, and relevant education, including an appropriate curriculum for the foundation stage and the National Curriculum

Figure 23.11   Fundamental principles in the Code of Practice

- The culture, practice, management and deployment of resources in a school or setting are designed to ensure **all children's needs are met**
- LEAs, schools and settings work together to ensure that any child's special educational needs are **identified early**
- LEAs, schools and settings exploit **best practice** when devising interventions
- Those responsible for special educational provision take into account **the wishes of the child concerned**, in the light of their age and understanding
- Special education professionals and **parents** work in **partnership**
- Special education professionals take into account the **views of individual parents** in respect of **their child's particular needs**
- Interventions for each child are **reviewed regularly** to assess their impact, the child's progress and the views of the child, their teachers and their parents
- There is close co-operation between all the agencies concerned and a **multi-disciplinary approach** to the resolution of issues
- LEAs make assessments in accordance with the **prescribed time limits**
- Where an LEA determines a child's special educational needs, statements are **clear and detailed**, made within **prescribed time limits, specify monitoring arrangements**, and are **reviewed annually**.

Figure 23.12 Critical success factors in the Code of Practice. LEAs, local educations authorities (bold as in the code of practice)

- his/her receiving the special educational provision which his/her learning difficulty calls for;
- the provision of efficient education for the children with whom he/she will be educated;
- the efficient use of resources.

Involvement of health authority

Section 322 places a duty upon the health authority or local authority to help the local education authority and specifies the action that they should take in specific circumstances.

Assessment of special educational needs

Bringing about an assessment

The parents can request an assessment of educational needs under Section 329 of the 1996 Act and the governing body of a grant-maintained school under Section 330.

The health authority or an NHS Trust has a duty to notify parents if they form the opinion in providing services for a child under 5 years that he/she has special educational needs (Section 332). After giving the parent an opportunity to discuss that opinion with an officer of the health authority or Trust, they have a duty to bring it to the attention of the appropriate local education authority. In addition, if the health authority or NHS Trust is of the opinion that a particular voluntary organisation is likely to be able to give the parent advice or assistance with any special educational needs that the child may have, they have a duty to inform the parent.

Carrying out the assessment

Where a local educational authority considers that a child has special educational needs and it is necessary for the authority to determine the special educational provision which any learning difficulty he/she has may call for, then the LEA must carry out an assessment. They must serve notice on the parents covering the following information:

- their intention to make an assessment;
- the procedure to be followed;
- the name of the officer from whom further information may be obtained; and
- the parents' right to make representations, and submit written evidence to the authority.

A Schedule of the Act covers the making of the assessments and enables regulations to be made and also requires the LEA to seek medical, psychological and educational advice in connection with the assessment.

Statement of special educational needs

If, in the light of the assessment, it is necessary for the LEA to determine the special educational provision which any learning difficulty the child may have calls for, the authority must make and maintain a statement of his special educational needs. The statement must set out the facts required. Schedule 27 of Education Act 1996 (as amended by the Special Educational Needs and Disability Act 2001) sets out the details of the parents' right to make representations and further regulations on statementing. Before making a statement, a local education authority shall serve on the parent of the child concerned a copy of the proposed statement.

Copy to the hospital school

The local education authority should give or provide on request a copy of the statement specifying certain special educational or non-educational provision to the hospital school or service. The LEA may have to make an amendment to the statement in order to name the hospital school where a child with special educational needs is likely to be a long-stay pupil. The parents have the right to comment on any such amendment in accordance with the provisions set out in Schedule 27 to the Education Act 1996 (replacing Schedule 10 of the Education Act 1993) (as amended by the Special Educational Needs and Disability Act 2001)

Parents' right of appeal

The parents can appeal both against an LEA decision not to make an assessment and/or statement and also against the description in the statement of the authority's assessment of the child's special educational needs (Section 326 of the 1996 Act), the special educational provision specified in the statement, or, if no school is named in the statement, that fact. The appeal must be made to a Special Educational Needs and Disability Tribunal (SENDIST) within 2 months of being told by the local authority in writing that they can appeal. The booklet *Special Education Needs and Disability Tribunal – How to Appeal* provides information for parents and is available on the teachernet website.[45] This booklet contains the form for a notice of appeal. The Special Educational Needs and Disability Act 2001 and the Special Education Needs Tribunal Regulations[46,47] can be obtained from the OPSI or SENDIST websites.[48]

Under the Special Educational Needs (Information) Act 2008 The Secretary of State has a duty to publicise anonymised information about SEN.

Special Educational Needs and Disability Tribunal

The Special Educational Needs Tribunal was established following the implementation of the Education Act 1993 (now consolidated in the Education Act 1996) and as a consequence of the Special Educational Needs and Disability Act 2001 became known as the Special Educational Needs and Disability Tribunal. From 1 April 2006 it became part of the Tribunals Service, an executive agency within the Ministry of Justice. It considers appeals against the decisions of the LEA about children's special educational needs if parents cannot reach agreement with the LEA.

The constitution of the SENDIST is set out in Sections 333 to 336 of the Education Act 1996 (as amended by the Special Educational Needs and Disability Act 2001). The Tribunal is independent. The Tribunals Service is responsible for the terms and conditions of tribunal judiciary, funding and the management of the secretariat and the design and operation of the Tribunal process. The chairman must be someone with a 7-year general qualification within the meaning of Section 71 of the Courts and Legal Services Act 1990 (i.e. a solicitor or barrister holding a right of audience, granted by the authorised body). Regulations cover the procedure to be followed and who can be panel members.

Powers

When an appeal is made to a SENT (Special Educational Needs Tribunal) under Section 326, it has the following powers:

- to dismiss the appeal;
- to order the authority to amend the statement, so far as it describes the authority's assessment of the child's special educational needs or specifies the special educational provision (and to make such other consequential amendments as the SENT thinks fit); or
- to order the authority to cease to maintain the statement.

The SENT cannot order the LEA to specify the name of any school in the statement unless the parent has expressed a preference or, in the proceedings, the parent, the LEA or both have proposed the school.

The local education authority cannot be obliged by a ruling in the Special Needs Tribunal to provide educational services that were surplus to meeting the special educational needs of the child.[49]

SENDISTs and the physiotherapist

The physiotherapist may be involved in providing reports for special education purposes and may consequently be called as a witness to hearings including the Special Educational Needs and Disability Tribunal. Reference should be made to Chapter 13 on giving evidence in court.

Consent by children

Chapter 7 covers the basic principles relating to trespass to the person and the importance of obtaining the consent of the patient. This section deals with the specific laws relating to consent by or on behalf of the child (i.e. a person under 18 years of age).

The young person of 16 and 17

A young person of 16 or 17 has the right to give consent to treatment under Section 8 of the Family Law Reform Act 1969. This is shown in Figure 23.13.

(1) The consent of a minor who has attained the age of 16 years, to any surgical, medical or dental treatment, which in the absence of consent, would constitute a trespass to the person, shall be as effective as it would be if he were of full age; and where a minor has by virtue of this section given an effective consent to any treatment it shall not be necessary to obtain any consent for it from his parent or guardian.

(2) In the section 'surgical, medical or dental treatment' includes any procedure undertaken for the purposes of diagnosis and this section applies to any procedures (including, in particular, the administration of an anaesthetic) which is ancillary to any treatment as it applies to that treatment.

(3) Nothing in the section shall be construed as making ineffective any consent which would have been effective if this section had not been enacted.

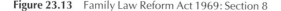

Figure 23.13   Family Law Reform Act 1969: Section 8

The definition of treatment under Section 8(2) would probably cover most treatments given by a physiotherapist where these are under the aegis of a doctor.

Section 8(3) has been interpreted as covering two situations – the giving of consent by a parent on behalf of the child of 16 or 17 and the giving of consent of a Gillick competent child (see below) under 16 years.

It does not, however, follow that a young person of 16 or 17 cannot be compelled to have treatment and the Court of Appeal in the case of *Re W*[50] upheld the decision of the High Court judge to order a child of 16 years who was suffering from anorexia nervosa to undergo medical treatment against her will.

The child under 16

The parent has a right at common law to give consent on behalf of the child. In addition, as a result of the House of Lords ruling in the Gillick case,[51] children under 16 years who have sufficient understanding and intelligence to be capable of making up their own minds can give a valid consent to treatment. As a result of this case we now have the term 'Gillick competent' (this is gradually being replaced by the phrase 'competent according to Lord Fraser's guidelines'), which signifies a child who has the maturity and competence to make a decision in the specific circumstances arising. The ruling in the Gillick case was followed by the High Court case brought by a mother who held that she should have been notified of the fact that her 14-year-old daughter was to have a termination of pregnancy. The judge upheld the right of a young person under 16 to keep information relating to a prospective abortion from the knowledge of the parents.[52] Mr Justice Silber followed the guidance given by Lord Fraser in the House of Lords in the Gillick case and maintained that it did not breach Article 8 of the ECHR

In life-saving situations, however, it is unlikely that the child under 16 years would be able to make a decision contrary to his or her best interests. Even where the child and parents both agree that treatment should not be given, as in the case of a Jehovah's Witness family, the court can order treatment to proceed if it is considered to be in the best interests of the child (case of *Re E* 1993).[53]

Supervision by parents

Can a child under 16 years be treated without parental supervision or presence or consent? A Gillick competent child under 16 years can give consent to treatment in his or her own right. However, where there are doubts about the capacity of the child to give consent to treatment, it would be advisable to ensure that a parent was present. In an emergency the person who is with the child can give consent to any immediately necessary treatment (S.3(5) Children Act 1989 – see below) and if no-one is present, the physiotherapist would be entitled to act in the best interests of the child.

Disputes between parents: parental responsibility

Even when parents are divorced or separated, under the Children Act 1989 Section 2(1), both parents retain parental responsibility for their children. Under Section 2(7) where more than one person has parental responsibility for a child each of them may act alone and without the other (or others) in meeting that responsibility. Even where one parent has a residence order in his or her favour, the other still retains parental responsibility and can exercise this to the full. One parent does not, therefore, have the right of veto over the other's actions. If, however, there has been a specific order by the court relating to a decision affecting the care or treatment of the child, then a single parent cannot change this or take any action that is incompatible with this order unless the approval of the court is obtained.

It therefore follows that if there is a dispute between parents who each have parental responsibilities over treatment decisions in respect of the child, either can go to court for a specific issue or prohibited steps order to be made. An unmarried father can obtain parental responsibility by registering the birth in his own name and completing the necessary forms. An unmarried father who fails to complete the requisite forms would not be seen by the courts as having parental responsibility even though he can be pursued for child benefit contributions. A White Paper published on 2 June 2008 puts forward proposals for a Welfare Reform Bill to change the law so that all unmarried fathers will be required to sign the baby's birth certificate. Registrars will be given the power to pursue reluctant fathers who do not want to be named. If the mother disputes the father's claim, the father can insist on a DNA test of paternity and if positive apply to register the birth.

Under the Children Act 1989 Section 3(5) a person who (a) does not have parental responsibility for a particular child, but (b) has care of the child may (subject to the provision of the Act) do what is reasonable in all the circumstances of the case for the purpose of safeguarding or promoting the child's welfare. It is suggested that this would include giving consent to necessary emergency treatment in the absence of the parents. In addition, professional staff would have a duty of care to take action to save life in such circumstances.

Situation: dispute between parents

A 14-year-old boy is brought into hospital by his father for surgery. During the premedication, the boy's mother called and staff realise that she is not aware of the planned surgery. The mother refuses to give consent. What action should the staff take?

Where both parents are married then either can give consent to treatment for the child. Divorce or separation does not end parental responsibilities. Unmarried fathers also have parental responsibilities, and therefore could give consent, where they have signed the appropriate forms as explained above. Where there is a dispute between parents over treatment for a child, then it must be determined what is in the child's best interests. If the parent who wishes to go against the clinical view of what is in the child's best interests refuses to accept the clinical judgment, then there could be an application to court for a specific issue order or prohibited steps order and a determination as to what is in the best interests of the child. Where the child is Gillick competent, then he or she could give consent.

Prohibited steps order

Where one parent wishes to prevent the other taking action that he or she does not consider is in the interests of the child, he or she may seek a prohibited steps order. This can be made under Section 8 of the Children Act 1989 and means that no step which could be taken by a parent in meeting his or her parental responsibility for a child and which is of a kind specified in the order shall be taken without the consent of the court. Thus, if one parent feared, for example, that the other was likely to agree to a mentally impaired daughter being sterilised, then that parent could obtain a prohibited steps order preventing consent being given without the consent of the court.

If the child is considered to be 'Gillick competent' and disagreed with actions which the parents were intending, he or she could seek the leave of the court to obtain a prohibited steps order. The court must be satisfied that the child has sufficient understanding to make the proposed application (Section 10(8)).

The health professional's first duty is to the interests of the child client and, while these would be in no way served by promoting discord between child and parent(s), it is possible that the health professional may become aware of situations where the Gillick competent child is in fundamental disagreement with how his or her parents are planning to proceed. This might be particularly so in carrying out treatments such as physiotherapy where talk and confidences are easily forthcoming. In such circumstances the physiotherapist should be aware of the help that is available and be able to steer her client in the right direction for legal assistance.

Specific issue order

This is the procedure where action is to be taken rather than prevented, for example in a dispute between parents over adaptations for a disabled child. A situation could arise where adaptations are required for a child under the Housing Acts (see Chapter 20); the parents live in different houses but the local authority is only prepared to pay for adaptations to one house. How is such a dispute resolved?

Either parent could take the case to court for a specific issue order and for a declaration from the court as to which parent was entitled to have the adaptations in his or her house. Obviously, account would be taken of where the child was likely to want to spend most time and which parent, if any, had a residence order. (It would of course be possible, funds permitting, for an individual parent to pay for the second house to be adapted as well.)

In the following case,[54] the father applied to the local authority for assistance as a homeless person, but the local authority decided that he was not in priority need of housing and that it was only in very exceptional cases that a child might be considered to reside with both parents.

Case: *Holmes-Moorhouse* v. *Richmond upon Thames London Borough Council* 2007

The father and mother had separated and a consent order was made by the family court that the father would leave the property of which the mother was the sole tenant. Both parents were to have a shared residence with the three younger children who would spend alternate weeks with the parents and half of each school holiday. The Court of Appeal held that once the court had made a residence order, it was not open to the local housing authority to take the view that the child was only staying with the father (as opposed to residing with him), even though the order was obtained by consent. The Court quashed the authority's decision and the father's application was to be reconsidered in the light of the court's decision.

Confidentiality of child information

The same principles apply in relation to maintaining the confidentiality of information provided by the child patient as apply to information provided by the adult patient (see Chapter 8). However, there may be situations where the interests of the child require confidential information to be passed on to an appropriate authority.

If possible, the consent of the child should be obtained to the disclosure. However, where the child refuses consent, or where the child lacks the capacity to give consent, the physiotherapist should notify the child of his/her view that the information should be passed on in the best interests of the child.

The physiotherapist should not make a commitment to the child that the confidential information will never be passed on. The physiotherapist should, however, ensure that he/she takes advice before breaching confidentiality. The physiotherapist should record the action he/she has taken and the reasons for it, and be prepared to justify his/her actions if subsequently challenged.

Situation: withholding information from a child

Parents of an 11 year old refuse to tell her that she is suffering from a serious heart condition and that she is to have cardiac surgery. She comes round in intensive care and is terrified. What could staff have done?

This situation raises the issue of what are the rights of the child to have information about their condition. Clearly the older the child, the more information about their condition should have been given to him or her. A child who is sufficiently mature and can appreciate the risks involved in any treatment can give a valid consent to treatment. However, if essential information is withheld from that young person, his or her ability to give consent and participate in the decision-making process will be severely restricted if not totally undermined. The British Medical Association[55] in its guidance on the law relating to consent by the child emphasises the importance of giving information to the child. Could therefore healthcare professionals override the parental requirement that no information should be given to the child? Hopefully, the healthcare professionals could use their persuasive powers to show the parents the importance of involving the child in the treatment and decision-making process. They must always act in the best interests of the child: the welfare of the child is the paramount consideration, and therefore if it is felt that the parents are acting contrary to the child's welfare, then ultimately the necessary information should be appropriately given to the child. Clearly, this is an issue which should be considered by the multi-disciplinary team and excellent records kept of the decision which is made and the reasons for it.

In the above scenario, the child has suffered considerable emotional harm in not being warned and prepared for what was to happen, and the parents have therefore acted contrary to her best interests even though they were of the belief that the child's ignorance was the best policy. Health professionals could have raised the issue with the parents at an earlier time and tried to persuade them of the advantage of being open and honest with the child.

Similar problems arise over the disclosure of diagnoses as in the following situation:

Situation: do I tell?

A girl of 13 is receiving palliative care for terminal stage cancer. Her parents have insisted that health professionals should not inform the girl that she is dying. Could the health professionals overrule the parents' wishes?

Parents cannot insist on acting contrary to the best interests of the child. If those health professionals caring for a child, are convinced that it is in the best interest of the child for certain information to be given to her, then, the parents should be persuaded of the advisability of the course of action. If they refuse to agree, then health professionals must act in accordance with the child's best interests. If necessary, an application could be made to court.

Where significant disputes with parents arise, it is important that an application to court should be made before the parents wishes are overruled. This is the principle that emerged from the long running Glass case, where the mother of a severely disabled boy refused to accept the clinicians' view that the boy should just be given palliative care. She eventually took the case to the European Court of Human Rights, which held that the failure of the NHS trust to seek a declaration from the court before administering diamorphine to her son without her consent and in writing him up for 'do not resuscitate' instructions without her knowledge was a breach of her Article 8 rights.[56]

Parents of a boy of 10 years who had a rare form of cancer decided to stop the treatment so that his final days should be filled with fun and not pain.[57]

Confidentiality and the statement of special educational needs

There are specific statutory provisions regulating the disclosure of the statement prepared on the special educational needs of the child.[41] Regulation 24 of the 2001 regulations restricts disclosure of the statement without the child's or parent's consent except in specific circumstances set down in the Regulations or the Act. These exceptions are set out in Figure 23.14. A child may consent to the disclosure of a statement for

The consent of the child is required for disclosure of the statement except:

● To persons to whom, in the opinion of the authority concerned, the statement should be disclosed in the interests of the child.
● For the purposes of any appeal under the Act.
● For the purposes of educational research which, in the opinion of the authority, may advance the education of children with special educational needs. This may be done if, but only if, the person engaged in the research undertakes not to publish anything contained in or derived from, a statement otherwise than in a form which does not identify any individual concerned, including in particular the child concerned and his or her parents.
● On the order of any court or for the purpose of any criminal proceedings.
● For the purposes of any investigation under the Local Government Act 1974 Part III (investigation of maladministration).
● To the Secretary of State when he requests disclosure to decide whether to give directions or make an order under Section 496, 497 or 497A of the Education Act 1996.
● For the purposes of an assessment of the needs of the child with respect to the provision of any statutory services for him being carried out by officers of a social services authority under section 5(5) of the Disabled Persons (Services, Consultation and Representation) Act 1986.
● For the purposes of a local authority performing its duties under the Children Act 1989.
● To Her Majesty's Inspectors.
● To the Connexions Service for the purposes of writing or amending a transition plan
● To a Young Offender institution for the purposes of the performance of its duties under rule 38 of the Young Offender Institution Rules 2001.

Figure 23.14   Exceptions to disclosure of statements of special educational needs requiring the consent of the child under the SEN Regulations 2001 Regulation 24

the purposes of Regulation 24 if his/her age and understanding are sufficient to allow him/her to understand the nature of that consent. If a child does not have sufficient age or understanding to allow him/her to consent to disclosure of his/her statement, the child's parent may consent on his/her behalf.

Access of the child to health records

Chapter 9 covers the basic principles that apply to access to records. Here we are concerned with access to records about children.

Access by child to records

Where the child has the capacity he/she can apply for access to his/her personal health data kept in computerised or manual form. Since the Data Protection Act 1998 covers non-computerised records, access to manually held personal health records comes under the provisions of that Act. The Department of Health recommended[58] that a certificate should be signed in which a responsible adult certifies that the child understands the nature of the application. Qualifications on the right of access to health records are set out in the 2000 regulations.[59] The procedure under the Data Protection Access provisions is considered in Chapter 9.

Right of the parent

A person with parental responsibilities can access the health records of his or her child. However, under Article 5(3), access would not be permitted to information:

- provided by the data subject in the expectation that it would not be disclosed to the person making the request;
- obtained as a result of any examination or investigation to which the data subject consented in the expectation that the information would not be so disclosed;
- which the data subject has expressly indicated should not be so disclosed.

Where a child has the capacity to consent to access, then he or she can give consent to parental access.

Exclusion of access

Whether the records are held in computerised or manual form, the application for access can be refused:

- if serious harm would be caused to the physical or mental health or condition of the data subject or another person (the data controller, who is not a health professional must consult the appropriate health professional before relying on this exemption);
- or would identify a third person (not being a health professional involved in the care of the child) who did not wish to be identified;
- if the data consists of personal data processed through the courts cannot be accessed if there is a prohibition on access by rules such as the Family Proceedings Courts (Children Act 1989) Rules 1991.[60]

Standards in the care of children and the National Service Framework

Chapter 10 sets out the principles of law that apply in ensuring that reasonable standards of professional care are provided. This will include multidisciplinary team working and the rational determination of priorities. Physiotherapists must ensure that they maintain their competence and that they keep up to date with developments in their field of specialisation. The Association of Paediatric Chartered Physiotherapists (APCP)

has prepared a document, *Standards of Practice for Paediatric Physiotherapists*, which is available from the CSP.[61]

National Service Frameworks for children, young persons and maternity services

The children's National Service Framework (NSF) was published in September 2004.[62] Five core standards are set in Part 1 for the NHS, local authorities and partner agencies to achieve high-quality service provision for all children and young people and their parents or carers.

Standard 1: promoting health and well-being, identifying needs and intervening early

The health and well-being of all children and young people is promoted and delivered through a coordinated programme of action, including prevention and early intervention wherever possible, to ensure long-term gain, led by the NHS in partnership with local authorities.

Standard 2: supporting parenting

Parents or carers are enabled to receive the information, services and support which will help them to care for their children and equip them with the skills they need to ensure that their children have optimum life chances and are healthy and safe.

Standard 3: child, young person and family-centred services

Children and young people and families receive high-quality services that are coordinated around their individual and family needs and take account of their views.

Standard 4: growing up into adulthood

All young people have access to age-appropriate services that are responsive to their specific needs as they grow into adulthood.

Standard 5: safeguarding and promoting the welfare of children and young people

All agencies work to prevent children suffering harm and to promote their welfare, provide them with the services they require to address their identified needs and safeguard children who are being or who are likely to be harmed. Part 2 sets standards for the following areas:

- children and young people who are ill;
- children in hospital;
- disabled children and young people and those with complex health needs;
- the mental health and psychological well-being of children and young people;
- medicines for children and young people.

Part 3 relating to maternity services

Part 3 of the NSF is concerned with Midwifery standards and Standard 11 is as follows:

> Women have easy access to supportive, high-quality maternity services, designed around their individual needs and those of their babies.

The expansion of that standard identifies:

- woman-centred care services;
- care pathways and managed care networks;
- improved pre-conception care;
- the identifying and addressing of mental health problems;
- choice of options in relation to place of birth;
- professional skilled in neonatal resuscitation at every birth;
- post-birth care based on a structured assessment provided by a multidisciplinary team;
- breastfeeding information and support for mothers.

The NSF should have a major impact on children's and maternity services in ensuring that minimum standards are implemented. Further information about the NSF is available from the Department of Health website.[63] The use made by the Healthcare Commission of NSFs in its inspections is discussed in Chapter 17 and on the Healthcare Commission website.[64]

The CSP has prepared a briefing paper on *The NSF for Children, Young People and Maternity Services.*[65]

Eventually the NSF standards should become part of the Bolam standard of reasonable care (see Chapter 10). In the same way, guidelines published by the National Institute for Health and Clinical Excellence (NICE) should become the norm. This does not mean however that the guidelines must be followed whatever the circumstances. If the individual circumstances of a particular patient/client suggest that the guidelines are not appropriate then the health professional must follow his or her professional judgment. Clearly clear documentation would be essential to record the justification for not following the national guidance.

Unorthodox treatments

Multidisciplinary care of the child may involve the use of unorthodox treatments. The physiotherapist must be aware that there is no legal concept of team liability, and if he/she acts contrary to the standards of professional competence of a reasonable physiotherapist, he/she could not use as a defence that he/she was carrying out the instructions of the team. If, therefore, a team member proposes an unorthodox treatment in the care of a child, the physiotherapist must be assured that this complies with the reasonable standards of care and that the parents/and or the child have given informed consent to the treatment, in the full knowledge that the proposed treatment is not of the usual kind but is in the circumstances justifiable.

Disputes with colleagues

- What is the legal situation if a physiotherapist is in dispute with his/her colleagues?

A physiotherapist is asked by a consultant to give specific clinical information to parents about the care and treatment of a son aged 10 years. The physiotherapist believes that this information should be imparted by the consultant since he/she would not be able to answer any questions raised by the parents.

It is a basic principle of law, that unless emergency circumstances exist, a health professional should not act outside the scope of his or her professional competence. This would apply to the giving of information as well as the carrying out of treatments or the diagnosis of a condition. Thus, a health professional could obtain the consent of parent or child (if competent) for treatment to be carried out by another health professional, but only if he/she understood what was involved and could answer the likely questions to be raised. In the above situation, if the physiotherapist considers that he/she does not have the requisite competence to give the necessary clinical information to the parents and son, then this should be explained to the consultant. Alternatively, he/she could give them the information which was within his/her competence, and then suggest that their further questions should be answered by the consultant personally. No person, employer, colleague or client, has the right to compel a health professional to act outside his or her competence.

Working with parents and others

It is clear that physiotherapists are unlikely to achieve major progress in the treatment of children unless they are able to secure and develop a partnership with parents and other healthcare professionals and other agencies such as schools. For example, in the care and treatment of dyspraxia Michele Lee and Graham Smith[66] were able to show through the use of outcome measures that physiotherapy had a positive effect on dyspraxia over 3 months. They hoped that, by giving parents and children a long-term management programme, the improved gain in muscle strength and skill abilities would be maintained. The authors emphasise the need for close liaison between physiotherapists, parents and schools. The programme involved the setting of goals by parents and child that they hoped to achieve by the review date.

The effectiveness of care in the community is often dependent upon the involvement of parents in the treatment of the child. The role of a domiciliary physiotherapist in the treatment of children with cystic fibrosis was reviewed by Diane Rogers and Mary Goodchild.[67] They show that the provision of a domiciliary physiotherapy service for cystic fibrosis has been a major development, allowing patients and their families increased access to physiotherapy both in the clinic and at home. Compliance with physiotherapy has been improved by discussion and demonstration in the home. They conclude that there is room for improvement in the service, but more detailed feedback is required from patients and their families.

Contributory negligence and the child

In Chapter 10 the defence of contributory negligence was discussed. This means that if the client is partly to blame for the harm which has occurred then there may still be liability on the part of the professional but the compensation payable might be reduced in proportion to the client's fault. However, where a child has been harmed, any defence of contributory negligence must take into account the fact that children are less capable than adults of taking care of themselves. The courts have been reluctant to find contributory negligence by a child, where an adult is at fault. The following case illustrates the law on contributory negligence in relation to children.

Case: *Gough* v. *Thorne*[68]

On 13 June 1962 a group of children were crossing the New Kings Road, Chelsea, London. They were Malcolm Gough, who was 17, his brother John, who was 10, and his sister Elizabeth, the plaintiff (claimant), who was 13½. They were coming from the Wandsworth Bridge Road, crossing the New Kings Road, and going to a swimming pool on the other side. They waited on the pavement for some little time to see if it was safe to cross. Then a lorry came up, coming up the Wandsworth Bridge Road and turning left into New Kings Road. The lorry driver had got pretty well half-way across the road, towards the bollards, and he stopped at about 5 feet from the bollards. He put his right hand out to warn the traffic which was coming up the road. He saw the children waiting he beckoned to them to cross, and they did. They had got across just beyond the lorry when a 'bubble' car, driven by the defendant, came through the gap between the front of the lorry and the bollard, about 5 feet, just missed the elder boy, and struck the young boy of 10, but ran into and seriously injured the plaintiff, Elizabeth, aged $13^{1}/_{2}$. The judge held that the 'bubble' car was going too fast in the circumstances, and that the driver did not keep a proper look-out because he ought to have seen the lorry driver's signal but did not see it. On the issue of contributory negligence, the trial judge found that she was 33% to blame for the accident. The plaintiff (i.e. claimant) appealed.

Lord Denning in the Court of Appeal disagreed with the finding of contributory negligence:

I am afraid that I cannot agree with the judge. A very young child cannot be guilty of contributory negligence. An older child may be; but it depends on the circumstances. A judge should only find a child guilty of contributory negligence if he or she is of such an age as reasonably to be expected to take precautions for his or her own safety: and then he or she is only to be found guilty if blame should be attached to him or her. A child has not the road sense or the experience of his or her elders. He or she is not to be found guilty unless he or she is blameworthy.

Lord Salmon expressed the situation in the following words:

The question as to whether the plaintiff [claimant] can be said to have been guilty of contributory negligence depends on whether any ordinary child of $13^{1}/_{2}$ could be expected to have done any more that this child did. I say, 'any ordinary child' I do not mean a paragon of prudence, nor do I mean a scatter-brained child, but the ordinary girl of $13^{1}/_{2}$.

Occupier's liability and a child

Case: J (a minor) v. Staffordshire County Council [69]

A 13-year-old pupil was injured when she pushed open the right hand door of double doors comprising glass panes. Her hand slipped from the push plate onto the adjacent panel of glass. The glass shattered causing severe injuries to her right hand and wrist. The County Council was found liable under the Occupier's Liability Act 1957 and at common law in failing to fulfil its duty of care. It had failed to comply with the BS standards for glass in doors. There was no finding of contributory negligence.

Where a child is allowed on to premises the duty of the occupier to ensure that the visitor is reasonably safe takes into account the fact that children will require a higher standard of care than an adult. Thus, the Occupier's Liability Act 1957, Section 2(3) as set out in Figure 23.15 states the position explicitly.

Physiotherapists must therefore take into account any reasonably foreseeable harm that could arise if children come into their departments or on to their premises. Children would also include those who may not be their patients,

The circumstances relevant for the present purpose include the degree of care, and of want of care, which would ordinarily be looked for in such a visitor, so that (for example) in proper cases . . . an occupier must be prepared for children to be less careful than adults . . .

Figure 23.15 Occupier's Liability Act 1957: Section 2(3)

but are the offspring of the patients. They would also come under the definition of visitors. In a case decided in May 2008, a mother won compensation on behalf of her child who was brain damaged following an accident at a bouncy castle party. The boy, who was 11 at the time, was kicked in the head by an older and taller boy on a bouncy castle. The couple who had hired the castle, and who were insured, were found liable because they had failed to supervise the children properly. However the Court of Appeal allowed the defendant's appeal and found that it was a freak accident, with no negligence on the part of the defendants.[70]

Midlands, Ofsted held that the Cafcass operation was inadequate and child safety was compromised on numerous occasions[71] and it had failed to protect children who are involved in divorce and separation cases.[72] Criticism has also been raised at a new protocol for managing child care cases, which have onerous requirements and the new court fee of £4000 (from £150) for taking children into care appears to have led to a fall in care order applications by a third.[73] Physiotherapists have some major challenges in this specialty.

Conclusions

Special care baby, paediatric and adolescent care can present considerable opportunities to the physiotherapist. Many lessons can be learnt from a clear and consistent monitoring of the service provided and a willingness to learn from complaints and criticisms. Physiotherapists should be aware of information provided by the CSP and its relevant Clinical Interest and Organisational Groups, the publications of the Department of Health, the Healthcare Commission and the Office for Standards in Education, Children's Services and Skills. In 2007 the government announced a £1-billion plan to improve children's welfare and education with better support for parents and families. The CSP welcomed this 10-year plan and said that physiotherapists would have a vital role to play in ensuring the objectives were met. Increasingly physiotherapists are working within multidisciplinary teams involved with the promotion of health lifestyles for children, including such initiatives as back care programmes and physical activity. Challenges in safeguarding the welfare of children continue however in spite of the Green Paper *Every Child Matters* and the subsequent legislative changes. The Children and Family Court Advisory Support Service (Cafcass) has been criticised in Ofsted inspection reports. In the first Ofsted inspection of Cafcass in the East

Questions and exercises

1   A parent brings to the out-patients department a child whom you suspect is subject to abuse. Outline the procedure which you would follow.

2   You are involved in the assessment of the special needs of a child, prior to his being statemented. You then discover that your recommendations are likely to be over-ruled by the local authority on resource grounds. What is the legal position?

3   You are involved in the care of a girl with learning disabilities and learn that her mother wishes her to be sterilised. You are of the view that her disability is not so severe that sterilisation would be justified. What action would you take? How would your answer differ if you discovered that the girl was over 18 years? (See also Chapter 22.)

4   A child that you are caring for tells you in confidence that she is being abused by her father. She emphasises that she does not want you to take any action. What is the legal situation? Does the age of the child make any difference and if so how?

References

1   Dimond, B.C. (1996) *The Legal Aspects of Child Health Care.* Mosby, London (provides an overview of child health law for all health professionals).

2   Pountney, T. (ed.) (2007) *Physiotherapy for Children.* Elsevier, Edinburgh.

3   Read, J., Clements, L., Ruebain, D. (2006) *Disabled Children and the Law,* 2nd edn. Jessica Kingsley Publishers, London.

4   The Association of Paediatric Chartered Physiotherapists (2007) *Information to Guide Good Practice for Physiotherapists Working with Children.* CSP, London.

5   http://www.dcsf.gov.uk/index.htm/

6   www.everychildmatters.gov.uk/

7   *In re B (Children) (Care orders: Standard of proof).* The Times Law Report, 12 June 2008 HL.

8   *R (on the application of BG)* v. *Medway Council* [2005] EWHC 1932 (Admin).

9   *R (on the application of A)* v. *Lambeth London Borough Council; R (on the application of G)* v. *Barnet London Borough Council* and *R (on the application of W)* v. *Lambeth Borough Council* [2003] UKHL 57; [2003] All ER (D) 385 (Oct).

10 *R (on the application of W.)* v. *Lincolnshire County Council* [2006] EWHC Admin 2365.

11 *Associated Provincial Picture Houses Ltd* v. *Wednesbury Corporation* [1948] 1 KB 223.[1947] 2 All ER 680.

12 Home Office, Department of Health, Department of Education and Science & Welsh Office (1991) *Working Together Under the Children Act 1989: a Guide to Arrangements for Inter-agency Co-operation for the Protection of Children from Abuse.* HMSO, London.

13 *D* v. *National Society for the Prevention of Cruelty to Children* [1977] 1 All ER 589.

14 *JD* v. *East Berkshire Community NHS Trust, North Staffordshire Hospital NHS Trust and Others,* Lloyd's Rep Med 1 [2003] 9, [2005] UKHL 23, [2005] 2 All ER 443.

15 Macaskill, M. (2008) Parents of Ill Vegan Girl May Face Police. *The Sunday Times,* 8 June.

16 http://www.victoria-climbie-inquiry.org.uk

17 Department of Health (2003) *Keeping Children Safe.* The Stationery Office, London.

18 Department of Health (2003) *What To Do if You're Worried a Child is Being Abused.* DH, London. www.dh.gov.uk

19 Department of Health (2003) Green Paper. *Every Child Matters.* DH, London.

20 HM Government (2006) *Working Together to Safeguard Children.* Stationery Office, London.

21 Council for Disabled Children (2006) *Safeguards for Disabled Children – a Resource for Local Safeguarding Children Boards.* DfES, London. Available from www.everychildmatters.gov.uk

22 HM Government (2008) *Safeguarding Children in Whom Illness is Fabricated or Induced.* Available from www.everychildmatters.gov.uk

23 Bennett, R. (2008) Abused Baby Might have Lived if 30 staff had Done Their Job. *The Times,* 14 February.

24 *R (M)* v. *Hammersmith and Fulham London Borough Council.* The Times Law Report, 3 March 2008.

25 *RP* v. *Nottingham City Council.* The Times Law Report, 10 June 2008.

26 www.ecm.gov.uk/resources-and-practice

27 *L.* v. *Reading BC* [2006] EWHC 2449 (QB); [2007] BLGR 576.

28 Chartered Society of Physiotherapy (2002) *Rules of Professional Conduct.* CSP, London.

29 www.everychildmatters.gov.uk/socialcare

30 Department of Health (1989) *An Introductory Guide to the Children Act for the NHS.* HMSO, London.

31 Bennett, R. (2008) Army of Amateurs Rides to the Rescue of Vulnerable Families. *The Times,* 31 May, p. 4.

32 www.interactivecsp.org.uk/network/

33 *R* v. *Gloucestershire County Council* [1997] 2 All ER 1.

34 *R.* v *E. Sussex CC ex parte Tandy* (1995) 95 LGR 745.

35 Housby Smith, N. (1994) A new era in education. *Paediatric Nursing* 6, 9, 6 and 14 (author public relations officer for the NAESC).

36 Department for Children, Education and Families (2004) Removing Barriers to Achievement: The Government's strategy for SEN. DfES, London.

37 *R* v. *Hampshire County Council, ex parte J* (1985) 84 LGR 547.

38 *R* v. *Lancashire County Council, ex parte Moore* (CA) (1985) 87 LGR 567.

39 Department of Education (1980) White Paper. *Special Needs in Education.* (Cmnd 7996). HMSO, London.

40 *R (M)* v. *Suffolk County Council* [2006] EWHC.

41 The Education (Special Educational Needs) (England) (Consolidated) Regulations 2001. SI No. 3455 Stationery Office, London.

42 Department of Education (2002) *Code of Practice on the Identification and Assessment of Special Educational Needs*. Department for Education, London.

43 The Association of Paediatric Chartered Physiotherapists (2003) *Special Education Needs the Code of Practice Guidelines for Paediatric Physiotherapists*. CSP, London.

44 Association of Paediatric Chartered Physiotherapists (2002) *Statutory Assessment of Children with Special Educational Needs*. CSP, London.

45 www.teachernet.gov.uk/wholeschool/sen

46 Special Education Needs Tribunal Regulations 2001 SI 600.

47 Special Education Needs and Disability Tribunal (General Provisions and Disability Claims Procedure) Regulations 2002 SI 1985.

48 www.opsi.gov.uk; www.sendist.gov.uk/Rules Legislation/index.htm.

49 *Hereford and Worcester County Council* v. *Lane* (CA) The Times Law Report, 10 April 1998; and reaffirmed in *Hackney London Borough Council* v. *Silyadin* The Times Law Report, 17 September 1998.

50 *Re W (a minor) (Medical Treatment)* [1992] 4 All ER 627.

51 *Gillick* v. *West Norfolk and Wisbech Area Health Authority* [1986] 1 AC 112.

52 *R (on the application of Axon)* v. *Secretary of State for Health* [2006] EWHC 37 admin.

53 *Re E (a Minor) (Wardship: Medical Treatment)* [1993] 1 FLR 386.

54 *Holmes-Moorhouse* v. *Richmond upon Thames London Borough Council* [2007] EWCA Civ 970; [2008] LGR 1.

55 British Medical Association (2001) *Consent, Rights and Choices in the Healthcare for Children and Young People*. BMA, London.

56 *Glass* v. *United Kingdom*, The Times Law Report, 11 March 2004, ECHR.

57 Nugent, H. (2008) Mother Stops Cancer Treatment for Son, 10. *The Times*, 3 January, p. 20.

58 HC(89)29 paragraph 4.

59 The Data Protection (Subject Access Modification) (Health) Order 2000 SI 413.

60 Family Proceedings Courts (Children Act 1989) Rules 1991 SI 1395 as amended.

61 Association of Paediatric Chartered Physiotherapists (2003) *Standards of Practice for Paediatric Physiotherapists*. CSP, London.

62 Department of Health (2004) *National Service Framework Children, Young People and Maternity Services*. DH, London.

63 www.dh.gov.uk/en/index.htm

64 www.healthcarecommission.org.uk

65 Chartered Society of Physiotherapists (2006) *The NSF for Children, Young People and Maternity Services. A Briefing Paper*. CSP, London.

66 Lee, M.G., Smith, G.N. (1998) The Effectiveness of Physiotherapy for Dyspraxia. *Physiotherapy* **84**, 6, 276–284.

67 Rogers, D., Goodchild, M.C. (1996) Role of a Domiciliary Physiotherapist in the treatment of Children with Cystic Fibrosis. *Physiotherapy* 82, 7, 396–402.

68 *Gough* v. *Thorne* [1966] 3 All ER 398.

69 *J (a Minor)* v. *Staffordshire County Council* (1997) 2 CLR 3783.

70 *Perry* v. *Samuel David Harris* EWCA [2008] 907.

71 Bennett, R. (2008) Protection Agency Staff Left Children at Risk from Abuse because of Errors. *The Times*, 15 February, p. 27.

72 Ford, R. (2008) Social Workers' Failings put Children at Risk. *The Times*, 28 May, p. 9.

73 Bennett, R. (2008) Fears for Children at Risk as Care Order Applications Fall by a Third. *The Times*, 6 May, p. 8.

24 Care of the Older Person

It would be a mistake to see older people as a clear client group. From a legal perspective there are no differences between the health care rights that apply to those over 75 or 85 or any other age level. However, from a clinical perspective the older people become the more likely it is that they have multiple health needs, and that these are likely to be exacerbated by economic and social problems. It is clear that the physiotherapist has a major role to play in the care of the older patient and that they are likely to form an increasing proportion of his/her case load. The Age Discrimination Regulations, which are discussed in Chapter 17, relate, at present, only to employment rights, but discrimination on grounds of age in the recognition of rights under the Human Rights Act 1998 by a public organisation or organisation exercising functions of a public nature would be unlawful (see below). The Equality Bill 2008/9 would if enacted extend the laws on age discrimination beyond the workplace to the provisions of goods, services and facilities and thus make discrimination by hospitals unlawful.

The basic principles of the law relating to patients' rights and to accountability and professional conduct cover adults of all ages. However, there are specific issues that can arise in the care of older people because:

- they may lack the competence to make decisions;
- they may require greater protection from risks;
- their economic and social situation may cause concerns for the physiotherapist.

The topics to be covered in this chapter are:

- Rights of older people: ageism
- Issues on consent and capacity
- Risk taking
- Restraint: the wanderer
- Exploitation by relatives and others
- Abuse of older people
- Use of volunteers
- Inter-agency cooperation
- Health and safety and manual handling
- Resources
- National Service Framework

Reference should also be made to the basic principles of law covered in other chapters and in particular to Chapter 25 on the law relating to death and dying. Information and guidance has been provided on the care of the older person by AGILE (Association of Chartered Physiotherapists working with older people) and by the Association of Chartered Physiotherapists in the Community (ACPC), which includes an undergraduate physiotherapy resource pack[1] and standards for physiotherapy practice.[2] AGILE has also prepared a manual of functional assessment tools and outcome measures for use with older people.[3]

Rights of the older person: ageism

There is a tendency for older clients to be treated differently because of their age. Thus, it is more likely that relatives will be told the diagnosis and prognosis before the patient; it is more likely that relatives will be asked for their consent for treatments to proceed and there is a danger that arbitrary age limits will be set, above which certain treatments will not take place. However, in law the basic principles of law of consent and confidentiality and rights to treatment do not change because a person is old. If the clients are competent then they alone are able to give consent and should be informed of any diagnosis, and they should have the right to decide whether or not they wish this information to be given to the relatives.

Similarly, there should be no cut-off points at which certain treatments are not made available. The criteria should be the physical ability of the patient to benefit from the specific treatment being discussed, whether that would be in his/her best interests and, if he/she is mentally competent, whether he/she gives consent. Article 14 of the European Convention on Human Rights (see Appendix 1) prohibits any discrimination in the implementation of the articles. It states that:

> The enjoyment of the rights and freedoms set forth in this Convention shall be secured without discrimination on any ground such as sex, race, colour, language, religion, political or other opinion, national or social origin, association with a national minority, property, birth or other status.

It follows therefore that if life-saving treatment or care is withheld from a person purely on the grounds of their age, then that could be a breach of Article 14 and Article 2. Article 3 and the right not to be subjected to inhuman or degrading treatment or punishment may also apply to older people. Article 8 and the right to private and family life, home and correspondence may also be breached where the dignity and privacy of an older person is not respected.

The Government launched a national dignity tour on 20 May 2008. It appointed Sir Michael Parkinson as National Dignity Ambassador to ensure that older people using care and health services are treated with dignity and respect at all times. The aim of the tour was to promote the Dignity in Care Campaign, which commenced in 2007. The campaign aims to eliminate tolerance of indignity in health and social care services through raising awareness and inspiring people to take action. In 2008 the campaign was extended from older people to include mental health needs. Information on the campaign, action which is being taken and the extension of the campaign can be obtained from the Department of Health (DH) social care website.[4]

The Age Discrimination Regulations only apply to employment. As a consequence, the aged now have remedies against employers who discriminate against them. In addition, they may be able to rely upon the Disability Discrimination Acts 1995 and 2005. However, a recent Spanish case has held that the Age Discrimination Directive does not apply to those over 65 years where the member country has a retirement age of 65[5] (see Chapter 17). Where older people are refused medical treatment, where the duty of confidentiality is broken and where consent is not obtained, older people have all the rights that the young adult has and which are described in earlier chapters in this book.

Issues on consent and capacity

Autonomy and intermittent incompetence

If the older client is competent then he or she has the right to give or withhold consent to treatment. The right of a mentally competent adult to refuse treatment has been reiterated by the Court of Appeal.[6] The court stated that it was the duty of the professional to ensure that the refusal was valid, i.e. that the adult had the requisite mental competence and was not under the undue influence of another nor suffering from any disability which impaired his or her capacity to give consent (see Chapter 7). The principles set out in the Mental Capacity Act 2005 now apply and replace the rulings at common law. Every adult is presumed to have the requisite mental capacity to give consent, unless there is evidence to rebut that presumption. The mentally competent adult is entitled to refuse treatment, even if the decision appears to others to be unwise (see Chapter 7).

One of the difficulties facing the physiotherapist is the possibility that the client is suffering from intermittent mental incapacity. This may be a feature of Alzheimer's disease. In such situations the physiotherapist would be advised to seek the assistance of others who could help to determine the mental capacity of the patient. Where the patient lacks the requisite mental capacity to make his or her own decisions, then the Mental Capacity Act 2005 would now apply. The fact that the mental capacity is only temporary does not prevent a person making treatment decisions during the time when they do have the requisite mental capacity.

Situation: refusal to accept residential care

A physiotherapist visits a patient at home for treatment following a stroke. She was extremely concerned about the patient's condition. It appeared that she was not able to care for herself properly and no one was helping her. The physiotherapist formed the view that the patient did not have the physical or mental competence to live on her own. What should the physiotherapist do?

This is not an unfamiliar situation to many physiotherapists. The physiotherapist would have to contact social services and arrange for a community care assessment to be made with interim assistance being provided until a residential placement could be arranged. Such a plan is of course dependent upon persuading the patient that to leave home is in her best interests. There are statutory powers under the Mental Health Act 1983 to remove the person to a place of safety but very specific conditions must be shown (see Chapter 21). In addition if there is no evidence of mental disorder to justify detention under mental health legislation, the principles of the Mental Capacity Act 2005 would apply, and if the person has the requisite mental capacity he or she is entitled to make his or her own decisions.

Powers under the National Assistance Act 1948

There are also statutory powers under the National Assistance Act 1948 for persons to be removed to a place of safety. The purpose of these powers is set out in Figure 24.1.

Such persons can be removed to a place of safety on an application by the community medical specialist (replacing the medical officer of health), who is required to give 7 days notice to a magistrates court. Because of the problems that could arise from this delay, an amending Act was passed in 1951 which enables an order to be made without notice in an emergency.

These provisions have been the subject of review by the Law Commission. The Law Commission in its Consultation Paper 130[7] has suggested that Section 47 of the National Assistance Act 1948 and the National Assistance (Amendment) Act 1951 should be repealed and replaced by a new scheme giving clearer and more appropriate powers to local social service

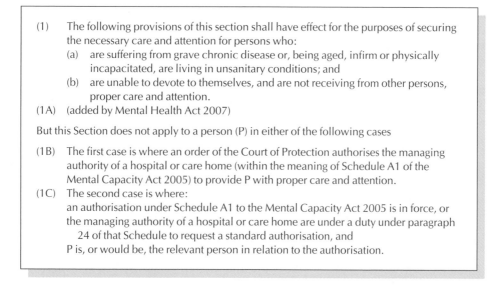

(1)   The following provisions of this section shall have effect for the purposes of securing
       the necessary care and attention for persons who:
       (a)   are suffering from grave chronic disease or, being aged, infirm or physically
              incapacitated, are living in unsanitary conditions; and
       (b)   are unable to devote to themselves, and are not receiving from other persons,
              proper care and attention.
(1A)   (added by Mental Health Act 2007)

But this Section does not apply to a person (P) in either of the following cases

(1B)   The first case is where an order of the Court of Protection authorises the managing
       authority of a hospital or care home (within the meaning of Schedule A1 of the
       Mental Capacity Act 2005) to provide P with proper care and attention.
(1C)   The second case is where:
       an authorisation under Schedule A1 to the Mental Capacity Act 2005 is in force, or
       the managing authority of a hospital or care home are under a duty under paragraph
           24 of that Schedule to request a standard authorisation, and
       P is, or would be, the relevant person in relation to the authorisation.

Figure 24.1   The National Assistance Act 1948: Section 47

authorities to intervene to protect incapacitated, mentally disordered or vulnerable people. Draft legislation was included in the final report of the Law Commission,[8] but the Mental Capacity Act 2005 did not include these provisions other than the introduction of a new criminal offence to ill treat or wilfully neglect a person who lacks capacity. The Mental Health Act 2007 made amendments to the Mental Capacity Act 2005 to enact the Bournewood safeguards (see Chapter 21) so that persons who are covered by those provisions do not come under the National Assistance Act 1948 Section 47 (see Sections 1A, 1B and 1C in Figure 24.1)

Under Section 48 of the National Assistance Act 1948 the local authority has a duty to provide temporary protection for property of those persons who are admitted to hospitals or care homes under the provisions of Section 47 or Part 111 of the Act. The section gives the council the power at all reasonable times to enter any premises which immediately before the removal of the person were his/her place of residence and deal with any movable property. The council can recover its expenses from the individual concerned or from any person liable to maintain him.

Where consent is refused

Where the client refuses to give consent to treatment and care, whatever the reason, the physiotherapist cannot usually compel the client to participate in therapy. Many therapies require the intentional involvement of the client. Where there appears to be a lack of mental capacity, it would be advisable for the physiotherapist to obtain the services of another health professional to determine the competence of the client to give consent. Forms are provided by the DH to cover the situation where treatment is given without consent in the case of a mentally incompetent person who is not under the Mental Health Act 1983,[9] and these are due to be updated as a consequence of the Mental Capacity Act 2005. The forms can be used by any health professional, and physio-therapists working in specialist areas may find it useful to adapt the forms for their specific purposes.

Situation: refusal of treatment

An older patient is admitted to hospital with confusion, secondary to an infection. Treatment with antibiotics is implemented. The patient makes a good recovery and the physiotherapist is asked to get her mobile. The patient refuses to even attempt to stand. The physiotherapist knows the importance of starting mobilisation as soon as possible to prevent loss of postural awareness, weakness and muscle and joint stiffness. What can the physiotherapist do in the face of such opposition?

This common situation requires all the physiotherapist's interpersonal skills. A good ploy would be for the physiotherapist to be on the ward when the patient is moved from bed to chair or when he needs the toilet, so that he is in a weight-bearing situation, and develop mobilisation from that point. If such tactics fail, then taking the patient off the ward to the physiotherapy department to unfamiliar surroundings, might assist in persuading the patient to commence mobilisation.

Restraint and the Mental Capacity Act 2005

Where a patient lacks the requisite mental capacity to make decisions about their care and treatment, then action can be taken in their best interests under the Mental Capacity Act 2005. The Act enables restraint to be used provided that certain conditions are present, i.e the first condition is that D reasonably believes that it is necessary to do the act in order to prevent harm to P. The second is that the act is a proportionate response to (a) the likelihood of P's suffering harm, and (b) the seriousness of that harm.

For the purposes of this section D restrains P if he/she (a) uses, or threatens to use, force to secure the doing of an act which P resists, or (b) restricts P's liberty of movement, whether or not P resists.

The mentally incompetent patient

Where the client is incompetent and unable to give consent, the physiotherapist can continue to provide care and treatment on the basis of the Mental Capacity Act 2005 (which replaces the common law right to provide care and treatment in the person's best interests on the basis of the House of Lord's ruling in the case of *Re F*[10]). The House of Lords confirmed this common law (i.e. judge made law) power to act out of necessity on behalf of a mentally incapacitated adult in the Bournewood case[11] but the European Convention on Human Rights (ECHR) held that there had been a breach of Article 5. As a consequence of the ECHR decision the Government introduced changes to the Mental Capacity Act 2005 that provide safeguards to persons who lacked the capacity to give consent to admission and had not been detained under the Mental Health Act 1983. (These safeguards, known as the Bournewood safeguards are considered in Chapter 21).

The Mental Capacity Act 2005 also placed on a statutory basis advance decisions that are also known as living wills or advance refusals of treatment. The statutory provisions are considered in the next chapter on death and dying. If a physiotherapist is aware that an older patient wishes to make an advance decision or living will, he/she should ensure that the mental competence of the patient to do so is established and that care is taken in recording their wishes. The Mental Capacity Act 2005 also established a lasting power of attorney (LPA) under which a person (known as the donor) could appoint a person, known as the donee, to act as his or her agent, making decisions on personal welfare and/or property and finance. The powers granted in relation to personal welfare decisions only come into force when the donor lacks the requisite mental capacity. LPAs are considered in more detail in the next section.

Lasting powers of attorney

A significant innovation of the Mental Capacity Act 2005 was the introduction of a lasting power of attorney. This will eventually replace the enduring power of attorney: new enduring powers of attorney cannot be created after October 2007, but those in existence remain valid until replaced with a lasting power of attorney by a mentally competent donor or until the donor dies. The lasting power of attorney, unlike the enduring power of attorney, can relate to both personal welfare decisions as well as to property and finance. (The enduring power of attorney can only relate to property and finance.) Sections 9–14 of the Mental Capacity Act 2005 set down the provisions for the creation and regulation of LPAs. The necessary forms can be obtained from the Office of the Public Guardian[12] and further information is available from the author's work.[13]

Risk taking

It is recognised that if vulnerable clients are to lead lives with a reasonable quality then certain risks must be faced. Thus, it would be less risky keeping clients in an institution rather than taking them out for walks or other activities. The Report[14] on the responses to the Government's Green Paper *Independence, Well-being and Choice*[15] (see below) points out that 'Care cannot and should not strive to be 100% risk free'. It recognised that there is a balance to be struck between enabling people to have control over their lives and ensuring that they are free from harm, exploitation and mistreatment. The Green Paper sought to encourage a more open debate about risk management. The feedback showed that there was support for the development of a risk management framework to include guidance and training to provide staff with the support they needed to operate in a new culture that favoured greater exposure to risk. The White Paper *Our Health, Our Care, Our Say*[16] published in 2006 emphasised choice and control as critical components of the future strategy for health and social care. It gave a commitment to developing a national approach to risk management. (The White Paper is considered more fully in Chapter 18.) Subsequently, the DH issued a guide to independence, choice and risk.[17] The guide can be downloaded from the DH website.[18] The guide provides a risk management framework for use by everyone involved in supporting adults using social care within any setting, including NHS staff working in multi-disciplinary or joint teams. It states that:

> The governing principle is that people have the right to live their lives to the full as long as that doesn't stop others from doing the same. By taking account of the benefits in terms of independence, well-being and choice, it should be possible for a person to have a support plan which enables them to manage risks and to live their lives in ways which best suit them.

The DH has also developed a supported decision tool template that is designed to guide and record the discussion when a person's choices involve an element of risk. This can be adapted to fit into local formats or used as a stand-alone tool.

The law requires that reasonable care should be taken to prevent the harm arising from reasonably foreseeable risks. This would necessitate a risk assessment not unlike that which would be required under the health and safety regulations (see Chapter 11).

In the event of harm actually arising to the client or another person, the health professional caring for the client would have to show:

- what risks were reasonably foreseeable;
- what reasonable action was taken to meet those risks;
- that this was in accordance with the reasonable standards of professional practice.

It follows that it is essential that records are kept of the basis of the decision making and any instructions given to others who are to care for the clients. This is a difficult area for the physiotherapist who may feel that he/she is squeezed between two principles of law – the right of the mentally competent adult to autonomy and the duty of care owed by the health professional to the client.

The risk of a fall and its consequences

A simple example of risk assessment and management can be seen in the risk of an older person falling. Thus, Adele Reece and Janet Simpson[19] discuss the need to teach older people how to cope after a fall. They suggest that older people are slightly more likely to learn successfully how to get up from the floor by the backward chairing method. Those who cannot learn to get up from the floor, should be helped by developing alternative strategies for summoning help and for preventing the consequences of the long lie.

In a subsequent article, Janet Simpson and others describe guidelines that have been developed for the collaborative rehabilitative management of older people who have fallen.[20] These guidelines are an example of multidisciplinary planning and working. They set out four aims:

- to improve older people's ability to withstand threats to their balance;
- to improve the safety of older people's surroundings;
- to prevent older people suffering the consequences of a long lie;
- to optimise older people's confidence and, whenever relevant, their carers' confidence, in their ability to move about as safely and as independently as possible.

At the heart of the philosophy of such guidelines are the basic principles of risk management – a fall is reasonably foreseeable, therefore simple measures can be introduced to minimise the risks.

Sometimes the patient might insist on walking unaided in spite of being advised against it. The physiotherapist would have to use all his/her persuasive powers to curb the patient's eagerness and to take all the reasonable means he/she can to protect the patient. The National Institute for Health and Clinical Excellence (NICE) has set a clinical practice guideline for the assessment and prevention of falls in older people that includes recommendations for research and audit criteria.[21] As with all NICE guidelines it emphasises that recommendations may not be appropriate for use in all circumstances. A limitation of a guideline is that it simplifies clinical decision making. A decision to adopt any particular recommendation must be made by the practitioner in the light of:

- available resources;
- local services, policies and protocols;
- the patient's circumstances and wishes;
- available personnel and devices;
- clinical experience of the practitioner;
- knowledge of more recent research findings;

The DH provided a progress report on the prevention of falls in 2007 and suggested that putting in place fully integrated falls prevention services could prevent up to 200 hip fractures annually in each Special Health Authority.[22] An update of the national clinical audit of falls and bone health for older people in 2007 has been provided by Carole MacGregor and Jackie Riglin.[23] An ageline database provides access to a wide range of resources relating to older people[24] as does Medline Plus.[25] AGILE, ACPC and OCTEP (Occupational Therapy with Elderly Persons) have jointly prepared guidelines for the collaborative rehabilitative management of people who have fallen which is available from the Chartered Society of Physiotherapy (CSP) website.

The risks of inactivity

The risk of wasting muscle power and loss of balance is also reasonably foreseeable among immobile older people. Rosemary Oddy[26] describes how the gymnastic ball offers excellent opportunities for strengthening muscle power and improving balance of older patients. When used with a retaining cuff, even those with dementia can sit on it and derive benefit from it.

All areas of clinical practice benefit from the adoption of the same principles of risk management that apply in health and safety situations (see Chapter 11).

Situation: risks in rehabilitation

A physiotherapist attempts to assist an older person to walk following a stroke. As she moves him from the chair he lets go his hold on her and falls to the floor, fracturing his pelvis. What is the legal situation of the physiotherapist?

The first question that must be asked is, what is the reasonable standard of the physiotherapist in this situation? Would any competent physiotherapist have acted as she did? Would a simple risk assessment not have suggested that a second person should be at hand to assist in the first steps of mobilisation? The physiotherapist is unlikely to face litigation personally, since her employer would be vicariously liable for her actions (see Chapter 10).

During the process of stroke rehabilitation the physiotherapist would try slowly to withdraw the level of support. The patient may progress from standing between two people, walking between two people, walking with one person, walking with an aid, and walking unaided. This progress is based on the clinical judgment of the physiotherapist. It has to be accepted that many patients never reach the point of walking unaided. Central to the clinical judgment at each stage in the progress is a risk assessment and management process.

Risk to others

Situation: too risky

A stroke patient, previously active with a full social life, is discharged having made a good recovery. He has been advised that he must contact the DVLA and his insurance company before thinking about driving again. He admits to the physiotherapist during a day hospital visit that he has driven but 'only around the village'. What is the physiotherapist's legal duty?

The physiotherapist should make it clear to the patient that in driving contrary to clinical advice he is committing an offence under Road Traffic legislation as well as putting at risk his own safety and that of others. Where she has considerable concerns about his mental and physical capacity to drive safely, there may well be justification in warning the patient that if he fails to notify the DVLA then she may feel obliged as part of her duty of care, to inform them herself. (See Chapter 8 on the exceptions to the duty of confidentiality.)

Restraint: the wanderer

Some older people can present special problems because of their disregard for their own health and safety and their inability to make rational decisions. In residential and nursing homes and also hospitals there is a temptation to lock doors or use forms of restraint to prevent the client wandering off into harm. Such forms of restraint are not lawful unless the provisions of the Mental Capacity Act 2005 as amended by the Mental Health Act 2007 are followed. Ideally there should be sufficient staff to prevent the need for doors to be locked or patients held under restraint. Sometimes it may be necessary to ensure that the client is protected by the Bournewood safeguards, which are discussed in Chapter 21.

Situation: wanderers

A physiotherapist visits a nursing home where a stroke patient is being cared for. She notes that many of the residents are sitting in seats with tables in front of them or with seats sloping down to the rear so that the resident is effectively trapped in them. She queries this with the home manager who tells her that that is the safest way of preventing them wandering off from the home, because they have been told they cannot lock the doors. The physiotherapist wonders if this is lawful.

Restraint can be a form of imprisonment. The provisions of the Mental Capacity Act discussed above in relation to restraint must be followed or the Bournewood safeguards be in place.

Restraint may be justified if it is reasonable, of short duration and in the best interests of a mentally incompetent person. However, permanent ongoing restraint through clothing or design of furniture is not lawful. The physiotherapist should discuss alternative systems of keeping the older person safe. If the managers of the home are not prepared to consider changes, then this may be raised with the registration body the Care Quality Commission (CQC). In addition, if the social services purchase places in the home they will also be concerned with standards of care and can issue notice if there appears to be a breach in the contract. Contractual conditions can be more demanding than the provisions of the Care Standards Act 2000.

Exploitation by relatives and others

The physiotherapist may occasionally encounter situations where it is apparent that an older client is being exploited financially. The physiotherapist should ensure that the Department of Social Security is notified if the exploitation relates to the use of social security funds. A new Court of Protection has been set up under the Mental Capacity Act 2005. This, unlike its predecessor, has jurisdiction not only in relation to property and financial affairs but also in matters relating to personal welfare.

Abuse of older people

'Granny bashing' and other forms of physical and mental abuse have been recognised as a danger of which all health and social services professionals should be aware. It is estimated by Help the Aged that 500 000 older people are believed to be abused at any one time in the UK. Should a physiotherapist suspect that his/her client is the victim of such action, he/she should take such care as is reasonable in all the circumstances to ensure that the older person is safe. This will probably necessitate referring the client

to the community health services such as the health visitor and also informing social services. Many charities offer guidance in recognising elder abuse and in taking action to prevent its occurrence. Counsel and Care has published a fact sheet giving advice on abuse and the risk to older people which is available from its website.[27] It covers the types, symptoms, location of abuse and the likely abusers and abused; the action to be taken if abuse is seen or suspected in a variety of locations and the law which applies. The Domestic Violence Crime and Victims Act (DVCV Act) 2004 requires persons living in a household where there is a child or vulnerable adult to take reasonable steps to prevent the unlawful death of that person. Reasonable steps suggested by Counsel and Care would include:

- reporting suspicions of abuse to the police;
- contacting local social services;
- making sure that any injuries are treated promptly;
- explaining concerns to the GP;
- contacting an organisation such as Action on Elder Abuse.

The DVCV Act defines a vulnerable person as:

> any person aged 16 or over whose ability to protect himself from violence, abuse or neglect is significantly impaired through physical or mental disability of illness, through old age or otherwise.

In addition, under the Mental Capacity Act 2005 it is a criminal offence under Section 44(2) to ill-treat or wilfully neglect a person who lacks capacity.

Action on Elder Abuse has a helpline number (0808 808 8141) and website.[28] It has recently launched a Safeguarding Adults Good Practice project together with the Practitioners Alliance for Vulnerable Adults. The project aims to provide practical methods of identifying and disseminating good practice from around the country and the data base is available from the Action on Elder Abuse website.

Age Concern[29] and Help the Aged[30] also provide information on elder abuse and the action that should be taken. For discussion on a new Independent Safeguarding Authority (ISA) see Chapter 17.

Use of volunteers

One of the principal philosophies of the community care policy is that provision of services for those in need should be based on a partnership between the statutory services, the private sector (including the voluntary sector) and the family. The physiotherapist should be aware of the contribution that voluntary groups and individual volunteers can make towards the care and quality of life of the patient/client, whether at home or in the hospital. She should, however, be alert to the legal implications of delegating tasks to volunteers and ensure that the principles set out in Chapter 10 on delegation and supervision are observed. A physiotherapist who delegated tasks to a volunteer who lacked the knowledge and experience to undertake that activity with reasonable safety could be liable for any harm that was caused.

Situation: volunteers

A volunteer borrows a wheelchair from the physiotherapy department to take a patient into the grounds for some fresh air (or a smoke!). He does not put the patient's foot securely onto the footrest of the chair and the foot is twisted back and injured when the chair is pushed forward. Who is liable?

There has clearly been negligence in the care of this patient. A duty of care is owed to the patient, reasonable care has not been taken and as a consequence the patient suffers harm. In order to assess who is responsible, the initial questions to be asked are:

- Who was responsible for delegating activities to the volunteer?

- Had the volunteer been taught how to ensure a patient was safe in a wheelchair?
- Had the volunteer been given clearly defined boundaries?

If faults can be shown in the delegation to and supervision of the volunteer, then that person delegating is liable and the employer would be vicariously liable for those failures. If the volunteer has had appropriate training, instructions and supervision, but disobeyed the rules, then he is liable. Although the volunteer is not an employee and so in strict law there is no employer to be vicariously liable for the volunteer, the NHS trust or other organisation would probably accept liability, in accordance with DH expectations, since it is directly liable for the patient's safety. Age Concern, which has an extensive programme for volunteers to befriend older persons, provides insurance cover for their volunteers. Many other charities using volunteers also provide cover.

Inter-agency cooperation

Statutory provisions require health authorities and local authorities to work closely together and with the private/voluntary sector in the performance of their statutory functions. Other organisations with which the physiotherapist may be involved include local authority housing departments, housing associations, care organisations, and many companies and firms that provide services for older people.

Physiotherapists should be aware of the resources available for the care of older people and from whom further information may be obtained. The CSCI publishes the reports of its inspections of care homes which are available on its website.[31] Its website can also be used to find a suitable care home in a particular location check the ratings of any home; and obtain advice and guidance. CSCI ratings are 3 stars excellent; 2 stars good, 1 star adequate and 0 star poor. CSCI has been replaced by CQC. Counsel and Care has also published a fact sheet Care Homes: What to Look For?, which is available on its website.[27]

Day hospitals

The physiotherapist should have a major role to play in the functioning of a day hospital and the assessment of clients. Jane Sword and Rod Lambert[32] provided a useful procedure and documentation for the assessment of domestic function in a day hospital for elderly mentally ill people. The form covers:

- comprehensive assessment of all areas of domestic function;
- a format that is easy to use and administer;
- information from which a consistent report format can be established;
- a high degree of correlation in the results obtained in the use of the form by a number of therapists;
- the highlighting of areas of ability and deficit, thereby enabling specific recommendations to be made and facilitating subsequent programme planning.

The value of multidisciplinary assessment is shown in the evaluation of the uniform data system for medical rehabilitation described by Arthur Peter.[33]

There is a danger that professionals in a day hospital are too over protective to a patient, providing the same level of physical support that they would give to a patient in hospital. It should be remembered that the patient is managing for him/herself at home and too much assistance in the hospital might undermine his/her confidence.

Health and safety and manual handling

The physiotherapist who cares for older people should ensure that he/she follows the principles set out in Chapter 11 in relation to manual handling and other health and safety regulations and be aware of the recent publication by the CSP on manual handling.[34] Even though the physiotherapist may see some manual handling in the care of his/her older clients as therapeutic, it still comes under the Manual Handling Regulations and he/she would be expected to carry out an appropriate risk assessment. The physiotherapist must also ensure that he/she receives regular updating of his/her training.

Situation: teaching the carers

A physiotherapist watches a husband demonstrate how he gets his wife out of a chair. The patient puts her arm around her husband's neck and pulls, putting him at considerable risk. The physiotherapist warns the husband of the dangers, but he says that he has always done it this way and sees no problem with it. Where does the physiotherapist stand if he later suffers harm?

It is quite likely in this situation that the husband will ignore the advice of the physiotherapist to introduce a different method of lifting his wife. If she arranges for the delivery of a hoist, he may well not use it. However, the physiotherapist has a duty to ensure that she gives the appropriate advice in such a way that he can see the serious dangers in his present method, and that she arranges the supply of any necessary equipment. If, having fulfilled her duty of care, the husband ignores her advice and does not use the equipment, then any harm which he suffers is at his own risk and he could not successfully hold the physiotherapist or her employers liable for it. CSP guidance on manual handling[34] and in particular Section 5 on education and continuing professional development can be used by the physiotherapist to develop her own professional skills in instructing others in manual handling.

Resources

Older people have not always received the priority in the allocation of resources which their needs require. Physiotherapists should beware of the dangers of using arbitrary age levels to deny services on a blanket basis, rather than assessing patients individually. It may be that a person in their 90s requires treatment that could be contra-indicated in a person much younger because their physical condition is much better.

Because of the mismatch between the demand for services and the resources available, physiotherapists have a duty to ensure that resources are used reasonably.

Situation: enough is enough

A physiotherapist considers that a stroke patient has reached her full potential and would now benefit from feeling 'in charge of her life'. The patient's husband disagrees and wants his wife to continue with regular rehabilitation. Should the physiotherapist provide further sessions?

No physiotherapist should accept instructions that are contrary to her professional judgment. This applies whoever is giving the instructions – patients, relatives or other professional colleagues. In this situation, it is a matter of professional judgment whether further sessions are clinically justified and if the physiotherapist has formed the view that progress will not be made, then she must make this clear to the patient and her husband. The latter has no legal right to enforce treatment that is not clinically indicated.[35] The physiotherapist should explain this sensitively, since the sessions may be seen by the relative as a necessary support, emotional as well as practical, and the physiotherapist may offer to review the situation after a specified time. It may be that day hospital attendance is appropriate. She should, of course, ensure that her record keeping is above reproach and should be prepared for the possibility of a complaint arising from the situation.

The Community Care (Residential Accommodation) Act 1998 requires local authorities to assist residents in the payment of fees for residential accommodation without undue delay, as soon as their capital resources fall below a specified sum which is updated. If the resources fall below this sum the council is obliged to pay all the fees. The Act reinforces the decision of the court in a case brought against Sefton Council by a resident who had had to contribute to the fees even though her resources were well below £10 000, the specified amount at that time. Sefton Council were following a policy of requiring older people to pay their own fees until all they had left was £1500, about the price of a funeral. The court declared Sefton's actions illegal and this decision is incorporated in the 1998 Act.[36]

Funding of long-term care

It is a principle of the NHS that health care is provided free at the point of service, unless there are statutory provisions that enable charges to be levied (as there are for prescriptions). In contrast, the provision of social services are in general subject to means testing. There are therefore considerable disputes in determining whether the NHS should provide specific services free, or whether they should be provided, on a means-tested basis, by social services. In the Grogan case,[37] the court had to determine whether a client was entitled to have services provided by the NHS. The case is considered in Chapter 18.

Following the decision in the Grogan case, the DH announced that new guidelines on determining eligibility for NHS continuing health care would be published in October 2007. Assessments for continuing NHS care were to be carried out by a multidisciplinary team using the concept of 'a primary health need' as the criteria for the receipt of continuing health care. The National Framework on *NHS Continuing Healthcare and NHS-funded Nursing Care* published in October 2007[38] set out the national framework, the legal framework, the primary health need, core values and principles, eligibility considerations, links to other policies, care planning and provision, review, dispute resolution and governance. It stated that primary health need should be assessed by looking at all of care needs and relating them to four key indicators:

- **nature**: the type of condition or treatment required and its quality and quantity;
- **complexity**: symptoms that interact, making them difficult to manage or control;

- **intensity**: one or more needs which are so severe that they require regular interventions;
- **unpredictability**: unexpected changes in condition that are difficult to manage and present a risk to the patient or to others.

The NHS would make decisions on eligibility for NHS continuing health care in collaboration with the local authority through a multidisciplinary team and with the full and active involvement of the patient and carers. Further information on the National Framework is available on the DH website.[39] Answers to frequently asked questions on continuing care are also available.[40]

A Royal Commission[41] was established to consider the funding of long-term care for older people and reported in March 1999. Its recommendations included the payment for some elements of care from public funds, and the establishment of a National Care Commission (Now the CSCI and now absorbed into the Care Quality Commission.)

Subsequently, there has been a divergence across the UK over the payment for personal and nursing services in care homes, with Scotland deciding that all personal and health costs of long-term care should be met from public funds.

The annual report for 2006–7 published by CSCI in January 2008[42] summarised the state of social care in England in 2006–7 and painted a picture of a society which was failing to meet the needs of older and disabled people. Local authorities under pressure from limited resources were tightening the eligibility criteria for receiving social services and were redefining more narrowly the 'core business' of adult social care and there was now a sharp divide between those people who benefit from the formal system of social care and those who are outside it. There is little consistency both within and between councils as to who is ineligible for care. People, who are lost to the system because they are not eligible for council-arranged services and cannot purchase their care privately, often struggle with fragile informal support arrangements and a poor quality of life. (The House of Lords decided in the Gloucester case[43] that resources could be taken into account when determining the assessment of and the level of social services to be provided by local authorities. This case is considered in Chapter 20.) Those who fund their own care are disadvantaged and lack advice and information about care options. The report saw the Government's proposed Green Paper on long-term care funding as an important opportunity to establish a fair and sustainable social care system, where people, whether they pay for their own care or not, as a minimum get good advice, an assessment of their situation, and access to high-quality services.

In 2008 the Government initiated a consultation on the future of care and support. It set up a care and support website[44] that can be accessed to take part in the debate. It points out given the longer life expectancy, the cost of disability benefits could increase by 50% in the next 20 years and there could be a £6 billion funding gap for social care. Since the proportion of people of working age in the population will decline, the Government will not be able to raise enough money through tax alone to meet the costs of care and support. A new insurance-based system was seen as a means of funding care for older people, which was forecast to reach £4 billion in the next 20 years. Feedback is invited in its efforts to find an affordable, fair and sustainable way of delivering and funding a first-class care and support system for the twenty-first century. A letter to *The Times*[45] from representatives of 12 organisations involved with the care of older and disabled people and their carers pointed out the fact that disabled and older people were being forced to end their support services because they could not afford them. It called for the government to conduct a thorough review of the impact of care charges and for these issues to be addressed in adult care reform.

Rationing care

Many local authorities have tightened their criteria for providing social care and are offering help only in critical cases. A legal challenge was brought against Harrow Council by several claimants who were in receipt of community care services. Harrow had proposed that owing to financial constraints it would limit provision of care services to people with need categorised as critical under the Fair Access to Care Services guidance issued by the Secretary of State. The judge decided that there was a general duty under Section 49A of the Disability Discrimination Act 1995 to have due regard to considerations listed therein. Those were important duties, which included the need to promote equality of opportunity and to take account of disabilities, even where that involved treating the disabled more favourably than others. There was no evidence that the legal duty and its implications were drawn to the attention of the decision makers who should have been informed, not just of the disabled as an issue, but of the particular obligations that the law imposed. Harrow's decision-making process had not complied with Section 49A of the Act.[46] The implications of this decision are still to be seen.

National Service Frameworks

The National Service Framework for Older People

The *National Service Framework (NSF) for Older People* was published in 2001[47] as a 10-year programme setting new national standards and service models of care across health and social services.

The NSF for older people covers the following standards:

- rooting out age discrimination
- person-centred care
- intermediate care
- general hospital care
- stroke
- falls
- mental health in older people
- the promotion of health and active life in older age.

It also considered the national support to underpin local action including: finance, workforce, research and development, clinical and practice decision support services and information. The NSF is available on the DH website. It was followed in 2004 by a publication of the CSP emphasising that independence was the top priority for older people.

More recently, the DH has published a strategy for long-term conditions setting five key outcomes for people with long-term conditions.[48] It points out that one in three of the population suffer from a long-term condition and the number of people with a long-term condition is expected to rise by 23% over the next 25 years. A revised edition of the compendium on long-term conditions first published in 2004 was published in 2008.[49]

The National Service Framework for long-term conditions

This NSF was published in 2005 sets out 11 quality requirements in health and social case services:

- a person-centred service
- early recognition followed by prompt diagnosis and treatment
- emergency and acute management
- early and specialist rehabilitation
- community rehabilitation and support
- vocational rehabilitation
- providing equipment and accommodation
- providing personal care and support
- palliative care
- support for family and carers
- care during admission to hospital.

The value of the NSF to the physiotherapist in securing resources and raising standards is considered by Jane Hobden and others in a public health supplement published in *Frontline* on 1 September 2005 and available on the CSP website. The CSP published a guide to the NSF on neurological long-term conditions in 2006.[50]

Stroke services

In 2005 the National Audit Office published a report on stroke services[51] which identified significant deficiencies in stroke services. Subsequently the Government has stated that a dedicated stroke care coordinator should be appointed in every local authority area in England to support survivors and their families. Additional ring-fenced funding has been made available to local authorities and to strategic health authorities. The CSP announced in May 2008 its support for the stroke project set up by the Stroke Association 'Step up for Stroke initiative'.[52]

Dementia

In January 2008 the Public Accounts Committee of the House of Commons published a report on improving services and support for people with dementia.[53] The report came to the following conclusions:

(1) Dementia affects over 560 000 people in England, costs about £14 billion a year but has not been a NHS priority. The National Dementia Strategy now being developed by the DH should have a clear timetable for implementation, and criteria for evaluation and reporting progress. It should also have an effective communication strategy to engage professionals, patient groups, the Royal Colleges, inspectorates and the voluntary sector.

(2) Unlike cancer and coronary heart disease, there is no single individual with responsibility or accountability for improving dementia services. The DH should appoint a Senior Responsible Officer.

(3) Between a half and two-thirds of people with dementia never receive a formal diagnosis. Diagnosis should always be made, regardless whether interventions are available and could be assisted if GP practices had greater support from mental health services; the Royal College of General Practitioners developed a dementia care pathway; and the Institute of Innovation and Improvement promulgated good diagnostic practice.

(4) There is a poor awareness among the public and some professionals of dementia and what can be done to help people with the disease. DH should commission a dementia awareness campaign.

(5) People with dementia require support from multiple health and social care providers but this is often difficult to manage. On diagnosis, people with dementia and their carers should be given a single health or social care professional contact point (e.g. a social worker or community psychiatric nurse) to improve the coordination of care.

(6) Carers save the taxpayer £5 billion a year, yet between a half and two-thirds of all carers do not receive the carer's assessment to which they are entitled. The DH should emphasise to local health organisations and their social care partners that they need to develop an action plan that gives priority to assessing and meeting the needs of carers and develop a commissioning tool-kit to demonstrate the cost benefits of the different options for providing support, including respite and domiciliary care.

(7) Sixty-two per cent of care home residents are currently estimated to have dementia but less than 28% of care home places are registered to provide specialist dementia care. CSCI should assess staff qualifications and training as part of its review of the quality of care for people with dementia, and local mental health teams should use the finding when allocating resources to community psychiatric teams.

(8) Hospital care for people with dementia is often not well managed, increasing the risk of longer stays, admission to a care home and deterioration in the patient's health. Hospitals should routinely undertake a mental health assessment. Care records should be shown to paramedicals, so that an informed decision on admission to hospital or to care home can be made.

Following the Public Accounts Committee report, the DH promised that a national dementia strategy will be developed. As part of an awareness campaign on dementia, the Alzheimer's Society has published in 2008 a booklet (*Worried about your Memory*) to assist in the identification of Alzheimer's which is available from its website.[54]

Conclusion

The demographic changes show that those over 65 will increase as a proportion of society and that the number of people over 85 will rise from 1 million in 2006 to 2.9 million in 2036. The resource implications for the provision of health and social care, as well as pensions and social security, are now coming on to the agenda of every political party. It can no longer be assumed that public expenditure can be the main source of assistance. In 2005 the CSP reported that older people were being let down by their local authority. Its research showed that 79 out of 150 social services departments in England have recorded a fall in the number of people aged 65+ that they help to continue living in their own homes.[55] It is apparent that resource issues in the care of older people will continue to be one of the principal challenges for the physiotherapist in the years to come. The results of the consultation on funding social care and support may have a major impact on the future direction of service provision for older people. A Management of Dementia in Care Homes Bill failed to get a second reading in Parliament. If enacted it would have:

- regulate the prescription of anti-psychotic drugs for people with dementia in care homes;
- introduced protocols for the prescribing, monitoring and review of such medication;
- made dementia training, including the use of anti-psychotics, mandatory for care home staff;
- required care homes to obtain support from specified external services.

Questions and exercises

1 A physiotherapist is concerned that an older person living on her own is refusing to accept any assistance and is neglecting herself. What legal powers exist in this situation?

2 An older person visiting a day hospital refuses to have post stroke exercises. What is the legal situation?

3 In a residential home, a physiotherapist discovers that all the doors are kept locked. When she enquires about this she is told that this is the only way in which the residents can be prevented from going out on to the main road. What action, if any, should she take?

References

1 Chartered Physiotherapists with Older People and Association of Chartered Physiotherapists in the Community (2005) *Information and Guidance on the Care of the Older Person*. CSP, London.

2 Association of Chartered Physiotherapists working with Older People (AGILE) (2004) *Physiotherapy with Older People: Standards of Physiotherapy Practice and Service Standards of Physiotherapy Practice*. CSP, London.

3 Association of Chartered Physiotherapists working with Older People (AGILE) (2005) *Manual of Functional Assessment Tools and Outcome Measures for use with Older People*. CSP, London.

4 www.dh.gov.uk/en/SocialCare/Socialcarereform/Dignityincare

5 *Felix Palacios de la Villa* v. *Cortefiel Servicios SA ECJ* [2007] 16 October Case C-411/05; The Times Law Report 23 October 2007.

6 *Re T* (Adult: Refusal of Medical Treatment) [1992] 4 All ER 649.

7 Law Commission (1993) *Mentally Incapacitated and Other Vulnerable Adults: Public Law Protection* (the third paper dealing with decision making and the mentally incapacitated adult). HMSO, London.

8   Law Commission (1995) Report No. 231. *Mental Incapacity*. HMSO, London.

9   Department of Health, London. Department of Health, Reference Guide to Consent for Examination or Treatment, DH, 2001; www.dh.gov.uk/ consent; Department of Health, Good Practice in Consent Implementation Guide, DH, November 2001.

10   *F v. West Berkshire Health Authority and Another* [1989] 2 All ER 545.

11   *R v. Bournewood Community and Mental Health NHS Trust* (HL) [1998] 3 All ER 289.

12   www.guardianship.gov.uk

13   Dimond, B. (2008) *Legal Aspects of Mental Capacity*. Blackwell Publishing, Oxford.

14   Department of Health (2005) *Responses to the Consultation on Adult Social Care in England: Analysis of Feedback from the Green Paper Independence, Well-being and Choice*. DH, London.

15   Department of Health (2005) *Green Paper. Independence, Well-being and Choice*. DH, London.

16   Department of Health (2006) *Our Health, Our Care, Our Say: A New Direction for Community Services*. DH, London.

17   Department of Health (2007) *Independence, Choice and Risk: a Guide to Best Practice in Supported Decision Making*. DH, London.

18   www.dh.gov.uk/en/SocialCare/ Socialcarereform/index.htm

19   Reece, A.C., Simpson, J.M. (1996) Preparing Older People to Cope after a Fall. *Physiotherapy* **82**, 4, 227–235.

20   Simpson, J., Harrington, R., Marsh, N. (1998) Guidelines for Managing Falls Among Elderly People. *Physiotherapy* **84**, 4, 173–177.

21   National Institute of Health and Clinical Excellence (2004) Clinical Practice Guideline for the Assessment and Prevention of Falls in Older People. NICE, London.

22   Philip, I. (2007) *A Recipe for Care – Not a Single Ingredient*. DH, London.

23   MacGregor, C., Riglin, J. (2007) Update on the National Clinical Audit of Falls and Bone Health for Older People. *Agility* **2**, 20–22.

24   www.aarp.org/research/ageline/about.html

25   www.nlm.nih.gov/medlineplus

26   Oddy R. (1996) Taming the Gymnastic Ball. *Physiotherapy* **82**, 8, 477–9.

27   www.counselandcare.org.uk

28   www.elderabuse.org.uk/index.htm

29   www.ageconcern.org.uk

30   www.helptheaged.org.uk

31   www.csci.org.uk

32   Sword, J., Lambert, R. (1989) Assessment of Domestic Function within a Day Hospital for Elderly Mentally Ill People. *British Journal of Occupational Therapy* **52**, 1, 16–17.

33   Peter, A. (1994) Evaluation of the Uniform Data System for medical Rehabilitation (including the functional independence measure) by Glenrothes Geriatric Day Hospital Team. *British Journal of Occupational Therapy* **57**, 3, 91–94.

34   Chartered Society of Physiotherapy (2008) *Guidance on Manual Handling*. CSP London.

35   *R. (on the application of Burke) v. General Medical Council and Disability Rights Commission and the Official Solicitor to the Supreme Court* [2004] EWHC 1879; [2004] Lloyd's Rep Med 451.

36   *R v. Sefton Metropolitan Borough Council ex parte Help the Aged* [1997] 4 All ER 532.

37   *R. (on the application of Grogan) v. Bexley NHS Care Trust* [2006] EWHC 44 (2006) 9 CCL 188.

38   Department of Health (2007) *National Framework for NHS Continuing Healthcare and NHS-funded Nursing Care*. DH, London.

39   www.dh.gov.uk/en/Publicationsandstatistics

40   www.dh.gov.uk/en/SocialCare/Deliveringadult socialcare/Continuingcare

41   Royal Commission on Long Term Care (1999) *With Respect to Old Age*. Cm 4192–1 1999. The Stationery Office, London.

42   Commission for Social Care Inspection (2008) *The State of Social Care in England 2006–7*. CSCI, London.

43   *R v. Gloucestershire County Council* [1997] 2 All ER 1.

44   www.careandsupport.direct.gov.uk

45   Mencap, Age Concern and others (2008) Adult Care Reform. Letter to the Editor. *The Times*, 5 June.

46   *R (on the application of Chavda) v. Harrow LBC* [2007] EWHC 3064 Admin; (2008) 11 C.C.L. Rep 187.

47   Department of Health (2001) *The National Service Framework for Older People*. DH, London.

48   www.dh.gov.uk/Healthcare/index.htm

49   Department of Health (2008) *Raising the Profile of Long Term Conditions Care: A Compendium of Information*. DH, London.

50   Chartered Society of Physiotherapists (2006) *NSF for Long Term Conditions – a Guide to the NSF on Neurological Long Term Conditions*. PA 66. CSP, London.

51 National Audit Office (2005) *Reducing Brain Damage: Faster Access to Better Stroke Care*. HC 452 Session 2005–6; www.nao.org.uk

52 www.stroke.org.uk

53 House of Commons Committee of Public Accounts (2008) *Improving Services and Support for People with Dementia*. Sixth Report of Session 2007–8 HC 228. Stationery Office, London.

54 www.alzheimers.org.uk

55 Chartered Society of Physiotherapy (2005) *Older People Being Let Down by their Local Authority*. CSP London.

25 Death and the Dying

It is an inevitable fact that physiotherapists across all specialisms will be involved in the care of dying patients. It is important that at such difficult times the physiotherapist has confidence in his/her knowledge of the law which applies. Very few books for physiotherapists deal directly with this topic, but help can be found in chapters in books dealing with certain conditions. For example chapter 11 in *Physiotherapy in Respiratory Care* covers communicating with and caring for patients who are dying.[1] See also the author's work on this subject.[2] This chapter discusses the law relating to the following topics:

- The extent of the duty to maintain life
- Involvement of the court
- Advance decisions/living wills
- Can the court order doctors to provide treatment?
- 'Not for resuscitation' orders
- Parents' refusal to consent to treatment
- Care of the dying patient
- Registration of death and the role of the coroner
- Organ transplants

The extent of the duty to maintain life

Healthcare professionals can be faced with the problem of whether there is a duty in law to carry out every possible procedure known to science in order to save the life of the patient or whether the law enables a person to be allowed to die. The law draws a distinction between withholding care and taking positive action to end life. The former may or may not be legally permissible, depending upon the condition and prognosis of the patient. The latter will always be illegal. It is not therefore the duty of the health professional to continue to provide high-technology care when the patient's prognosis is considered hopeless, and the patient can be allowed to die. Mr Burke, a patient suffering from a chronic debilitating condition, had challenged the General Medical Council (GMC) guidelines on withholding treatment arguing that he could insist on being treated even when it was contrary to professional judgment. He succeeded in the High Court, but the appeal of the GMC was allowed by the Court of Appeal.[3] (The case is discussed below and in Chapter 6.)

Human rights and the right to life

Article 2 of the European Convention of Human Rights (see Appendix 1) recognises the right to life. However, arguments that this right was breached when people were allowed to die have failed. In a case[4] in 2000, parents lost their attempt to ensure that a severely handicapped baby born prematurely was resuscitated if necessary. The judge ruled that the hospital should provide him with palliative care to ease his suffering, but should not try to revive him as that would cause unnecessary pain. In another case, the President of the Family Division, Dame Elizabeth Butler-Sloss, held that the withdrawal of life-sustaining medical treatment was not contrary to Article 2 of the Human Rights Convention and the right to life where the patient was in a persistent vegetative state (PVS). The ruling was made on 25 October 2000 in cases involving Mrs M, a 49-year-old woman who suffered brain damage during an operation abroad in 1997 and was diagnosed as being in a PVS in October 1998, and in the case of Mrs H, aged 36, who fell ill in America as a result of pancreatitis during Christmas 1999.[5] In the light of these decisions, it would appear that failure to resuscitate a patient, when circumstances justify the decision, would not amount to a breach of Article 2.

In a case to determine whether a hospital was in breach of Article 2 following the suicide of a detained mental patient, it was held that the claimant had to show that at the time of the suicide the hospital knew or ought to have known of the existence of a real and immediate risk to her life from self-harm and that it failed to take measures which reasonably might have been expected to avoid that risk.[6] The Court of Appeal did not accept the Trust's argument that the claimant had to establish gross negligence by the defendant. The facts of the case were that the claimant's mother, who had a long history of mental illness had been detained under Section 3 of the Mental Health Act 1983. She had made frequent attempts to leave and eventually succeeded and walked to a railway station and jumped in front of train. The Court of Appeal compared the situation of a detained mentally ill patient to that of a prisoner, who were both under the control of a state in a way in which ordinary patients were not.

Breach of Article 2 has also been claimed in cases where it had been alleged that an inadequate inquiry had been held in relation to a death or serious harm in custody. Thus, in a case where a young man attempted suicide in Feltham Young offenders Institution and was left brain damaged, the Court of Appeal held that in such a situation Article 2 rights required that there was a clear obligation on the Secretary of State to ensure that there was an effective inquiry into the near death.[7]

An application for an inquest to be held was granted in the case of *Bicknell* v. *HM Coroner for Birmingham and Solihull* in 2007.[8] The daughter of a man who had died in a care home applied for judicial review of the coroner's decision not to hold an inquest. The father had been suffering from mental health problems and had died soon after admission to the home. Despite the daughter's concern about his treatment, the death was not reported to the coroner and the funeral and cremation took place. The National Care Standards Commission (predecessor to the Commission for Social Care Inspection) carried out an inquiry and the owners voluntarily closed the home. The daughter gave the coroner the report of a medical expert who criticised the medical records in the home and raised concerns about the increased dose of medication and the bucket chair in which he was placed. The coroner held that there was no evidence of unnatural death and refused the request for an inquest. The High Court held that the medical evidence and the daughter's observations gave rise to a reasonable cause to suspect that he had died an unnatural death. In addition, the results of the National Care Standards Commission inquiry revealed concerns about his death.

Murder and manslaughter

To kill a patient may be murder or manslaughter.

Murder is when a man of sound memory, and of the age of discretion, unlawfully killeth within any country of the realm any reasonable creature *in rerum natura* under the King's peace, with malice aforethought, either expressed by the party or implied by law, so as the party wounded, or hurt, etc. die of the wound or hurt etc. (within a year and a day after the same). (Words in parentheses subsequently deleted.)

This definition of murder was given in a court case in the seventeenth century by Sir Edward Coke. In 1996 the limitation of time was removed, so that it is not now required that the person dies within a year and a day of the act which caused the death.

Manslaughter is divided into two categories – voluntary and involuntary. Voluntary covers the situation where there is the mental intention to kill or complete indifference to the possibility that death could arise from one's actions, i.e. the mental requirement of a crime (*mens rea*) but there are extenuating factors:

- provocation
- death in pursuance of a suicide pact
- diminished responsibility.

The effect of these extenuating factors is that a murder verdict would not be obtained but the defendant could be guilty of voluntary manslaughter.

Involuntary manslaughter exists when the *mens rea* for murder is absent. Such circumstances would include:

- gross negligence;
- killing recklessly where the recklessness may be insufficient for it to be murder;
- an intention to escape from lawful arrest.

Defences to a charge of murder or manslaughter include:

- killing in the course of preventing crime or arresting offenders;
- killing in the defence of one's own person or that of another;
- killing in defence of property.

Use of excessive force will negate these defences.

Where the accused is convicted of manslaughter the judge has complete discretion over sentencing. In contrast, where there is a murder conviction, at present the sentence is a mandatory one of life imprisonment. The Law Commission published a consultation paper in 2006 for a new Homicide Act.[9] It put forward the proposal that the structure of a reformed law of homicide should comprise three general offences plus specific offences: first-degree murder would have a mandatory life sentence, second-degree murder would have a discretionary life sentence, manslaughter would have a fixed term of years maximum imprisonment and specific offences such as assisting suicide and infanticide should have a fixed term of years maximum imprisonment. Provisions have been included in the Coroners and Justice Bill currently before Parliament.

In February 2008 a husband who had suffocated his sick wife was given a 12-month suspended prison sentence and escaped prison.[10] He had admitted manslaughter on grounds of diminished responsibility and aiding and abetting his wife's suicide. His wife suffered from multiple sclerosis. In another case a woman who tried repeatedly to kill her disabled husband was given 100 hours of community service. The judge was satisfied that her attempts were a cry for help and not a serious attempt to kill her husband.[11] Her husband was crippled by arthritis and she had looked after him every day for 5 years at her home while working full time. The judge accepted that she was unable to cope with the strain of caring for him.

Voluntary euthanasia

By this is meant the killing of a person with that person's consent. This is unlawful. It could amount to murder, punishable on conviction

> A person who aids, abets, counsels or procures the suicide of another or an attempt by another to commit suicide, shall be liable on conviction on indictment to imprisonment. [up to 14 years]

Figure 25.1   The Suicide Act 1961: Section 2(1)

by life imprisonment, or it could be seen as manslaughter with the discretion over sentencing. Alternatively, if the act amounts to assistance in a suicide bid, then it is illegal under Section 2(1) of the Suicide Act 1961, which is shown in Figure 25.1.

Situation: asking for help

The wife of a patient who was in the terminal stages of a respiratory disease was concerned that the patient found breathing difficult in spite of constant oxygen and no longer wished to carry on living. She asked the physiotherapist if she would provide her with some medicines to help her husband out of his misery. What right of action does the physiotherapist have?

There is no grey area of law here. Any action on the part of the physiotherapist to assist the wife in ending her husband's misery would constitute a criminal wrong and they could both face murder or manslaughter proceedings or prosecution for an offence under the Suicide Act.

Case of Diane Pretty[12]

In a well-publicised case, Diane Pretty, a sufferer of motor neurone disease, appealed to the House of Lords that her husband should be allowed to end her life, and not be prosecuted under the Suicide Act 1961. The House of Lords did not allow her appeal. It held that if there were to be any changes to the Suicide Act to legalise the killing of another person, then these changes should be made by Parliament. As the law stood, the Suicide Act made it a criminal offence to aid

and abet the suicide of another person and the husband could not be granted immunity from prosecution were he to assist his wife to die. The House of Lords held that there was no conflict between the human rights of Mrs Pretty as set out in the European Convention on Human Rights. Mrs Pretty then applied to the European Court of Human Rights in Strasbourg, but lost. The Court held that there was no conflict between the Suicide Act 1961 and the European Convention of Human Rights. The Council of Europe issued a press release entitled Chamber judgement in the case of *Pretty* v. *the United Kingdom* published on April 29 2002.[13]

An MS sufferer Debbie Purdy was permitted to bring an action to clarify the law on assisted suicide. She wished her husband to take her to a Belgian clinic or Switzerland to commit suicide if her condition became unbearably painful and wants to ensure that he would not be prosecuted for aiding and abetting her suicide.[14]

However, she failed in her application. The High Court held that it had great sympathy for Ms Purdy, her husband and others in a similar position to know in advance whether they will face prosecution for doing what many would regard as something that the law should permit, namely to help a loved one to go abroad to end their suffering when they are unable to do it on their own. However, the court said that this would involve a change in the law. The offence of suicide is very widely drawn to cover all manner of different circumstances: only Parliament can change it. The court also said that the Code of Practice for Crown Prosecutors issued by the Director of Public Prosecutions, coupled with the general safeguards of administrative law, satisfied human rights convention standards and met the need for clarity and foreseeability and there was no breach of Article 8 of the European Convention on Human Rights and the right to private and family life.

Ms Purdy was given leave to appeal to the Court of Appeal.[15]

Even where the parents wish a grossly handicapped baby to die, any professional who intentionally speeds up the process of death could be guilty of causing the death of the child.

Case: *R v. Arthur*[16]

A paediatrician was prosecuted for attempting to cause the death of a grossly handicapped baby who was suffering from Down's syndrome and who had other disabilities. He had prescribed dihydrocodeine and nursing care only.

The judge had stated that:

There is no special law in this country that places doctors in a separate category and gives them extra protection over the rest of us ... Neither in law is there any special power, facility or license to kill children who are handicapped or seriously disadvantaged in an irreversible way.

Dr Arthur was however acquitted by the jury.

In contrast, at the other end of life, Dr Nigel Cox[17] was convicted when he prescribed potassium chloride to a terminally ill patient and was sentenced to a year's imprisonment which was suspended for a year. He also had to appear before disciplinary proceedings of the Regional Health Authority, his employers and before the GMC.

The Select Committee of the House of Lords[18] has reported that there should be no change in the law to permit euthanasia. This is also the view put forward by the Law Commission in a report in 1995.[19] Lord Joffe has introduced several Bills into the House of Lords to legalise assisting in a suicide. However, none has ever obtained Parliamentary approval and assisting another person to die still remains unlawful.

Letting die

Do these cases mean that it is never lawful to permit patients to die whatever the circumstances of their condition? The answer is that the law does not expect constant medical intervention whatever the prognosis and, in certain circumstances, it is legally permissible to let a patient die. A distinction is however drawn between letting die and killing.

Adults

Where an adult wishes to die and refuses treatment, then crucial to the decision making and withholding treatment is their mental capacity to make a decision or the existence of a living will (now known as an advance decision) (see below).

Situation: coming off a ventilator

A tetraplegic patient attended by the physiotherapist told her that he wished to be allowed to die and come off the ventilator. What is the legal situation?

This is the situation that arose in the Karen Quinlan case in the USA, where an extremely long court case resulted in a decision being made that she could come off the ventilator. Once off, ironically, she survived for several years. More recently in the UK a patient who had become paralysed following a haemorrhage was ventilated against her wishes. She applied to court for a declaration that she could lawfully refuse ventilation. The only issue before the judge was whether she had the mental capacity to make such a decision. After hearing evidence of two psychiatrists as to her mental competence the judge had no alternative other than to make the declaration she sought and to find that she had been subjected to a trespass to her person.[20] The case of Ms B is considered in more detail in Chapter 7.

A mentally competent person has the right to refuse treatment. However, in this situation the physiotherapist should be careful not to undertake any action which could be interpreted as aiding or abetting a suicide attempt. The physiotherapist should also obtain independent advice on the mental competence of the patient to refuse treatment (see Chapter 7 and the law relating to consent).

Children

The following is an example of the court permitting a child to be allowed to die.

Case: *Re C*[21]

In this case a baby was born suffering from congenital hydrocephalus and had been made a ward of court for reasons unconnected with her medical condition. The local authority sought the court's determination as to the appropriate manner in which she should be treated in the event of her contracting a serious infection or her existing feeding regimes becoming unviable. A specialist paediatrician assessed C's condition as severely and irreversibly brain damaged, the prognosis of which was hopeless. He recommended that the objective of any treatment should therefore be to ease suffering rather than prolong life. While not specifying the adoption or discontinuance of any particular procedures, he further advised consultation with C's carers as to the appropriate method of achieving that objective. The judge accepted this report and approved the recommendations as being in her best interests. However, he made a very restrictive order to treat the child 'to die'.

The official solicitor who had been appointed *guardian ad litem* (see Glossary) of the child, appealed to the Court of Appeal on the ground that the judge had not jurisdiction and was plainly wrong in the exercise of his discretion to make an order that the hospital be at liberty to treat the minor to die.

The Court of Appeal varied the judge's order and the words 'to die' were changed to 'to allow her life to come to an end peacefully and with dignity'. The court emphasised that the decisions on treatment rested with the medical professionals:

The hospital do continue to treat the minor within the parameters of the opinion expressed by [the specialist paediatrician] in his report of 13.4.1989 which report is not to be disclosed to any person other than the health authority.

In *Re J*[22] (1990) the baby was a ward of court and in contrast with the case of *Re C* the baby was not at the point of death.

Case: *Re J* 1990

J's prognosis was not good and, although he was expected to survive a few years, he was likely to be blind, deaf, unable to speak and have serious spastic quadriplegia. The judge made an order that he should be treated with antibiotics if he developed a chest infection but if he were to stop breathing he should not receive artificial ventilation. The official solicitor on behalf of the child appealed against the order on the grounds that unless the situation was one of terminal illness or it was certain that the child's life would be intolerable, the court was not justified in approving the withholding of life saving treatment.

The Court of Appeal held that the court can never sanction positive steps to terminate the life of a person. However, the court could direct that treatment without which death would ensue need not be given to prolong life, even though the child was neither on the point of death nor dying. The court had to undertake a balancing exercise in assessing the course to be adopted in the best interests of the child, looked at from his point of view and giving the fullest possible weight to his desire, if he were in a position to make a sound judgment, to survive, but also taking into account the pain and suffering and quality of life which he would experience if life were prolonged and the pain and suffering involved in the proposed treatment.

The parents do not have the final say, though their wishes must be taken into account in determining the outcome for the child. Ultimately the courts, as is seen in the case of *Re J* (1992) (see below), have made it clear that the decision should be in the hands of the health professionals, i.e. the doctors. In recent years there have been several contested cases between parents and paediatricians as to whether active treatment should be given to a very severely disabled child. One example is that of the case of Charlotte Wyatt, where several applications were made to court for a declaration as to what was in the child's best interests.[23]

The Royal College of Paediatrics and Child Health (RCPCH)[24] has published a framework for practice in determining whether life-saving treatment should be withheld or withdrawn. These proposals cover the following situations.

Situations where withholding or withdrawal of treatment could be considered:

- brain dead
- persistent vegetative state
- the 'no chance' situation
- the 'no purpose' situation
- the 'unbearable' situation.

The principles, put forward in the first edition have been reaffirmed in the second edition, and are set out in Figure 25.2. Figure 25.3 shows the axioms that flow from the fundamental principles set out in the United Nations Convention on the Rights of the Child (1989).

Involvement of the court

When should the consent of the court be obtained to taking action? There are probably many occasions in practice when a patient is allowed to die without court approval being obtained.

Children and young persons

In the case of a young person under 18 years, if there is a dispute with clinicians it is advisable for there to be an application to the court rather than the clinicians ignore the views of the parents as to what is in the best interests of the child. This is the conclusion from the dispute between the parent of Glass and the paediatricians.[25] The case eventually went to the European Court of Human Rights, which held that the failure of the NHS trust to seek a declaration from the court before administering diamorphine to her son without her consent and in writing him up for 'do not resuscitate' instructions without her knowledge was a breach of her Article 8 rights.

---

(1) To act always in the child's best interests
(2) It is unrealistic to expect a complete consensus – aim to seek as much ethical common ground as possible
(3) Seek court intervention if disputes between the health care team, the child, the parents and carers cannot be resolved
(4) Consider each situation on its merits
(5) There is no ethical difference between the withdrawal and the withholding of treatment.
(6) The duty of care is not absolute
(7) Redirection of care from life sustaining to palliation is not withdrawal of care
(8) It is never permissible to withdraw pain relief or contact
(9) Treatments the primary aim of which is the relief of suffering, but which may incidentally hasten death, may be justified

Figure 25.2 Principles set by the Royal College of Paediatrics and Child Health

- There is no significant ethical difference between withdrawing (stopping) and withholding treatments, given the same ethical objective.
- Optimal ethical decision making concerning children requires open and timely communication between members of the Health Care Team and the child and family respecting their values and beliefs and the fundamental principles of ethics and human rights.
- Parents may ethically and legally decide on behalf of children who are unable, for whatever reason, to express preferences, unless they are clearly acting against the child's best interest or are unable, unwilling or persistently unavailable to make decisions on behalf of their child.
- The wishes of a child who has obtained sufficient understanding and experience in the evaluation of treatment options should be given substantial consideration in the decision-making process.
- The antecedent wishes and preferences of the child, if known, should also carry considerable weight given that conditions at the time for action match those envisaged in advance.
- In general, resolution of disagreement should be by discussion, consultation and consensus.
- The duty of care is not an absolute duty to preserve life by all means. There is no obligation to provide life sustaining treatment if:
  - its use is inconsistent with the aims and objectives of an appropriate treatment plan
  - the benefits of that treatment no longer outweigh the burden to the patient.
- It is ethical to withdraw life sustaining treatment if refused by a competent child; or from children who are unable to express wishes and preference when the Health Care Team and parent/carers agree that such treatment is not in the child's best interests.
- A redirection of management from life-sustaining treatment to palliation represents a change in beneficial aims and objectives and does not constitute a withdrawal of care.
- The range of life-sustaining treatments is wide and will vary with the individual circumstances of the patient. It is never permissible to withdraw procedures designed to alleviate pain or promote comfort.
- There is a distinction to be drawn between treatment of the dying patient and euthanasia. When a dying patient is receiving palliative care, the underlying cause of death is the disease process. In euthanasia, the intended action is to cause death.
- It follows that use of medication and other treatments which may incidentally hasten death may be justified if their primary aim is to relieve suffering. The EAC–RCPCH does not support the concept of euthanasia.
- Legal intervention should be considered when disputes between the Health Care Team, the child, parents and carers cannot be resolved by attempts to achieve consensus.

Figure 25.3   Axioms put forward by the Ethics Advisory Committee (EAC) of the Royal College of Paediatrics and Child Health (RCPCH)

Mentally competent adults

If a patient refuses treatment and it is determined that the patient has the capacity to refuse to give consent, then the patient's refusal cannot be overruled (see Chapter 7 and the case of *Re C*).

Adults lacking the requisite mental capacity

Where the patient lacks mental competence, if the doctors, the parents and the rest of the multidisciplinary team are agreed that the prognosis of the patient is extremely poor and that aggressive treatment is inappropriate there is unlikely to be a court hearing. The patient will be allowed to die and 'nature to take its course'. Under the Mental Capacity Act 2005, where the patient lacks the requisite mental capacity to make his or her own decision, in the absence of an advance decision or living will, decisions must be made in his or her best interests. However, it is a specific requirement of Section 4(5) that 'where the determination relates to life-sustaining treatment (the person making the decision) must not, in considering whether the treatment is in the best interests of the person concerned, be motivated by a desire to bring about his death'.

If there are disputes over what is in the best interests of a mentally incapacitated patient, an application could be made to the Court of Protection, which since October 2007 has jurisdiction over issues of the personal welfare as well as the property and finance of those lacking mental capacity. The following case preceded the establishment of the new Court of Protection but the same principles would apply under the Mental Capacity Act 2005.

The Tony Bland case

Case: *Airedale NHS Trust* v. *Bland* [26]

> The patient was a victim of the football stadium crush at Hillsborough and it was established that, although he could breathe and digest food independently, he could not see, hear, taste, smell or communicate in any way and it appeared that there was no hope of recovery or improvement. Given the importance of the issues involved the matter was referred to the House of Lords, which had to decide if it was lawful to permit artificial feeding to be discontinued in the case of a patient in a persistent vegetative state.

The House of Lords held that it would be in the best interests of the patient to discontinue the nasal gastric feed and he was later reported as having died. It specifically recommended that if any similar decisions were required to be made in the future there should be application before the courts and a court in Bristol gave consent in

a similar case [27] a few months after the House of Lords decision on Tony Bland.

Court guidance

A practice note was issued by the Official Solicitor [28] following the case and in due course further directions will be issued in the light of the Mental Capacity Act 2005 and hearings before the Court of Protection.

Advance decisions or Living wills

A living will (also known as an advance refusal of treatment or advance decision or an advance directive) is a statement, made when a person is mentally competent, over what treatments and care they would wish to refuse at a later time, when they no longer have the mental capacity to make decisions. Statutory provision has been made for advance decisions by the Mental Capacity Act 2005 (MCA), which came into force in October 2007.

An advance decision is defined in Section 24(1) as being a decision made by a person ('P'), after he has reached 18 and when he has capacity to do so, that if:

(a) at a later time and in such circumstances as he may specify, a specified treatment is proposed to be carried out or continued by a person providing health care for him, and

(b) at that time he lacks capacity to consent to the carrying out or continuation of the treatment,

the specified treatment is not to be carried out or continued.

Although the MCA in general covers those over 16 years, 18 years is the minimum age for making a valid advance decision because of the present power of the court to overrule the refusal of life-saving treatment by a young person under 18 years. (See Chapter 23 and the case of *Re W*. [29])

There is no necessity for the advance decision to be written in a particular format (except for refusal of life-sustaining treatment – see below), since Section 24(2) states that a decision may be regarded as specifying a treatment or circumstances even though expressed in layman's terms. However, clearly it is essential that the treatment which is being refused is unambiguous and therefore there are considerable advantages if professional help is obtained on its wording.

The Act permits the person who drew up the advance decision to withdraw it or alter it at any time provided that he has the mental capacity to do so. This withdrawal (including a partial withdrawal) need not be in writing. Nor need an alteration be in writing unless as a result of the alteration it now refers to the refusal of life-sustaining treatment, since special statutory provisions apply to life-sustaining treatments.

Life-sustaining treatments

An advance decision is not applicable to life-sustaining treatment unless:

(a)   the decision is verified by a statement by P to the effect that it is to apply to that treatment even if life is at risk, and
(b)   the decision and statement comply with the conditions set down in Section 24(6).

These conditions for an advance decision covering life-sustaining treatments are as follows:

(a)   it is in writing,
(b)   it is signed by P or by another person in P's presence and by P's direction,
(c)   the signature is made or acknowledged by P in the presence of a witness, and
(d)   the witness signs it, or acknowledges his signature, in P's presence.

The effect of an advance decision

An advance decision does not come into effect until the maker has lost the mental capacity to make his/her own decisions. To be valid it must relate to the treatment in question and to the circumstances envisaged by the maker. If there are reasonable grounds for believing that circumstances exist which the maker of the advance decision (P) did not anticipate at the time of the advance decision and which would have affected his/her decision had he/she anticipated them, then the advance decision would not apply.

If the advance decision is valid and the circumstances are as envisaged and the treatment is as specified, then health professionals and others must accept the refusal of the patient, if they have no reason to believe it to be invalid or inapplicable. If a person is satisfied that an advance decision exists which is valid and applicable to the treatment, then he or she could incur liability for carrying out or continuing the treatment contrary to the wishes expressed in the advance decision. On the other hand, a person does not incur liability for the consequences of withholding or withdrawing a treatment from P if, at the time, he reasonably believes that an advance decision exists which is valid and applicable to the treatment.

If however

(a)   the maker has withdrawn the decision at a time when he/she had capacity to do so, or
(b)   has under a lasting power of attorney created after the advance decision was made, conferred authority on the donee (or, if more than one, any of them) to give or refuse consent to the treatment to which the advance decision relates, or
(c)   has done anything else clearly inconsistent with the advance decision remaining his/her fixed decision,

then the advance decision will not apply to the situation and is not binding upon those caring for the patient. As an advance statement however it should be taken into account in determining the patient's best interests since this statement is an expression of the patient's views (see Chapter 7 and determination of best interests).

In the event of reasonable doubt about the validity of an advance decision, an application can be made to the Court of Protection for a declaration as to its existence, its validity and its applicability to the treatment in question. In the meantime life-sustaining treatment can be provided or anything which is reasonably believed to be necessary to prevent a serious deterioration in P's condition, while a decision is sought from the court.

Situation: refusing treatment

A patient, on hearing that he was suffering from motor neurone disease, wrote an advanced refusal of treatment indicating that he would not wish to receive any artificial feeding. He is now finding it more and more difficult to swallow and artificial feeding is seen as the only option. The consultant has stated that this should be commenced and refuses to accept that the living will has any significance to his clinical judgment. What is the law?

Since October 2007 if an advance decision is to cover a refusal of life-sustaining treatment, then the statutory provisions set out above must be satisfied. If these are satisfied, then there is an obligation upon all health professionals to respect the wishes of the patient. If the consultant treats the patient contrary to the wishes expressed in a valid and applicable advance decision, then he is guilty of trespass to the person (see Chapter 7) and those acting on behalf of the patient could instigate an action against him.

Can the court order doctors to provide treatment?

Case: *Re J* (1992)[30]

J was born in January 1991 and suffered an accidental fall when he was a month old, with the result that he was profoundly handicapped both mentally and physically. He was severely microcephalic, his brain not having grown sufficiently following the injury. He also had severe cerebral palsy, cortical blindness and severe epilepsy. He was in general fed by a nasal gastric tube. Medical opinion was unanimous that J was unlikely to develop much beyond his present functioning, that that level might deteriorate and that his expectation of life, although uncertain, would be short. The paediatrician's report stated that, given J's condition, it would not be medically appropriate to intervene with intensive procedures such as artificial ventilation if he were to suffer a life-threatening event.

The baby was in the care of foster parents with whom the local authority shared responsibility. The local authority applied to the court under Section 100 of the Children Act 1989 to determine whether ventilation should be given to the child. The mother supported the requirement that the hospital and doctors should be forced to put the baby on a life support machine.

The judge regarded J's best interests as well as the interests of justice in preserving his life as both pointing in favour of the grant of an interim injunction requiring such treatment to take place. The hospital appealed.

In the Court of Appeal Lord Donaldson, Master of the Rolls, stated that he could not at present conceive of any circumstances in which requiring a medical practitioner (or a health authority acting by a medical practitioner) to adopt a course of treatment, which in the *bona fide* clinical judgment of the practitioner was contra-indicated as not being in the patient's best interests, would be other than an abuse of power, as directly or indirectly requiring the practitioner to act contrary to the fundamental duty he owed to his patient.

Lord Donaldson said that the order of the judge, ordering specific treatment to take place, was wholly inconsistent with the law as stated in *Re J*[22] (see above) and in *Re R*[31] and could not be justified on the basis of any known authority. It was also erroneous on two other substantial grounds:

- its lack of certainty as to what was required of the health authority; and
- its failure adequately to take account of the sad fact of life that health authorities might on occasion find that they had too few

resources, either human or material or both, to treat all the patients whom they would like to treat in the way they would like to treat them.

It was the health authority's duty to make choices. The court would have no knowledge of competing claims to resources and was in no position to express any view on their deployment of these resources.

The Court of Appeal thus held that where a paediatrician caring for a severely handicapped baby considered that mechanical ventilation procedures would not be appropriate the court would not grant an injunction requiring such treatment to take place.

The effect of the Court's decision to set aside the judge's ruling was to leave the health authority and its medical staff free, subject to consent not being withdrawn, to treat J in accordance with their best clinical judgment. That did not mean that in no circumstances should J be subjected to mechanical ventilation.

The reluctance of the court to interfere with the decision making of the doctors in the interests of the patient was seen in a recent case in very different circumstances. In a case[32] where the father of a girl of 10 suffering from leukaemia brought an action against the health authority for its refusal to fund a course of chemotherapy followed by a second bone marrow transplant operation, the Court of Appeal took the view that the courts should not intervene in such a decision but that the health authority should follow medical advice as to what was in the best interests of the child. (See Chapter 6 for a fuller discussion of the case.)

In the Burke case the Court of Appeal held that a patient could not insist on being provided with treatment when it was contrary to professional discretion (see below).

Under the MCA decisions relating to extremely serious treatment decisions would now go before the Court of Protection. The Code of Practice on the MCA[33] states that:

Cases involving any of the following decisions should therefore be brought before a court:

- chemotherapy and surgery for cancer
- electroconvulsive therapy
- therapeutic sterilisation
- major surgery (such as open-heart surgery or brain/neurosurgery)
- major amputations (for example, loss of an arm or leg)
- treatments which will result in permanent loss of hearing or sight
- withholding or stopping artificial nutrition and hydration, and
- termination of pregnancy.

'Not for resuscitation' orders

A joint statement from the British Medical Association, Resuscitation Council (UK) and the Royal College of Nursing[34] provided guidance on decisions relating to cardiopulmonary resuscitation in 1999 (updated in 2001 and 2007). The original guidance was commended to NHS trusts in September 2000 by the NHS Executive[35] in an NHS Circular. Every trust should have in place a policy relating to the use of Not For Resuscitation instructions.

What is the legal significance of such orders?

Competent adults

If patients have the mental competence to understand the situation they are entitled to refuse to give consent to any treatment, even though the treatment is life saving (see Chapter 7 and in particular the case of *Re Ms B*[20]).

Children and young persons

Although a child of 16 or 17 has a statutory right to give consent to treatment, a case in 1992 decided that children cannot refuse treatment that is in their best interests. In the case of *Re W*[36] a girl of 16 years refused to be treated for anorexia nervosa, but her refusal was overruled by the court (see Chapter 23). If, however, the decision made by the minor is considered to be in his or her best interests, then it would be valid for all professional carers of that patient to accept that refusal of care and the instructions that the patient is not to be resuscitated.

Mental incapacity

Where the patient is mentally incapacitated, then the Mental Capacity Act 2005 applies and action must be taken in the best interests of that person, unless the person has, when he or she had the requisite mental capacity, drawn up an advance decision or appointed a lasting power of attorney. If the consultant in charge of the care of the patient decides that it is in the best interests of the patient that he or she should not be resuscitated then this decision would stand. In the event of a dispute over the best interests of the patient, an application could be made to the Court of Protection for a declaration as to what was in the best interests of the patient. The steps laid down in Section 4 of the MCA should be followed in determining what are the best interests (see Chapter 7 and Box 7.2).

Relatives and carers

- Could the relatives give 'not for resuscitation' (NFR) or 'do not resuscitate' instructions?

Relatives are able to make day-to-day decisions on behalf of a mentally incapacitated adult, provided that they make them in the best interests of the patient and follow the statutory principles and steps set down under Section 4 of the MCA. Where there is no binding advance decision

or lasting power of attorney, the clinical team would normally make serious medical decisions. In the absence of persons who could be consulted, an independent mental capacity advocate should be appointed and would report on the best interests of the patient, according to the statutory provisions. If there are relatives, then the MCA requires full consultation with them in order to satisfy the statutory provisions. If a relative has been appointed under a lasting power of attorney, which gives to the donee the power to make decisions about life-sustaining treatment, then that donee would have the right to make a decision as to whether the patient is to be resuscitated. The statutory provisions must however have been complied with. Similarly if the patient had, when competent, drawn up an advance decision that covers resuscitation in the circumstances which now exist, then provided the statutory provisions relating to advance decisions refusing life-sustaining treatment (see above) are complied with, then these NFR instructions must be followed.

An NFR matrix

Figure 25.4 provides a matrix showing how the factors of mental competence and prognosis impact on each other in NFR decisions.

The Burke case in the middle box on the bottom line, where the mentally competent patient is asking for treatment when the prognosis is bad, applies where a patient asks for treatment contrary to clinical judgment. A mentally competent patient does not have an absolute right to insist on treatment when it is not clinically indicated.

Is the patient competent?	No	Yes – and the patient asks for treatment	Yes – but the patient refuses treatment
Good prognosis	**resuscitate**	**resuscitate**	**NFR**
Bad prognosis	**NFR**	**The Burke case**[62]	**NFR**

Figure 25.4 A matrix for 'not for resuscitation' (NFR)

However, it depends upon the detailed circumstances – resuscitation may or may not be clinically indicated and if it is not clinically indicated, a mentally competent person cannot compel such treatment to be given. The ruling in the Court of Appeal in the Burke case.[3,37] would apply. The case is set out in Chapter 6.

Parents' refusal to consent to treatment

An example of where the courts refused to uphold the parents' wish to allow the child to die is seen in the following case.

Case: *Re B*[38]

> In *Re B* a child was born suffering from Down's syndrome and an intestinal blockage. She required an operation to relieve the obstruction if she was to live more than a few days. If the operation were performed, the child might die within a few months but it was probable that her life expectancy would be 20–30 years. Her parents, having decided that it would be kinder to allow her to die rather than live as a physically and mentally handicapped person, refused to consent to the operation. The local authority made the child a ward of court and, when a surgeon decided that the wishes of the parents should be respected, they sought an order authorising the operation to be performed by other named surgeons.

The judge decided that the parents' wishes should be respected and refused to make the order.

The local authority appealed to the Court of Appeal, which allowed the appeal. It stated that:

(1)   The question for the court was whether it was in the best interests of the child that she should have the operation and not whether the parents' wishes should be respected.
(2)   Since the effect of the operation might be that the child would have the normal span of life of a Down's syndrome person; and

(3)   Since it had not been demonstrated that the life of a person with Down's syndrome was of such a nature that the child should be condemned to die;
(4)   The court would make an order that the operation be performed.

Crucial to the decision in this case was the prognosis of the child. In a contrasting case the parents' refusal was upheld by the courts.

Case: *Re T (a minor)* (wardship: medical treatment[39])

> A child was born with a life-threatening liver defect. After unsuccessful treatment, the prognosis was that he would not live beyond two and a half years without a liver transplant. The mother refused to give consent to the operation because she was not willing to permit the child to undergo the pain and distress of invasive surgery. She later moved out of the country. The local authority, at the consultants' instigation, applied to the court for permission to carry out the operation and for the child to be returned to the jurisdiction in order that the operation could be carried out. The High Court judge held that the mother's refusal was unreasonable and it was in the child's best interests to undergo the liver transplant. The mother appealed.

The Court of Appeal upheld that appeal. The paramount consideration was the welfare of the child and not the reasonableness of the parent's refusal of consent. However, since the welfare of the child depended upon the mother, her views were relevant. The judge had failed to assess the relevance or the weight of the mother's concern as to the benefits to her child of the surgery and post-operative treatment, the dangers of failure both long term as well as short term, the possibility of the need for further transplants, the likely length of life and the effect on her child of all those concerns, together with the strong reservations expressed by one of the consultants about coercing the mother into playing a crucial part in the aftermath of the operation and thereafter.

It must be stressed, however, that *Re T* is an unusual case and there were very special circumstances that led to the court upholding the wishes of the parents over those of the doctors.

The right to insist on treatment

Parents

Parents do not have the right to insist upon care or treatment that the doctors consider is not in the best interests of the child. As has been discussed above, the court would not order the doctors to carry out treatment on a child, which the doctors considered was not in the best interests of the child. (See also the case of Jamie Bowen[32] discussed in Chapter 6.)

Mentally competent adults

Nor do any adults have an absolute right to insist upon treatment. A health professional would be failing in his/her obligations if he/she provided treatment, on the patient's insistence, knowing that it was professionally contra-indicated, or even just of no effect. If a patient purported in a living will to direct that treatment be given rather than just refusing treatment in anticipation, this direction is likely to be of little effect if it is not supported by professional judgment as to its appropriateness (see Figure 25.4, the Burke case and also Chapter 6).

Care of the dying patient

Children

The Association for Children's Palliative Care (ACT) (formerly the Association for children with life-threatening or terminal conditions and their families) has been active in developing a charter for their care. Its clauses are set out in Figure 25.5.

The Department of Health has prepared guidance for health service organisations on caring for the dying patient, which can be accessed on its website.[40] In July 2008 the Government published an end of life strategy for the following 10 years. This stated that patients with terminal conditions should have a care plan setting out how they might be supported with pain relief; that patients should have more choice over where they die and should be encouraged to make their wishes known. 'Rapid response' nursing teams should be available to provide care to those who wish to die in the setting they choose. Medical staff should be trained to speak to the patient about his or her prognosis. An extra £286 million would be allocated to support the strategy.

General application

The Chartered Society of Physiotherapy (CSP) has identified the role of the physiotherapist in palliative care in its response to the Health Select Committee's Inquiry into hospice and palliative care.[41] The National Council of Palliative Care (NCPC) has published a bulletin on the palliative care needs of older people which would be useful for physiotherapists.[42] The National Service Framework (NSF) on long-term conditions published in 2005 contains a section on palliative care which could be used to ensure that the resources are provided to maintain the required standard. The NSF is available on the DH website (see also Chapter 24).

Situation: am I dying?

A community physiotherapist was asked by a patient suffering in the terminal stages of motor neurone disease 'How much longer do I have?' The physiotherapist knew that he was dying but found it difficult to answer since the patient's wife refused to acknowledge to the patient the true position.

The answer to the question may require all the physiotherapist's skills and sensitivity. On the one hand, she cannot lie to the patient, although in fact she would probably not know the exact

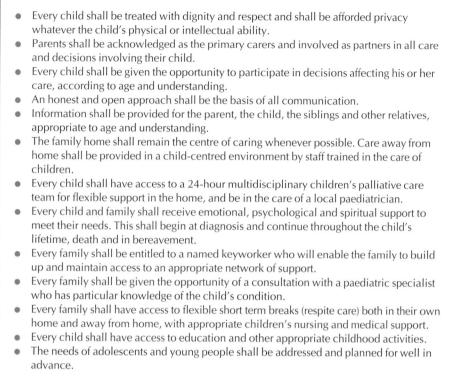

- Every child shall be treated with dignity and respect and shall be afforded privacy whatever the child's physical or intellectual ability.
- Parents shall be acknowledged as the primary carers and involved as partners in all care and decisions involving their child.
- Every child shall be given the opportunity to participate in decisions affecting his or her care, according to age and understanding.
- An honest and open approach shall be the basis of all communication.
- Information shall be provided for the parent, the child, the siblings and other relatives, appropriate to age and understanding.
- The family home shall remain the centre of caring whenever possible. Care away from home shall be provided in a child-centred environment by staff trained in the care of children.
- Every child shall have access to a 24-hour multidisciplinary children's palliative care team for flexible support in the home, and be in the care of a local paediatrician.
- Every child and family shall receive emotional, psychological and spiritual support to meet their needs. This shall begin at diagnosis and continue throughout the child's lifetime, death and in bereavement.
- Every family shall be entitled to a named keyworker who will enable the family to build up and maintain access to an appropriate network of support.
- Every family shall be given the opportunity of a consultation with a paediatric specialist who has particular knowledge of the child's condition.
- Every family shall have access to flexible short term breaks (respite care) both in their own home and away from home, with appropriate children's nursing and medical support.
- Every child shall have access to education and other appropriate childhood activities.
- The needs of adolescents and young people shall be addressed and planned for well in advance.
- Every family shall have timely access to practical support, including clinical equipment, financial grants, suitable housing and domestic help.

Figure 25.5   The ACT (Association for Children's Palliative Care) charter for children with life-threatening conditions and their families.

answer to the question. Nor should she collude with the spouse in keeping information from the patient. On the other hand, she needs to attempt to create some understanding between patient and spouse and should be aware of organisations that could assist in this dilemma.

Registration of death and the role of the coroner

The doctor who attended the patient during the last illness must certify the death and give the cause unless the circumstances are such that the death should be reported to the coroner. These would include the following:[43]

- where the deceased was not attended in his last illness by a doctor;
- where the deceased was not seen by a doctor either after death or within the 14 days prior to death;
- where the cause of death is unknown;
- where death appears to be due to industrial disease or poisoning;
- where death may have been unnatural or caused by violence or neglect or abortion or attended by suspicious circumstances;
- where death has occurred during an operation or before recovery from an anaesthetic.

The following causes of death would therefore be reportable to the coroner:

- deaths following from a criminal offence such as murder, manslaughter or causing death by dangerous driving;
- suicide;
- deaths arising from road traffic accidents, industrial accidents, domestic accidents, etc.;
- death in custody: prison or police custody;
- deaths associated with medical treatment;
- sudden death;
- deaths following abortion, drug dependence or alcoholism;
- infant deaths where no midwife or doctor was present, cot deaths.

Usually the individual coroners will make known their requirements in respect of the notification of deaths occurring in hospital. Some, for example, may require reporting of all deaths occurring within 24 hours of emergency admission.[44]

Until the coroner has formally notified the doctor of his/her decision in relation to the deceased, the body remains under the control of the coroner, i.e. under his/her jurisdiction. The coroner has the right to request a post-mortem and there can be no action taken in respect of the body without his/her consent.

Situation: unnatural death

A physiotherapist visits a patient who is terminally ill. When she arrives, she is met by a distraught partner who says that he has just found the patient unconscious in bed with empty bottles of painkillers beside her. He does not know whether the doctor should be called.

It would appear from the few facts given here that the patient has made a suicide attempt. The duty of care owed to the patient would require the physiotherapist to ensure that emergency medical care was summoned. Were the patient to die, the doctor might be unable to certify the cause of death and would need to notify the coroner.

- Can relatives view the body?

Once the coroner has jurisdiction over the body, his or her consent must be obtained before the body can be viewed by the relatives.[45]

Post-mortem

If the coroner orders a post-mortem, the relatives have no right to refuse this. This is so even when the religious views of the deceased would be against a post-mortem.[46] On the other hand, if the doctor requests a post-mortem where the body is not under the jurisdiction of the coroner the person in charge of the body, usually a spouse or relative, could refuse to give consent. The requirements of the Human Tissue Act 2004 must be followed.

Inquest

Where a death has been reported to the coroner he/she will decide whether or not an inquest will be held. The coroner is obliged by law to hold an inquest:

- where there are reasons to suspect a criminal offence has caused the death;
- in cases of industrial accidents and diseases;
- on deaths in prison or police custody.

The existence of a general discretion to hold an inquest has been doubted.[47] The purpose of the inquest is to ascertain:

(1) who the deceased was;
(2) how, when and where the deceased came by his/her death.[48]

Possible verdicts are:

- natural causes
- unlawful killing
- killed lawfully
- suicide
- accidental death
- misadventure
- dependence upon a drug
- non-dependent abuse of drugs

- industrial disease
- neglect
- want of attention at birth
- attempted/self-induced abortion

An open verdict indicates that there is insufficient evidence to determine the nature of the death, i.e. the evidence did not further or fully disclose the means whereby the cause of death arose. A narrative verdict is sometimes given where it is necessary to explain the cause of death. For example, where an operation took place which of necessity would lead to the death of one conjoined twin, the coroner gave a narrative verdict.[49] Rule 43 of the coroner's rules was amended[50] from 17 July 2008 to require a coroner to report circumstances in which further deaths could occur if action is not taken to prevent them. The agency receiving such a report will be required to give the coroner a written response within 56 days stating what action has been taken. The amendment also allows the coroner to share relevant information with Local Safeguarding Children Boards to enable them to carry out their statutory functions of conducting child death reviews. Copies of the coroners' reports would be sent to other interested parties (including the bereaved families) and to the Lord Chancellor and to be published. This means that reports and responses will be centrally collated for the first time so that any trends can be identified, monitored and lessons learned can be shared widely.

Once completed the inquest cannot be resumed but the High Court has the power under Section 13(1)(b) of the Coroners Act 1988 to order another inquest to be held.

The physiotherapist and the coroner's court

A physiotherapist might be required to give evidence at an inquest on the events that preceded death. The physiotherapist should be alert to this possibility, for example the physiotherapist may know that a child who has died in an apparent cot death suffered from certain symptoms prior to his death. This information from the physiotherapist may be vital at any inquest.

It is essential that the physiotherapist obtains assistance from a senior manager or lawyer on the preparation of a statement that the coroner's office will require from him/her. If the physiotherapist is subsequently asked to attend the inquest he/she should have assistance in preparation for giving evidence. One means of preparation is for the physiotherapist to attend a different inquest so that he/she can have an understanding of the geography of the court, the procedure that is followed and the level of formality required at a time when he/she is not personally involved (see Chapter 13 on giving evidence).

The physiotherapist should note that the coroner's court is known as an 'inquisitorial' one. This means that, unlike the magistrates', crown courts and civil courts, where an action is brought by one person or organisation against another and the judge controls the proceedings – an 'adversarial' system – the coroner determines the witnesses who will give evidence, the course of the proceedings and he/she will disallow any question that in his/her opinion is not relevant or otherwise not a proper one. The coroner can himself examine the witnesses, often asking leading questions where information is not disputed to speed up the hearing. Hence the words 'inquisitorial' and 'inquest' (see Glossary).

Where the death has been reported to the coroner, no certificate can be issued or registration take place until he/she has made a decision. If the coroner decides that a post-mortem should be carried out, but no inquest is needed, he/she will issue Form B, which is sent or taken to the Registrar. The Registrar will then issue the death certificate and the certificate for disposal which is required by the undertaker before burial can take place. Authorisation for cremation requires an additional medical certificate or the certificate issued by the coroner.

The Registrar General for England and Wales has the right to supply information contained in any register of deaths to a person or body specified in the order for use in the prevention, detection, investigation or prosecution of offences.[51]

Death and miscarriage

Born alive

If a baby is born alive and then dies, there must be a registration of both the birth and the death.

Stillbirth

A stillbirth is defined as:

> Where a child issues forth from its mother after the 24th week of pregnancy, and which did not at any time after being completely expelled from its mother breathe or show any signs of life. (Section 41 of the Births and Deaths Registration Act 1953, as amended by Section 1 of the Still Birth Act 1992)

The stillbirth has to be registered as such and the informant has to deliver to the Registrar a written certificate that the child was not born alive. This must be signed by the registered medical practitioner or the registered midwife who was in attendance at the birth or who has examined the body. The certificate must state, to the best of the knowledge and belief of the person signing it, the cause of death and the estimated duration of the pregnancy (Section 11(1)(a)). Alternatively, a declaration in the pre-scribed form giving the reasons for the absence of a certificate and that the child was not born alive could be made (Section 11(1)(b)).

A stillbirth should be disposed of by burial in a burial ground or churchyard or by cremation at an authorised crematorium. A health authority should not dispose of a stillbirth without the consent of the parents.

Fetus of less than 24 weeks

If the fetus was delivered without any signs of life, then no registration is necessary. The fetus may be disposed of without formality in any way which does not constitute a nuisance or an affront to public decency. If the fetus, after expulsion, shows signs of life and then dies, it would have to be treated as both a birth and a death.

Health professionals should be sensitive to the fact that parents may suffer the same feelings of bereavement whatever the period of gestation and should therefore arrange for counselling and support as they would if the baby were full term.

Future changes

An inquiry was set up after the conviction of Harold Shipman for the murder of 15 patients (and possibly another 200). The third report[52] considered the present system for death and cremation certification and for the investigation of deaths by coroners, together with the conduct of those who had operated those systems in the aftermath of the deaths of Shipman's victims. The report noted that the present system of death and cremation certification failed to detect that Shipman had killed any of his 215 victims. The report made significant recommendations for the reform of the coroner's system and the cer-tification of death. Following the Third Shipman Report, a position paper was published by the Home Office[53] in March 2004 and constituted the Government's response to the Fundamental Review of Death Certification and Coroner Services[54] and the Shipman Inquiry. In February 2006 the Minister of State for Constitutional Affairs announced the implementation of the first set of reforms: those relating to the coroners' service,[55] a draft coroners bill, together with a draft charter for the bereaved were published in June 2006 to enable pre-legislative scrutiny to be undertaken by the Select Committee for the Department of Constitutional Affairs (DCA). The draft Bill was scrutinised by the DCA Select Committee,[56] which made strong criticisms about the fact that many of the proposals contained in the Shipman Report and in the position paper were omitted from the Bill, in particular the changes to the death certification system and a national system for the office of coroner. The Select Committee was also concerned that there was inadequate resourcing of the coronial service. The Government responded to these recom-mendations in November 2006.[57] A Coroners and Justice Bill is currently being discussed in Parliament.

Research by Bruce Guthrie at the University of Dundee suggests that even if the reforms were implemented, another Dr Shipman would probably not be identified till after he had committed about 30 murders.[58]

Organ transplants

The donation of organs from a deceased person and from a living person are both regulated by the Human Tissue Act 2004.

Human Tissue Act 2004

This Act covers the use of tissue and organs from the living and the dead.

Transplants from dead donors

If the dying person has been registered as an organ donor with the NHS organ donor register[59] or is carrying a donor card, then that would count as a valid consent for the removal of the organs. Where the deceased person had made it clear that he/she would wish his/her organs to be donated, relatives cannot overrule this request unless there is evidence that the deceased changed his/her mind. In contrast, where the deceased has not indicated any views about donation, then consent can be given by any person whom he/she has nominated to act on his/her behalf. Where there has been no such nomination, then a person in a qualifying relationship such as a partner or other relative or friend can give consent. The Act sets out the order of precedence of such persons. The Government is at present reviewing the law on organ donation and there are calls for an opt-out system to be adopted, i.e. unless the deceased person had made a specific request not to be regarded as an organ donor, organs could be taken.

New guidelines are to be published which will allow transplant surgeons to begin removing organs 5 minutes after a donor's heart has stopped in order to tackle the shortage of transplant donors.[60] The new guidelines will give doctors permission to omit a complex set of tests to establish brain stem death, which can take 20 minutes. The guidelines have met with concern and considerable debate.

Donation from live donors

Situation: live donation

A physiotherapist cares for a renal patient aged 23 years. She has been on dialysis for a number of years but has been advised that a kidney transplant is urgently required. Her mother has offered to be a donor and seeks the advice of the physiotherapist over whether such an offer would be accepted.

This situation would now come under the Human Tissue Act 2004. Donations from living donors can now take place provided strict statutory specifications are followed. These statutory provisions include information being given to the donors and recipients before consent is given. There can be paired donors so that where relatives are not a match they can be linked with a similar couple or couples who are equally unmatched so that pairings of matched donor/ donee can be created. Where the statutory provisions are satisfied, approval to the transplantation from a live donor can be given by the Human Tissue Authority.

Conclusions

In their care of terminally ill patients, physiotherapists need to be confident in their knowledge about the laws that apply. They may, for example, feel great empathy for a tetraplegic patient who no longer has the desire to live. They must be aware, however, that to assist in the death would be to commit a crime under the Suicide Act. Similarly, in the care of patients suffering from motor neurone disease they must keep a clear distinction between the right of the mentally capacitated patient to refuse to be treated, including the right of the patient to make an advance decision or appoint a donee under a lasting power of attorney, and the criminal act of killing the patient. They are also required to develop the skills to assist the bereaved in a practical way as the guidance provided by the Association of Chartered Physiotherapists in Women's Health (ACPWH) on those who have lost a baby or had a still birth illustrates.[61]

✏️ Questions and exercises

1   In what circumstances could a patient facing a terminal illness refuse treatment? (See also Chapter 7.)

2   Draw up the requirements for a valid advance decision which is intended to relate to life-sustaining treatment.

3   Parents of a child suffering from cystic fibrosis have suggested to you that physiotherapy and antibiotic treatment should be stopped. What are the legal considerations in this request and what action would you take?

4   Following the death of a patient in hospital who had been receiving physiotherapy treatment you are asked to provide a statement for the coroner. What principles would you bear in mind in preparing the statement? (See also Chapter 13.)

References

1   Hough, A. (2001) *Physiotherapy in Respiratory Care*, 3rd edn. Nelson Thornes, Cheltenham.

2   Dimond, B. (2008) *Legal Aspects of Death*. Quay Publications Dinton.

3   *R (on the application of Burke)* v. *General Medical Council and Disability Rights Commission and the Official Solicitor to the Supreme Court* [2004] EWHC 1879; [2004] Lloyd's Rep Med 451.

4   *A National Health Service Trust* v. *D* (2000) The Times Law Report, 19 July; [2000] Lloyd's Rep Med 411.

5   *NHS Trust A* v. *Mrs M and NHS Trust B* v. *Mrs H Family Division. The Times*, 25 October 2000; [2001] 1 All ER 801; [2001] 2 F.L.R. 367.

6   *Savage* v. *South Essex Partnership NHS Foundation Trust*. The Times Law Report, 9 January 2008; [2007] EWCA Civ 1375.

7   *R (on the application of JL)* v. *Secretary of State for the Home Department* [2007] EWCA Civ 767.

8   *Bicknell* v. *HM Coroner for Birmingham and Solihull* [2007] EWHC 2547 (Admin) (2008) 99 B.M.L.R 1.

9   Law Commission (2006) A new Homicide Act for England and Wales. Consultation paper 177.

10 Fletcher, H. (2008) Husband is Spared Jail for Suffocating Sick Wife who Wanted to Die. *The Times*, 2 February.

11 de Bruxelles, S. (2008) Freedom for Woman who Kept Trying to Kill her Husband. *The Times*, 13 May.

12 *R (on the application of Pretty)* v. *DPP* [2001] UKHL 61, [2001] 3 WLR 1598.

13 *Pretty* v. *United Kingdom* [2002] 35 EHRRI; [2002] 2 FLR 45.

14 Gibb, F. (2008) MS Sufferer Wins Right to Hearing on Assisted Suicide. *The Times*, 12 June.

15 *R (on the application of Purdy)* v. *DPP* [2008]. The Times Law Report, 17 November 2008.

16 *R* v. *Arthur* reported in *The Times*, 6 November 1981.

17 *R* v. *Cox* [1993] 2 All ER 19.

18 House of Lords: Committee on Medical Ethics, Session 1993–4 (31 January 1994) HMSO, London.

19 Law Commission (1995) Report No. 231. *Mental Incapacity*. HMSO, London.

20 *Re B* (Consent to treatment: capacity), The Times Law Report, 26 March 2002; [2002] 2 All ER 449.

21 *Re C* (a minor) (Wardship; medical treatment) [1989] 2 All ER 782.

22 *Re J* (a minor) (wardship; medical treatment) [1990] 3 All ER 930.

23 *Wyatt* v. *Portsmouth Hospital NHS Trust* [2004] EWHC Civ 2247; [2005] EWHC 117; [2005] EWHC 693; [2005] EWCA Civ 1181; [2005] EWHC 2293,.

24 Royal College of Paediatrics and Child Health (2004) *Withholding or Withdrawing Life Saving Treatment in Children. A Framework for Practice*, 2nd edn. RCPCH, London.

25 *R* v. *Portsmouth Hospitals NHS Trust ex parte Glass* [1999] 2 FLR 905; [1999] Lloyds RM 367; *Glass* v. *UK*, TLR, 11 March 2004, ECHR.

26 *Airedale NHS Trust* v. *Bland* [1993] 1 All ER 821.

27 *Frenchay Healthcare NHS Trust* v. *S* [1994] 2 All ER 403.

28 Practice Note [1996] 4 All ER 766.

29 *Re W* (a minor) (Medical Treatment) [1992] 4 All ER 627.

30 *Re J* [1992] 4 All ER 614; The Times Law Report, 12 June 1992.

31 *Re R* [1991] 4 All ER 177.

32 *R* v. *Cambridge and Huntingdon Health Authority ex parte B*. The Times Law Report, 15 March 1995. [1995] 2 All ER 129.

33 Ministry of Constitutional Affairs (2007) Code of Practice on Mental Capacity Act 2005 paragraph 10.45; www.justice.gov.uk.

34 British Medical Association, Resuscitation Council (UK) and the Royal College of Nursing (1999) *Decisions Relating to Cardiopulmonary Resuscitation*, BMA, London. Updated March 2001 and October 2007.

35 NHS Executive, Resuscitation Policy HSC 2000/028, September 2000.

36 *Re W* (a minor) (medical treatment) [1992] 4 All ER 206.

37 *R. (on the application of Burke)* v. *General Medical Council and Disability Rights Commission and Official Solicitor to the Supreme Court* [2004] EWHC 1879; [2004] Lloyd's Rep. Med 451; [2005] EWCA Civ 1003, 28 July 2005.

38 *Re B* (a minor) (wardship; medical treatment) [1981] 1 WLR 1421.

39 *Re T* (a minor) (wardship: medical treatment) [1997] 1 All ER 906; *Re C* (sic) (a minor; refusal of parental consent) [1997] 8 Med LR 166.

40 Department of Health (2005) *When a Patient Dies: Advice on Developing Bereavement Services in the NHS*. DH, London; http://www.dh.gov.uk/en/index.htm.

41 Chartered Society of Physiotherapists (2004) *Health Select Committee Inquiry into Hospice and Palliative Care – Response by the CSP*. CSP, London.

42 National Council of Palliative Care (2006) *The Palliative Care Needs of Older People*. Briefing bulletin Number 14. NCPC, London.

43 List taken from The Registration of Births and Deaths Regulations 1987 SI No. 2088; see further Knight, B. (1992) *Legal Aspects of Medical Practice*, 5th edn. pp 95–102, Churchill Livingstone, Edinburgh.

44 Knight, B. (1992) *Legal Aspects of Medical Practice*, 5th edn. p. 96, Churchill Livingstone, Edinburgh.

45 Dimond, B.C. (1995) Death in the Accident and Emergency Department. *Accident and Emergency Nursing* 3, 1, 38–41.

46 *R* v. *Westminster City Coroner, ex parte Rainer* (1968) 112 Solicitors Journal 883.

47 *R* v. *Poplar Coroner, ex parte Thomas* (CA) (1993) 2 WLR 547.

48 Coroners Act 1988 Section 11(5)(b).

49 *In re A (Minors: conjoined twins: medical treatment)*. The Times Law Report, 10 October 2000.

50 The Coroners (Amendment) Rules 2008 SI No 1652.

51 Supply of Information (Register of Deaths) (England and Wales) Order 2008 SI 570.

52 Shipman Inquiry Third Report: Death and Cremation Certification, 14 July 2003; www.the-shipman-inquiry.org.uk/reports.asp.

53 Home Office Reforming the Coroner and Death Certification Service. A Position Paper CM 6159 March 2004 Stationery Office.

54 Tom Luce Chair Fundamental Review of Death Certification and the Coroner Services in England, Wales and Northern Ireland Home Office 2003.

55 Department for Constitutional Affairs Coroners Service Reform Briefing Note February 2006 DCA.

56 Department for Constitution Affairs Select Committee's Report on the Reform of the Coroners' System and Death Certification 2006.

57 Government Response to the Report by the Constitutional Affairs Select Committee (Cm 6943, Session 2005-6) November 2006.

58 Hawkes, N. (2008) No Method in Place to Stop Killing Spree by New Shipman. *The Times*, 3 May.

59 www.uktransplant.org.uk/uk

60 Rogers, L. (2008) Brain-death Test Dropped to Boost Organ Donation. *The Sunday Times*, 29 June.

61 Association of Chartered Physiotherapists in Women's Health (2007) *Exercise and Advice after the Still Birth or Death of Your Baby*. CSP, London.

62 *R. (on the application of Burke)* v. *General Medical Council and Disability Rights Commission and the Official Solicitor to the Supreme Court* [2004] EWHC 1879; [2004] Lloyd's Rep Med 451.

Section F
Specialist Topics

26 Teaching and Research

This chapter looks at the specific problems which face the physiotherapist who is involved in teaching and research. Reference should also be made to Chapter 5, which considers the educational issues and the role of the Health Professions Council (HPC) and the Chartered Society of Physiotherapy (CSP).

The following topics will be considered:

- Liability in connection with education and training
- Legal issues arising from the conduct of research
- Conclusions

Liability in connection with education and training

Failure to maintain professional competence

Every physiotherapist has a duty to maintain his/her professional competence; failure to do so could lead to being called to account in several different forums:

- civil proceedings for negligence if a person is harmed as a result of this failure;
- professional conduct proceedings of the HPC, which could result in the physiotherapist being struck off the HPC register;
- disciplinary proceedings if the physiotherapist is an employee;
- criminal proceedings if serious harm or death has occurred.

An example of the problems that can be faced by inadequate post-registration training can be seen from the survey carried out by Lesley Silcox[1] on training for wheelchair prescribing. The results of the survey showed that the situation on training had only slightly improved since the McColl Report,[2] which criticised the number of people in unsuitable wheelchairs showing inadequate standards of wheelchair assessment, prescription and advice. If harm arose to a client as the result of a physiotherapist failing to ensure that his/her competence to practise was maintained and that he/she was up to date with relevant information, the physiotherapist or his/her employer could be liable for that harm. The HPC has published standards for continuing professional development (CPD), which are available from the CSP.[3] These are considered in

Chapter 5. The CSP has also published resources for CPD which aim to assist members in securing resources to undertake CPD.[4]

Liability of the instructor

Failures in teaching

This duty to maintain competence applies equally to the physiotherapist lecturer/tutor as it does to the practitioner. Even an instructor could be held liable in negligence for failures as a teacher. It would have to be proved that a student, in reliance on negligent advice from the instructor, caused harm to a colleague or client and that this harm could be seen as a reasonably foreseeable result of that negligent advice. The causation element (see Chapter 10) may be difficult to establish, since the instructor could argue that there are many sources of advice for the student who should not rely entirely upon the instructor. The CSP has provided guidance on assessment processes for learners that is aimed at contributing to the development of learning.[5]

Administrative failures

However, if the instructor were to give the student the wrong information about the syllabus which was being studied or the timetable or place of the examinations, and as a result the student failed the examination, then liability of the instructor and his/her employer could be established. In addition, if students pay the fees for the tuition themselves, there could be liability in contract law for any failure to provide tuition in accordance with the contract stipulations.

For developments in the law of negligence relating to the giving of references see Chapter 10. For the principles of contract law see Chapter 19.

Lecturers and other educationalists should be aware that administrative weaknesses or inefficiencies could give rise to court hearings and complaints. Thus, in one case a would-be physiotherapy student was wrongly informed through the admissions system by the University of Salford that he was being offered a place. He wrote accepting the offer, and then learnt later that a mistake had been made and there had never been a place for him. His application for specific performance of the contract and a mandatory injunction compelling the University to give a place was dismissed. He appealed to the Court of Appeal,[6] which held that there probably was a binding agreement that the university would accept him for the degree course in physiotherapy, but it was not prepared to order an injunction on the grounds that it was not just to compel the university to provide a place for a student whose academic record was not good enough. His appeal was therefore dismissed. Even though the prospective student failed on the facts in this case, the fact remains that a contract is created between student and institution with obligations on both sides.

The Court of Appeal held that overseas students could change their course, but if they wanted an extension of stay in the UK, they had to be able to produce evidence of satisfactory progress whether or not on the course named in the application for entry clearance or on another recognised course.[7]

Teaching intimate procedures

Teachers on post-graduate training courses should be particularly diligent to follow the guidelines issued by the CSP when providing instruction in intimate examinations, such as pelvic floor and vaginal assessment. The CSP has issued guidance[8] on instruction to post-graduate physiotherapists in these assessments. Where fellow students are used to practise such examinations it recommends that:

- full information should be given to the students in advance;
- students should be given the option to opt in or out;
- consent forms should be used that would include information as to what would be involved in such a practical session.

Teaching manipulation

The CSP has also issued guidance on the safe teaching of manipulation to undergraduates.[9] It emphasises the importance of undertaking an assessment of the student who is to be used as a model and the facilities available. It also sets out the principles for safe teaching and practice, stressing the importance of obtaining consent from the student and ethical approval from the institution.

Supervision of students in clinical placements

The same principle would apply in the supervision of students in clinical placements. The student is entitled to receive a reasonable standard of care from the clinical instructor, and, if harm were to occur to the student or to others in the failure to provide the appropriate level of supervision or in delegating inappropriate activities to the student, the instructor and his/her employer would be liable in negligence. The CSP has provided guidance on how to complete the experiential route for accreditation of clinical educators.[10]

Reference should be made to Chapter 10 on negligence and in particular the section on supervision and delegation. The CSP has prepared guidance for developing student placements in the community.[11]

One interesting initiative is the use of learning contracts in physiotherapy clinical education. Vinette Cross[12] describes the approach used with one group of undergraduates and the relevance of learning contracts to CSP initiatives on CPD. The approach is based on three key requirements. Learning contracts should:

- provide a structure for clinical education experiences;
- foster a supportive learning climate for both students and clinical educators;
- facilitate reflective practice.

Legal responsibility for the clinical education remains with the clinical instructors who define the boundaries of the learning decisions and decide on non-negotiable aspects of the learning process.

Liability for harm to students or harm caused by students

If harm arises to the student, then the student would have to show that a reasonable standard of care was not provided. The student would not be an employee and could not therefore point to the duty of care owed by employer to employee at common law (see Chapter 11). Instead the student could rely upon the duty of care owed in the law of negligence or upon statutory duties set out in the Health and Safety Regulations or the Occupier's Liability Act 1957.

The following is an example of breach of Health and Safety Regulations by a further education college.

Case: *Anderson v. Newham College of Further Education* 2002[13]

Anderson, a mobile site supervisor who worked for Newham College of Further Education, received two severe fractures at work when he fell. While he was checking premises he noted a broken window in a lecture room and fell over a frame containing a white board which was propped against the wall, the wrong way round with the feet sticking into the gangway. The judge held that there had been no negligence at common law but that there had been a breach of Regulation 12(3) of the Workplace (Health Safety and Welfare) Regulations 1992, but held the claimant 90% to blame for the accident because of his contributory negligence (see Chapter 10). The Court of Appeal dismissed the defendant's appeal but reduced the level of contributory negligence to 50%.

If the student caused harm to another person, it depends upon the facts whether there was negligence and who was at fault. Thus the tutor might assess the student as competent to carry out a particular activity and ensure that he/she was receiving the appropriate supervision. However, in spite of this appropriate delegation and supervision, the student might still act negligently and therefore be to blame for causing harm to another person. In such an event, compensation would be paid out by the college or the Trust, depending on the memorandum of agreement between the college and those offering the clinical placement. This agreement should lay down provisions as to which party is responsible vicariously for the negligence of the student.

Information on insurance cover for physiotherapy students is discussed in a publication prepared by Graybrook Ltd for the CSP.[14] It considers in what circumstances students would need to have individualised cover for practice-based learning and seeks to answer common queries raised about insurance and students. It states that it is impossible to generalise about higher education cover for students and recommends that both placement organisers and physiotherapy programme organisers should check with the higher education provider on the insurance situation and if necessary ensure that students have individualised insurance cover.

Duty of employer to provide facilities for post-registration training or continuing professional development

It could be argued that, since the healthcare employer has a duty of care at common law to its patients and/or clients it must therefore as part of this duty ensure that its staff are competent. In addition, as part of the contractual duty that it owes to its employees, it must provide competent fellow staff. Should the employer fail to fulfil this duty, and harm befall a patient/client or employee as a result, then the employer could be directly liable in negligence. Thus, one can assume that the employer's duty includes the duty to ensure that staff are kept competent and that paid study leave should be made available as an implied condition of the contract of employment.

This logic has not, however, so far been categorically established in the courts. The uncertainty has meant that there is wide variation across the country as to the rights of employees in obtaining paid study leave. Practitioners registered with the Nursing and Midwifery Council now have to prove that they have undertaken at least 5 study days (or comparable training) every 3 years in order that they can be re-registered. Similarly, the HPC has laid down requirements for CPD and the duty of each registrant to keep a record and to be prepared to submit to audit. There is no agreement that NHS Trusts will automatically fund CPD and practice varies from Trust to Trust.

Physiotherapists have an obligation to maintain competence under the HPC Standards of Conduct, Performance and Ethics. Clause 4 requires registrants to keep high standards of performance and Clause 5 requires registrants to keep their professional knowledge and skills up to date. A similar duty is set out in the Rule 2 of the CSP Rules, which requires members to

> only practise to the extent that they have established, maintained and developed their ability to work safely and competently and shall ensure that they have appropriate professional liability cover for that practice.

This duty to maintain competence would also be implied at common law as part of ensuring that they practise according to the accepted approved practice of reasonable practitioners in that field (the Bolam test). It is clearly of interest to physiotherapists to use local collective bargaining to ensure that provision is made in their contracts for paid study leave, secondment and other forms of post-registration training and education. When demand for physiotherapists exceeds the supply then, in order to retain or attract their services, NHS Trusts may be prepared (or forced) to compile attractive packages. (At the time of writing, only half of those who qualified in 2007 were able to obtain employment within the NHS, so at present the supply of physiotherapists would appear to exceed the availability of funded posts.)

Training of assistants

It must not be forgotten that as the dependence on assistants increases so resources must be allocated to ensure that they are appropriately trained. There appears little doubt that the skill-mix ratio in physiotherapy is changing as increasing numbers of assistants are being employed compared to registered physiotherapists.

In Chapter 10 the legal issues relating to delegation and supervision are discussed. A prior requirement of delegation is that the assistant should be properly trained. A joint paper by the College of Occupational Therapy and the CSP in 2005[15] sets out a national framework for the education and development of support workers. It follows up the Modernisation Agenda of the NHS (see Chapter 17), which plans for support workers to develop their roles supported by relevant education and development opportunities. The Allied Health Professionals published a joint statement on foundation degrees for support workers in 2006.[16] The CSP published in 2005 details of sources of funding for physiotherapy assistants undertaking formally accredited programmes of study.[17] More recently in 2007 the CSP has published an information paper on support worker education and development.[18]

Legal issues arising from the conduct of research

Research-based practice

The Bolam test (which is discussed in Chapter 10) is the accepted test for defining acceptable professional practice. As was discussed, what a reasonable body of responsible practitioners would accept as appropriate practice will change as standards of care improve and develop. The findings from substantiated research will therefore eventually become integrated into accepted practice and it is essential that the professional keeps abreast of changes in recommended practice. Evidence-based practice (EBP) should become the norm. Should the physiotherapist

fail to follow accepted practice and there is no reasonable justification (e.g. particular circumstances of the individual patient) for him/her not to do so and should harm occur to the client as a result, then the physiotherapist or his/her employer could face an action for negligence (see Chapter 10). A definition of EBP quoted by the CSP in its website on effective practice is as follows:

> Conscious, explicit and judicious use of current best evidence in making decisions about the care of individual patients.[19]

Further, with pressures on resourcing, physiotherapists need to justify their activities in terms of clinical effectiveness. Only research can establish that the service they can provide in different clinical situations justifies its use (see Chapter 17). Both the HPC and the CSP recognise the importance and significance of research in the development of health care and treatment. The HPC in its standards of proficiency for physiotherapists requires registrants to be able to use research, reasoning and problem solving skills to determine appropriate actions. It also requires registrants to be able to draw on appropriate knowledge and skills in order to make professional judgments.

In 2002 the CSP published priorities for research across a wide diversity of clinical specialities including older people; neurology; women's health; musculoskeletal; mental health and learning disabilities. This was followed by a research and clinical effectiveness strategy in 2004, which was built on the overall aims of the CSP strategy for 2005–10. The National Physiotherapist Research Network (NPRN) was established in 2005. It aims to encourage and facilitate physiotherapy-related research across the UK and the integration of research into practice. Its aims are shown in Figure 26.1. The NPRN has developed 20 regional clusters or hubs through which to develop research. Involvement by individual physiotherapists is discussed by Philippa Lyon,[20] who works full time in support of the NPRN. Its annual report is available from the CSP. The importance of evidence-based

- Develop the physiotherapy scientific knowledge base
- Provide access to the knowledge base to the physiotherapy profession and likeminded researchers
- Support the implementation of the knowledge base within physiotherapy practice
- Encourage and facilitate the engagement of physiotherapists nationally in research activity, both at a professionl and interprofessional level
- Encourage growth in research capacity
- Encourage the use of evidence within physiotherapy practice
- Encourage the identification of relevant research questions within physiotherapy and healthcare practice generally
- Encourage an increase in phsyiotherapy research output at a national level
- Encourage the growth of the profile of physiotherapy research in healthcare
- Encourage the uptake of research funding opportunities by members of the physiotherapy profession
- Identify a wider range of funding opportunities for physiotherapy and physiotherapy-related research
- Increase the knowledge within the physiotherapy profession of a wide range of funding opportunities.

Figure 26.1   General Aims of the National Physiotherapy Research Network

health care for the personal development of the physiotherapist is emphasised by Ann Moore[21] and explained in relation to physiotherapy practice by Jean Kelly.[22]

Protecting the patient from the researcher

Consent

Consent must be obtained from adult mentally competent patients/clients or the Gillick competent child (see Chapter 23) or from parents of children before research is carried out. It is also essential that all relevant information should be given about any risks of harm from the research.

A distinction should, however, be made between therapeutic and non-therapeutic research in the discussion of consent in relation to research. Where the patient/client stands to benefit personally from the research, then it could be argued that the research on adults incapable of giving consent could be conducted as part of their treatment plan. However, if the individual has no personal benefit from it, research to which

any risks, however slight, were attached would not be justified. This would also apply to research on children. Reference should be made to Chapter 23 and the law relating to consent by a child (i.e. a person under 18 years).

The information that is given to the patient/client and the consent form to be signed should be approved by the Local Research Ethics Committee (see below) before the research commences.

Consent to research and the mentally incapacitated adult

The Mental Capacity Act (MCA) 2005 has introduced stringent provisions in relation to research involving those who are over 16 years and who are unable to give consent. The statutory provisions apply to research other than clinical trials. Clinical trials come under separate EU regulations drawn up as a consequence of the European Directive[23] (see below).

Under Sections 30–34 of the MCA the provisions relating to research and the mentally incapacitated adult are set out.

Conditions for intrusive research

The MCA prohibits intrusive research being carried out on, or in relation to a person who lacks the capacity to consent unless certain conditions are met. These conditions are shown in Box 26.1. Intrusive research is defined in Section 30(2) as 'research which would be unlawful if carried out on a person capable of giving consent, but without that consent'.

Box 26.1   Conditions required for research on those lacking the requisite mental capacity to give consent.

- That the research is part of a research project
- Which is approved by an appropriate body as defined in Section 31
- Complies with the conditions laid down in Section 31 (see Box 26.2) and
- Complies with conditions relating to the consulting of carers and additional safeguards (i.e. Sections 32 and 33 see below)

The Code of Practice[24] notes that the Act does not have a specific definition for 'research' and it quotes the definitions used by the Department of Health and National Assembly for Wales Publications Research Governance Framework for Health and Social Care:

research can be defined as the attempt to derive generalisable new knowledge by addressing clearly defined questions with systematic and rigorous methods.[25]

The Code of Practice points out that research may:

- provide information that can be applied generally to an illness, disorder or condition
- demonstrate how effective and safe a new treatment is
- add to evidence that one form of treatment works better than another
- add to evidence that one form of treatment is safer than another, or
- examine wider issues (for example, the factors that affect someone's capacity to make a decision).

The Code of Practice[26] notes that:

It is expected that most of the researchers who ask for their research to be approved under the Act will be medical or social care researchers. However, the Act can cover more than just medical and social care research. Intrusive research which does not meet the requirements of the Act cannot be carried out lawfully in relation to people who lack capacity.

Non-intrusive research

Non-intrusive research could include research of anonymised records or the use of anonymous tissue or blood left over after it had been collected for use in other procedures. Although such research is excluded from the provisions of the Mental Capacity Act 2005, it could come under other legislative provisions such as the Data Protection Act 1998 and regulations under the Data Protection Act and the Human Tissue Act 2004.

Requirements for approval

The appropriate body (i.e. the person, committee or other body specified by the Secretary of State in regulations[27]) may not approve a research project relating to a person lacking the capacity to consent unless the conditions shown in Box 26.2 are present.

(2)   The research is connected with an impairing condition affecting P (the person lacking mental capacity) or its treatment

(3)   An impairing condition is defined in Section 31(3) as a condition which is (or may be) attributable to, or which causes or contributes to, the impairment of, or disturbance in the functioning of, the mind or brain

(4)   There must be reasonable grounds for believing that the research would not be as effective if carried out only on, or only in relation to, person who have the capacity to consent to taking part in the project

(5)   The research must (a) have the potential to benefit P without imposing on P a burden that is disproportionate to the potential benefit to P or (b) be intended to provide knowledge of the causes or treatment of, or of the care of persons affected by, the same or a similar condition

(6)   If (b) applies and not (a), there must be reasonable grounds for believing (a) that the risk to P from taking part in the project is likely to be negligible, and (b) that anything done to, or in relation to, P will not (i) interfere with P's freedom of action or privacy in a significant way, or (ii) be unduly invasive or restrictive

(7)   There must be reasonable arrangements in place for ensuring that the requirements of Section 32 and 33 are in place. [Consulting carers and additional safeguards (see below)]

Consulting of carers

The researcher 'R' is required to take reasonable steps to identify a person who is not engaged in a professional capacity nor receiving remuneration but is engaged in caring for P or is interested in P's welfare and is prepared to be consulted by the researcher under Section 32.

Subsection (7) makes it clear that the fact that a person is the donee of a lasting power of attorney given by P, or is P's deputy, does not prevent him/her from being the person consulted under Section 32.

If such a person cannot be identified, then R must in accordance with guidance issued by the Secretary of State or the Welsh Assembly nominate a person who is prepared to be consulted by R but has no connection with the project.

R must provide the carer or nominee with information about the project and ask him for advice as to whether P should take part in the project and what, in his opinion, P's wishes and feelings about taking part in the project would be likely to be if P had capacity in relation to the matter. If the person consulted advises R that in his/her opinion P's wishes and feelings would be likely to lead him to decline to take part in the project (or to wish to withdraw from it), if he had the capacity, then R must ensure that P does not take part, or if he is already taking part, ensure that he is withdrawn from it.

If treatment has commenced it is not necessary to discontinue the treatment if R has reasonable grounds for believing that there would be a significant risk to P's health if it were discontinued.

Urgent research (S.32(8)(9))

Special provisions apply where treatment is to be provided as a matter of urgency and R considers that it is also necessary to take action for the purposes of the research as a matter of urgency, but it is not reasonably practicable to consult under the above provisions of this section.

In these circumstances R must have the agreement of a registered medical practitioner who is not concerned in the organisation or conduct of the research project or where it is not reasonably practicable in the time available to obtain that agreement, he/she acts in accordance with a procedure approved by the appropriate body at the time when the research project was approved under Section 31. When R has reasonable grounds for believing that it is no longer necessary to take the action as a matter of urgency, he/she cannot continue to act in reliance on these urgent provisions (S.32(10)).

Additional safeguards

There are additional safeguards to protect the interests of the person lacking the requisite mental capacity:

Nothing may be done to, or in relation to a person taking part in the research project who is incapable of giving consent,

- to which he appears to object (whether by showing signs of resistance or otherwise) except where what is being done is intended to protect him from harm or to reduce or prevent pain or discomfort, or
- which would be contrary to an advance decision of his which has effect or any other form of statement made by him and not subsequently withdrawn and R is aware of this.

The MCA expressly states (S.33(3)) that the interests of the person must be assumed to outweigh those of science and society.

Loss of capacity during research project

Section 34 applies if P had consented to take part in a research project, begun before the commencement of Section 30 (1 April 2007), but before the conclusion of the project loses capacity to consent to continue to take part in it. In such a situation regulations may provide that despite his/her loss of capacity, research of a prescribed kind may be carried out on, or in relation to, P if:

- the project satisfies the prescribed requirements;
- any information or material relating to which is used in the research is of a prescribed

description and was obtained before P's loss of capacity;
- the person conducting the project takes in relation to P such steps as may be prescribed for the purpose of protecting him/her.

Regulations[28] covering the situation where an adult who had given consent to participation in research lost the requisite mental capacity during the research project were enacted in 2007. They provide that in such circumstances, despite P's loss of capacity, research for the purposes of the project may be carried out using information or material relating to him/her if certain specified conditions exist:

(a) the project satisfies the requirements set out in Schedule 1;
(b) all the information or material relating to P that is used in the research was obtained before P's loss of capacity;
(c) the person conducting the project (R) takes in relation to P such steps as are set out in Schedule 2.

Schedule 1 is shown in Box 26.3.

Box 26.3   Schedule 1 to the Regulations on loss of capacity during the research project. Requirements that the project must satisfy

(1) A protocol approved by an appropriate body and having effect in relation to the project makes provision for research to be carried out in relation to a person who has consented to take part in the project but loses capacity to consent to continue to take part in it.
(2) The appropriate body must be satisfied that there are reasonable arrangements in place for ensuring that the requirements of Schedule 2 will be met. (See Box 26.4 for Schedule 2.)

Schedule 2 of the Regulations is shown in Box 26.4

Box 26.4 Schedule 2 to the Regulations on loss of capacity during the research project. Steps which the person conducting the project must take.

(1) R must take reasonable steps to identify a person who— (a) otherwise than in a professional capacity or for remuneration, is engaged in caring for P or is interested in P's welfare, and (b) is prepared to be consulted by R under this Schedule.

(2) If R is unable to identify such a person he must, in accordance with guidance issued by the Secretary of State, nominate a person who— (a) is prepared to be consulted by R under this Schedule, but (b) has no connection with the project.

(3) R must provide the person identified under paragraph 1, or nominated under paragraph 2, with information about the project and ask him— (a) for advice as to whether research of the kind proposed should be carried out in relation to P, and (b) what, in his opinion, P's wishes and feelings about such research being carried out would be likely to be if P had capacity in relation to the matter.

(4) If, any time, the person consulted advises R that in his opinion P's wishes and feelings would be likely to lead him to wish to withdraw from the project if he had capacity in relation to the matter, R must ensure that P is withdrawn from it.

(5) The fact that a person is the donee of a lasting power of attorney given by P, or is P's deputy, does not prevent him from being the person consulted under paragraphs 1 to 4.

(6) R must ensure that nothing is done in relation to P in the course of the research which would be contrary to (a) an advance decision of his which has effect, or (b) any other form of statement made by him and not subsequently withdrawn, of which R is aware.

(7) The interests of P must be assumed to outweigh those of science and society.

(8) If P indicates (in any way) that he wishes the research in relation to him to be discontinued, it must be discontinued without delay.

(9) The research must be discontinued without delay if at any time R has reasonable grounds for believing that one or more of the requirements set out in Schedule 1 is no longer met or that there are no longer reasonable arrangements in place for ensuring that the requirements of this Schedule are met in relation to P.

(10) R must conduct the research in accordance with the provision made in the protocol referred to in paragraph 1 of Schedule 1 for research to be carried out in relation to a person who has consented to take part in the project but loses capacity to consent to take part in it.

It is hoped that the implementation of these provisions of the MCA are monitored to assess their effectiveness in protecting those incapable of giving consent to participation in a research project and at the same time enabling important research into the underlying conditions of mental incapacity to take place.

Consent and clinical trials

Clinical trials that come under the clinical trials regulations,[29.] enacted in 2004, are excluded from the statutory provisions of the MCA 2005. Article 5 makes provisions for clinical trials on incapacitated adults not able to give informed legal consent.

Confidentiality

Exactly the same principles of confidentiality apply in relation to the personal information obtained from undertaking research as apply to information obtained in respect of treatment. It is probable, however, that the exceptions to the duty to maintain confidentiality recognised by the law in relation to personal information obtained in the course of caring for patients (see Chapter 8) would also apply to information obtained through research.

In 1996 three doctors were brought before professional conduct proceedings of the General Medical Council as a result of the publication of a case study on a patient which she claimed was recognised as being about her and which she alleged to have been published without her consent. The doctors were not struck off the Register. It was emphasised, however, that the rules were now that it is necessary to get the specific consent of the patient to the publication of a case study.

The physiotherapist as researcher

Physiotherapy should be a research-based profession and it is therefore essential that care and treatments are research based. There is encouragement for individual physiotherapists to take part in research projects. The CSP has provided details of the organisations that provide resources for funding research.[30] It also has a charitable trust, which through the Physiotherapy Research Foundation provides research funding for CSP members to undertake research.

Local Research Ethics Committees

New arrangements relating to the establishment of Local Research Ethics Committees and multi-centre research ethics committees have been published by the Department of Health in August 2001.[31]

An ad hoc advisory group was set up to review the operation of NHS Research Ethics Committees. Its report[32] was published in June 2005. Its conclusions ranged widely over the need for change in the system of Research Ethics Committees (RECs), the need to address perceived weaknesses in the REC system, and provide better support for Chairs, members and administrative staff. The aim of its recommendations was to raise the status and profile of RECs, and lay the firm foundation for a REC system that can be more responsive to changing requirements in the future in a UK wide context. It recommended that significant changes to the NHS research-ethics committee system should be made which are shown in Box 26.5. The Government stated that these changes would be phased in from spring 2006.

Box 26.5   Recommendations of the Advisory Group on the Operation of NHS Research Ethics Committees (RECs).

(1)   The remit of NHS RECs should not include surveys or other non-research activity if they present no material ethical issues for human participants. COREC should develop guidelines to aid researchers and committees in deciding what is appropriate or inappropriate for submission to RECs.

(2)   RECs should not reach decisions based on scientific review. In the unusual situation of a REC having reservations about the quality of the science proposed, they should be able to refer to COREC for scientific guidance.

(3)   The recently introduced managed operating system has been well received. Its use of IT points the way to further efficiency and quality improvements. We believe that responsibility for site specific assessment should be transferred to NHS hosts as soon as acceptable mechanisms for quality assurance are in place.

(4)   The application form and application process call for improvement. The form should take more explicit account of differences between types of research and should also give more space and attention to ethical issues.

(5)   We strongly encourage NHS research hosts to adopt common national systems. Substantial improvement to local R&D procedures and their interaction with ethical review including the ability to make multiple use of information supplied once is required in order to reduce bureaucracy and timescales. This is the most pressing of all our recommendations.

(6)   We believe that a smaller number of RECs perhaps one for each Strategic Health Authority, with a limited number of exceptions would be more appropriate. Their operations would be more intense than at present, with a greater use of electronic communications. The time commitment required of members and support staff for training should be more formally recognised, as should the time taken in committee hearings and preparation. This implies paying REC members appropriately, either directly or through compensating their employers.

(7)   Research Ethics Committees must represent the public interest as well as patient perspectives on research. This means that membership needs to be drawn from a wider mix of society and that all members need to be supported by appropriate training. We believe that our recommendation that we move towards a system of fewer, paid RECs will support this objective.

(8)   The issue of excessive inconsistency amongst committees should be addressed by concentrating on the provision of appropriate training, and on capturing and sharing good practice where issues and arguments have been already explored. The newly introduced system of quality assurance by peer review amongst committees and their members should assist this process and should be further developed.

(9)   We propose the creation of 'Scientific Officers' in COREC to support the work of committees. They might undertake much of the preliminary assessment required, and review reports. Chairs, for whom it is a major burden, currently undertake this work.

The CSP published an information paper on Research Ethics and Ethics Committees (RES 7) in October 2001.

Publication

As indicated above, it is now the policy of the General Medical Council (GMC) that publication of individual case studies requires the prior consent of the patient and it may be prudent for other health professionals to work on this basis too.

It is also extremely wise for researchers to discuss and agree arrangements for possible publication of the research before it is undertaken in order to prevent disputes arising over censorship and control once the outcome is known. Some funding bodies who have sponsored the research may require that they see the findings before they permit publication. This may be seen, however, as an unjustified restraint on the dissemination of the results.

Often research results are publicised at conferences by way of poster displays. An extremely useful article in *Physiotherapy* gives guidance on the preparation of posters for display.[33]

Accuracy

It is possible that if research is published that contains errors of design and interpretation and persons suffer harm as a result of dependence upon the conclusions drawn, then there could be liability in negligence. A centre for cancer treatment in women in Bristol suffered financial loss as the result of a research report which suggested that the centre achieved worse results than other treatment centres. It was later learnt that the researchers had failed to take account of the fact that the Bristol centre took patients at a much later stage in their illness than other centres and therefore like was not being compared with like.

Physiotherapists who knowingly take part in research that is not sound could face professional conduct proceedings. There is a useful chapter on the sources of error in research in Carolyn Hicks' book *Research for Physiotherapists*.[34]

Intellectual property and copyright

Sometimes research projects can lead to lucrative rewards – the design of a new piece of equipment or an innovative idea for supporting disabled persons.

- If a physiotherapist is fortunate enough to have a commercially valuable idea, who should get the rewards?

The answer depends upon the circumstances in which the project was conceived. Thus, if the physiotherapist is undertaking research and development as part of his/her work as a full-time employee, then the employer would be seen as the owner of the research, though a generous employer may well develop an income-sharing scheme with the employee. If, on the other hand, the research has been developed by the physiotherapist entirely on his/her own, with no involvement from the employer or its resources, he/she would be the owner of the intellectual property. The physiotherapist should take advice on patenting the design so that his/her ownership is legally recognised.[35]

Involvement of users in research

Carol Thomas and Anne Perry[36] reported on research to examine the health needs of persons with strokes and the place of the user's views in healthcare planning. They conclude that in order to give users more opportunity to direct knowledge that is generated, there should be more partnership at every stage – before the design of any research project is agreed, in validating the results of the research, and also in identifying how the results can be disseminated to users as well as purchasers and providers.

Another means of using consumers in research is by means of the focus group. Julius Sim and Jackie Snell[37] point out the advantages of using focus group techniques in comparison with other methods of data collection in physiotherapy research. However, there are dangers, for example the moderator can unconsciously or subconsciously lead the group to endorse a preconceived hypothesis and careful planning is necessary before the focus group convenes.

Conclusions

Physiotherapy practice must be based on knowledge obtained through research. Evidence-based practice will be essential in the twenty-first century. Ultimately the Bolam test (see Chapter 10) as to what is the accepted approved practice of the reasonable physiotherapist should be supported by clinical evidence. The work of the National Institute for Health and Clinical Excellence, the National Service Frameworks and the Healthcare Commission are leading to standards being developed across all health specialities and professions. Research should be encouraged to underpin practice and the CSP is playing a major role in these developments.

Questions and exercises

1 A physiotherapy student reports to you, her tutor, that she was aware that a client in a home for those with learning disabilities was being abused by a member of staff. What action would you take and what action would you advise her to take?

2 Obtain a copy of the memorandum of agreement between your college and the NHS Trust that takes your students on placements. To what extent does it determine responsibility for the negligence of the student or responsibility for harm to the student whilst on clinical placement?

3 You are wishing to carry out a research project. Draw up a schedule setting out the initial tasks you should undertake before you actually begin the data collection.

4. You wish to conduct research that will involve adults who are incapable of giving consent to participation. What statutory provisions must you take into account?

References

1 Silcox, L. (1995) Assessment for the Prescription of Wheelchairs: What Training is Available to Therapists. *British Journal of Occupational Therapy* **58**, 3, 115–118.

2 McColl, I. (1986) *Review of the Artificial Limb and Appliance Centres*. HMSO, London.

3 Chartered Society of Physiotherapy (2006) *Standards for CPD*. CPD 39. CSP, London.

4 Chartered Society of Physiotherapy (2005) *Resources for Continuing Professional Development*. CPD 11. CSP, London.

5 Chartered Society of Physiotherapy (2005) *Developing Effective Assessment Procedures*. CSP, London.

6 *Moran v. University of Salford* (CA) reported in *The Times*, 23 November 1993; 12 November 1993, Lexis Transcript.

7 *GO and others* v. *Secretary of State for the Home Department*. The Times Law Report, 23 July 2008.

8 Chartered Society of Physiotherapy (1996) *Pelvic Floor and Vaginal Assessment*. Information Paper No. PA 19. CSP, London.

9 Chartered Society of Physiotherapy (1997) *Guidance on the Safe Teaching of Manipulation to Undergraduates*. Professional Affairs Department Information Paper No 40. CSP, London.

10 Chartered Society of Physiotherapy (2004) *Accreditation of Clinical Educators Experiential Route: Guidance Notes for Applicants*. ACE 02. CSP, London.

11 Chartered Society of Physiotherapy (2006) *Guidance for Developing Student Placements in the Community and other Non-traditional Settings*. Information Paper PA 10. CSP, London.

12 Cross, V. (1996) Introducing learning contracts into physiotherapy clinical education. *Physiotherapy* **82**, 1, 21–27.

13 *Anderson v. Newham College of Further Education* [2002] EWCA Civ 505.

14 Chartered Society of Physiotherapy/Graybrook Ltd (2008) *Students and Insurance Cover*. CSP, London.

15 College of Occupational Therapists and Chartered Society of Physiotherapists (2005) *A National Framework for Support Worker Education and Development*. CSP and COT, London.

16 Chartered Society of Physiotherapy and Allied Health Professionals (2006) *Joint Statement on Foundation Degrees for Support Workers*. CSP, London.

17 Chartered Society of Physiotherapy (2005) *Sources of Funding for Physiotherapy Assistants*. CPD 27. CSP, London.

18 Chartered Society of Physiotherapy (2007) *Support Worker Education and Development: Learning Opportunities*. CSP London.

19 Sackett, D.L. *et al.* (1996) British Medical Journal **312**, 71–72.

20 Lyon, P. (2005) Growing and Supporting Physiotherapy Related Research: The National Physiotherapy Research Network. *In Touch* **113**, 31–33.

21 Moore, A. (2001) Evidence-based Healthcare – One of the Biggest Buzzwords in Health Services. *In Touch* **98**, 3–9.

22 Kelly, J. (2003) Evidence Based Practice. *In Touch* **104**, 24–31.

23 EC Directive 2001/20/EC.

24 Code of Practice Mental Capacity Act 2005 Department of Constitutional Affairs February 2007 paragraph 11.2.

25 www.dh.gov.uk/en/Publicationsandstatistics/index.htm and www.word.wales.gov.uk/content/governance/governance-e.htm

26 Code of Practice Mental Capacity Act 2005 Department of Constitutional Affairs February 2007 paragraph 11.5.

27 Mental Capacity Act 2005 (Appropriate Body) (England) Regulations 2006 SI No 2810; Mental Capacity Act 2005 (Appropriate Body) (England) (Amendment) Regulations 2006 SI No 3474.

28 The Mental Capacity Act 2005 (Loss of Capacity during Research Project) (England) Regulations 2007 SI No 679.

29 The Medicines for Human Use (Clinical Trials) Regulations 2004 SI 2004 No 1031.

30 Chartered Society of Physiotherapy (2001) *Sources of Research Funding*. RES 03. CSP, London.

31 Department of Health Governance arrangements for NHS Research Ethics Committees 3 August 2001.

32 Department of Health Report of the Ad Hoc Advisory Group on the Operation of NHS Research Ethics Committees June 2005.

33 Murray, R., Thaw, M., Strachan, R. (1998) Visual Literacy: Designing and Presenting a Poster. *Physiotherapy* **84**, 7, 319–327.

34 Hicks, C. (1995) *Research for Physiotherapists: Project Design and Analysis.* Churchill Livingstone, Edinburgh.

35 McKeough, J. (1996) Intellectual Property and Scientific Research. *Australian Journal of Physiotherapy* **42**, 3, 235–242.

36 Thomas, C., Perry, A. (1996) Research on Users' Views about Stroke Services. *Physiotherapy* **82**, 1, 6–12.

37 Sim, J., Snell, J. (1996) Focus Groups in Physiotherapy Evaluation and Research. *Physiotherapy* **82**, 3, 189–198.

27 Complementary Medicine

Growth of interest in complementary and alternative medicines

There is no doubt about the interest that now exists in complementary or alternative therapies.[1] It was estimated that a third of the population have tried its remedies or visited its practitioners.[2] The Health Education Authority has published an *A to Z Guide*, which covers 67 therapies.[3] A book on complementary therapies for physical therapists has been written by Robert Charman.[4] A chair in complementary therapy has been provided at Exeter University.

The Prince of Wales suggested the setting up of a group to consider the current positions of orthodox, complementary and alternative medicine in the UK and how far it would be appropriate and possible for them to work more closely together. Four working groups looking at

- research and development
- education and training
- regulation
- delivery mechanisms

were established under a steering group chaired by Dr Manon Williams, Assistant Private Secretary to HRH the Prince of Wales. It reported in 1997 and made extensive recommendations.[5] These included:

- encouraging more research and the dissemination of its results;
- emphasising the common elements in the core curriculum of all healthcare workers, both in orthodox medicine and in complementary or alternative medicine;
- establishing statutory self-regulatory bodies for those professions that could endanger patient safety;
- identifying areas of conventional medicine and nursing which are not meeting patients' needs at present.

It also recommended the establishment of an Independent Standards Commission for Complementary and Alternative Medicine. In 2003 it published *National Guidelines for the Use of Complementary Therapies in Supportive and Palliative Care Services.*[6]

In December 2004 the Prince of Wales Foundation for Integrated Health was given £900 000 by the Department of Health (DH) to support its work in developing robust systems for regulation for the main complementary healthcare professions. The work and progress of the Prince's Foundation for Integrated Health in the establishment of the Complementary and Natural Healthcare Council can be seen on its website.[7] In 2000, the House of Lords Select Committee on Science and Technology reviewed the field of complementary and alternative medicines and made significant recommendations on their control and use within the NHS.[8] It divided such therapies into three groups:

(1) Professionally organised therapies, where there is some scientific evidence of their success, although seldom of the highest quality, and there are recognised systems for treatment and training of practitioners. This group includes acupuncture, chiropractic, herbal medicine, homoeopathy and osteopathy.

(2) Complementary medicines where evidence that they work is generally lacking, but which are used as an adjunct rather than a replacement for conventional therapies, so that lack of evidence may not matter so much. Included in this group are the Alexander technique, aromatherapy, nutritional medicine, hypnotherapy and Bach and other flower remedies.

(3) Techniques that offer diagnosis as well as treatment, but for which scientific evidence is almost completely lacking. This group cannot be supported and includes naturopathy, crystal therapy, kinesiology, radionics, dowsing and iridology.

The Select Committee of the House of Lords considered that some remedies such as acupuncture and aromatherapy should be available on the NHS and NHS patients should have wider access to osteopathy and chiropractic. The report can be accessed from the UK Parliamentary website.[9]

Registration of complementary therapies

The DH established working groups to consider the regulation of herbal medicine practitioners and acupuncturists.[10] Proposals that herbalists will have to register with a new governing body to be eligible to practise and some herbal treatments will only be available from licensed practitioners were put out to consultation, and an analysis of responses to the consultation was published in February 2005.[11] The DH intended to publish a draft Section 60 (Health Act 1999) order for consultation on a new Complementary and Alternative Medicine Council for the regulation of herbal medicine and acupuncture in the latter part of 2005. However, this has not yet taken place. At the request of the DH, the Prince of Wales's Foundation for Integrated Health has established a Complementary and Natural Healthcare Council (see below).

A study was carried out on the use of complementary or alternative therapies among people undergoing cancer treatment. It reported in January 2006[12] and is available on the DH website.[13]

A report of the working group looking at chronic fatigue syndrome (CFS/ME) considered patients' views on the use of complementary and alternative medicines and their value in the management of the illness.[14]

Implications for physiotherapists

Physiotherapists are affected by the growing popularity of complementary and alternative therapies in two ways. The physiotherapist may be aware that patients are consulting practitioners in complementary medicine therapies and may be taking medicines, or other treatment, for the same conditions for which the physiotherapist him/herself is giving advice. Conversely, some physiotherapists are themselves undertaking training in a therapy regarded as complementary to conventional medicine. The Chartered Society of Physiotherapy (CSP) drew up guidance on physiotherapy and complementary medicines in 2002.[15] The guidance defines complementary medicines and looks at the scope of professional practice and then at the integration of complementary medicine and physiotherapy.

This chapter therefore looks at the following topics:

- Definition of complementary therapies
- The clients receiving complementary therapy
- disclosure to the physiotherapist
- ignorance on the part of the physiotherapist
- The physiotherapist as complementary therapist
- Agreement of employer
- Consent of patient
- Defining standards
- Examples of therapies undertaken by physiotherapists

Definition of complementary therapies

Complementary is defined as: completing: together making up a whole, ... of medical treatment, therapies, etc. ... (l. Complementum – *com-*, intens. and *plere* to fill).[16]

It is thus seen to work in parallel with orthodox medicine. The BCMA therefore states that therapy groups which are represented by the BCMA should advise and encourage patients to see their doctor wherever appropriate.

The client receiving complementary therapy

Disclosure to the physiotherapist

When a patient is referred to a physiotherapist in the NHS, then information relating to that person's care within the NHS would also be given. In addition, where there is a referral within social services, then the person referring, whether GP or social worker, would provide the physiotherapist with the information required in order to determine priorities. Thus, the physiotherapist should have basic information about the client in order to determine the care that is required by the client. In addition, the physiotherapist would usually have access to health records kept on the patient, to ensure that his/her care is compatible with other treatment the patient is receiving.

In contrast, where the patient is receiving treatment from a complementary therapist, there is usually no official way in which this information can be made known to the physiotherapist other than through the patient. The physiotherapist therefore relies upon the openness of the patient in disclosing information that may be relevant to the treatment and care which the physiotherapist is offering.

Clearly, the importance of this communication between patient and physiotherapist will depend upon the relevance of the complementary therapy to the treatment and care which the physiotherapist provides. Some therapies may have little effect; others, such as acupuncture, may have a significant effect on the recommendations the physiotherapist may make.

The CSP has given guidance on patients who seek treatment both within and outside the NHS,[17] emphasising the importance of good communication between the practitioners and discussing their spheres of responsibility. If there is a conflict between the two treatments, then the therapists need to discuss this with the patient who should be given the choice over which course to pursue, with a reassurance that they can return to the other, when the chosen course has ended.

Ignorance on the part of the physiotherapist

- Does it matter that the physiotherapist has no knowledge of the complementary therapy that the patient is undergoing?

The answer is that it may have an important effect and, had the physiotherapist been aware of certain information about the therapy, he/she may have advised the patient differently.

Situation: complementary therapy

A physiotherapist employed by an NHS Trust is caring for a patient with chronic back pain. The physiotherapist is not aware that the patient is also visiting an acupuncturist for his condition and is also considering consulting a chiropractor or osteopath. If harm occurs to the patient, how can the physiotherapist show that it was not her treatment which caused the harm?

In this situation it would have been of value to the client if the work of the physiotherapist had been undertaken in the light of the methods, effects and intentions used by the acupuncturist, so that her work complemented this rather than possibly conflicted with it. Unless, however, the physiotherapist has a basic understanding of the practice of acupuncture, she would be unable to work in parallel.

Where harm has occurred, expert evidence on causation would be required to show whether anything the physiotherapist had done could have caused that harm. It is hoped that, in reviewing the practice of the physiotherapist, it would be revealed that the patient had been receiving treatment from other persons. In the light of this any liability on the part of each of these persons could be analysed.

Situation: working together

A patient informs the physiotherapist that she is also receiving treatment from an osteopath. The physiotherapist recommends that the patient gives her the details so that she can contact the osteopath with a view to working in tandem. The patient refuses to give that information.

The patient's attitude makes it very difficult for the physiotherapist to ensure that there is harmony in the practice of the two therapists. It may be that the physiotherapist would find it difficult to provide appropriate treatment not knowing what the other therapist is doing. However, she should not automatically refuse the patient NHS physiotherapy care. She should seek advice and

discuss further with the patient her objections to her having contact with the osteopath.

Osteopathy and chiropractic have now received state registered status and the popularity and availability of their services within the NHS might increase. It is important for physiotherapists to understand the benefits and limits of the treatments offered by these other therapies, so that they can understand how their practice as physiotherapists fits into the service which these others provide.

The physiotherapist as complementary medicine therapist

Agreement of employer

It is recognised that many physiotherapists are considering the use of complementary therapies in the treatment of clients. If a physiotherapist obtains a training in a complementary therapy, the physiotherapist should ensure that he/she obtains the agreement of the employer before he/she uses this skill as part of his/her practice as a physiotherapist. If the physiotherapist fails to do this and causes harm to the patient while using his/her complementary therapy skills, then his/her employer could argue that the physiotherapist was not acting in course of employment when he/she caused the harm. The employer is therefore not vicariously liable (see glossary and Chapter 10) and the physiotherapist must accept personal liability for the harm that has been caused. The following example explains the legal position.

Situation: acupuncture

A physiotherapist following her basic training developed skills in acupuncture. One of her NHS patients was suffering from considerable pain and the physiotherapist offered to provide acupuncture to relieve the pain. It was arranged that the patient would come to the hospital at the end of the day's clinic. Unfortunately, the physiotherapist placed the needle in a nerve and caused permanent damage to the patient. The patient is claiming compensation.

If the NHS trust gave expressed or implied consent to this work by the physiotherapist then her work as an acupuncturist could be seen as being in the course of employment. In this case the NHS Trust would be vicariously liable for the harm that has been caused and pay any compensation due. On the other hand, if the NHS Trust was unaware of the work as an acupuncturist then it may refuse to accept vicarious liability for her work as an acupuncturist, arguing that the work was not performed in the course of her employment as a physiotherapist (see Chapter 10 on vicarious liability). In this case the physiotherapist would have to accept personal liability for the harm done and be responsible for payment of the compensation due. It is therefore crucial that the physiotherapist ensures that she has her own insurance cover for such work.

It is also essential for the physiotherapist to obtain the consent of the employer if he/she intends to practice privately during working hours. In the case of *Watling* v. *Gloucester County Counci*[18] (the full facts are discussed in Chapter 17) an occupational therapist was dismissed when he saw private patients for alternative therapy during working hours. His application for compensation for unfair dismissal failed.

Consent of the patient

It is also essential that the patient should explicitly give consent before the physiotherapist is allowed to use any complementary therapies on him/her. The basic principles of obtaining consent apply (see Chapter 7) but, since a patient would not normally expect a physiotherapist to be providing complementary therapies, it is imperative that the physiotherapist gives full details of all that is involved and makes it absolutely clear that the patient is fully entitled

to receive the treatment usually provided by the physiotherapist even though he or she refuses the complementary therapy and care. It is preferable to obtain the consent in writing and to put in a leaflet the information that the patient should be told about the treatment.

An information leaflet on the risks of acupuncture was prepared from a consensus gathering in 2001.[19] Although the risks in acupuncture are seen as minimal, it was emphasised that it was insufficient for the consent form to be handed to the patient by a receptionist for signature without any opportunity for the patient to discuss it with the practitioner. It is important that the practitioner ensures that the patient has fully understood all of the risks and taken them into consideration in giving consent.

Defining standards

One of the difficulties of some complementary therapies is that there may not be a clear definition of the expected standard of care. If harm were to occur, to succeed in a claim for compensation the patient would have to establish that the therapist failed to use the reasonable standard of care which he, the patient, was entitled to expect. This may not be easy to prove. In a case in 2000[20] a practitioner of traditional Chinese herbal medicine was held not to be liable when a patient who took nine doses of a herbal remedy became ill and later died of acute liver failure. The illness and death was attributable to a rare and unpredictable reaction to the remedy. His widow failed in her action against the practitioner. The High Court held that on the evidence before it the actions of the practitioner had been consistent with the standard of care appropriate to traditional Chinese herbal medicine in accordance with established requirements. In a recent case in July 2008 there was no agreement on the standard which should have been applied and the claimant won an out of court settlement. Mrs Page, 52 years, won more than £800 000 after she claimed that a radical detox diet left her brain-damaged and epileptic. She said that she had been told to drink four extra pints of water a day and reduce her salt intake to prevent fluid retention and reduce weight.[21] The nutritional therapist and life coach denied any fault and the claim was settled by her insurance company, without any admission of liability. Solicitors for the defendant stated that all allegations of substandard practice were denied and the settlement was less than half the amount claimed.

Guidance is provided by the Acupuncture Association of Chartered Physiotherapists on safe practice, which includes guidelines for the treatment of musculoskeletal pain.[22] It covers the treatment records and medico-legal requirements; safe needling and potentially hazardous acupoints; the safe workplace; and needlestick injuries. The appendices include a specimen patient consent form, which includes a questionnaire on potential contra-indications. Further information on acupuncture in physiotherapy can be obtained from Val Hopwood's book.[23]

Examples of therapies undertaken by physiotherapists

On its website the CSP states that physiotherapists can be seen as pioneers of complementary (or alternative) approaches to health care. The Society currently has four such recognised groups. Three of them have an overt focus on one treatment modality – acupuncture, craniosacral and reflex therapy groups – and the energy medicine group embraces underlying principles behind many complementary techniques.

Acupuncture

The Acupuncture Association of Chartered Physiotherapists (AACP) gives advice and guidance to members on the practice of acupuncture by physiotherapists and acts as a forum for the interchange of information and research. Contact details are available through the CSP. The AACP has a regional network and publishes a journal twice a year and is an associate member of the British Medical Acupuncture Society and the British Acupuncture Council. The CSP has issued guidance on the licensing of acupuncture,[24] explaining the provisions of the Local Government (Miscellaneous Provisions) Act 1982 in relation to the licensing of premises in England and Wales but outside of London.

Val Hopwood and George Lewith[25] discuss how acupuncture can be used in the motor recovery of the upper limb after a stroke, but emphasise the importance of additional case studies to confirm their results. Research has also suggested that a course of acupuncture may increase success in IVF treatment by 65%.[26]

In 2006 the AACP emphasised the importance of physiotherapists who practise acupuncture registering with the new Council which was being planned at that time. In preparation for the new regulation regime, the AACP tightened up its accreditation by physiotherapists wishing to practise acupuncture and planned to publish a framework regulating all aspects of education and training.[27] Physiotherapists form the largest group of registered health professionals offering acupuncture.

Energy medicine

The Association of Chartered Physiotherapists in Energy Medicine (ACPEM) is a recognised clinical interest group which has a regional network and a biannual newsletter. Formal courses in myofascial release, subtle touch and energy medicine are offered or recommended. The Association encourages its members to maintain and update their personal continuing professional development portfolio and take part in ongoing discussions on outcome measures.

A physiotherapist, Steve Gibbs, has set up the British Healing Energy Therapy Association (BHETA). It aims to focus upon the theories regarding Healing Energy Therapy (HET) and will take a multidisciplinary approach. He hopes to see healing energy accepted from the scientific angle, so that it can be incorporated into mainstream practice.[28] BHETA conducted two pilot studies into the use of HET to aid recovery from chronic fatigue syndrome and for pain relief in arachnoiditis and is putting forward theories based on scientific research to suggest how the mechanisms behind traditional 'laying on of hands' may work.[29]

Craniosacral therapy

This is described by Susan Hollenbery[30] as

> about the ability to perceive, acknowledge, allow, enhance and facilitate the patient's own healing process without the necessity to judge, intervene or perform. Treatment is the art of being, not of doing.

In contrast to physiotherapy which seeks to treat the symptoms that the patient is complaining about, craniosacral therapy looks at the patient as a whole.

> Any attempt to treat only the local disorder with localised treatments, may shift the problem, sooner or later, to another part of the body.

Reflextherapy and massage

The Association of Chartered Physiotherapists in Reflextherapy provides information, support and training to chartered physiotherapists and other health professionals in reflextherapy. The Association of Chartered Physiotherapists in Massage (ACPIM) considers the relationship between physiotherapy and aromatherapy as practised by a physiotherapist.

Where a physiotherapist practices as an aromatherapist, he/she is practicing outside the scope of physiotherapy (see CSP PA 21 and 32) The subtle difference is when a patient consults the physiotherapist as an aromatherapist, rather than when a physiotherapist integrates his/her aromatherapy skills or massages with essential oils.

The ACPIM has published guidance on massage with essential oils within physiotherapy.[31]

In Chapter 16 of *Learning Disabilities* a book edited by Jeanette Rennie,[32] Libby Davies and Jane Bruce[33] explore the use of complementary therapies with those with learning disabilities, taking case studies as examples of their use. Thus, the use of aromatherapy with David a 21-year-old client with multiple handicaps including epilepsy and severe learning disabilities led to a reduction in chest infections and therefore less use of antibiotics.

Aromatherapy

A sub-group of the Association for Chartered Physiotherapists with an Interest in Massage (ACPIM) is the aromatherapy group, i.e. physiotherapists who have trained in aromatherapy. At the present time, this activity is seen as beyond the scope of the professional practice of a chartered physiotherapist and the CSP does not consider that a chartered physiotherapist working in aromatherapy is covered by the professional protection of the CSP or by its insurers. However, this was written before the publication of the *Scope of Physiotherapy Practice*, 2008, by the CSP and many would see aromatherapy as coming under 'kindred activities' the fourth pillar of activities recognised by the Royal Charter (see Chapter 1).

This is a serious issue for chartered physiotherapists practising in this area. If they do not have confirmation in writing that they are covered by the CSP, then they must ensure that they obtain personal insurance cover from an aromatherapy organisation or one of the umbrella groups for complementary therapies.[34] If they are using aromatherapy during their employment, they should also ensure that they have the approval (preferably in writing) of their employer/senior manager for that activity.

Chinese medicine, physiotherapy and psychiatry

John Tindall examined traditional Chinese medicine (TCM) and natural medicine in psychiatry[35] and concluded that physiotherapists are in a good position to use various natural healthcare models within psychiatry, but that it is important to receive full and comprehensive training in those particular areas. In his clinic they were developing a Chinese herbal medicine pharmacy and wrote more than 3000 prescriptions a year for various ailments from substance abuse, to HIV, mental health problems, dermatology, etc.

Yoga

A clinical interest group on yoga has been established which aims to bring together physiotherapy professionals to explore and investigate yoga techniques and their integration into clinical practice. It does not as yet have CSP status as a recognised group.

Complementary and Natural Healthcare Council

The Prince's Foundation for Integrated Health set up a Federal Working Group, which spent 12 months considering the formation of a new council. Its report was published in February 2008.[36] It recommended developing a federal structure for the voluntary self-regulation of complementary healthcare professions, i.e. a single regulatory body rather than a series of regulators for each complementary healthcare profession. The new body is to be called the Complementary and Natural Healthcare Council and will be made up of four elements:

- Federal Regulatory Council
- Profession Specific Boards
- Functional Boards
- Practice Advisory Panel.

The members of the council and the functional boards will be lay people, appointed independently; each profession-specific board (one for each profession) will have a lay Chair and four registrants from the appropriate profession. Each Profession Specific Board will select one of its practitioner members to sit on the Practice Advisory Panel, which will provide a pool of expertise to support the Council. The report recommended robust procedures for handling complaints and fitness to practise issues, along with a code of conduct and ethics based on the code used by the Health Professions Council. The complementary healthcare professions that are, or have been, part of the Foundation for Integrated Health's regulation programme have developed, or are developing, the competencies necessary for entry to the Register. Full public and professional liability insurance will be mandatory, as will continuing professional development. The Federal Working Group has suggested that an independent, external organisation be invited to review the work of the Complementary and Natural Healthcare Council from time to time, to ensure that it remains fit for purpose and that it meets the needs of all who have an interest in its work. The Department of Health has provided start-up funding but the aim is for the Complementary and Natural Healthcare Council to be financed solely by registration fees. The Department of Health will also ensure that the principles underpinning professional regulation as set out in its White Paper *Trust, Assurance and Safety*[37] are implemented (see Chapter 3) The intention was that the Council's register should be in place and operative by June 2008. To be eligible for registration, a practitioner must be a member of a therapy that is itself a member of the Council. Those therapy associations which are already members include: the Alexander technique, aromatherapy, the Bowen technique, cranial therapy, homeopathy, massage therapy, naturopathy, nutritional therapy, reflexology, reiki, shiatsu and yoga therapy. The overall intention is that the Council will provide enhanced consumer confidence and safety through a credible, robust and professional voluntary regulatory structure for the practice of complementary health care in the UK.

The NHS spends £50 million a year on therapies that will come under the Council. It was reported that NHS homoeopathy, which will come under the Council, is in sharp decline with only 37% of Trusts offering homoeopathic treatment.[38]

Conclusions

A turning point for many complementary and alternative therapies has now arrived with the establishment of the Complementary and Natural Healthcare Council and the emphasis on research-based effective treatments. Those therapists whose treatments which are not proven to be effective on the basis of research evidence will not be registered by the Council nor will they obtain funding from the NHS. The involvement of physiotherapists in alternative and complementary therapies is likely to continue but they will be involved in research to establish their effectiveness. The greater the use by and training of physiotherapists in additional therapies, the more likely that they are to become concerned at the meaning and direction of physiotherapy itself. It is possible that eventually some of the therapies at present seen as complementary could become an integral part of physiotherapy practice. Further information on complementary therapies can be obtained from the website of the Complementary Healthcare Information Service.[39] The CSP also has set up a complementary health website.[40]

References

1   Dimond, B.C. (1998) *The Legal Aspects of Complementary Therapy Practice*. Churchill Livingstone, Edinburgh.
2   Laurance, J. (1996) Alternative Health: An Honest Alternative or just Magic? *The Times*, 5 February, p. 11.

Questions and exercises

1   You have decided that you would like to undertake training in aromatherapy and eventually use it as part of your practice as a physiotherapist. What actions would you take to ensure that your plans are compatible with your role as a physiotherapist and as an employee?

2   You are visiting a patient in the community and become concerned that she appears to be paying a lot of money to a chiropractor and her condition does not seem to be improving; in fact, you consider that it is deteriorating. What action, if any, would you take?

3   Do you consider that those complementary therapies which so wished, should be permitted to have registered status under either the Health Professions Council or the Complementary and Natural Healthcare Council and if so, do you consider the criteria laid down by the HPC suitable and sufficient to protect the patient? (Refer also to Chapter 3.)

3   Health Education Authority (2006) *A–Z guide on Complementary Therapies*. Available from www.internethealthlibrary.com.
4   Charman, R. (2000) *Complementary Therapies for Physical Therapists*. Butterworth Heinemann, Oxford.
5   Foundation for Integrated Medicine (1997) *Integrated Healthcare: A Way Forward for the Next Five years*. FIM, London
6   Tavares, M. (2003) *National Guidelines for the Use of Complementary Therapies in Supportive and Palliative Care*. The Prince of Wales's Foundation for Integrated Health and the National Council for Hospice and Specialist Palliative Care, London.
7   www.fih.org.uk/
8   House of Lords Select Committee on Science and Technology, 6th Report: complementary and alternative medicine, Session 1999–2000, 21 November 2000.
9   www.parliament.uk
10   www.dh.gov.uk/en/index.htm

11 Statutory regulation of herbal medicine and acupuncture: Report of the consultation 2005; available on the DH website.

12 Professor Jessica Corner and others. A study of the use of complementary and alternative therapists among people undergoing cancer treatment: A quantitative and qualitative study. Final Report Department of Health and University of Southampton January 2006.

13 www.dh.gov.uk/en/Researchanddevelopment/index.htm

14 www.dh.gov.uk/en/Aboutus/Ministersand DepartmentLeaders/ChiefMedicalOfficer/index.htm

15 Chartered Society of Physiotherapy (2002) *Physiotherapy and Complementary Medicines*. PA 48 CSP, London.

16 Pamphlet of the British Complementary Medicine Association BCMA. Further information can be obtained from www.bcma.co.uk

17 Chartered Society Physiotherapy (2004) CSP 0065. *Patients Seeking Treatment in the Public & Private Sector*. CSP, London.

18 *Watling* v. *Gloucester County Council*. EAT/868/94, 17 March 1995, 23 November 1994, Lexis transcript.

19 White, A., Cummings, M., Hopwood, V., MacPherson, H. (2001) *Informed Consent for Acupuncture – An Information Leaflet Developed by Consensus. Acupuncture in Medicin*e 2001; 19(2): 123–129.

20 *Shakoor (Deceased)* v. *Situ* [2000] 4 All ER 181.

21 Mostrous, A. (2008) £800,000 for Brain Injury 'caused by high-fluid diet'. *The Times*, 23 July, p. 16.

22 Acupuncture Association of Chartered Physiotherapists (2007) *Guidelines for Safe Practice*, revised edition CSP London.

23 Hopwood, V. (2004) *Acupuncture in Physiotherapy*. Butterworth Heinemann, Oxford.

24 CSP Professional Affairs Department (1995) No. PA 24. *Licensing of Acupuncture*. CSP, London.

25 Hopwood, V., Lewith, G. (1997) The Effect of Acupuncture on the Motor Recovery of the Upper Limb after Stroke. *Physiotherapy* **83**, 12, 614–619.

26 Hawkes, N. (2008) Course of Acupuncture may Increase Success of IVF Treatment by 65%. *The Times*, 6 February, p. 11.

27 Stevenson, P. (2006) *Frontline* 15 February www.csp.org.uk/director/newsandevents/frontline.

28 Gibbs, S. (1996) The British Healing Energy Therapy Association. *In Touch* **81**, 24.

29 Gibbs, S. (1997) Healing Energy Therapy. *Physiotherapy* **83**, 2, 73–4.

30 Hollenbery, S. (1995) Touching is Believing: Treatment with Craniosacral Therapy. *In Touch* **74**, 12–3.

31 ACPIM (2007) *Massage with Essential Oils Within Physiotherapy*. CPS, London.

32 Rennie, J. (ed.) (2001) *Learning Disability Physical Therapy, Treatment and Management. A Collaborative Approach*. Whurr Publishers, London.

33 Davies, L., Bruce, J. Complementary Therapies. In: Rennie J. (ed.) *Learning Disability Physical Therapy, Treatment and Management. A Collaborative Approach*. Chapter 16. Whurr Publishers, London 2001.

34 See Dimond, B.C. (1998) *The Legal Aspects of Complementary Therapy Practice*. Churchill Livingstone, Edinburgh.

35 Tindall, J. (1994) Traditional Chinese Medicine (TCM) and Natural Medicine in Psychiatry. *Journal of the Association of Chartered Physiotherapists in Psychiatry* XI, 8–13.

36 The Prince's Foundation for Integrated Health (2008) *A Federal Approach to Professionally-Led Voluntary Regulation for Complementary Healthcare: A Plan for Action*. The Prince's Foundation for Integrated Health, London.

37 Department of Health (2007) White Paper. *Trust, Assurance and Safety: the Regulation of Health Professionals in the 21st Century*. Cmnd 7013. DH, London.

38 Rose, D. (2008) NHS Homoeopathy in Sharp Decline. *The Times*, 30 January.

39 www.chisuk.org.uk

40 www.csp.org.uk

Conclusion

28 The Future

In July 2008, to link in with the sixtieth anniversary of the establishment of the NHS on 5 July 1948, the final report of Professor Lord Darzi, *High Quality of Care for All* on the future of the NHS was published.[1] It had been preceded by an interim report in October 2007, which set out the vision of an NHS which was fair, personalised, effective and safe and that outlined the immediate steps to be taken before the final report, which included the primary care trusts ensuring greater access to GP services at weekends and out of hours. The interim report was followed on 9 May 2008 by a review *Leading Local Change*, in which 74 local clinical working groups had developed models of care for their regions. This document set out five pledges for the changes to the NHS:

(1) Changes will always be to the benefit of patients.
(2) Change will be clinically driven.
(3) All change will be locally led.
(4) Patients, carers, the public and other key partners will be involved.
(5) Existing services will not be withdrawn until new and better services are available to patients so they can see the difference.

The final report was the culmination of extensive consultation and review with over 60 000 people participating, including 2000 clinicians, and other health and social care professionals from every NHS region in England. Its aim was to create an NHS that is focused on helping people to stay healthy. The publication of the final report was preceded by an announcement that 150 large health centres, known as polyclinics, were to be established which will be run by nurses. Nurses will be encouraged to set up not-for-profit firms to run the practices by being allowed to opt out of the NHS without losing pension rights.

The review saw the immediate steps as being:

(a) Every primary care trust will commission comprehensive well-being and prevention services, in partnership with local authorities, with the services offered personalised to meet the specific needs of their local populations.
(b) A Coalition for Better Health, with a set of new voluntary agreements between the Government, private and third sector organisations on actions to improve health outcomes.
(c) Raised awareness of vascular risk assessment through a new 'Reduce Your Risk' campaign.

(d)   Support for people to stay healthy at work.
(e)   Support GPs to help individuals and their families stay healthy.

Patients are to be given more rights and control over their own health by:

- extending choice of GP practice;
- introducing a new right to choice in a NHS constitution;
- ensuring everyone with a long-term condition has a personalised care plan;
- piloting personal health budgets;
- guaranteeing patients access to the most clinically and cost-effective drugs and treatments.

High-quality care is to be at the centre of the NHS and to secure this the following measures will be taken:

- new enforcement powers for the Care Quality Commission;
- independent quality standards and clinical priority setting;
- systematic publications on quality of care, including reports from patients on the quality of their experience; accounts to be provided by law by all registered healthcare providers;
- funding to reflect quality of care that patients receive;
- strengthening clinical excellence awards scheme for doctors;
- easy access for NHS staff to information about high-quality care;
- measures to ensure continuous improvement in the quality of primary and community care;
- new best practice tariffs focused on areas for improvement.

Other measures will be taken to strengthen the involvement of clinicians in decision making in the NHS, including the appointment of medical directors and quality boards at regional and national level

A new Quality Observatory is to be established in every region of the NHS to inform local quality improvement efforts. Innovation and advances in the NHS are to be encouraged:

Strategic Health Authorities will have a new legal duty to promote innovation; with new funds and prizes being made available; clinically and cost-effective innovation in medicines and medical technologies is to be encouraged with new partnerships between the NHS, universities and industry.

Frontline staff are to be empowered with reinvigorated practice-based commissioning, encouragement of social enterprise organisations and easy transfer of NHS staff with protected pension rights; improvements in the quality of NHS education and training; a three-fold increase in investment in nurse and midwife preceptorships and doubling investment in apprenticeships for healthcare support staff

The NHS constitution

The Darzi report includes a NHS constitution,[2] which can be seen in Appendix 2 of this book. The constitution sets out the seven key principles that guide the NHS, the rights and responsibilities of patients, the rights and responsibilities of staff and the values underpinning the NHS. It thus attempts to consolidate all the existing legal rights of patients, staff and public in one document and to set down some pledges such as:

> The NHS will strive to provide all staff with personal development, access to appropriate training for their jobs, and line management support to succeed. (Pledge)

The NHS Constitution is to be accompanied by a statement of accountability. All organisations providing NHS services will be obliged by law to take account of the Constitution and its principles and values in their decisions and actions.

The NHS Constitution is underpinned by statutory provision in the Health Bill currently being debated in Parliament. This places a duty on NHS organisations to have regard to the Constitution. A Handbook on the Constitution is to be published by the Secretary of State.

The Darzi proposal to establish an NHS constitution was welcomed by several senior figures in mental health in a letter to *The* Times,[3] who saw the opportunity of committing the NHS to treat mental and physical health problems with equality. One danger resulting from a constitution is the possibility of increasing litigation within the NHS. Most of the rights of the patients are to be found in statute or common law (as this book shows). The rights of staff are also embodied in health and safety legislation and are terms of the contract of employment. However, many of the pledges such as the staff development one set out above are not an implied term of the contract nor an explicit statutory right. Does a pledge mean that it is actionable in a court of law? Is there a danger that it could become smooth talk with no substance? The extent to which more laws can provide the answer to problems within the NHS is highly questionable.

Other criticisms of the report are that the new powers intended for the Care Quality Commission and the amalgamation of the existing inspectorates in the new body are unnecessary and will not decrease costs nor lead to greater efficiency. The Darzi review and draft constitution were subject to consultation, which ended on 17 October 2008. The finalised NHS Constitution was published on 21 January 2009.

It is inevitable that any major proposals for change within the NHS will lead to controversy and debate and the DH website published the reaction on the media. One major criticism from the chief executive of King's Fund health think-tank, who welcomes a new era where patients will be able to check on the quality of the services, was that there are no estimates of how much all this will cost. The absence of financial costings is serious in view of the proposal that all patients will have access to the drugs approved by the National Institute for Health and Clinical Excellence. Nor is there any indication of just how different the government expects the quality of health services to be in 5 or 10 years' time.

Nor is there any indication of the timescale within which the proposals will be implemented. The report proposes that both individual trusts and individual staff will be rewarded for quality service, but there is no discussion of how low quality providers will be treated.

However, the Darzi review does set out a strategy which can be used by health professionals to develop their own services according to established values and clear standards. For example, it is planned that about 15 million clients with long-term conditions will have individual care plans. Physiotherapists should already have individual care plans for each of their clients and can ensure that they are developed on a multidisciplinary basis including social services.

The implementation of the final Darzi proposals will constitute a significant development in the future. In addition many Bills are in the process of enactment in Parliament and may come into force in April 2009. The Chartered Society of Physiotherapy in its seminal paper on the scope of professional practice has also paved the way in which physiotherapy practice can develop safely and effectively beyond its present boundaries.

It is hoped that this second edition will continue to assist physiotherapists in developing their awareness of the legal context within which they practice and in meeting the many challenges to come.

References

1   Department of Health (2008) *High Quality of Care for All*. CM 7432. DH, London.
2   Available on the DH website with supporting documents; dh.gov.uk
3   Paul Farmer, Chief Executive Mind, and others (2008) Letter to the Editor: Inequitable Illnesses. *The Times*, 22 February.

Appendix 1
Schedule 1 to Human Rights Act 1998

Schedule 1 to Human Rights Act 1998
  Articles of the European Convention on Human Rights

Part I
The Convention Rights and Freedoms

Article 2
Right to life

(1) Everyone's right to life shall be protected by law. No one shall be deprived of his life intentionally save in the execution of a sentence of a court following his conviction of a crime for which this penalty is provided by law.

(2) Deprivation of life shall not be regarded as inflicted in contravention of this Article when it results from the use of force which is no more than absolutely necessary:
   (a) in defence of any person from unlawful violence;
   (b) in order to effect a lawful arrest or to prevent the escape of a person lawfully detained;
   (c) in action lawfully taken for the purpose of quelling a riot or insurrection.

Article 3
Prohibition of torture

No one shall be subjected to torture or to inhuman or degrading treatment or punishment.

Article 4
Prohibition of slavery and forced labour

(1) No one shall be held in slavery or servitude.

(2) No one shall be required to perform forced or compulsory labour.

(3) For the purpose of this Article the term 'forced or compulsory labour' shall not include:
   (a) any work required to be done in the ordinary course of detention imposed according to the provisions of Article 5 of this Convention or during conditional release from such detention;
   (b) any service of a military character or, in case of conscientious objectors in countries where they are recognised, service exacted instead of compulsory military service;
   (c) any service exacted in case of an emergency or calamity threatening the life or well-being of the community;

(d)   any work or service which forms part of normal civic obligations.

Article 5
Right to liberty and security

(1)   Everyone has the right to liberty and security of person. No one shall be deprived of his liberty save in the following cases and in accordance with a procedure prescribed by law:

(a)   the lawful detention of a person after conviction by a competent court;

(b)   the lawful arrest or detention of a person for non-compliance with the lawful order of a court or in order to secure the fulfilment of any obligation prescribed by law;

(c)   the lawful arrest or detention of a person effected for the purpose of bringing him before the competent legal authority on reasonable suspicion of having committed an offence or when it is reasonably considered necessary to prevent his committing an offence or fleeing after having done so;

(d)   the detention of a minor by lawful order for the purpose of educational supervision or his lawful detention for the purpose of bringing him before the competent legal authority;

(e)   the lawful detention of persons for the prevention of the spreading of infectious diseases, of persons of unsound mind alcoholics or drug addicts or vagrants;

(f)   the lawful arrest or detention of a person to prevent his effecting an unauthorised entry into the country or of a person against whom action is being taken with a view to deportation or extradition.

(2)   Everyone who is arrested shall be informed promptly, in a language which he understands, of the reasons for his arrest and of any charge against him.

(3)   Everyone arrested or detained in accordance with the provisions of paragraph 1(c) of this Article shall be brought promptly before a judge or other officer authorised by law to exercise judicial power and shall be entitled to trial within a reasonable time or to release pending trial. Release may be conditioned by guarantees to appear for trial.

(4)   Everyone who is deprived of his liberty by arrest or detention shall be entitled to take proceedings by which the lawfulness of his detention shall be decided speedily by a court and his release ordered if the detention is not lawful.

(5)   Everyone who has been the victim of arrest or detention in contravention of the provisions of this Article shall have an enforceable right to compensation.

Article 6
Right to a fair trial

(1)   In the determination of his civil rights and obligations or of any criminal charge against him, everyone is entitled to a fair and public hearing within a reasonable time by an independent and impartial tribunal established by law. Judgment shall be pronounced publicly but the press and public may be excluded from all or part of the trial in the interest of morals, public order or national security in a democratic society, where the interests of juveniles or the protection of the private life of the parties so require, or to the extent strictly necessary in the opinion of the court in special circumstances where publicity would prejudice the interests of justice.

(2)   Everyone charged with a criminal offence shall be presumed innocent until proved guilty according to law.

(3)   Everyone charged with a criminal offence has the following minimum rights:

(a)   to be informed promptly, in a language which he understands and in detail, of the nature and cause of the accusation against him;

(b) to have adequate time and facilities for the preparation of his defence;

(c) to defend himself in person or through legal assistance of his own choosing or, if he has not sufficient means to pay for legal assistance, to be given it free when the interests of justice so require;

(d) to examine or have examined witnesses against him and to obtain the attendance and examination of witnesses on his behalf under the same conditions as witnesses against him;

(e) to have the free assistance of an interpreter if he cannot understand or speak the language used in court.

Article 7
No punishment without law

(1) No one shall be held guilty of any criminal offence on account of any act or omission which did not constitute a criminal offence under national or international law at the time when it was committed. Nor shall a heavier penalty be imposed than the one that was applicable at the time the criminal offence was committed.

(2) This Article shall not prejudice the trial and punishment of any person for any act or omission which, at the time when it was committed, was criminal according to the general principles of law recognised by civilised nations.

Article 8
Right to respect for private and family life

(1) Everyone has the right to respect for his private and family life, his home and his correspondence.

(2) There shall be no interference by a public authority with the exercise of this right except such as is in accordance with the law and is necessary in a democratic society in the interests of national security, public

safety or the economic wellbeing of the country, for the prevention of disorder or crime, for the protection of health or morals, or for the protection of the rights and freedoms of others.

Article 9
Freedom of thought, conscience and religion

(1) Everyone has the right to freedom of thought, conscience and religion; this right includes freedom to change his religion or belief and freedom, either alone or in community with others and in public or private, to manifest his religion or belief, in worship, teaching, practice and observance.

(2) Freedom to manifest one's religion or beliefs shall be subject only to such limitations as are prescribed by law and are necessary in a democratic society in the interests of public safety, for the protection of public order, health or morals, or for the protection of the rights and freedoms of others.

Article 10
Freedom of expression

(1) Everyone has the right to freedom of expression. This right shall include freedom to hold opinions and to receive and impart information and ideas without interference by public authority and regardless of frontiers. This Article shall not prevent States from requiring the licensing of broadcasting, television or cinema enterprises.

(2) The exercise of these freedoms, since it carries with it duties and responsibilities, may be subject to such formalities, conditions, restrictions or penalties as are prescribed by law and are necessary in a democratic society, in the interests of national security, territorial integrity or public safety, for the prevention of disorder or crime, for the protection of health or morals, for the protection of the reputation

or rights of others, for preventing the disclosure of information received in confidence, or for maintaining the authority and impartiality of the judiciary.

Article 11
Freedom of assembly and association

(1)   Everyone has the right to freedom of peaceful assembly and to freedom of association with others, including the right to form and to join trade unions for the protection of his interests.
(2)   No restrictions shall be placed on the exercise of these rights other than such as are prescribed by law and are necessary in a democratic society in the interests of national security or public safety, for the prevention of disorder or crime, for the protection of health or morals or for the protection of the rights and freedoms of others. This Article shall not prevent the imposition of lawful restrictions on the exercise of these rights by members of the armed forces, of the police or of the administration of the State.

Article 12
Right to marry

Men and women of marriageable age have the right to marry and to found a family, according to the national laws governing the exercise of this right.

Article 14
Prohibition of discrimination

The enjoyment of the rights and freedoms set forth in this Convention shall be secured without discrimination on any ground such as sex, race, colour, language, religion, political or other opinion, national or social origin, association with a national minority, property, birth or other status.

Article 16
Restrictions on political activity of aliens

Nothing in Articles 10, 11 and 14 shall be regarded as preventing the High Contracting Parties from imposing restrictions on the political activity of aliens.

Article 17
Prohibition of abuse of rights

Nothing in this Convention may be interpreted as implying for any State, group or person any right to engage in any activity or perform any act aimed at the destruction of any of the rights and freedoms set forth herein or at their limitation to a greater extent than is provided for in the Convention.

Article 18
Limitation on use of restrictions on rights

The restrictions permitted under this Convention to the said rights and freedoms shall not be applied for any purpose other than those for which they have been prescribed.

Part II
The First Protocol

Article 1
Protection of property

Every natural or legal person is entitled to the peaceful enjoyment of his possessions. No one shall be deprived of his possessions except in the public interest and subject to the conditions provided for by law and by the general principles of international law.

The preceding provisions shall not, however, in any way impair the right of a State to enforce such laws as it deems necessary to control the use of property in accordance with the general interest or to secure the payment of taxes or other contributions or penalties.

Article 2
Right to education

No person shall be denied the right to education. In the exercise of any functions which it assumes in relation to education and to teaching, the State shall respect the right of parents to ensure such education and teaching in conformity with their own religious and philosophical convictions.

Article 3
Right to free elections

The High Contracting Parties undertake to hold free elections at reasonable intervals by secret ballot, under conditions which will ensure the free expression of the opinion of the people in the choice of the legislature.

Part III
The Sixth Protocol

Article 1
Abolition of the death penalty

The death penalty shall be abolished. No one shall be condemned to such penalty or executed.

Article 2
Death penalty in time of war

A State may make provision in its law for the death penalty in respect of acts committed in time of war or of imminent threat of war; such penalty shall be applied only in the instances laid down in the law and in accordance with its provisions. The State shall communicate to the Secretary General of the Council of Europe the relevant provisions of that law.

Appendix 2
NHS Constitution

The NHS belongs to us all

Constitution

The NHS belongs to the people. It is there to improve our health, supporting us to keep mentally and physically well, to get better when we are ill and, when we cannot fully recover, to stay as well as we can. It works at the limits of science – bringing the highest levels of human knowledge and skill to save lives and improve health. It touches our lives at times of basic human need, when care and compassion are what matter most.

The NHS is founded on a common set of principles and values that bind together the people who it serves – patients and public – and the staff who work for it.

This Constitution establishes the **principles** and **values** of the NHS in England. It sets out the patients, public and staff the **rights** to which they are entitled and **pledges** which the NHS is committed to achieve, together with **responsibilities** which the public, patients and staff owe to one another to ensure that the NHS operates fairly and effectively. All NHS bodies and private and third sector providers supplying NHS services will be required by law to take account of this Constitution in their decisions and actions.

The Constitution will be renewed every ten years, with the involvement of patients, public and staff. It will be accompanied by the *Handbook to the NHS Constitution*, to be renewed at least every three years, setting out current guidance on the rights, pledges, duties and responsibilities established by the Constitution. These requirements for renewal will be made legally binding. They will guarantee that the principles and values which underpin the NHS are subject to regular review and recommitment; and that any government which seeks to alter the principles or values of the NHS, or the rights, pledges, duties and responsibilities set out in this Constitution, will have to engage in a full and transparent debate with the public, patients and staff.

1. Principles that guide the NHS

Seven key principles guide the NHS in all it does. They are underpinned by core NHS values which have been derived from extensive discussions with staff, patients and the public. These values are set out at the back of this document.

1. The NHS provides a comprehensive service, available to all irrespective of gender, race, disability, age, sexual orientation religion or belief. It has a duty to each and every individual that it serves and must respect their human rights. At the same time, it has a wider social duty to promote equality through the services it provides and to pay particular attention to groups or sections of society where improvements in health and life expectancy are not keeping pace with the rest of the population.

2. Access to NHS services is based on clinical need, not an individual's ability to pay. NHS services are free of charge, except in limited circumstances sanctioned by Parliament.

3. The NHS aspires to the highest standards of excellence and professionalism – in the provision of high-quality care that is safe, effective and focused on patient experience; in the planning and delivery of the clinical and other services it provides; in the people it employs and the education, training and development they receive; in the leadership and management of its organisations; and through its commitment to innovation and to the promotion and conduct of research to improve the current and future health and care of the population.

4. NHS services must reflect the needs and preferences of patients, their families and their carers. Patients, with their families and carers, where appropriate, will be involved in and consulted on all decisions about their care and treatment.

5. The NHS works across organisational boundaries and in partnership with other organisations in the interest of patients, local communities and the wider population. The NHS is an integrated system of organisations and services bound together by the principles values and now reflected in the Constitution. The NHS is committed to working jointly with local authorities and a wide range of other private, public and third sector organisations at national and local level to provide and deliver improvements in health and wellbeing.

6. The NHS is committed to providing best value for taxpayers' money and the most effective and fair use of finite resources. Public funds for healthcare will be devoted solely to the benefit of the people that the NHS serves.

7. The NHS is accountable to the public, communities and patients that it serves. The NHS is a national service funded through national taxation, and it is the Government which sets the framework for the NHS and which is accountable to Parliament for its operation. However, most decisions in the NHS, especially those about the treatment of individuals and the detailed organisation of services, are rightly taken by the local NHS and by patients with their clinicians. The system of responsibility and accountability for taking decisions in the NHS should be transparent and clear to public, patients and staff. The Government will ensure that there is always a clear and up-to-date statement of NHS accountability for this purpose.

2a. Patients and the public – your rights and NHS pledges to you

Everyone who uses the NHS should understand what legal rights they have. For this reason, important legal rights are summarised in this Constitution and explained in more detail in the *Handbook to the NHS Constitution*, which also explains what you can do if you think you have not received what is rightfully yours. This summary does not alter the content of your legal rights.

This Constitution also contains **pledges** that the NHS is committed to achieve. Pledges go above and beyond legal rights. This means that pledges are not legally binding but represent a commitment by the NHS to provide high quality services.

Access to health services:

You have the right to receive NHS services free of charge, apart from certain limited exceptions sanctioned by Parliament.

You have the right to access NHS services. You will not be refused access on unreasonable grounds.

You have the right to expect your local NHS to assess the health requirements of the local community and to put in place the services to meet those needs as considered necessary.

You have the right in certain circumstances to go to other European Economic Area countries or Switzerland for treatment which would be available to you through your NHS Commissioner.

You have the right not to be unlawfully discriminated against in the provision of NHS services including on grounds of gender, race, religion, sexual orientation, disability (including learning disability or mental illness or age).[1]

The NHS also commits:

- to provide convenient, easy access to services within the waiting times set out in the Handbook to the NHS Constitution. (pledge);
- to make decisions in a clear and transparent way, so that patients and the public can understand how services are planned and delivered. (pledge); and
- to make the transition as smooth as possible when you are referred between services, and to include you in relevant discussions. (pledge).

Quality of care and environment:

You have the right to be treated with a professional standard of care, by appropriately qualified and experienced staff, in a properly approved or registered organisation that meets required levels of safety and quality.[2]

You have the right to expect NHS organisations to monitor, and make efforts to improve the quality of healthcare they commission or provide.

The NHS also commits:

- to ensure that services are provided in a clean and safe environment that is fit for purpose, based on national best practice. (pledge); and

- continuous improvement in the quality of services you receive, identifying and sharing best practice in quality of care and treatments. (pledge).

Nationally approved treatments, drugs and programmes:

You have the right to drugs and treatments that have been recommended by NICE[3] for use in the NHS, if your doctor says they are clinically appropriate for you.

You have the right to expect local decisions on funding of other drugs and treatments to be made rationally following a proper consideration of the evidence. If the local NHS decides not to fund a drug or treatment you and your doctor feel would be right for you, they will explain that decision to you.

You have the right to receive the vaccinations that the Joint Committee on Vaccination and Immunisation recommends that you should receive under an NHS-provided national immunisation programme.

The NHS also commits:

- to provide screening programmes as recommended by the UK National Screening Committee (pledge).

Respect, consent and confidentiality:

You have the right to be treated with dignity and respect in accordance with your human rights.

You have the right to accept or refuse treatment that is offered to you, and not to be given any physical examination or treatment unless you have given valid consent. If you do not have the capacity to do so, consent must be obtained from a person legally able to act on your behalf, or the treatment must be in your best interests.[4]

You have the right to be given information about your proposed treatment in advance, including any significant risks and any alternative treatments which may be available, and the risks involved in doing nothing.

You have the right to privacy and confidentiality and to expect the NHS to keep your confidential information safe and secure.

You have the right to access your own health records. These will always be used to manage your treatment in your best interests.

The NHS also commits:

- to share with you any letters sent between clinicians about your care. (pledge).

Informed choice:

You have the right to choose your GP practice, and to be accepted by that practice unless there are reasonable grounds to refuse, in which case you will be informed of those reasons.

You have the right to express a preference for using a particular doctor within your GP practice, and for the practice to try to comply.

You have the right to make choices about your NHS care and to information to support these choices. The options available to you will develop over time and depend on your individual needs. Details are set out in the *Handbook to the NHS Constitution*.

The NHS also commits:

- to inform you about what healthcare services are available to you, locally and nationally. (pledge); and
- to offer you easily accessible, reliable and relevant information to enable you to participate fully in your own healthcare decisions and to support you in making choices. This will include information on the quality of clinical services where there is robust and accurate information available. (pledge).

Involvement in your healthcare and in the NHS:

You have the right to be involved in discussions and decisions about your healthcare, and to be given information to enable you to do this.

You have the right to be involved, directly or through representatives, in the planning of healthcare services, the development and consideration of proposals for changes in the way those services are provided, and in decisions to be made affecting the operation of those services.

The NHS also commits:

- to provide you with the information you need to influence and scrutinise the planning and delivery of NHS services. (pledge); and
- to work in partnership with you, your family, carers and representatives (pledge).

Complaint and redress:

You have the right to have any complaint you make about NHS services dealt with efficiently and to have it properly investigated.

You have the right to know the outcome of any investigation into your complaint.

You have the right to take your complaint to the Health Service Ombudsman, if you are not satisfied with the way your complaint has been dealt with by the NHS.

You have the right to make a claim for judicial review if you think you have been directly affected by an unlawful act or decision of an NHS body.

You have the right to compensation where you have been harmed by negligent treatment.

The NHS also commits:

- to ensure you are treated with courtesy and you receive appropriate support thoughout the handling of a complaint; and the fact that you have complained will not adversely affect your future treatment (pledge);

- when mistakes happen, to acknowledge them, apologise, explain what went wrong and put things right quickly and effectively (pledge); and
- to ensure that the organisation learns lessons from complaints and claims and use these to improve NHS services (pledge).

2b. Patients and the public – your responsibilities

The NHS belongs to all of us. There are things that we can all do to help it work effectively and to ensure resources are used responsibly:

You should recognise that you can make a significant contribution to your own, and your family's, good health and well-being, and take some personal responsibility for it.

You should register with a GP practice – the main point of access to NHS care.

You should treat NHS staff and other patients with respect and recognise that causing a nuisance or disturbance on NHS premises could result in prosecution.

You should provide accurate information about your health, condition and status.

You should keep appointments, or cancel within reasonable time. Receiving treatment within the maximum waiting times may be compromised unless you do.

You should follow the course of treatment which you have agreed with your clinician if you find this difficult.

You should participate in important public health programmes such as vaccination.

You should ensure that those closest to you are aware of your wishes about organ donation.

You should give feedback – both positive and negative – about the treatment and care you have received, including any adverse reactions you may have had.

3a. Staff – your rights and NHS pledges to you

It is the commitment, professionalism and dedication of staff working for the benefit of the people the NHS serves which really make the difference. High quality care requires high quality workplaces, with commissioners and providers aiming to be employers of choice.

All staff should have rewarding and worthwhile jobs, with the freedom and confidence to act in the interest of patients. To do this, they need to be trusted, actively listened to. They must be treated with respect at work, have the tools, training and support to deliver care, and opportunities to develop and progress.

The Constitution applies to all staff, doing clinical or non-clinical NHS work, and their employers. It covers staff wherever they are working, whether in public, private or third sector organisations.

Staff have extensive **legal rights**, embodied in general employment and discrimination law. These are summarised in the *Handbook to the NHS Constitution*. In addition, individual contracts of employment contain terms and conditions giving staff further rights.

The rights are there to help ensure that staff:

- have a good working environment with flexible working opportunities, consistent with the needs of patients and with the way that people live their lives;
- have a fair pay and contract framework;
- can be involved and represented in the workplace;
- have healthy and safe working conditions and an environment free from harassment, bullying or violence;
- are treated fairly, equally and free from discrimination; and
- can raise an internal grievance and if necessary seek redress, where it is felt that a right has not been upheld.

In addition to these legal rights, there are a number of **pledges** which the NHS is committed to achieve. Pledges go above and beyond your legal rights. This means that they are not legally binding but represent a commitment by the NHS to provide high-quality working environments for staff.

The NHS also commits:

- to provide all staff with clear roles and responsibility and rewarding jobs for teams and individuals that make a difference to patients, their families and carers and communities (pledge);
- to provide all staff with personal development, access to appropriate training for their jobs, and line management support to succeed. (pledge);
- to provide support and opportunities for staff to maintain their health well-being and safety (pledge); and
- to engage staff in decisions that affect them and the services they provide, individually and through representatives organisations and through local partnership working arrangement. All staff will be empowered to put forward ways to deliver better and safer services for patients and their families (pledge).

3b. Staff – your responsibilities

All staff have responsibilities to the public, their patients and colleagues.

Important legal duties are summarised below.

You have a duty to accept professional accountability and maintain the standards of professional practice as set by the appropriate regulatory body, applicable to your profession or role.

You have a duty to take reasonable care of health and safety at work for you and others, and to co-operate with employers to ensure compliance with health and safety requirements.

You have a duty to act in accordance with the express and implied terms of your contract of employment.

You have a duty not to discriminate against patients or staff and to adhere to equal opportunities and equality and human rights legislation.

You have a duty to protect the confidentiality of personal information that you hold unless to do so would put anyone at risk of significant harm.

You have a duty to be honest and truthful in applying for a job and in carrying out that job.

The Constitution also includes **expectations** that reflect how staff should play their part in ensuring the success of the NHS and delivering high-quality care.

You should aim:

- to maintain the highest stand-ards of care and service, taking responsibility not only for the care you personally provide, but also for your wider contribution to the aims of your team and the NHS as a whole;
- to take up training and development opportunities provided over and above those legally required of your post;
- to play your part in sustainably improving services by working in partnership with patients, the public and communities;
- to be open with patients, their families, carers or representatives, including if anything goes wrong; welcoming and listening to feedback and addressing concerns promptly and in a spirit of co-operation. You should contribute to a climate where the truth can be heard and the reporting of, and learning from, errors is encouraged; and
- to view the services to provide from the standpoint of a patient, and involve patients, their families and carers in the services you provide, working with them, their communities and other organisations, and making it clear who is responsible for their care.

NHS values

Patients, public and staff have helped develop this expression of values that inspire passion in the NHS and should guide it in the 21st century. Individual organisations will develop and refresh their own values, tailored to their local needs. The NHS values provide common ground for co-operation to achieve shared aspirations.

Respect and dignity. We value each person as an individual, respect their aspirations and commitments in life, and seek to understand their priorities, needs, abilities and limits. We take what others have to say seriously. We are honest about our point of view and what we can and cannot do.

Commitment to quality of care. We earn the trust placed in us by insisting on quality and striving to get the basics right every time: safety, confidentiality, professional and managerial integrity, accountability, dependable service and good communication. We welcome feedback, learn from our mistakes and build on our successes.

Compassion. We respond with humanity and kindness to each person's pain, distress, anxiety or need. We search for the things we can do, however small, to give comfort and relieve suffering. We find time for those we serve and work alongside. We do not wait to be asked, because we care.

Improving lives. We strive to improve health and well-being and people's experiences of the NHS. We value excellence and professionalism wherever we find it – in the everyday things that make people's lives better as much as in clinical practice, service improvements and innovation.

Working together for patients. We put patients first in everything we do, by reaching out to staff, patients, carers, families, communities, and professionals outside the NHS. We put the needs of patients and communities before organisational boundaries.

Everyone counts. We use our resources for the benefit of the whole community, and make sure nobody is excluded or left behind. We accept that some people need more help, that difficult decisions have to be taken – and that when we waste resources we waste others' opportunities. We recognise that we all have a part to play in making ourselves and our communities healthier.

References

1 The Government intends to use the Equality Bill to make unjustifiable age discrimination against adults unlawful in the provision of services and exercise of public functions. Subject to Parliamentary approval, this right not to be discriminated against will extend to age when the relevant provisions are brought into force for the health sector.

2 The registration system will apply to some NHS providers in respect of infection control from 2009, and more broadly from 2010. Further detail is set out in the Handbook to the NHS Constitution.

3 NICE (the National Institute for Health and Clinical Excellence) is an independent NHS organisation producing guidance on drugs and treatments. 'Recommended' means recommended by a NICE technology appraisal. Primary care trusts are normally obliged to fund NICE technology appraisals from a date no later than three months from the publication of the appraisal.

4 If you are detained in hospital or on supervised community treatment under the Mental Health Act 1983 different rules may apply to treatment for your mental disorder. These rules will be explained to you at the time. They may mean that you can be given treatment for your mental disorder even though you do not consent.

(Produced by the Department of Health. © Crown Copyright 2008.)

Table of Cases

Table of Statutes

Glossary

acceptance – an agreement to the terms of an offer which leads to a binding legal obligation, i.e. a *contract*.

accusatorial – a system of court proceedings where the two sides contest the issue (contrast with *inquisitorial*).

Act of Parliament – *statute*.

action – legal proceedings.

actionable per se – a court action where claimant does not have to show loss, *damage* or harm to obtain compensation, e.g. an action for *trespass to the person*.

actus reus – essential element of a crime that must be proved to secure a conviction, as opposed to the mental state of the accused (*mens rea*).

acute care – care for a disease or illness with rapid onset, severe symptoms and brief duration.

advance decision – is when someone who has mental capacity (is able to make and understand a decision) decides that they do not want a particular type of treatment if they lack capacity in the future. A doctor must respect this decision if it is valid and applicable. An advance decision must be about treatment a person wants to refuse and when that person wants to refuse it.

adversarial – approach adopted in an *accusatorial* system.

advocate – a person who pleads for another: it could be paid and professional, such as a *barrister* or *solicitor* – or it could be a lay advocate either paid or unpaid; a witness is not an advocate.

affidavit – a statement given under oath.

Agenda for Change – the system of pay put in place in 2004 for most NHS-employed staff. Pay is linked to job content, and the skills and knowledge staff apply to perform jobs. The system is underpinned by a job evaluation scheme.

alternative dispute resolution – methods to resolve a dispute without going to court such as mediation.

alternative provider – this is one type of contract primary care trusts of *medical services* can have with primary care providers. This contract is *(APMS) contracts* particularly designed to bring in new types of provision, such as social enterprise and the voluntary sector. See also *general medical services (GMS)* and *personal medical services (PMS) contracts*.

approved social worker (ASW) – a social worker qualified for the purposes of the Mental Health Act 1983. The Mental Health Act 2007 replaces the ASW with an approved mental health professional.

arrestable offence – an offence defined in Section 24 of the Police and Criminal Evidence Act 1984 that gives to the citizen the power of arrest in certain circumstances without a warrant.

assault – a threat of unlawful contact (*trespass to the person*).

Audit Commission – an independent body responsible for ensuring that public money is spent economically, efficiently and effectively in the areas of local government, housing, health, criminal justice and fire and rescue services.

balance of probabilities – standard of proof in *civil* proceedings.

barrister – a lawyer qualified to take a case in court.

battery – an unlawful touching (*see* trespass to the person).

bench/magistrates – *justices of the peace.*

best interests – anything done for people without capacity must be in their best interests (there is no legal definition of best interests but the criteria to be used is in Section 4 of the Mental Capacity Act 2005). Best Interests means thinking about what is best for the person, not about what anyone else wants.

Bolam test – test laid down by Judge McNair in the case of *Bolam* v. *Friern HMC* on the standard of care expected of a professional in cases of alleged *negligence*.

burden of proof – duty of a party to litigation to establish the facts or, in criminal proceedings, the duty of the prosecution to establish both *actus reus* and *mens rea.*

Care Quality Commission (CQC) – Inspection body set up April 2009 for health and social case.

Care Services Improvement Partnership (CSIP) – the Care Services Improvement Partnership (CSIP), part of the Care Services Directorate at the Department of Health, was set up on 1 April 2005 to support positive changes in services and in the well-being of people with mental health problems, people with learning disabilities, people with physical disabilities, older people with health and social care needs, children and families with health and social care needs and people in the criminal justice system with health and social care needs .

cause of action – facts that entitle a person to sue.

certiorari – an *action* taken to challenge an administrative or judicial decision (literally: to make more certain).

Child and adolescent mental health services (CAMHS) – specific mental health services for children and young people.

Children's Centres – are local facilities designed to help families with young children by providing access to a range of key services under one roof such as health, social care and parenting support .

Children's Trusts – are organisational arrangements which bring together strategic planners from relevant sectors to identify where children and young people need outcomes to be improved in a local area and to plan services accordingly.

choose and book – currently being introduced throughout England, choose and book is an NHS initiative that allows people to make their first outpatient appointment, after discussion with their GP, at a time, date and place that suits them .

choose and book menu – the choose and book menu is the list of services available to be chosen by a patient following a search by a GP for a particular specialty or clinic.

Choosing Health – a White Paper published on 16 November 2004 that set out proposals for supporting the public to make healthier and more informed choices in regard to their health.

citizens' summit – the final stage in the *Your Health, Your Care, Your Say* listening exercise which involved almost 1000 people from across the country and from all walks of life discussing and agreeing priorities for community health and care services. They deliberated policy options and prioritised them, including options raised spontaneously by people in four previous regional events. See also *Your Health, Your Care, Your Say.*

civil action – proceedings brought in the civil courts.

civil wrong – an act or omission which can be pursued in the civil courts by the person who has suffered the wrong (*see tort*).

claimant – person bringing a civil *action* (originally *plaintiff*).

Commission for Social Care Inspection (CSCI) – the replaced inspectorate for all social care services in England by CQC.

commissioning – the full set of activities that local authorities and Primary Care Trusts undertake to make sure that services funded by them, on behalf of the public, are used to meet the needs of the individual fairly, efficiently and effectively.

committal proceedings – hearings before the *magistrates* to decide if a person should be sent for *trial* in the Crown Court.

common law – law derived from the decisions of judges, case law, judge-made law.

community care – care or support provided by social services departments and the NHS to assist people in their day-to-day living.

community hospitals – local hospitals serving relatively small populations (less than 100 000), providing a range of clinical services but not equipped to handle emergency admissions on a 24/7 basis.

community matrons – community matrons are case managers with advanced level clinical skills and expertise in dealing with patients with complex long-term conditions and high intensity needs. This is a clinical role with responsibility for planning, managing, delivering and co-ordinating care for patients with highly complex needs living in their own homes and communities.

community strategies – plans that promote the economic, environmental and social well-being of local areas by local authorities as required by the Local Government Act 2000.

conditional fee system – a system whereby client and lawyer can agree that payment of fees is dependent on the outcome of the court *action*; also known as 'no win, no fee'.

conditions – terms of a contract (*see* warranties).

constructive dismissal – the employer has shown an intention of no longer abiding by the contract of employment and this therefore gives the employee the right either to see the contract as ended by this breach of contract or of treating the contract as continuing but being able to claim damages or compensation for this breach of contract.

constructive knowledge – knowledge that can be obtained from the circumstances.

continuing professional development (CPD) – the means by which professionals demonstrate to their professional body that they are updating and maintaining their skills.

continuous service – length of service an employee must have served to be entitled to receive certain statutory or contractual rights.

contract – an agreement enforceable in law.

contract for services – an agreement enforceable in law whereby one party provides services, not being employment, in return for payment or other consideration from the other.

contract of service – a contract for employment.

contributory negligence – the claimant is partly to blame for the harm that has occurred.

coroner – a person appointed to hold an inquiry (inquest) into a death that occurred in unexpected or unusual circumstances.

counter-offer – a response to an offer that suggests different terms and is therefore counted as an offer, not an **acceptance**.

criminal wrong – an act or omission which can be pursued in the criminal courts.

crisis resolution teams – teams providing intensive support for people with severe mental illness to help them through periods of crisis and breakdown.

cross-examination – questions asked of a witness by the lawyer for the opposing side: leading questions may be asked.

damages – a sum of money awarded by a court as compensation for a *tort* or breach of contract.

declaration – a ruling by the court setting out the legal situation.

Directgov – a website (www.directgov.uk) that provides a first stop for a wide range of information on national and local government and associated services, including education and learning, travel and transport and health and well-being.

direct payments – payments given to individuals so that they can organise and pay for the social care services they need, rather than using the services offered by their local authority.

disabled facilities grants (DFG) – grants issued by councils towards meeting the cost of providing adaptations and facilities (such as bath grab rails) to enable disabled people to continue to remain independent in their own homes.

disclosure – documents made available to the other party.

dissenting judge – a judge who disagrees with the decision of the majority of judges.

distinguished – (of cases) rules of precedent require judges to follow decisions of judges in previous cases, where these are binding on them. However, in some circumstances, it is possible to come to a different decision, because the facts of the earlier case are not comparable to the case now being heard and therefore the earlier decision can be 'distinguished'.

district general hospital (DGH) – a hospital which provides a range of clinical services sufficient to meet the needs of a defined population of about 150 000 or more for hospital care but not necessarily including highly specialised services.

examination in chief – witness is asked questions in court by the lawyer of the party that has asked the witness to attend. Leading questions may not be asked.

ex gratia – as a matter of favour, e.g. without admission of *liability*, of payment offered to a claimant.

ex parte – an application made to the court (usually on an urgent matter) without the other side being present or represented.

expert patient programme (EPP) – the expert patient programme (EPP) is an NHS programme designed to spread good self care and self-management skills to a wide range of people with long-term conditions. Using trained non-medical leaders as educators, it equips people with arthritis and other long-term conditions with the skills to manage their own conditions.

expert witness – evidence given by a person whose general opinion, based on training or experience, is relevant to some of the issues in dispute (contrast with *witness of fact*).

fair access to care services (FACS) – guidance issued by the Department of Health to local authorities about eligibility criteria for adult social care.

framework contract – a contract listing a range of suppliers who have demonstrated that they are able to supply specified goods or services. Once in place, the contract enables organisations to call upon one or more of the suppliers to supply the goods or services as they are required.

frustration – (of contracts) ending of a contract by operation of law, because of the existence of an event not contemplated by the parties when they made the contract, e.g. imprisonment, death, blindness.

General Medical Council (GMC) – the statutory body responsible for licensing doctors to practise medicine in the UK. It protects, promotes and maintains the health and safety of the public by ensuring proper standards in the practice of medicine.

general medical services (GMS) – this is one type of contract primary care trusts can have with primary care providers. It is a nationally negotiated contract that sets out the core range of services provided by family doctors (GPs) and their staff. See also *Alternative Provider of Medical Services (APMS) contracts* and *Personal Medical Services (PMS) contracts*.

General Social Care Council (GSCC) – the social care workforce regulator. It registers social care workers and regulates their conduct, education and training.

Gershon Review – an independent review of public sector efficiency commissioned by HM Treasury and conducted by Sir Peter Gershon. The report, *Releasing resources to the front line*, was published in July 2004 and was incorporated into the 2004 Spending Review. To support implementation, the Department of Health established the Care Services Efficiency Delivery programme.

GPwSI (general practitioners with special interests) supplement –their generalist role by delivering a clinical service beyond the normal scope of general practice They may undertake advanced procedures or develop specific services. They do not offer a full consultant service. See also *practitioners with special interests (PwSI)*.

Green Paper – a preliminary discussion or consultation document often issued by the government in advance of the formulation of policy.

guardian *ad litem* – a person with a social work and child care background who is appointed to ensure that the court is fully informed of the relevant facts which relate to a child and that the wishes and feelings of the child are clearly established. The appointment is made from a panel set up by the local authority.

guilty – a finding in a criminal court of responsibility for a criminal offence.

Health Direct Online – the Health Direct Online service is being developed to promote people's understanding of health and provide advice, information and practical support to encourage healthier ways of living that improve the quality of all our lives and communities.

Healthcare Commission (Commission for Health Audit and Inspection) – the independent inspectorate in England and Wales that promotes improvement in the quality of the NHS and independent health care replaced by CQC.

hearsay – evidence that has been learnt from another person.

hierarchy – recognised status of courts that results in lower courts following the decisions of higher courts (see *precedent*). Thus decisions of the House of Lords must be followed by all lower courts unless they can be *distinguished*.

independence well-being and choice – *Independence, Well-being and Choice: Our Vision for the Future of Social Care for Adults in England* is a Green Paper setting out the Government's proposals for the future direction of social care for adults of all ages in England.

independent sector – an umbrella term for all non-NHS bodies delivering health care, including a wide range of private companies and voluntary organisations.

indictment – a written accusation against a person, charging him with a serious crime, triable by jury.

individual budgets – individual budgets bring together a variety of income streams from different agencies to provide a sum for an individual, who has control over the way it is spent to meet his or her care needs .

integrated service improvement programme (ISIP) – an NHS programme that integrates the planning and delivery of benefits from the investment in workforce reform, Connecting for Health and best practice from the Modernisation Agency and NHS Institute. The programme aims to drive delivery of efficiency through effective commissioning and integrated planning. The programme supports the delivery of savings as set out in Sir Peter Gershon's report on public service efficiencies to the Chancellor. See also *Gershon Review*.

informal – of a patient who has entered hospital without any statutory requirements.

injunction – an order of the court restraining a person.

inquisitorial – a system of justice whereby the truth is revealed by an inquiry into the facts conducted by the judge, e.g. coroner's court.

invitation to treat – early stages in negotiating a contract, e.g. an advertisement or letter expressing interest. An invitation to treat will often precede an offer that, when accepted, leads to the formation of an agreement that, if there is consideration and an intention to create legal relations, will be binding.

judicial review – an application to the High Court for a judicial or administrative decision to be reviewed and an appropriate order made, e.g. *declaration*.

justice of the peace (JP) – a lay **magistrate**, i.e. not legally qualified, who hears *summary* (minor) *offences* and sometimes indictable (serious) offences in the magistrates' court in a group of three (*see bench magistrates*).

liable/liability – responsible for the wrong doing or harm in civil proceedings.

litigation – civil proceedings.

local area agreements (LAAs) – a local area agreement (LAA) is a 3-year agreement that sets out the priorities for a local area in certain policy fields as agreed between central government, represented by the Government Office, and a local area, represented by the local authority and local strategic partnership (LSP) and other partners at local level. The agreement is made up of outcomes, indicators and targets aimed at delivering a better quality of life for people through improving performance on a range of national and local priorities.

local authority – local authorities are democratically elected local bodies with responsibility for discharging a range of functions as set out in local government legislation.

local delivery plan (LDP) – a plan that every primary care trust (PCT) prepares and agrees with its Strategic Health Authority (SHA) on how to invest its funds to meet its local and national targets, and improve services. It allows PCTs to plan and budget for delivery of services over a three-year period.

local strategic partnerships (LSPs) – LSPs bring together representatives of all the different sectors (public, private, voluntary and community) and thematic partnerships. They have responsibility for developing and delivering the sustainable community strategy and local area agreement.

long-term conditions – those conditions (for example, diabetes, asthma and arthritis) that cannot, at present, be cured but whose progress can be managed and influenced by medication and other therapies.

Lyons Review – an independent inquiry by Sir Michael Lyons which is examining the future role and function of local government before making recommendations on funding reforms

to inform the 2007 Comprehensive Spending Review.

magistrate – a person (*see justice of the peace* and *stipendiary magistrate*) who hears summary (minor) offences or indictable offences that can be heard in the magistrates' court.

mens rea – mental element in a crime (contrast with *actus reus*).

mental health services – a range of specialist clinical and therapeutic interventions across mental health and social care provision, integrated across organisational boundaries.

minimum practice income guarantee (MPIG) – introduced as part of the new general medical services (MPIG) contract (introduced from April 2004) to provide income protection to general practices moving from the previous contract to the new, to prevent a reduction in income. It applies to those practices which hold general medical services contracts. See *General Medical Services (GMS)*.

National Institute for Health and Clinical Excellence (NICE) – the independent organisation responsible for providing national guidance on the promotion of good health and the prevention and treatment of ill health.

National Minimum Standards (NMS) – standards set by the Department of Health for a range of services, including care homes, domiciliary care agencies and adult placement schemes. The Care Quality Commission (CQC) must consider the NMS in assessing social care providers' compliance with statutory regulations.

National Service Framework (NSF) – Department of Health guidance that defines evidence-based standards and good practice in a clinical area or for a patient group. Examples include mental health, coronary heart disease and older people.

NHS Connecting for Health – an agency of the Department of Health that delivers new, integrated IT systems and services to help modernise the NHS and ensure care is centred around the patient.

NHS Direct – provides 24-hour access to health information and clinical advice, via telephone

(0845 46 47 in England), as well as a website (NHS Direct Online www.nhsdirect.nhs.uk) and an interactive digital TV service (NHS Direct Interactive). A printed *NHS Direct Healthcare Guide* is also available.

NHS Electronic Care Records (NHS Care Records Service) – this service is being developed to provide a secure, live, interactive NHS Care Record for every patient in England, which will be accessible to all health and care professionals, whichever NHS organisation they work in .

NHS Employers – the employers' organisation for the NHS in England, giving employers throughout the NHS an independent voice on workforce and employment matters.

NHS Foundation Trusts (FT) – NHS hospitals that are run as independent, public benefit corporations, controlled and run locally. Foundation Trusts have increased freedoms regarding their options for capital funding to invest in delivery of new services.

NHS Improvement Plan – a Government plan, published in June 2004, that sets objectives for the NHS and related agencies.

NHS Plan – a Government plan for the NHS, published in July 2000, that set out a 10-year programme of investment and reform for the NHS.

NHS walk-in centres – centres staffed by nurses that offer fast and convenient access to treatment and information without needing an appointment .

negligence – a civil *action* for compensation, also a failure to follow a reasonable standard of care.

next friend – a person who brings a court action on behalf of a minor.

offer – a proposal made by a party that, if accepted, can lead to a *contract*. It often follows an *invitation to treat*.

Office for Standards in Education (Ofsted) – the inspectorate for children and learners in England. It is their job to contribute to the provision of better education and care through effective inspection and regulation.

Ombudsman – a commissioner (e.g. health, local government) appointed by the government to hear complaints.

ongoing need – a defined health and care need that continues over time, although the intensity of care and support needed will fluctuate.

opportunity age – cross-government strategy, published by the Department for Work and Pensions on 24 March 2005. The strategy aims to improve older people's access to public services, and make it possible for them to exercise more choice, and promote independence, enabling older people to remain in their own homes.

Organisation for Economic Co-operation and Development (OECD) – international organisation with a core membership of 30 countries which promotes democratic government and the market economy. It is best known for its publications on economic issues and its statistics.

Overview and Scrutiny Committee (OSC) – a committee made up of local government councillors that offers a view on local NHS and social care matters.

partnerships for older people projects (POPPs) – a 2-year programme of work led by the Department of Health with £60 million ring fenced funding (£20 million in 2006/07 and £40 million in 2007/08) for local authority-based partnerships to lead pilot projects to develop innovative ways to help older people avoid emergency hospital attendance and live independently longer. The overall aim is to improve the health, wellbeing and independence of older people.

patients' forums (or patient and public involvement forums) – patient-led organisations, established by the NHS Reform and Healthcare Professions Act 2002, for every trust (including NHS Foundation Trusts) and primary care trusts. Their functions include monitoring the quality of services and seeking the views of patients and carers about those services.

payment into court – an offer to settle a dispute at a particular sum, which is paid into court.

The claimant's failure to accept the offer means that the claimant is liable to pay costs, if the final award is the same or less than the payment made.

pedagogic – of the science of teaching.

personal medical services (PMS) contracts – this is one type of contract primary care trusts can have with primary care providers. This contract is locally negotiated with practices. See also *general medical services (GMS)* and *alternative provider of medical services (APMS) contracts*.

plaintiff – term formerly used to describe one who brings an action in the civil courts. Now the term *claimant* is used.

plea in mitigation – a formal statement to the court aimed at reducing the sentence to be pronounced by the judge.

practice-based commissioning (PBC) – GPs have direct responsibility for managing the funds that the Primary Care Trust (PCT) has to pay for hospital and other care for the GP practice population.

practice direction – guidance issued by the head of the court to which they relate on the procedure to be followed.

practitioners with special interests (PwSI) – the term covering all primary care professionals working with an extended range of practice. A PwSI will specialise in a particular type of care in addition to their normal role, e.g. a PwSI in dermatology would see patients with more complex skin ailments. See also *GPwSI*.

pre-action protocol – rules of the Supreme Court that provide guidance on action to be taken before legal proceedings commence.

precedent – a decision that may have to be followed in a subsequent court hearing (*see hierarchy*).

prima facie – at first sight; sufficient evidence brought by one party to require the other party to provide a defence.

primary care – the collective term for all services which are people's first point of contact with the NHS.

primary care trusts (PCTs) – free-standing statutory NHS bodies with responsibility for delivering health care and health improvements to their local areas. They commission or directly provide a range of community health services as part of their functions.

privilege – in relation to evidence, being able to refuse to disclose it to the court.

privity – relationship that exists between parties as the result of a legal agreement.

professional misconduct – conduct of a registered health practitioner that could lead to conduct and competence proceedings by the registration body.

proof – evidence that secures the establishment of a claimant's, prosecution's or defendant's case.

prosecution – pursuing of criminal offences in court.

public service agreement (PSA) – an agreement between each government department and HM Treasury which specifies how public funds will be used to ensure value for money.

quality and outcomes framework (QOF) – part of the contract primary care trusts have with GPs. It is nationally negotiated and rewards best practice and improving quality.

quantum – amount of compensation, or the monetary value of a claim.

Queen's Counsel (QC) – a senior barrister, also known as a 'silk'.

reasonable doubt – to secure a conviction in criminal proceedings the prosecution must establish 'beyond reasonable doubt' the guilt of the accused.

Re F ruling – a professional who acts in the best interests of an incompetent person who is incapable of giving consent does not act unlawfully if he follows the accepted standard of care according to the *Bolam Test*.

rescission – where a contract is ended by the order of a court or by the cancellation of the contract by one party entitled in law to do so.

scope of practice – a health professional's scope of practice is the area or areas of their profession in which they have the knowledge, skills and experience to practise lawfully, safely and effectively.

secondary care – the collective term for services to which a person is referred after first point of contact. Usually this refers to hospitals in the NHS offering specialised medical services and care (outpatient and inpatient services).

secondary prevention – secondary prevention aims to limit the progression and effect of a disease at as early a stage as possible. It includes further primary prevention.

single assessment process (SAP) – an overarching assessment of older people's care needs to which the different agencies providing care contribute.

Skills For Care – responsible for the strategic development of the adult social care workforce in England. It supports employers in improving standards of care through training and development, workforce planning and workforce intelligence. Alongside the new Children's Workforce Development Council, it is the English component of Skills for Care and Development, the UK-wide Sector Skills Council for social care, children and young people.

Skills for Health – the Sector Skills Council for the health sector in the UK, covering all roles and functions within the NHS and independent sectors. It helps the sector develop solutions that deliver a skilled and flexible workforce to improve health and health care.

Social Care Institute for Excellence (SCIE) – an independent registered charity established in 2001 to develop and promote knowledge about good practice in social care .

social enterprise – businesses involved in social enterprise have primarily social objectives. Their surpluses are reinvested principally in the business or community.

social exclusion – social exclusion occurs when people or areas suffer from a combination of linked problems including unemployment, poor skills, low incomes, poor housing, high-crime environments, bad health and family breakdown. It involves exclusion from essential services or aspects of everyday life that most others take for granted.

Social Exclusion Unit (SEU) – part of the Office of the Deputy Prime Minister, the Social Exclusion Unit provides advice and produces reports with recommendations on tackling specific social exclusion issues .

solicitor – a lawyer who is qualified on the register held by the Law Society.

standards for continuing professional development – the standards for continuing professional development link a health professional's ongoing learning and development with their continued registration.

standards of proficiency – these are the standards for safe and effective practice in each profession. Health professionals must meet these standards to become registered.

statute law (statutory) – law made by Acts of Parliament.

step-down care – part of intermediate care facilities that are outside acute hospitals, enabling people who strongly value their independence to leave acute hospital and get ready to return home.

step-up care – part of intermediate care facilities that are outside acute hospitals, enabling people who strongly value their independence to receive more support than is available at home.

Strategic Health Authority (SHA) – the local headquarters of the NHS, responsible for ensuring that national priorities are integrated into local plans and for ensuring that primary care trusts are performing well. They are the link between the Department of Health and the NHS.

stipendiary magistrate – a legally qualified magistrate who is paid (i.e. has a stipend).

strict liability – liability for a criminal act where the mental element does not have to be proved; in civil proceedings liability without establishing *negligence*.

subpoena – an order of the court requiring a person to appear as a witness (*subpoena ad testificandum*) or to bring records/documents (*subpoena duces tecum*).

summary judgment – a procedure whereby the claimant can obtain judgment without the defendant being permitted to defend the action.

summary offence – a lesser offence that may only be heard by *magistrates*.

supporting people programme – a grant programme providing local housing-related support to services to help vulnerable people move into or stay independently in their homes.

Sure Start – Sure Start is a government programme to achieve better outcomes for children and parents through increased availability to childcare, improved health and emotional development for young people, and better parental support.

Telecare – a combination of equipment, monitoring and response that can help individuals to remain independent at home. It can include basic community alarm services able to respond in an emergency and provide regular contact by telephone as well as detectors which detect factors such as falls, fire or gas and trigger a warning to a response centre. Telecare can work in a preventative or monitoring mode, for example, through monitoring signs, which can provide early warning of deterioration, prompting a response from family or professionals. Telecare can also provide safety and security by protecting against bogus callers and burglary.

third sector – includes the full range of non-public, non-private organisations which are non-governmental and 'value-driven'; that is, motivated by the desire to further social, environmental or cultural objectives rather than to make a profit.

tort – a civil wrong excluding breach of contract. It includes: *negligence, trespass (to the person,* goods or land), nuisance, breach of statutory duty and defamation.

trespass to the person – a wrongful direct interference with another person. Harm does not have to be proved.

trial – a court hearing before a judge.

ultra vires – outside the powers given by law (e.g. of a statutory body or company).

universal services – services provided for the whole community, including education and health, housing, leisure facilities and transport.

Valuing People Support Team – a Department of Health team working to improve services for people with learning disabilities through regional programmes of events, networks and support for groups and partnership boards. Its work is underpinned by national programmes designed to support local implementation.

vicarious liability – liability of an employer for the wrongful acts of an employee committed while in the course of employment.

volenti non fit injuria – to the willing there is no wrong; voluntary assumption of risk.

voluntary and community sector – an 'umbrella term' referring to registered charities as well as non-charitable non-profit organisations, associations, self-help groups and community groups, for public or community benefit.

Wanless Report/Wanless Review – an evidence-based assessment of the long-term resource requirements for the NHS. Commissioned by HM Treasury and conducted by Derek Wanless, the report, *Securing Our Future Health: Taking a Long-TermView,* was published in April 2002.

ward of court – a minor placed under the protection of the High Court, which assumes responsibility for him or her and all decisions relating to his or her care must be made in accordance with the directions of the court.

warranties – terms of a *contract* that are considered to be less important than the terms described as **conditions**: breach of a condition entitles the innocent party to see the contract as ended, i.e. repudiated by the other party (breach of warranties entitles the innocent party to claim damages).

Wednesbury principle – court will intervene to prevent or remedy abuses of power by public authorities if there is evidence of unreasonableness or perversity. Principle laid down by the Court of Appeal in the case of *Associated Provincial Picture House Ltd* v. *Wednesbury Corporation* [1948] 1 KB 233.

White Paper – documents produced by the government setting out details of future policy on a particular subject.

without prejudice – without detracting from or without disadvantage to. The use of the phrase prevents the other party using the information to the prejudice of the one providing it.

witness of fact – a person who gives evidence of what they saw, heard, did or failed to do (contrast with *expert witness*).

writ – a form of written command, e.g. the document that used to commence civil proceedings. Now a claim form is served.

'year of care' approach – describes the ongoing care a person with a long-term condition should expect to receive in a year, including support for self-management, which can then be costed and commissioned. It involves individual patients through the care planning process, enabling them to exercise choice in the design of a package to meet their individual needs.

Your Health, Your Care, Your Say – the listening exercise with the public about what their priorities are for future health and social care services. It comprised four regional events, a range of local events and other activities including questionnaires. The process culminated in a national Citizens' Summit. The events were deliberative, with a *Citizens' guide* given to participants beforehand to introduce the key issues.

Further Reading

Allen, R., Crasnow, R., Beale, A. (2007) *Employment Law and Human Rights*, 2nd edn. Oxford University Press.

Appelbe, G.E., Wingfield, J. (eds) (2005) *Dale and Appelbe's Pharmacy: Law and Ethics*, 8th edn. Pharmaceutical Press.

Atkinson, J. (2007) *Advance Directives in Mental Health – Theory, Practice and Ethics*. Jessica Kingsley Publications.

Barrett, B., Howells, R. (2000) *Occupational Health and Safety Law Text and Materials*. Cavendish.

Beale, H.G. (ed.) (2006) *Chitty on Contracts*, 3rd cumulative supplement to 29th edn. Sweet & Maxwell.

Beauchamp, T.L., Childres, J.F. (2001) *Principles of Biomedical Ethics*, 5th edn. Oxford University Press.

Benny, R., Sargeant, M., Jefferson, M. (2006) *Employment Law Questions and Answers*, 2nd edn. Oxford University Press.

Blom-Cooper, L., *et al.* (1996) *The Case of Jason Mitchell: Report of the Independent Panel of Inquiry*. Duckworth.

Blom-Cooper, L., Hally, H., Murphy, E. (1996) *The Falling Shadow – One Patient's Mental Health Care 1978–1993* (Report of an Inquiry into the Death of an Occupational Therapist at Edith Morgan Unit, Torbay 1993), Duckworth.

Brazier, M. (2007) *Medicine, Patients and the Law*, 4th edn. Penguin.

British Medical Association (1998) *Medical Ethics Today*. BMJ Publishing.

Britton, A. (2004) *Health Care Law and Ethics*. W . Green.

Carey, P. (2004) *Data Protection – a Practical Guide to UK and EU Law*, 2nd edn. Oxford University Press.

Clements, L. (2004) *Community Care and the Law*, 3rd edn. Legal Action Group.

Clerk, J.F. (2006) *Clerk and Lindsell on Torts*, 19th edn. Sweet & Maxwell.

Committee of Experts Advisory Group on AIDS (1994) *Guidance for Health Care Workers' Protection against Infection with HIV and Hepatitis*. HMSO.

Connolly, M. (2006) *Discrimination Law*. Thomson Sweet & Maxwell.

Cooper, J. (ed.) (2000) *Law, Rights and Disability*. Jessica Kingsley.

Deakin, S., Johnston, A., Markensinis, B. (2007) *Markensinis and Deakin's Tort Law*, 6th edn. Clarendon Press.

Denis, I.H. (1999) *The Law of Evidence*. Sweet & Maxwell.

Department of Health (1993) *AIDS/HIV Infected Health Care Workers*. DH.

Dimond, B.C. (1992) *Accountability and the Nurse*, Distance Learning Pack. South Bank University.

Dimond, B.C. (1996) *Legal Aspects of Child Health Care*. Mosby.

Dimond, B.C. (1997) *Legal Aspects of Care in the Community*. Macmillan.

Dimond, B.C. (1998) *Legal Aspects of Complementary Therapy Practice*. Churchill Livingstone.

Dimond, B.C. (1999) *Patients' Rights, Responsibilities and the Nurse*, 2nd edn. Central Health Studies, Quay Publications.

Dimond, B.C. (2002) *Legal Aspects of Pain Management.* Quay Publications/Mark Allen.

Dimond, B.C. (2002) *Legal Aspects of Patient Confidentiality.* Quay Publications/Mark Allen.

Dimond, B.C. (2009) *Legal Aspects of Consent*, 2nd edn. Quay Publications/Mark Allen.

Dimond, B.C. (2004) *Legal Aspects of Health and Safety.* Quay Publications/Mark Allen.

Dimond, B.C. (2005) *Legal Aspects of Medicines.* Quay Publications/Mark Allen.

Dimond, B.C. (2005) *Legal Aspects of Midwifery*, 3rd edn. Books for Midwives Press.

Dimond, B.C. (2005) *Legal Aspects of Occupational Therapy*, 2nd edn. Blackwell Scientific.

Dimond, B.C. (2007) *Legal Aspects of Mental Capacity* Blackwell Scientific.

Dimond, B.C. (2008) *Legal Aspects of Death.* Quay Publications/Mark Allen.

Dimond, B.C. (2009) *Legal Aspects of Nursing*, 5th edn. Pearson Education.

Dimond, B.C., Barker, F. (1996) *Mental Health Law for Nurses.* Blackwell Science.

Eliot, C. (2007) *The English Legal System,* 8th edn. Pearson Education.

Fraser, J., Nolan, M. (2004) Child Protection: a guide for midwives, 2nd edn. Books for Midwives.

Glynn, J., Gomez, D. (2005) *Fitness to Practise: Healthcare Regulatory Law, Principles and Process.* Sweet & Maxwell.

Grainger, I., Fealy, M., Spencer, M. (2000) *Civil Procedure Rules in Action*, 2nd edn. Cavendish.

Harris, D.J. (2005) *Cases and Materials on the European Convention on Human Rights*, 2nd revised edn. Butterworth.

Harris, P. (2007) *An Introduction to Law*, 7th edn. Butterworth.

Health and Safety Commission (1999) *Management of Health and Safety at Work Regulations: Approved Code of Practice.* HMSO.

Health and Safety Commission (1992) *Guidelines on Manual Handling in the Health Services.* HMSO.

Health and Safety Commission (1992) *Manual Handling Regulations: Approved Code of Practice.* HMSO.

Hendrick J. (2006) *Law and Ethics in Nursing and Healthcare*, 2nd edn. Nelson Thornes Publishers.

Herring, J. (2006) *Medical Law and Ethics* Oxford University Press.

Heywood-Jones, I. (ed.) (1999) *The UKCC Code of Conduct: A Critical Guide.* Nursing Times Books.

Hockton, A. (2002) *The Law on Consent to Treatment.* Sweet & Maxwell.

Hoggett, B. (2005) *Mental Health Law*, 5th edn. Sweet & Maxwell.

Holland, J., Burnett, S. (2006) *Employment Law.* Oxford University Press.

Howarth, D.R., O'Sullivan, J.A. (2000) *Hepple, Howarth and Matthews Tort: Cases and Materials*, 5th edn. Butterworths.

Howells, G., Weatherill, S. (2005) *Consumer Protection Law*, 2nd edn. Dartmouth.

Humphreys, N. (2005) *Trade Union Law and Collective Employment Rights.* 2nd edn. Jordans.

Hunt, G., Wainwright, P. (eds) (1994) *Expanding the Role of the Nurse.* Blackwell Scientific.

Hurwitz, B. (1998) *Clinical Guidelines and the Law.* Oxford Radcliffe Medical Press.

Hurwitz, B., de Zulueta, P. (2006) *Everyday Ethics in Primary Care.* BMJ.

Ingman, T. (2006) *The English Legal Process*, 11th edn. Blackstone Press.

Jay, R. (2007) *Data Protection Law and Practice*, 3rd revised edn. Sweet & Maxwell.

Jones, M.A. (2003) *Medical Negligence*, 3rd edn. Sweet & Maxwell.

Jones, M.A. (2007) *Textbook on Torts*, 9th edn. Oxford University Press.

Jones, M.A., Morris, A.E. (2005) *Blackstone's Statutes on Medical Law*, 4th edn. Oxford University Press.

Jones, R. (2006) *Mental Health Act Manual*, 10th edn. Sweet & Maxwell.

Keenan, D. (2004) *Smith and Keenan's English Law*, 14th edn. Longman.

Kennedy, I., Grubb, A. (2000) *Medical Law*, 3rd edn. Butterworth.

Kennedy, T. (1998) *Learning European Law.* Sweet & Maxwell.

Kidner, R. (2003) *Blackstone's Statutes on Employment Law*, 13th edn. Oxford University Press.

Kloss, D. (2005) *Occupational Health Law*, 4th edn. Blackwell Scientific.

Leach, P. (2005) *Taking a Case to the European Court of Human Rights*, 2nd edn. Blackstone Press Ltd.

Lee, R. (2007) *Tolley's Health and Safety at Work Handbook.* 19th edn. Tolley.

Lee, R.G., Morgan, D. (2001) *Human Fertilisation and Embryology.* Blackstone Press Ltd.

Lewis, T. (2005) *Employment Law*, 6th edn. Legal Action Group.

Lockton, D. (2007) *Employment Law 2007–8*, 5th edn. Routledge-Cavendish.

McHale, J., Fox, M. (2007) *Health Care Law*, 2nd edn. Sweet & Maxwell.

McHale, J., Tingle, J. (2007) *Law and Nursing*, 2nd edn. Elsevier Health Sciences.

McLean, S. (2007) *Impairment and Disability: Law and Ethics at the Beginning and End of Life*. Routledge-Cavendish.

Mandelstam, M. (1998) *An AZ of Community Care Law*. Jessica Kingsley.

Mandelstam, M. (2005) *Community Care Practice and the Law*, 3rd edn. Jessica Kingsley.

Mason, J.K., McCall-Smith, R.A., Laurie, G.T. (2002) *Law and Medical Ethics*, 6th edn. Butterworth.

Metzer, A., Weinberg, J. (1999) *Criminal Litigation*. Legal Action Group.

Miers, D., Page, A. (1990) *Legislation*, 2nd edn. Sweet & Maxwell.

Miles, A., Hampton, J., Hurwitz, B. (2000) *NICE, CHI and the NHS Reforms. Enabling Excellence or Imposing Control?* Aesculapius.

Montgomery, J. (2003) *Health Care Law*, 2nd edn. Oxford University Press.

Murphy, J. (2006) *Street on Torts*, 12th edn. Butterworths.

Nairns, J. (2006) *Discrimination Law: Text, Cases and Materials* Oxford University Press.

Painter, R.W., Holmes, A. (2006) *Cases and Materials on Employment Law*, 6th edn. Oxford University Press.

Pitt, G. (2007) *Employment Law*, 6th edn. Sweet & Maxwell.

Pyne, R.H. (1998) *Professional Discipline in Nursing, Midwifery and Health Visiting*, 3rd edn. Blackwell Scientific Publications.

Richardson, P.J. (ed.) (2007) *Archbold: Criminal Pleadings, Evidence and Practice*, 55th revised edn. Sweet & Maxwell.

Rogers, W.V.H. (2006) *Winfield and Jolowicz on Tort*, 17th edn. Thomson, Sweet & Maxwell.

Rose, W. (ed.) (2008) *Blackstone's Civil Practice*. Oxford University Press.

Rowson, R. (1990) *An Introduction to Ethics for Nurses*. Scutari Press.

Rowson, R. (2006) Working *Ethics – How to be Fair in a Culturally Complex World*. Jessica Kingsley.

Rubenstein, M. (2002) *Discrimination – Guide to Relevant Case Law*. 15th edn. Eclipse Group.

Rumbold, G. (1999) *Ethics in Nursing Practice*, 3rd edn. Baillière Tindall.

Salvage, J. (1998) *Nurses at Risk: Guide to Health and Safety at Work*, 2nd edn. Heinemann.

Sellars, C. (2002) *Risk Assessment with People with Learning Disabilities*. Blackwell.

Selwyn, N. (2006) *Selwyn's Law of Employment*, 14th edn. Butterworth.

Sime, S. (2006) *Practical Approach to Civil Procedure*, 9th edn. Blackstone Press.

Skegg, P.D.G. (1998) *Law, Ethics and Medicine*, 2nd edn. Oxford University Press.

Slapper, G., Kelly, D. (2006) *The English Legal System*, 8th edn. Routledge-Cavendish.

Social Security Inspectorate, Department of Health (1993) *No Longer Afraid: Safeguard of Older People in Domestic Settings*. HMSO.

Stauch, M. (2005) *Text and Materials on Medical Law*, 3rd edn. Cavendish.

Steiner, J. (2006) *Textbook on EC Law*, 9th edn. Oxford University Press.

Stone, J., Matthews, J. (1996) *Complementary Medicine and the Law*. Oxford University Press.

Storch, J. (2004) *Towards a Moral Horizon: Nursing Ethics for Leadership and Practice*. Pearson Education.

Taylor, S. Emir, A. (2006) *Employment Law: An introduction* Oxford University Press.

Tingle, J. Cribb, A. (2007) *Nursing law and ethics* 3rd edn Blackwell Publishers.

Tingle, J., Foster, C. (2002) *Clinical Guidelines: Law, Policy and Practice*. Cavendish.

Tschudin, V. (2002) Ethics in Nursing: the caring relationship, 3rd edn. Butterworth-Heinemann.

Vincent, C. (ed.) (1995) *Clinical Risk Management*. BMJ Publishing.

Wheeler, J. (2006) *The English Legal System*, 2nd edn. Pearson Education.

White, R., Carr, P., Lowe, N. (2002) *A Guide to the Children Act 1989*, 3rd edn. Butterworth.

Wilkinson, R., Caulfield, H. (2000) *The Human Rights Act: A Practical Guide for Nurses*. Whurr Publishers.

Zander, M. (2005) *Police and Criminal Evidence Act*, 1st supplement to 5th edn. Sweet & Maxwell.

Useful Websites

Action for Advocacy	www.actionforadvocacy.org
Action on Elder Abuse	www.elderabuse.org.uk
Advisory Conciliation and Arbitration Service	www.acas.org.uk
Age Concern	www.ageconcern.org.uk
Alert	www.donoharm.org.uk
Alzheimer's Research	www.alzheimers-research.org.uk
Alzheimer's Society	www.alzheimers.org.uk
Association of Contentious Trust and Probate Solicitors	www.actaps.com
Audit Commission	www.audit-commission.gov.uk
Bailii (case law resource)	www.bailii.org/ew/cases
CARERS UK	www.carersuk.org
Care Services Improvement Partnership	www.csip.org.uk
Citizens Advice Bureaux	www.bailii.org/databases.htm
Citizen Advocacy Information and Training	www.citizenadvocacy.org.uk
Civil Procedure Rules	www.direct.gov.uk/en/index.htm
Clinical Negligence Scheme for Trusts	www.nhsla.com/Claims/Schemes/CNST
Equality and Human Rights Commission	www.equalityhumanrights.com.
Commission for Racial Equality	www.cre.gov.uk
Commission for Social Care and Inspection	www.csci.gov.uk
Community Legal Service Direct	www.clsdirect.org.uk
Complementary Healthcare Information Service	www.chisuk.org.uk
Contact the Elderly	www.contact-the-elderly.org
Convention on the International Protection of Adults	www.hcch.net/index_en.php?
Council for Healthcare Regulatory Excellence	www.chre.org.uk
Commission for Patient and Public Involvement in Health	www.cppih.org
Counsel and Care	www.counselandcare.org.uk
Court Funds Office	www.hmcourts-service.gov.uk/infoabout/cfo/index.htm

Court of Protection	via the Office of Public Guardian or HM Courts Services
Central Office for Research Ethics Committees	www.corec.org
Dementia Care Trust	www.patient.co.uk
Department for Business Enterprise and Regulatory Reform	www.berr.gov.uk/employment
Department for Education and Skills	www.dcsf.gov.uk
Department for Work and Pensions	www.dwp.gov.uk
Department of Health	www.dh.gov.uk
Department of Trade and Industry	www.berr.gov.uk
Disability Law Service	www.dls.org.uk
Domestic Violence	www.crimereduction.homeoffice.gov.uk/dv
Down's Syndrome Association	ww.downs-syndrome.org
Family Carer Support Service	www.familycarers.org.uk
Family Mediation Helpline	www.familymediationhelpline.co.uk
Foundation for People with Learning Disabilities	www.learningdisabilities.org.uk
General Medical Council	www.gmc-uk.org
Headway – brain injury Association	www.headway.org.uk
Health and Safety Commission	www.hse.gov.uk
Health and Safety Executive	www.hse.gov.uk
Help the Aged	www.helptheaged.org.uk
Help the Hospices	www.hospiceinformation.info
Healthcare Commission	www.healthcarecommission.org.uk
Health Professions Council	www.hpc-uk.org
HM Courts Service	www.hmcourts-service.gov.uk
Home Farm Trust	www.hft.org.uk
Human Fertilisation and Embryology Authority	www.hfea.gov.uk
Human Genetics Commission	www.hgc.gov.uk
Human Rights	www.humanrights.gov.uk
Independent Mental Capacity Advocate	www.dh.gov.uk/imca
Information Commissioner's Office	www.ico.gov.uk
Law Centres Federation	www.lawcentres.org.uk
Law Society	www.lawsociety.org.uk
Legal cases (England and Wales)	www.bailli.org/ew/cases
Legislation	www.opsi.gov.uk/legislation or www.legislation.hmso.gov.uk
Linacre Centre for Healthcare Ethics	www.linacre.org
Making Decisions Alliance	www.makingdecisions.org.uk
Manic Depression Fellowship	www.mdf.org.uk
MedicAlert Foundation	www.medicalert.org.uk
Medicines and Healthcare Products Regulatory Agency	www.mhra.gov.uk
MENCAP	www.mencap.org.uk
Mental Capacity Implementation Programme	www.dca.gov.uk/legal-policy/mental-capacity/index.htm
Mental Health Act Commission	www.mhac.org.uk
Mental Health Foundation	www.mentalhealth.org.uk
Mental Health Lawyers Assoc	www.mhla.co.uk
Mental Health Matters	www.mentalhealthmatters.com
Mind	www.mind.org.uk
Ministry of Justice	www.justice.gov.uk
Motor Neurone Disease Association	www.mndassociation.org.uk
National Audit Office	www.nao.gov.uk

National Autistic Society	www.nas.org.uk
	www.autism.org.uk
National Care Association	www.nca.gb.com
National Family Carer Network	www.familycarers.org.uk
National Health Service Litigation Authority	www.nhsla.com
National Mediation Helpline,	www.nationalmediationhelpline.com
National Patient Safety Agency	www.npsa.nhs.uk
National Perinatal Epidemiology Unit	www.npeu.ox.ac.uk
National Treatment Agency	www.nta.nhs.uk
NHS website	www.nhs.uk
NHS Direct	www.nhsdirect.nhs.uk
NHS Professionals	www.nhsprofessionals.nhs.uk
NICE	www.nice.org.uk
Nursing and Midwifery Council	www.nmc-uk.org
Office of Public Guardian	www.publicguardian.gov.uk
Office of Public Sector Information	www.opsi.gov.uk
Official Solicitor	www.officialsolicitor.gov.uk
Open Government	www.open.gov.uk
Pain website	www.pain-talk.co.uk
Patient's Association	www.patients-association.org.uk
Patient Concern	www.patientconcern.org.uk
People First	www.peoplefirst.org.uk
Prevention of Professional Abuse Network	www.popan.org.uk
Princess Royal Trust for Carers	www.carers.org
Relatives and Residents Association	www.relres.org
RESCARE (The National Society for mentally disabled people in residential care)	www.rescare.org.uk
Respond	www.respond.org.uk
Rethink (formerly the National Schizophrenia Fellowship)	www.rethink.org
Royal College of Nursing	www.rcn.org.uk
Royal College of Psychiatrists	www.rcpsych.ac.uk
SANE	www.sane.org.uk
Scope	www.scope.org.uk
Sense	www.sense.org.uk
Solicitors for the Elderly	www.solicitorsfortheelderly.com
Speaking Up	www.speakingup.org
Speakability	www.speakability.org.uk
Shipman Inquiry	www.the-shipman-inquiry.org.uk/reports.asp
Solicitors for the Elderly	www.solicitorsfortheelderly.com
Stroke Association	www.stroke.org.uk
Together: Working for Wellbeing	www.together-uk.org
Turning Point	www.turning-point.co.uk
UK Homecare Association	www.ukhca.co.uk
UK Parliament	www.parliament.uk
United Response	www.unitedresponse.org.uk
Values into Action	www.viauk.org
Veterans Agency	www.veteransagency.org.uk
VOICE UK	http://voiceuk.org.uk
Voluntary Euthanasia Society	www.ves.org.uk
Welsh Assembly Government	www.wales.gov.uk
World Medical Association	www.wma.net/e/policy/b3.htm

Index